INTERVENTIONAL CARDIOLOGY: FUTURE DIRECTIONS

John H.K. Vogel, MD, FACC
Director of Cardiology, Goleta Valley Community Hospital;
Director, Santa Barbara Heart and Lung Institute, Santa Barbara;
Clinical Professor of Medicine, University of Southern California School of Medicine, Los Angeles, California

Spencer B. King, III, MD, FACC
Professor of Medicine and Radiology
Director, Andreas Gruentzig Cardiovascular Center, Emory University School of Medicine, Atlanta, Georgia

with 362 illustrations

The C. V. Mosby Company

ST. LOUIS • BALTIMORE • PHILADELPHIA • TORONTO 1989

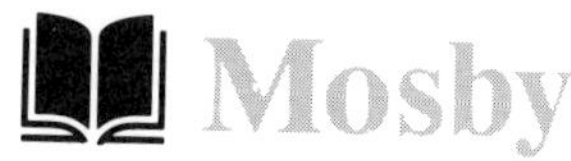

Editor: Richard A. Weimer
Editorial Project Manager: Lisa G. Cunninghis
Design: Todd Gast
Production: Editing, Design and Production, Inc.

This book is dedicated to the memory of Dr. Andreas M. Gruentzig.

Only those who
will risk going too far
can possibly find out how
far they can go.
T.S. Eliot

Printed in the United States of America

The C.V. Mosby Company
11830 Westline Industrial Drive, St. Louis, Missouri 63146

Library of Congress Cataloging in Publication Data
Interventional cardiology: future directions/[edited] by John H.K. Vogel.
p. cm.
Includes bibliographies and index.
ISBN 0-8016-5320-7
1. Heart—Diseases—Treatment. I. Vogel, John H.K., 1932-
[DNLM: 1. Cardiovascular Diseases—therapy. WG 166 I615]
RC683.8.I59 1989
617'.412—dc19
DNLM/DLC
for Library of Congress

88-39188
CIP

CL/MV/MV 9 8 7 6 5 4 3 2 1

CONTRIBUTORS

JOHN W. ALLEN, MD
Associate Clinical Professor of Medicine, University of Southern California, White Memorial Medical Center, Los Angeles, California

DAVID AUTH, PhD
Department of Medicine, University of Washington School of Medicine and the Seattle Veterans Administration Hospital, Seattle, Washington

ROSA M. AVOLIO, RN
Head Nurse, Cardiology, Goleta Valley Community Hospital, Santa Barbara, California

LINA BADIMON, PhD
Mayo Clinic, Rochester, Minnesota

JEAN PIERRE BASSAND, MD
Centre Hospitalier, Besancon, France

JACQUES BERLAND, MD
Hopital Charles Nicolle, Rouen, France

MICHEL E. BERTRAND, MD
Service de cardiologie B et Héurodynamique, Hopital Cardiologique, Lille Cedex, France

PETER BLOCK, MD, FACC
Associate Professor of Medicine, Harvard Medical School; Director, Cardiac Catheterization Laboratory, Massachusetts General Hospital, Boston, Massachusetts

JACQUES BOCHAT, MD
Unite d'hémodynamique, Centre Hospitalier Regional Morvan, Brest, France

NICOLAAS BOM, PhD
The Thoraxcenter, Erasmus University and University Hospital, Rotterdam, The Netherlands

RAOUL BONAN, MD, FACC
Assistant Professor of Medicine, University of Montreal Faculty of Medicine; Director, Cardiac Catheterization Laboratory, Montreal Heart Institute, Montreal, Quebec

ROBERT F. BONNER, PhD
Senior Investigator, Biomedical Engineering and Instrumentation Branch, Division of Research Services, National Institutes of Health, Bethesda, Maryland

TASSILO R. BONZEL, MD
Cardiologist, Director of Cardiology, Medical Clinic I, Fulda, Federal Republic of Germany

JEAN M. BRUNETAUD, M.D.
Division of Cardiology B and Hemodynamic University Hospital of Lille, France

YVES CHABRILLAT, MD
Clinique de la Résidence du Parc, Marseilles, France

JAMES H. CHESEBRO, MD
Associate Professor of Medicine and Consultant in Cardiovascular Diseases, Mayo Clinic, Rochester, Minnesota

FRÉDÉRIC COLLET, MD
Centre Jules Cantini, Marseilles, France

BARRY J. COUGHLIN, MD
Cardiologist, Medical Director, Non-Invasive Diagnostic Laboratory, Valley Medical Group, Lompoc, California

ALAIN CRIBIER, MD
Professor, Division of Cardiology, University of Rouen; Rouen Cedex, France

ANTHONY N. DeMARIA, MD, FACC
Chief of Cardiology and Professor of Medicine, University of Kentucky College of Medicine; President, American College of Cardiology, Lexington, Kentucky

JOHN S. DOUGLAS, Jr., MD
Andreas Gruentzig Cardiovascular Center of Emory University, Departments of Medicine and Radiology, Emory University School of Medicine, Atlanta, Georgia

GERARD DROBINSKI, MD
Hopital de la Pitié Salpetrière, Paris, France

MICHAEL S. FELD, PhD
Professor of Physics and Director, G.R. Harrison Spectroscopy Laboratory, Massachusetts Institute of Technology, Cambridge, Massachusetts

JAMES S. FORRESTER, MD, FACC
Professor of Medicine, University of California, Los Angeles, School of Medicine; Director of Cardiovascular Research, Cedars-Sinai Medical Center, Los Angeles, California

JEAN L. FOURRIER, MD
Division of Cardiology B and Hemodynamics, University Hospital of Lille, France

BEAT FRIEDLI, MD
Professor of Pediatric Cardiology, Department of Pediatrics, University Hospital, Geneva, Switzerland

VALENTIN FUSTER, MD
Mayo Clinic, Rochester, Minnesota

ROBERT GINSBURG, MD
Clinical Assistant Professor of Medicine and Chief, Center for Interventional Vascular Therapies, Stanford University Medical Center, Stanford, California

ANTOINE GOMMEAUX, MD
Service de Cardiologie B et Hémodynamique, Hopital Cardiologique, Lille Cedex, France

WARREN S. GRUNDFEST, MD
Assistant Clinical Professor of Surgery, University of California, Los Angeles, School of Medicine; Assistant Director of Surgery and Director of Laser Surgery and Surgical Research, Cedars-Sinai Medical Center, Los Angeles, California

STEVEN R. GUNDRY, MD
Division of Thoracic and Cardiovascular Surgery, University of Maryland School of Medicine, Baltimore, Maryland

MARGARET HALL, MD
Department of Medicine, University of Washington School of Medicine and the Seattle Veterans Administration Hospital, Seattle, Washington

D. DENNIS HANSEN, MD
Department of Medicine, University of Washington School of Medicine and the Seattle Veterans Administration Hospital, Seattle, Washington

GEOFFREY O. HARTZLER, MD, FACC
Consulting Cardiologist, Mid-America Heart Institute; Clinical Professor of Medicine, University of Missouri at Kansas City, Kansas City, Missouri

MAGDALENA HERAS, MD
Mayo Clinic, Rochester, Minnesota

ANN HICKEY, MD
University of California, Los Angeles, School of Medicine; Cedars-Sinai Medical Center, Los Angeles, California

KIYOSHI INOUE, MD, FACC
Chief, Cardiovascular Disease Center, Tokyo Metropolitan Police Hospital, Tokyo, Japan

MICHAEL INTLEKOFER, MD
Department of Medicine, University of Washington School of Medicine and the Seattle Veterans Administration Hospital, Seattle, Washington

JOSEPH A. IZATT, PhD
G.R. Harrison Spectroscopy Laboratory, Massachusetts Institute of Technology, Cambridge, Massachusetts

ANDREW JAKUBOWSKI, MD
University of California, Los Angeles, School of Medicine; Cedars-Sinai Medical Center, Los Angeles, California

YVES JUILLIÈRE, MD
Catherization Laboratory and Laboratory for Clinical and Experimental Image Processing, Centre Hospitalier Regional et Universitaire de Nancy, Hôpiteaux de Brabois, Vandoeuvre Cedex, France

HANJÖRG JUST, MD
Professor of Medicine, Director, Medical Clinic III, Cardiology, Freiburg, Federal Republic of Germany

PAMELA J. KAISER, MPH
Research Coordinator, White Memorial Medical Center, Los Angeles, California

MARTIN KALTENBACH, MD
Professor of Internal Medicine and Cardiology, Leiter Department of Cardiology, Center of Internal Medicine, Klinikum der Johann Wolfgang Goethe-Universitaet, Frankfurt, Germany

WOLFGANG KASPER, MD
Cardiologist, Medical Clinic III, Freiburg, Federal Republic of Germany

KENNETH R. KENSEY, MD
Assistant Professor of Cardiology, Temple University/Einstein Medical Center, Philadelphia, Pennsylvania

SPENCER B. KING III, MD, FACC
Professor of Medicine, Cardiology, and Radiology, Director, Andreas Gruentzig Cardiovascular Center, Emory University School of Medicine, Emory University Hospital, Atlanta, Georgia

CARTER W. KITTRELL, PhD
G.R. Harrison Spectroscopy Laboratory, Massachusetts Institute of Technology, Cambridge, Massachusetts

GISBERT KOBER, MD
Professor of Internal Medicine and Cardiology, Department of Cardiology, Center of Internal Medicine, Klinikum der Johann Wolfgang Goethe-Universitaet, Frankfurt, Germany

RENE KONING, MD
Catheterization Laboratory and Laboratory for Clinical and Experimental Image Processing, Hopital Charles Nicolle, Rouen Cedex, France

JOHN R. KRAMER, MD
Department of Cardiology, Cleveland Clinic Foundation, Cleveland, Ohio

KEIICHI KUWAKI, MD
Tokyo, Japan

JEAN M. LABLANCHE, MD
Division of Cardiology B and Hemodynamic, University Hospital of Lille, Lille Cedex, France

CHARLES T. LANCÉE, PhD
The Thoraxcenter, Erasmus University and University Hospital, Rotterdam, The Netherlands

FRANCIS Y.K. LAU, MD
Clinical Professor of Medicine, Loma Linda University, Los Angeles, California

MARTIN B. LEON, MD
Senior Investigator, Cardiology Branch, National Heart, Lung, and Blood Institute, National Institutes of Health, Bethesda, Maryland

B. LETAC, MD
Professor, Director of Cardiology, University of Rouen, Rouen Cedex, France

FRANK LITVACK, MD
Assistant Professor of Medicine, University of California, Los Angeles, School of Medicine; Associate Director of Cardiac Catheterization Laboratories, Cedars-Sinai Medical Center, Los Angeles, California

JAMES J. LIVESAY, MD, FACC
Associate Surgeon, Texas Heart Institute and St. Luke's Episcopal Hospital, Houston, Texas; Clinical Associate Professor of Surgery, University of Texas Medical School at Houston, Houston, Texas

PHILLIPE MARACHE, PhD
Division of Cardiology B and Hemodynamic, University Hospital of Lille, Lille Cedex, France

R. BRUCE McFADDEN, MD, FACC
Cardiologist, Clinical Assistant Professor of Medicine, University of Southern California School of Medicine, Los Angeles, California

R. HARDWIN MEAD, MD
Attending Cardiologist, Sequoia Hospital, Redwood City, California; Clinical Instructor of Medicine, Stanford University Medical Center, Stanford, California

BERNHARD MEIER, MD
Cardiology Center, University Hospital, Geneva, Switzerland

THOMAS MEINERTZ, MD
Professor of Medicine, Cardiologist, Medical Clinic III, Freiburg, Federal Republic of Germany

HISATOSHI MINATO, MT
Tokyo, Japan

FREDERICK W. MOHR, MD
Koenitswinter, West Germany

SERGE MORDON, PhD
Division of Cardiology B and Hemodynamics, University Hospital of Lille, Lille Cedex, France

CHARLES E. MULLINS, MD
Professor of Clinical Pediatrics, Baylor College of Medicine; Associate Director of Pediatric Cardiology, Texas Children's Hospital, Houston, Texas

ALLEN B. NICHOLS, MD, FACC
Associate Professor of Clinical Medicine, College of Physicians and Surgeons, Columbia University, New York, New York; Associate Director, Cardiac Catheterization Laboratory, Columbia-Presbyterian Medical Center, Catheterization Laboratory, Columbia-Presbyterian Medical Center, New York, New York

MICHAEL R. NIHILL, MD
Associate Professor of Pediatrics, Baylor College of Medicine; Associate Pediatric Cardiologist, Texas Children's Hospital, Houston, Texas

LEONARD A. NORDSTROM, MD
Clinical Assistant Professor of Medicine, University of Minnesota Medical School, Minneapolis; Chief, Department of Cardiology, Parke-Nicollet Clinic, St. Louis Park, Minnesota

HIDENOBU OCHIAI, MD
Tokyo, Japan

THANASSIS PAPAIOANNOU, MSc
Laser Laboratory, Los Angeles, California

FIROOZ PARTOVI, PhD
G.R. Harrison Spectroscopy Laboratory, Massachusetts Institute of Technology, Cambridge, Massachusetts

WILLIAM J. PENNY, MD
Mayo Clinic, Rochester, Minnesota

JÉROME PETIT, MD
Hopital Marie Lannelongues, Le Plessis Robinson, France

LOUIS D. PREVOSTI, MD
Research Fellow, Cardiology Branch, National Heart, Lung, and Blood Institute, National Institutes of Health, Bethesda, Maryland

JAMES L. RITCHIE, MD, FACC
Professor of Medicine, University of Washington School of Medicine, Seattle; Chief, Cardiovascular Disease Section, Veterans Administration Medical Center, Seattle, Washington

KEITH A. ROBINSON, PhD
Andreas Gruentzig Cardiovascular Center of Emory University, Departments of Medicine and Radiology, Emory University School of Medicine, Atlanta, Georgia

ALLAN M. ROSS, MD, FACC
Professor of Medicine and Director, Division of Cardiology, George Washington University Medical Center, Washington, DC

GARY S. ROUBIN, MB, PhD
Andreas Gruentzig Cardiovascular Center of Emory University, Departments of Medicine and Radiology, Emory University School of Medicine, Atlanta, Georgia

MICHAEL A. RUDER, MD
Attending Cardiologist, Sequoia Hospital, Redwood City, California; Clinical Instructor of Medicine, Stanford University Medical Center, Stanford, California

CARLOS E. RUIZ, MD
Associate Professor, Interventional Laboratory Heart Institute, Good Samaritan Hospital; Associate Professor of Medicine-Cardiology, Loma Linda University, Los Angeles, California

TIMOTHY A. SANBORN, MD
Associate Professor of Medicine; Director, Interventional Cardiology, Research and Laser Angioplasty Program, Mount Sinai Medical Center, New York, New York

JOHAN C.H. SCHUURBIERS
The Thoraxcenter, Erasmus University and University Hospital, Rotterdam, The Netherlands

MATTHEW R. SELMON, MD
Staff Cardiologist, Sequoia Hospital, Redwood City, California; Assistant Clinical Professor of Medicine, Stanford University School of Medicine, Stanford, California

PATRICK W. SERRUYS, MD
The Thoraxcenter, Erasmus University and University Hospital, Rotterdam, The Netherlands

RAMACHANDRA K. SETTY, MD, FACC
Medical Director, Cardiovascular Laboratory at Marion Medical Center, Santa Maria, California

ULRICH SIGWART, MD, FACC
Associate Professor of Medicine, Centre Hospitalier Universitaire Vaudois, Lausanne, Switzerland

JOHN B. SIMPSON, MD, FACC
Staff Cardiologist, Sequoia Hospital, Redwood City, California; Assistant Clinical Professor of Medicine, Duke University Medical Center, Durham, North Carolina

CORNELIS J. SLAGER, MSc
The Thoraxcenter, Erasmus University and University Hospital Rotterdam-Dijkzigt, Rotterdam, The Netherlands

MIKEL SMITH, MD
Associate Professor of Medicine, Division of Cardiology, University of Kentucky Medical Center, Lexington, Kentucky

NELLIS A. SMITH, MD
Attending Cardiologist, Sequoia Hospital, Redwood City, California

PAUL D. SMITH, PhD
Senior Physicist, Biomedical Engineering and Instrumentation Branch, Division of Research Services, National Institutes of Health, Bethesda, Maryland

J. RICHARD SPEARS, MD, FACC
Associate Professor, Wayne State University School of Medicine; Director, Cardiac Laser Laboratory, Harper Hospital, Detroit, Michigan

SIPKE STRIKWERDA, MD
Department of Cardiology, Leiden University Hospital, Leiden, The Netherlands

H.J.C. SWAN, MD, PhD, FACC
Professor of Medicine, University of California, Los Angeles, UCLA School of Medicine; Senior Consultant, Cedars-Sinai Medical Center, Los Angeles, California

ETSUKO TAKANO, MT
Tokyo, Japan

CARL L. TOMMASO, MD
Director, Cardiac Catheterization Laboratory, University of Maryland School of Medicine, Baltimore, Maryland

KEIKO UEDA, MD
Tokyo, Japan

ALEC VAHANIAN, MD
Hopital TENON, Paris, France

CHRISTIAN VALLBRACHT, MD
Department of Cardiology, Center of Internal Medicine, Klinikum der Johann Wolfgang Goethe-Universitaet, Frankfurt, Federal Republic of Germany

WALDINA V.A. VANDENBROUCKE, MD
The Thoraxcenter, Erasmus University and University Hospital, Rotterdam, The Netherlands

JOHN H.K. VOGEL, MD, FACC
Director of Cardiology, Goleta Valley Community Hospital and Director, Santa Barbara Heart and Lung Institute, Santa Barbara; Clinical Professor of Medicine, University of Southern California School of Medicine, Los Angeles, California

ROBERT A. VOGEL, MD, FACC
Director, Division of Cardiology, University of Maryland School of Medicine, University of Maryland Hospital, Baltimore, Maryland

ROGER A. WINKLE, MD
Director, Cardiac Surveillance Unit and Electrophysiology Laboratory, Sequoia Hospital, Redwood City, California; Clinical Associate Professor of Medicine, Stanford University Medical Center, Stanford, California

THOMAS WISENBAUGH, MD
Associate Professor of Medicine, Division of Cardiology, University of Kentucky Medical Center, Lexington, Kentucky

HELMUT WOLLSCHLÄGER, MD
Cardiologist, Medical Clinic III, Frieburg, Federal Republic of Germany

MUAYED AL ZAIBAG, MBChB, FRCP, FACC
Head, Adult Cardiology Division, Riyadh Armed Forces Hospital, Saudi Arabia

FELIX ZIJLSTRA, MD
Catheterization Laboratory and Laboratory for Clinical and Experimental Image Processing, The Thoraxcenter, Erasmus University and University Hospital Rotterdam-Dijkzigt, Rotterdam, The Netherlands

FOREWORD

H.J.C. Swan, MD, PhD, MACP

A decade ago, saphenous vein coronary bypass grafting had gained broad acceptance as an effective treatment for selected cases of severe coronary disease in the hands of skilled and experienced cardiologists and cardiovascular surgeons. Prosthetic cardiac valves also were in general use, with dramatic reductions in morbidity and mortality compared to earlier experiences. This account of recent developments in catheter-based interventional cardiology presents a radical departure from those accepted practices, particularly in the case of coronary artery disease.

Coronary grafting by saphenous vein or internal mammary artery is based on the principle of bypassing and not disturbing the existing intracoronary pathology. Thus, anastomosis into a healthy or moderately diseased distal coronary artery allows for partial or complete restoration of blood flow. The excellent overall results of these procedures on short- and long-term mortality and life quality in optimally managed patients are tempered by the requirements of a major operative procedure with the attendant short and intermediate term morbidity, and high costs to the patient in particular and to society in general. Catheter-based interventional cardiology approaches obstructive coronary artery disease in a completely different manner. The objective is to "remodel" the area of primary pathology with restoration of blood flow through the epicardial coronary circulation. The potential advantages include low short-term morbidity and a significant reduction in costs, although a substantive one-year reocclusion rate requires restudy in as many as 40% to 50% of cases and repeat dilatation in 25% to 30% of the cases.

In 1978, after carefully honing technical skills in patients with peripheral vascular disease, Andreas Gruentzig applied the principle of catheter-based dilatation to the much smaller coronary arteries. His initial experience[1] demonstrated that the symptoms of coronary artery disease could be substantively relieved by high pressure inflation of a small bladder borne on a cardiac catheter. Initial procedures were carried out on symptomatic patients with single- and double-vessel coronary disease. A five- to eight-year follow-up report on all surviving patients demonstrated continued benefits from this direct procedure.[2,3] In recent years, these principles have been applied to more complex vascular anatomy.

While newer guidewire guidance systems and improved catheter construction have facilitated broader applications of the basic principle, it seems less likely that the excellent results in simpler vascular disease will be consistently achieved in more complex cases. Not only does severe atherosclerotic disease extend to several vessels, but several lesions may occur in series in a single vessel. Branch points are particularly susceptible to atherosclerosis and present technical difficulties to the invasive cardiologist. Further, the composition of the obstructive lesions is highly variable between patients from essentially cholesterol-containing plaques, complex fissured plaques with partial or extensive thrombosis formation, to diffuse generalized atherosclerosis of a length of epicardial coronary vessel with increases in local segmental stenoses. Application of angioplasty in patients with unstable angina and following thrombolysis in evolving myocardial infarction is now proposed. Endothelial disruption is present and the potential for additional localized thrombosis and severe vasoconstriction are a consequence of disorder in endothelial function.[4] Recent angioscopy studies have demonstrated that these conditions—unstable angina, acute myocardial infarction and, more importantly,

PTCA itself—results in a crude distortion of the coronary vessel wall. Angioplasty may be effective by distortion of the relatively normal vessel structure without modifying the area of primary pathology.

This text reviews many of these problems. It proposes an intraluminal approach to the removal of obstructive intravascular atherosclerosis by a variety of ingenious techniques. It addresses the issue of downstream embolization and attention is given to facilitating the repair of the endothelium with consideration of anticoagulation and the use of antiplatelet agents.

Application of coronary balloon angioplasty in clinical practice and the need for study of current efficacy of angioplasty techniques have not been critically assessed by cardiologists. In spite of the small procedure-related mortality and morbidity, decisions as to selection of appropriate treatment in the more complex cases should not be made by an invasive cardiologist acting alone. Analysis of many complex factors must precede the election by an individual cardiologist for angioplasty as the optimal treatment for an individual patient. Anatomical changes must be implicated in the genesis of myocardial ischemia by the presence of symptoms and demonstration of hypoperfusion. Decisions based on coronary angiogram alone are totally unjustified; the occasional complications can result in serious penalties to all concerned—and especially to the patient.

Balloon valvuloplasty may consist of a "bridging" intervention in certain patients with aortic valvular disease. The greatest application of the techniques may be in mitral valve stenosis of rheumatic origin. It brings to mind the use of the "finger fracture" technique used more than three decades ago to relieve mitral stenosis. Double balloon techniques may be highly effective on the mitral valve provided that the valve tissue is flexible and that cordial pathology is minimal. This may be of greatest significance in Third World countries in which the availability of sophisticated surgical techniques and prosthetic cardiac valves (and the associated need for anticoagulation) is minimal. Rheumatic heart disease is still near epidemic levels in many parts of the world; balloon angioplasty for mitral valve stenosis in the younger patient could provide dramatic relief for a substantial number of these patients. Balloon angioplasty of the initial mitral valve in patients with an enlarged left atrium, or calcific change in the valve, does not appear to have the same likelihood of success and may carry a very considerable risk.

Valvuloplasty for aortic stenosis has stimulated both support and criticism. The actual alteration in valve mobility and acute hemodynamics appears to be small. Nevertheless, significant improvements in symptomatology and relief of heart failure has been demonstrated in the elderly critically ill patient with severe aortic stenosis. Although calcific emboli may occur in this situation, reported incidences have been surprisingly small.

These contributions by the many distinguished cardiologists to Dr. Vogel's text represent an intermediate rather than a definitive report in the application of these new techniques in invasive cardiology. Problems in angioplasty that might have been predicted a decade ago seem less than might be anticipated and clinical results are better. The next major advance appears to be "remodeling" by removal of abnormal tissue from the areas of pathology rather than relief of obstruction by techniques based on compressive distortion. These are but logical developments based on the fundamental observation by Andreas Gruentzig that it is possible to remodel obstructive coronary atherosclerosis by intracoronary manipulations. Would that he were still with us, to continue to provide his imaginative, considered, and outstanding leadership in invasive cardiology in these exciting times.

REFERENCES

1. Gruentzig, A.: Transluminal dilatation of coronary-artery stenosis, Lancet **1:**263, 1978.
2. Gruentzig, A., King, I.I.I., S.B. Schlumpf, M., Siegenthaler, W.: Long-term follow-up after percutaneous transluminal coronary angioplasty: The early Zurich experience, N. Engl. J. Med. **316:**183-1127, 1987.
3. Kent, K.M.: Coronary angioplasty: A decade of experience, N. Engl. J. Med. **316**(18):1148-1149, 1987.
4. Forrester, J.S., Litvack, F., Grundfest, W., Hickey, A.: Perspective of coronary disease seen through the arteries of living man, Circulation, **75:**505-513, 1987.

PREFACE

This book focuses on future directions in interventional therapies in the rapidly expanding field of cardiovascular disease. A broad interaction between the various approaches relating to aggressive interventional therapy is presented. The specific approaches to therapy, including the techniques and results of major cardiologists from around the world involved in the development of laser angioplasty, balloon valvuloplasty, balloon angioplasty and other mechanical devices for improving coronary blood flow and improving valvular and mechanical function are presented. In addition, methodology for the interpretation of hemodynamic and metabolic function is presented.

I would like to offer my deepest appreciation to my friend and co-editor, Dr. Spencer B. King, without whose help this textbook would not have been possible. I am deeply grateful for the continued help and understanding of my wife, Cynthia M. Vogel, and my daughter, Kristen Marie Richmond, for their understanding of the time necessary to make this book a reality, having been pursued during a continued, active private practice of medicine.

J.H.K. Vogel, MD, FACC

CONTENTS

Chapter 1

Percutaneous Transluminal Coronary Angioscopy as the Guiding Therapy for Intracoronary Thrombolysis and Angioplasty

Kiyoshi Inoue, MD, FACC
Keiichi Kuwaki, MD
Hidenobu Ochiai, MD
Keiko Ueda, MD
Etsuko Takano, MT
Hisatoshi Minato, MT

Thrombus formation occurring at the site of a disrupted coronary plaque is considered to be the precipitating event resulting in acute coronary syndrome.[1-4] The early removal of such thrombi has been demonstrated to be advantageous in both short- and long-term mortality studies. For this reason, therapy aimed at preventing, limiting, or removing such thrombi is gaining interest.[5-8]

The immediate objective of thrombolysis or emergency angioplasty in acute myocardial infarction is to produce a rapid and hemodynamically effective recanalization of the occluded infarct-related artery. Currently, coronary cineangiography is the method for demonstrating the immediate outcome of these interventions. However, whether the recanalization was effective or incomplete, the degree of residual atherosclerosis lining the wall cannot be clearly judged by means of contrast arteriography. However, coronary angioscopy should permit precise intraluminal evaluation.[9-12] Since 1983 we have been reporting our attempts to develop percutaneous transluminal coronary angioscopy (PTCA).[13-16] Recently we have gained experience with simplified PTCA techniques during routine coronary arteriography.[17]

This chapter discusses the results of our attempts to develop a technique to obtain more accurate visual characterization of thrombolytic recanalization and coronary balloon angioplasty.

EXPERIMENTAL PREPARATION

Direct visualization of the dynamic intravascular events following experimental procedures to cause injury to the endothelial covering and to give partial stenosis by external constriction were studied in canine coronary arteries in vivo. Endothelial abrasion usually causes rapid production of mural thrombi which is further accelerated by temporary ligation. Intravascular images of the intimal injury and partial stenosis, thrombus formation and its growth are repeatedly monitored by our PTCAS system. These experiments tested the technical feasibility of PTCAS and evaluated the significance of direct visualization of the intraluminal events.

We have been using a relatively straight portion of the left circumflex (LCX) of the canine coronary artery as an experimental setting for creating thrombus for endoscopy (Fig. 1-1). The transluminal angioscopic catheter is introduced antegrade via the carotid artery using guiding catheters. In the open heart preparation, positioning of the angioscopic catheter in the LCX can be confirmed by its inner illumination. In addition, contrast arteriograms through the guiding catheter within the LCX are made for determining the position of the catheter and the coronary anatomy. Intimal abrasion of the coronary artery is performed under fluoroscopy using a bronchial biopsy brush through the guiding catheter. The images during both intracoronary thrombolysis and balloon angioplasty are also compared with serial angiographic findings. A power injector was used to obtain a transient bloodless visual field by flushing saline solution at a rate ranging from 0.5 ml/sec to 3 ml/sec depending on the size or rate of flow in the circulation. A total of 3 to 10 ml of saline was flushed intermittently to obtain transient bloodless visual fields for 10 to 20 beats.

In Vivo Visualization of the Intact Canine Coronary Artery

Figure 1-2 shows images of the intact inner wall of the proximal portion of the LCX. The smooth intima of the LCX is clearly visualized. These serial photographic images are taken using high-speed 35-mm film during the flushing with saline solution. The bloodless visual fields are seen in the top right two and middle three. The endothelium of the intact canine LCX coronary artery is seen as smooth in these panels. The bottom three images show reopacification by backflow.

In Vivo Visualization of Coronary Arterial Thrombus

The left panel in Fig. 1-3 is the control and the right is the intraluminal appearance immediately after the intimal abrasion. In Fig. 1-4, the endothelial damage and the intimal flap created by abrasion are clearly seen. Focal hemorrhage, mixed mural thrombi, red thrombi, and fibrin netting are shown. These changes cannot normally be detected by contrast arteriography. The abraded area is highly thrombogenic. The abraded area is externally ligated and approximately 90% stenosis is created to reduce blood flow and to facilitate thrombus formation. This situation is similar to the thrombotic events occurring in association with coronary plaque fissuring at the site of high-grade stenotic atherosclerotic lesions. Repeated angioscopy is performed to follow the in vivo spontaneous growth of thrombi. Approximately 45 minutes following ligation, thrombotic occlusion is created as shown in Fig. 1-5. In a proximal view, one can see flushing of the thrombotic area, while thick tomato-puree-like red thrombi develop following the total thrombotic occlusion and fill the visual field (Fig. 1-6, B). Usually, large amounts of occlusive thrombus are created around the abrazed and partially stenosed area. The thrombotic occlusion was composed

Text continues on page 8.

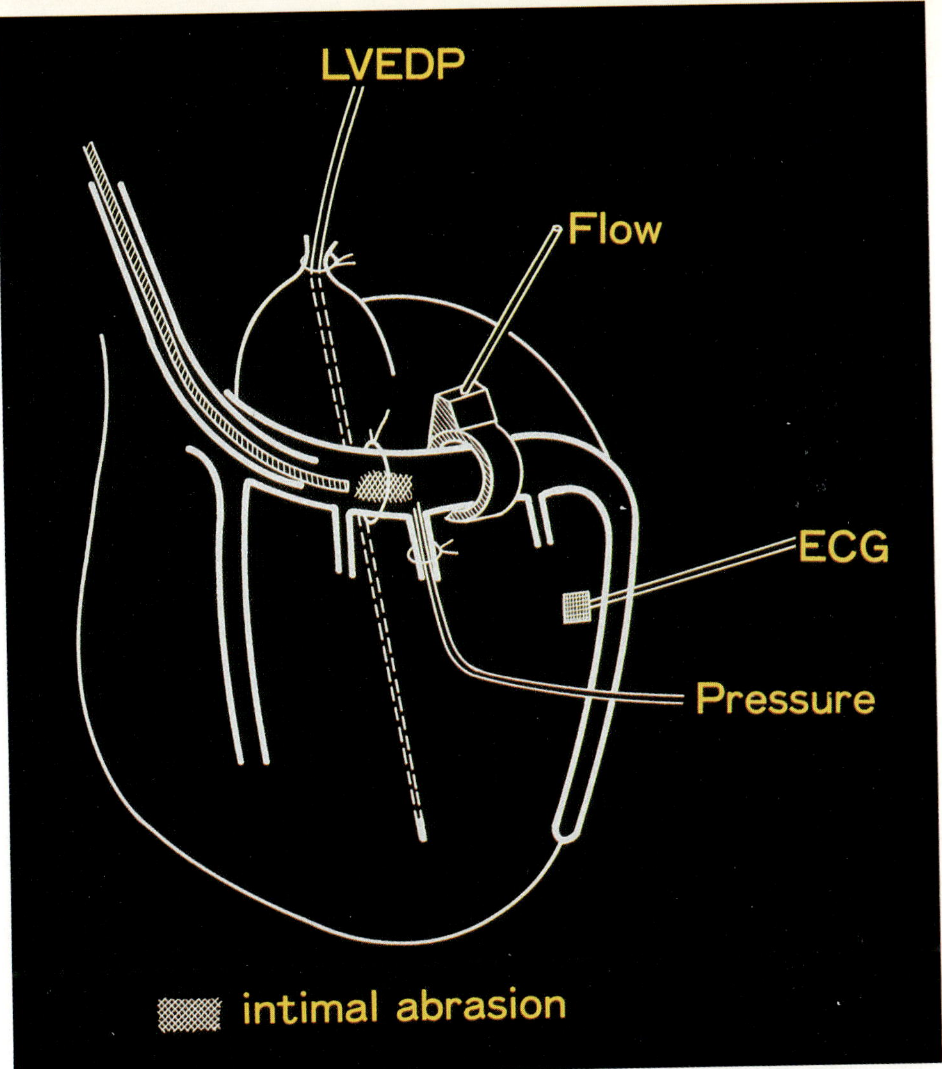

Fig. 1-1. Schema of an experimental setting for creating canine coronary arterial thrombus as the observational target for endoscopy. In the canine, the heart is exposed by means of a pericardial sling under pentobarbital anesthesia and room-air ventilation. A small plastic constrictor and a Doppler flow probe are placed around the relatively straight portion of the proximal left circumflex (LCX) artery. Phasic and mean flows, a pressure through the distal catheter, left ventricular (LV) pressure through the left artrial (LA) appendage, surface electrocardiogram, and heart rate are monitored. The angioscopic catheter is inserted into the area just proximal to the constrictor using a guiding catheter that is delivered by way of the right carotid artery. In this preparation, the positioning in the LCX artery of the angioscopic catheter can easily be made by its inner illumination. Following successful visualization of the intact inner wall, an abrasion of the endothelial covering using a biopsy brush available for bronchial biopsy and 75 to 90% intraluminal narrowing by the constrictor are made at the site just proximal to the Doppler flow probe under fluoroscopic guidance. Totally obliterative coronary arterial thrombus is usually created within 40 to 50 minutes. Angioscopy and arteriography are repeated throughout the experimental PTCR and PTCA.

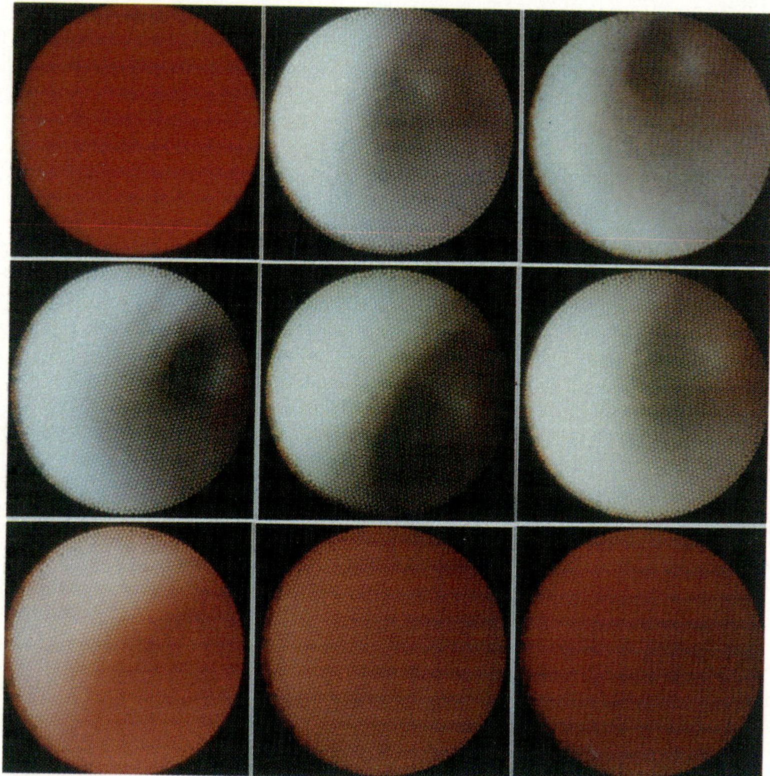

Fig. 1-2. In-vivo endoscopy of the intact canine coronary artery. *Top left,* Pulsating blood can be seen. *Top, middle and left panels,* By flushing the pressurized warm saline solution to create a transient bloodless field, the smooth endothelium of the intact proximal left circumflex (LCX) artery is visualized, as seen also in the pictures in the middle panels. The dimple in the inner LCX wall itself is due to the nature of the tortuous coronary arterial tree. The bottom three panels show the process of reopacification by backflow.

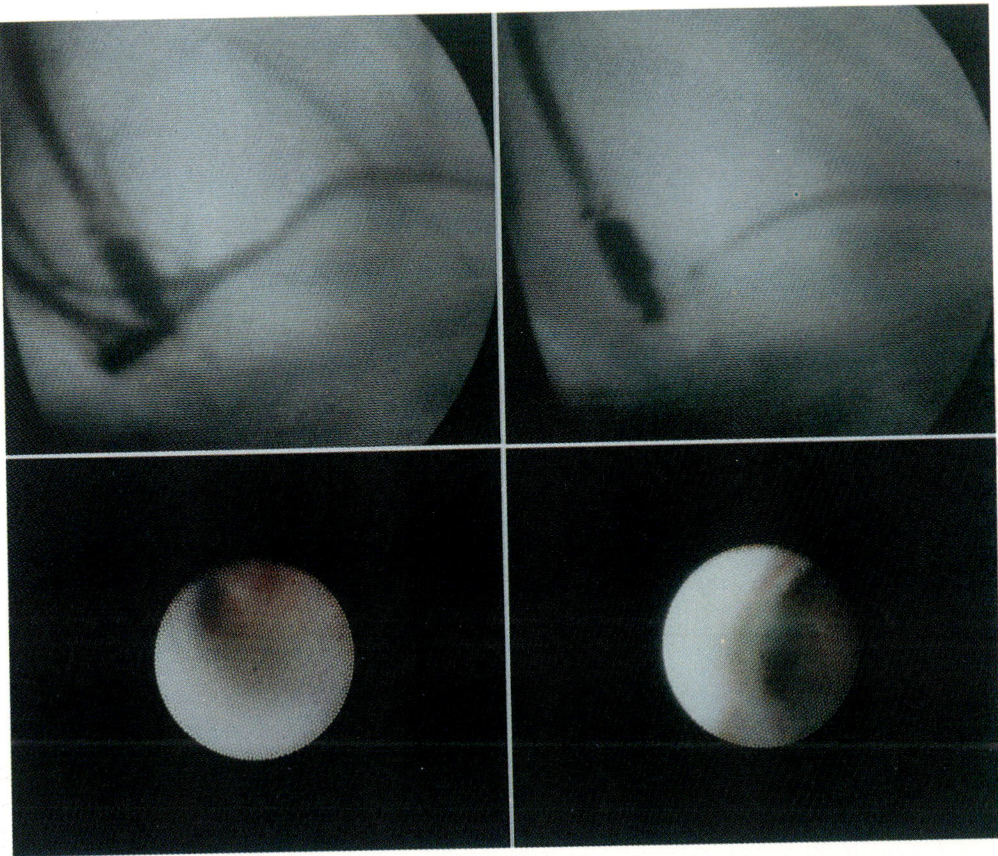

Fig. 1-3. Coronary arteriography and angiography to compare intact and abraded endothelium. The left panel shows the contrast arteriography *(upper left)* and angioscopy *(lower left)* of the intact proximal LCX and the right panel are those following abrasion. A frayed endothelial covering and focal hemorrhages are clearly visualized in the angioscopy *(lower right panel)* but not by contrast arteriography *(upper right panel.)*

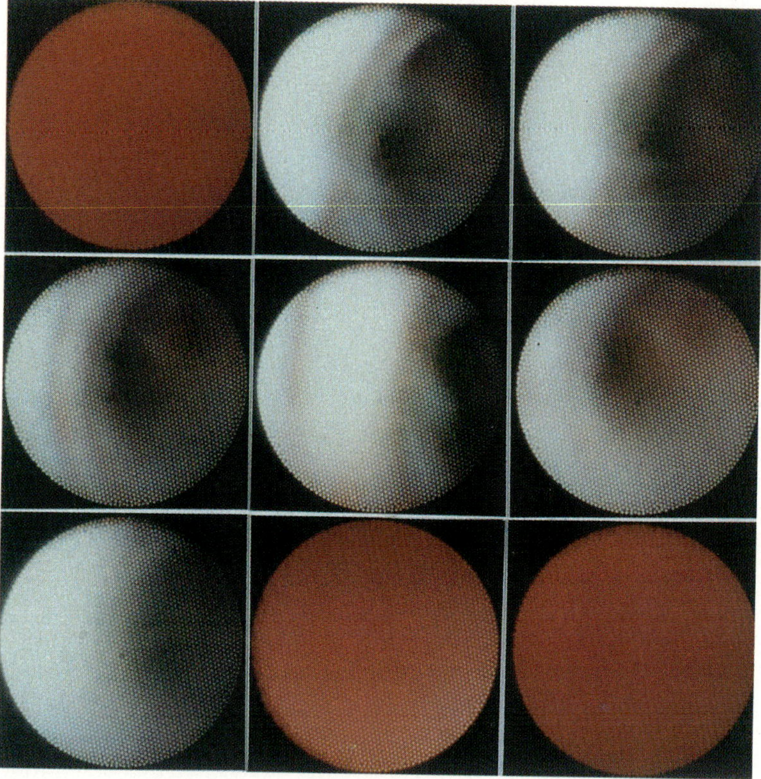

Fig. 1-4. Angioscopic images of the abraised endothelium of the proximal LCX. Serial photographic images taken by high-speed 35 mm films during saline flushing. The frayed intimal flap, focal hemorrhages, and rapidly appearing mural thrombi are clearly visualized by flushing of pressurized saline solution *(top, middle and right panel; middle panel;* and *bottom left panel).*

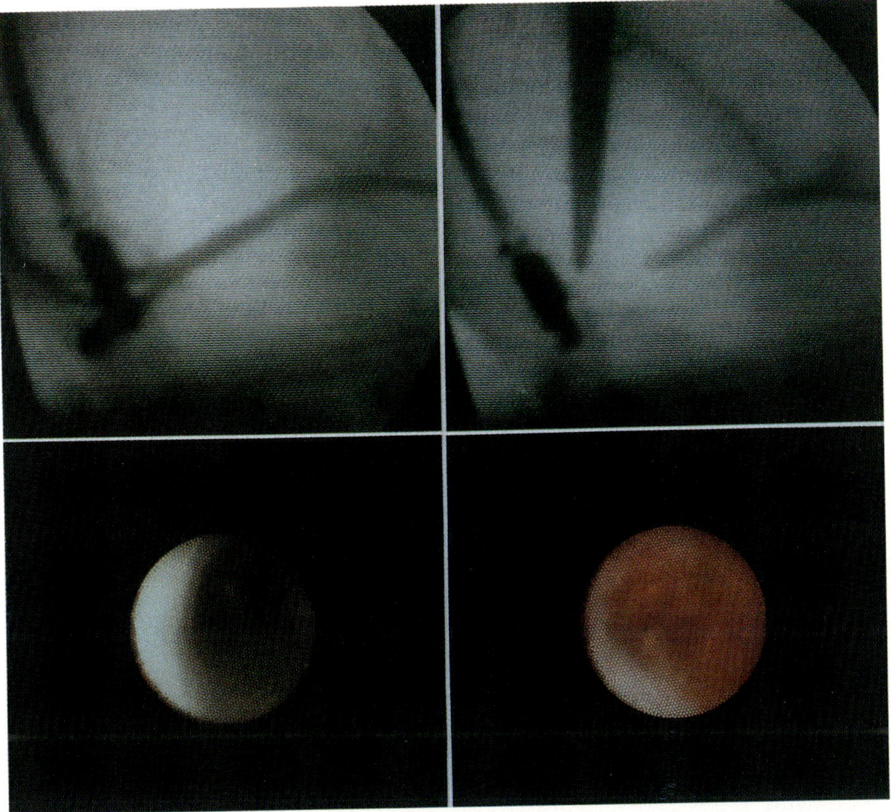

Fig. 1-5. Angioscopy of in-vivo occlusive coronary arterial thrombi. The abraded area is seen to be highly thrombogenic. A portion of the abraded area is externally ligated and approximately 75 to 90% stenosis is created to reduce blood flow and to facilitate thrombus formation *(lower left)*. Approximately 45 minutes following ligation, total thrombotic occlusion is created. In a proximal view, after flushing of the thrombotic area, thick tomato puree–like red thrombi occur as a result of nonflow *(lower right)*.

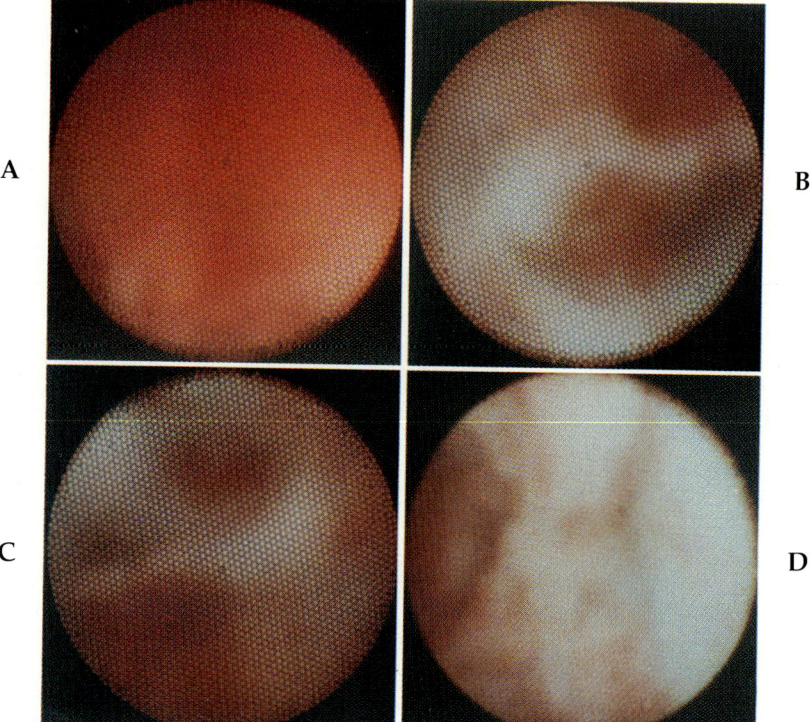

Fig. 1-6. Angioscopy of in-vivo occlusive coronary arterial thrombi. *Top left panel,* In a proximal view seen after flushing of the thrombotic area, thick tomato puree—like red thrombi develop following the total thrombotic occlusion and fill the visual field. *Top right panel,* Proximal view of subtotal thrombotic occlusion. The central lumen created by the concentric development of mural thrombi is corked by the spongy red thrombi. The well-developed mixed mural thrombi, fibrin clots, and spongy red thrombi are seen in the lower panels. *Bottom left panel,* The surface is uneven, because growth occurs against flow. *Bottom right panel,* By repeated flushing with saline solution, the red spongy thrombi covering up the mural thrombi are partially washed out, revealing the uneven surface of the maturing mixed mural thrombi.

of a firm mural thrombus and a solid red thrombus being spongy in nature. The central lumen created by the concentrical development of the mural thrombi is corked by the spongy red thrombi. The well developed mixed mural thrombi, fibrin clots, and spongy red thrombi are seen in the lower panels of Fig. 1-6. Mixed mural thrombi usually develop concentrically. The surface is uneven because it grows up against the flow (bottom left panel).

By repeated flushing with saline solution, the red spongy thrombi covering up the mural thrombi are partially washed out, revealing the uneven surface of the maturing mixed

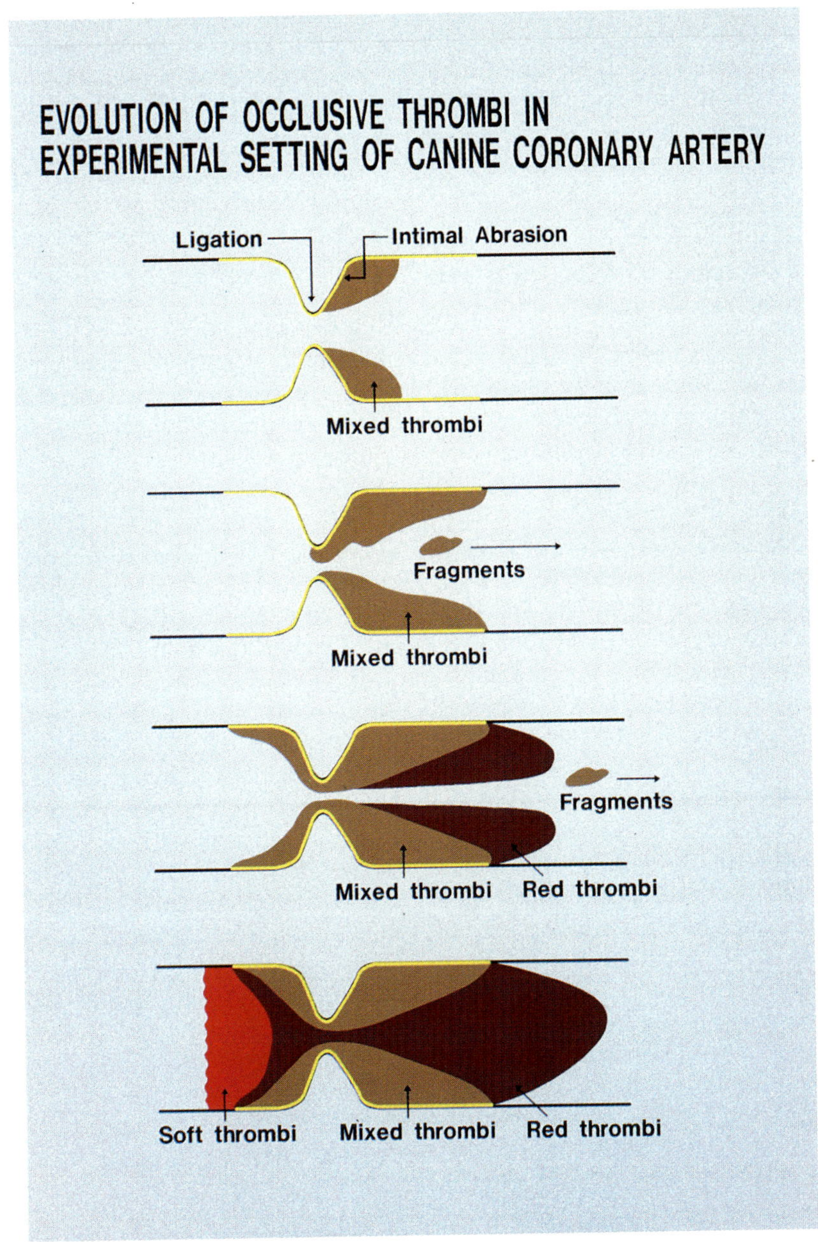

Fig. 1-7. Schema of the evolution of occlusive thrombi in experimental setting of canine coronary artery. Cross-sectional anatomy of the abraded and stenosed area show the process of natural development of the occlusive thrombi following intimal abrasion plus external constriction, charted from our series of angioscopic observations.

mural thrombi (bottom right panel). This solid spongy red thrombi covers up the mixed mural thrombi which are created concentrically around the abraded and stenosed area. The matured occlusive thrombi are in fairly large amounts, being composed of firm mixed thrombi, fibrin nettings, and red thrombi with long tails.

Proposed Evaluation of the Coronary Arterial Thrombus (Fig. 1-7)

Figure 1-6 illustrates the cross-sectional anatomy of the abraded and stenosed area and the process of the natural development of the occlusive thrombi, charted from our series of angioscopic observations. Mural thrombi, initially created on the proximal side of the stenosis, gradually develop in size, while small fragments of mixed thrombi or fibrin clots are carried into the distal site and may produce thrombotic occlusion of smaller arteries. Actually, we saw these fragments by passing the angioscope through the stenosed area. Sudden ventricular fibrillation can occur in this situation. This process may be responsible for sudden cardiac death in the clinical setting. The concentrically developed mixed mural thrombi gradually reduce the lumen and produce the subtotal obstruction; then the red spongy thrombi cover up the central lumen to create total thrombotic occlusion. In this situation, the cyclic flow variations in distal flow and pressure are frequently observed. We believe that the red spongy thrombi covering the central lumen might be responsible for this phenomenon.[15] Subsequently, a matured thrombus is created, with total thrombotic occlusion (Fig. 1-6, bottom right panel).

Angioscopy-Guided Intracoronary Thrombolysis

Figure 1-8 illustrates the process of thrombolysis by t-PA intracoronary infusion. The top left panel shows the occlusive thrombi before lysis, and from top middle to bottom right shows the process dissolution. Lysis of red thrombi is initiated, then gradual denudation, splitting, and lysis of mixed thrombi occur during t-PA infusion. After 15 minutes of t-PA intracoronary infusion, thrombolysis is occurring as shown in the top middle and right panels. Tomato-puree-like thrombi are no longer present. After 30 minutes, solid, spongy red thrombi are being dissolved as in the top right and bottom left panels.

Splitting of red thrombi due to dissolution and partial denudation of the mural mixed thrombi are seen in the bottom middle panel. Although cineangiographically we can confirm the partial restoration of blood flow in these situations, the complex interior process of thrombolysis cannot be perceived in the routine contrast arteriogram.

With continuing t-PA infusion, slow but progressive thrombus dissolution, cracking of red thrombus, and denudation of mural thrombi continue. As flow is restored, judged by measuring distal flow and pressures, thrombolysis seemed to be almost complete after 45 minutes of t-PA infusion. However, the residual mixed thrombi and a large amount of fibrin netting are still present (Fig. 1-8, bottom right panel). With these direct interior views using the angioscope, the exact degree to which thrombolysis has occurred can easily be confirmed. These changes normally cannot be detected by routine contrast arteriography. With continuing t-PA infusion and poking with the guide wire, the residue is further cleared. Now, the abraded wall with small attached mural thrombi is clearly visible due to further passive clearing. But the thrombus begins to redevelop around mural thrombi after stopping the t-PA infusion.

Angioplasty During PTCA

Using a similar technique, complete thrombotic occlusion is created, and the external constriction is removed in a canine model. Balloon dilatation is applied to the occluded area (Fig. 1-9). Two images in Fig. 1-10 compare the interior views before and after balloon angioplasty applied for the total throm-

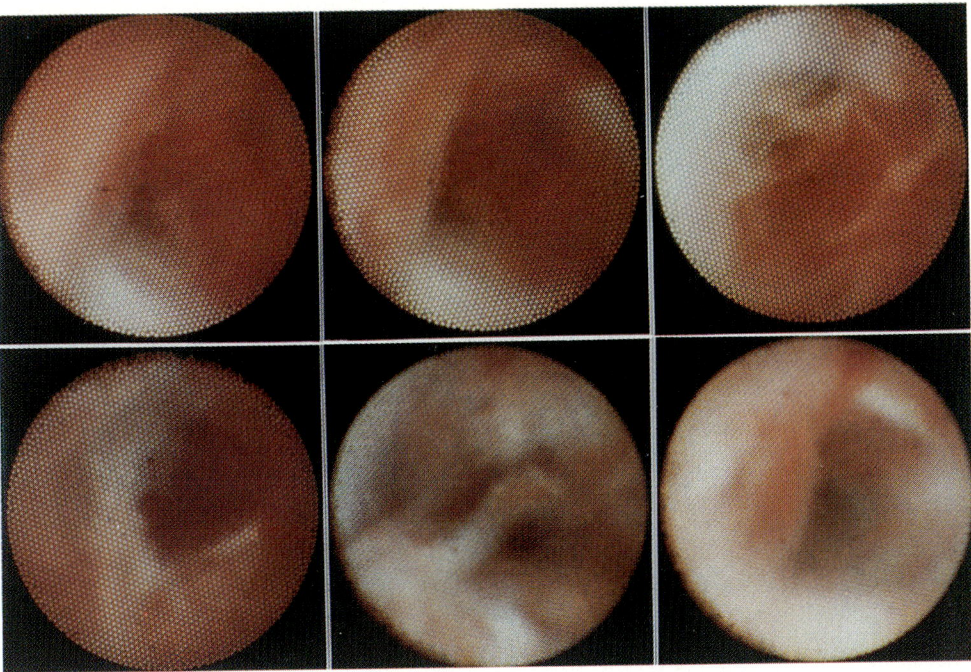

Fig. 1-8. Angioscopy during thrombolysis. With TPA intracoronary infusion, thrombolysis can be accomplished. The tomato puree–like thrombi are no longer present. A solid spongy red thrombus are being percoleted. The splitting of red thrombi caused by its dissolution and the partial denudation of the mural mixed thrombi are seen.

botic occlusion. Balloon dilatation was applied only once. The left panel is the control, and the right panel is the outcome immediately after the angioplasty. As shown in Fig. 1-10, the recanalized lumen is occluded immediately after angioplasty because of the spongy nature of the red thrombi covering the mixed mural thrombi. Figure 1-11 demonstrates the process of effective balloon dilatation being repeated. The top left panel is the control, and the top middle and right panels are the outcome of a single dilatation. The cracked and dilated lumen is immediately reoccluded as in the middle and right panels. The rest of the images are the outcomes of repeated dilatation. The cracking of the mural thrombi and focal hemorrhaging of the endothelium are results of the interventions.

In other words, the mixed mural thrombi, denudated and split residual thrombus, fibrin clots, and focal hemorrhage are results of balloon angioplasty. These lesions are highly thrombogenic. Figure 1-12 illustrates in vivo angioscopic mechanism applied for the thrombotic coronary occlusion in this experimental setting. As shown in this schema, with balloon dilatation, the cracking of both firm mural and spongy red thrombi is produced. This results in the silhouette of contrast arteriography as shown in the middle panel. The cracking occurs eccentrically without causing serious intimal damage when the thrombi develop concentrically.

However, rupture of intact intimal lining and hemorrhage can be caused when the development of thrombus occurs in an uneven fashion. These observations indicate the importance of the interrelationships between the

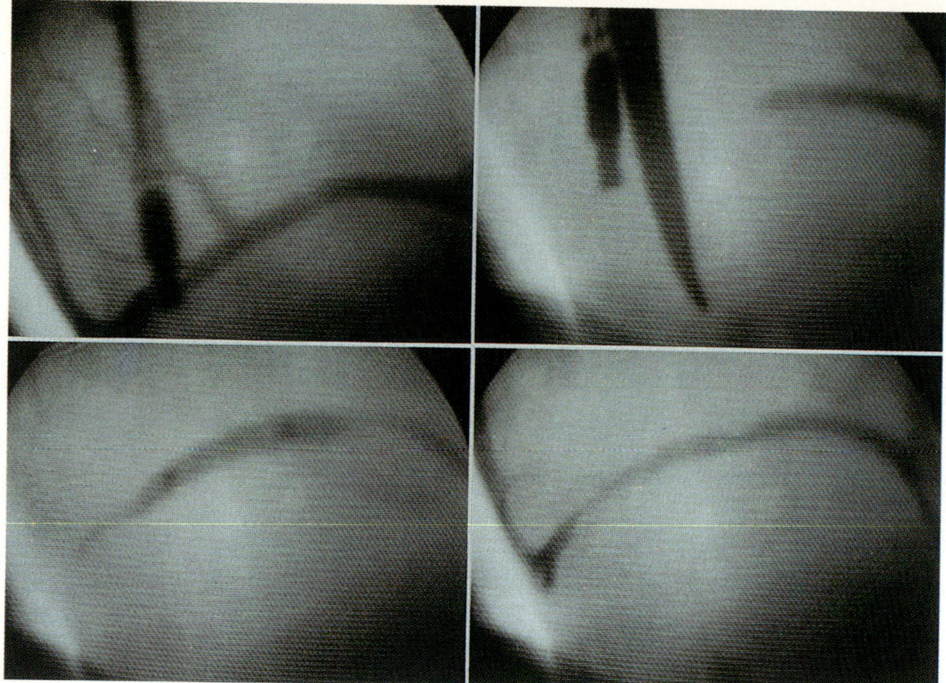

Fig. 1-9. Balloon angioplasty. *Upper right,* Using similar technique, a complete thrombotic occlusion is created in another canine model. Thrombi have totally obliterated the lumen owing to nonflow. *Lower left,* Balloon dilatation is applied to the occluded area, and the area of occlusion is recanalized *(lower right).*

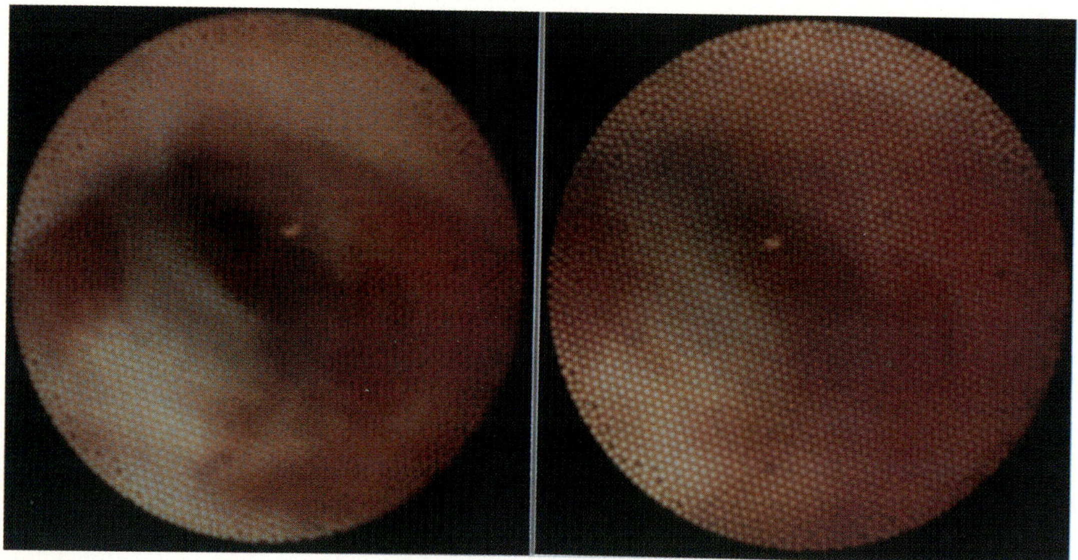

Fig. 1-10. Angioscopic outcome of ineffective balloon angioplasty. Control *(left)* and outcome *(right)* immediately after a single angioplasty. As can be seen, the recanalized lumen is occluded immediately after the angioplasty, because of the spongy nature of the red thrombi covering up the mixed mural thrombi.

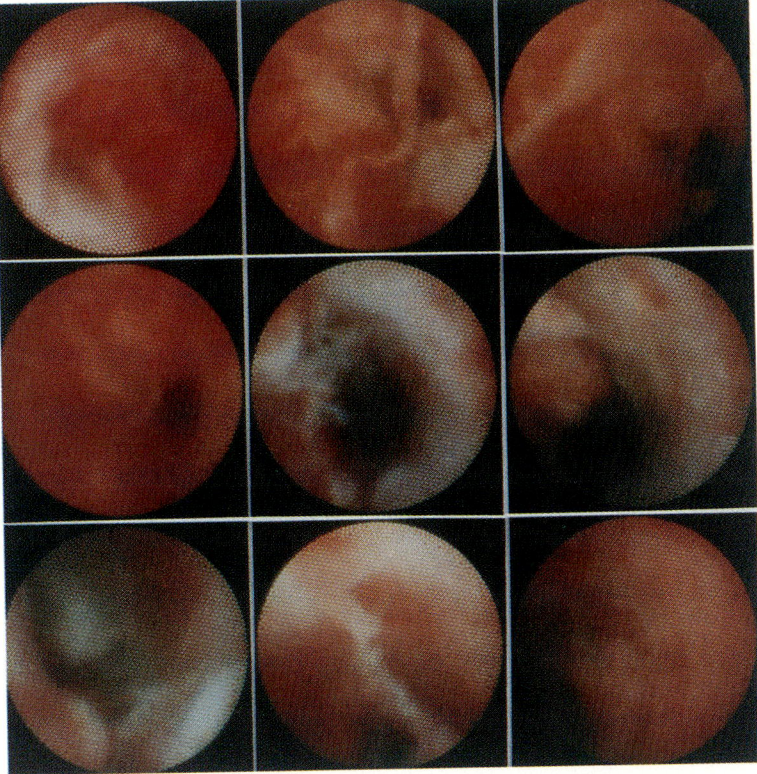

Fig. 1-11. Angioscopy during effective balloon angioplasty. The process of effective balloon dilatation is being repeated. Control *(top left)* and outcome *(top, middle and right)* of a single PTCA. After the procedure, the cracked and dilated lumen is immediately reoccluded again, as shown in the middle and right panel. The rest of the illustrations are those of repeated dilatation. The cracking of the mural thrombi and focal hemorrhaging of the endothelium following the repeated balloon angioplasty are clearly visualized.

inside appearance of the thrombotic occlusion and the method of angioplasty.

Through these experiences in canine preparations, and with direct macropathologic observations during percutaneous transluminal coronary reperfusion (PTCR) and PTCA, we have gained further insight into the complex mechanisms of thrombus formation, thrombolysis, and thrombus reformation. We believe percutaneous transluminal angioscopy is a useful technique in thrombolysis and angioplasty in a clinical setting.

CLINICAL APPLICATION

The technical feasibility of PTCA as a guiding therapy during intracoronary thrombolysis or angioplasty was tested using an angioscopic catheter we developed for the intraluminal visualization of the infarct-related artery. The results of recanalizing interventions during coronary arteriography were studied within a few hours from the onset of acute myocardial infarction.

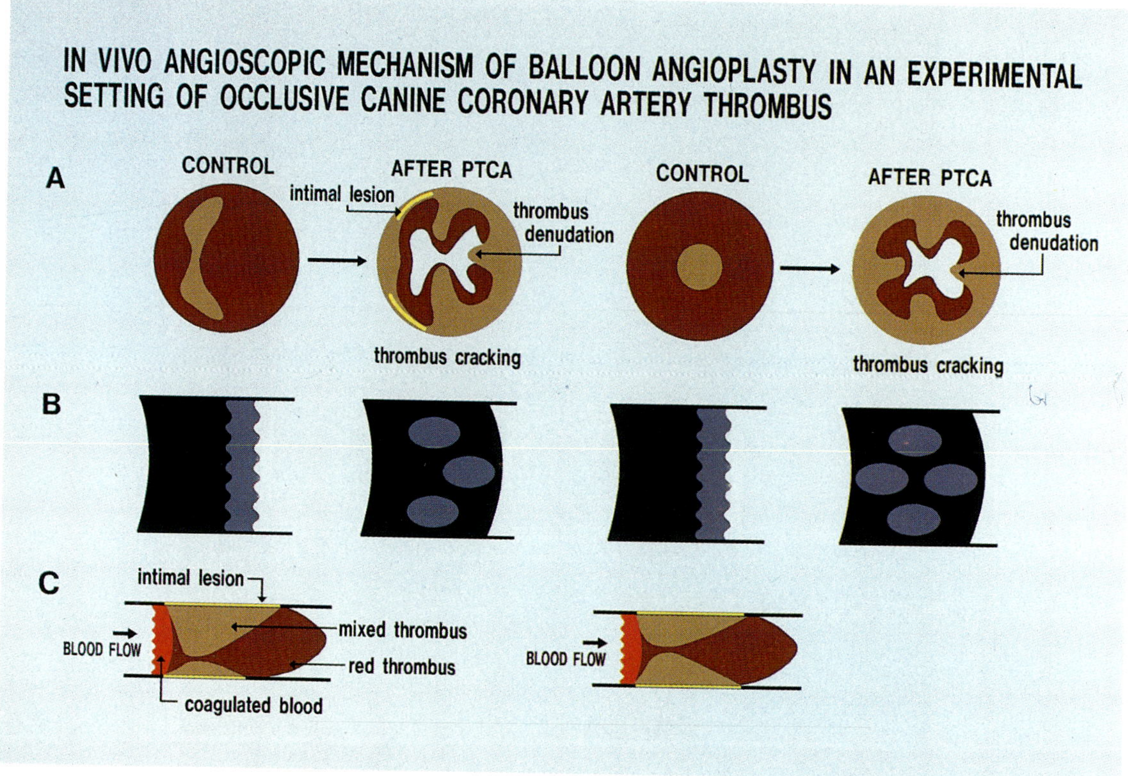

Fig. 1-12. In-vivo angioscopic mechanism of balloon angioplasty in an experimental setting of occlusive canine coronary artery thrombus.

Angioscopic Catheter and Its Imaging System

The angioscopic catheter and its insertion technique in patients are similar to those explained in the experimental setting. A sterile and disposable angioscopic catheter (outer diameter 0.75 mm, and 210 cm in length) (Fig. 1-13A) we developed is applied for this purpose. The light guide is connected to the Xenon lamp, and the image guide is connected to the CCD camera head. The image is recorded, stored, and displayed on a VTR system (Fig. 1-13B). Figure 1-14 shows how the catheter is delivered by a double guiding catheter system into the coronary artery using the percutaneous Judkins approach through the femoral artery. We developed several variations of angioscopic catheters, with and without the fabricated tip angulation mechanism, ranging from 0.7 to 1.4 mm in outer diameter. The catheter contains 3000 pixels of imaging fibers plus 50 illuminating bundles. The model in this photograph has a tip 0.75 mm in diameter and 210 cm in length. The tiny tip of this catheter is turned on in the model in the upper panel and used as a radiopaque silhouette in the proximal LAD as shown in the lower panel of Fig. 1-14.

Double Guiding Catheter System

The double guiding catheter system used for angioscopy is composed of a regular F#8 for PTCA and the thin-wall soft tip #5. The inner guiding catheter is introduced proximal to the coronary artery through the outer guid-

A

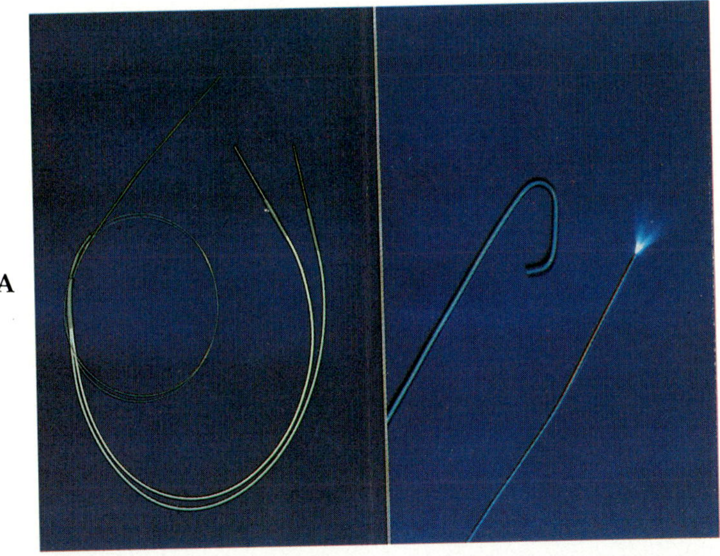

B

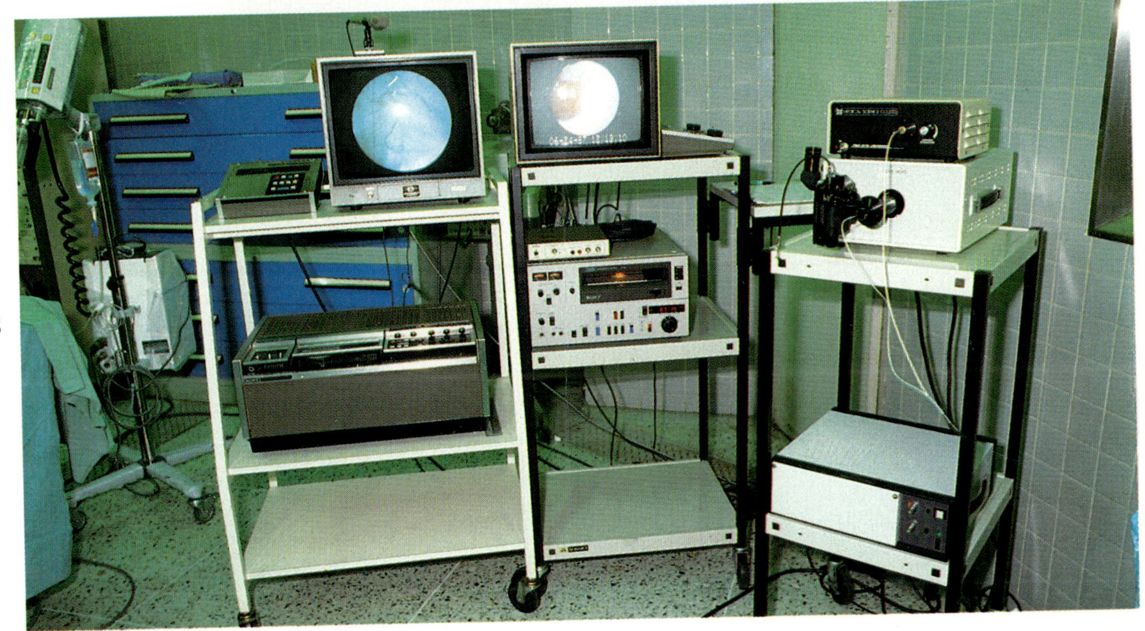

Fig. 1-13. A, disposable angioscopic catheter. We developed a sterile and disposable angioscopic catheter. The outer diameter of 0.75 mm, and it is 220 cm in length. On the left is the regular 7F Swan-Ganz catheter. Although we developed four variations of the disposable angioscopic catheter with or without the tip angulation device, ranging in outer diameter from 0.3 to 14.0 mm, a 0.75 mm model is mainly used in this series. **B,** angioscopic imaging system used in our catheterization laboratory. The light guide is connected to the xenon lamp and the image guide is connected to the CCD camera head. The image is recorded, stored, and displayed on a VTR system.

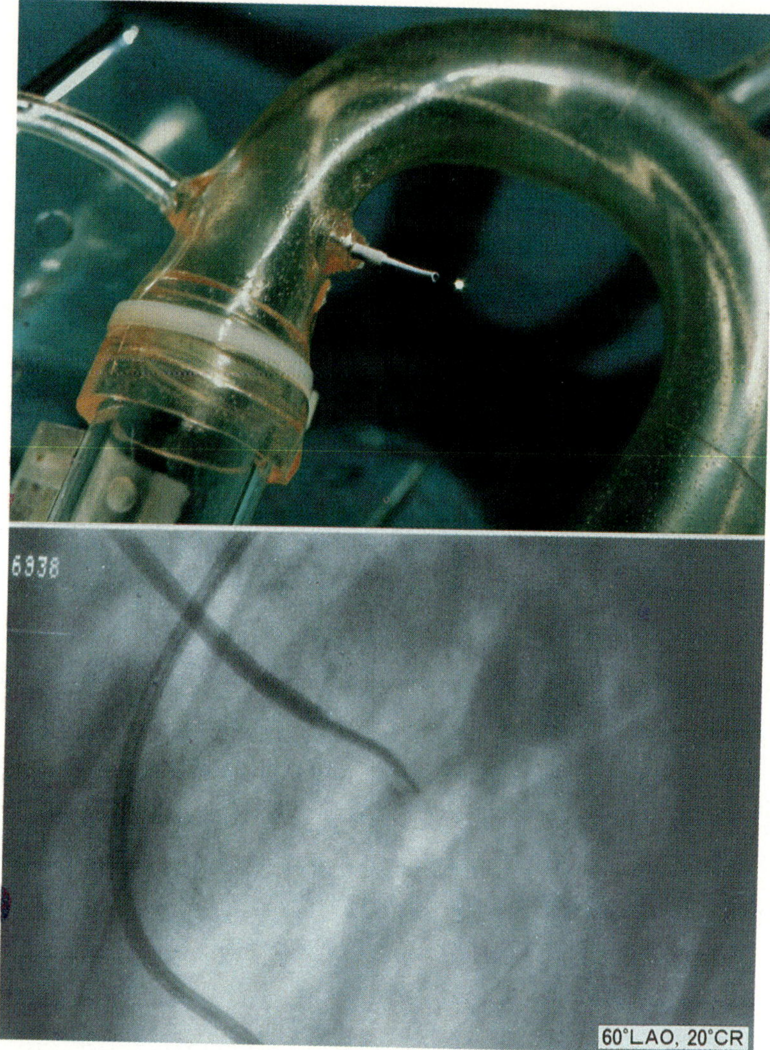

Fig. 1-14. Catheter is delivered by a double guiding catheter system into the left coronary artery by the percutaneous transluminal approach via the femoral artery. The tiny tip of the angioscopic catheter is shown turned on in a model in the upper panel and as a radiopaque silhouette in the lower panel.

ing catheter and is left in place. It is then used for inserting the angioscopic catheter and flushing dextrose solution to obtain a visible field. Initially, a regular F#8 guiding catheter for PTCA is introduced into the coronary artery by way of the femoral artery, and diagnostic arteriography is performed. A regular F#5 thin-wall soft tip guiding catheter is introduced into the proximal coronary artery using a guide wire by way of the outer guiding catheter. Then, the guide wire is removed, and the inner guiding catheter is locked. The tip end of the inner guiding catheter is positioned just proximal to the occlusion. The surface of the angioscopic catheter is wiped with heparin gauze to prevent clot-

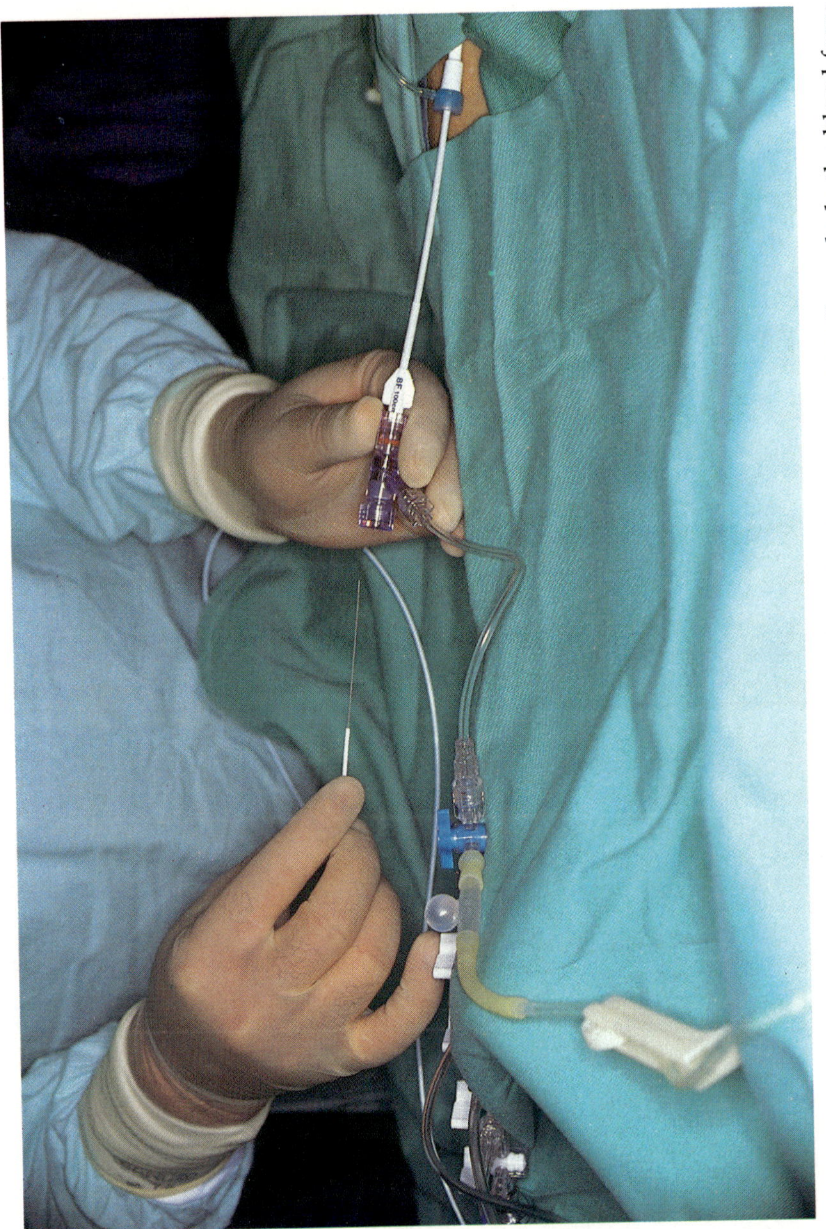

Fig. 1-15. Insertion technique of angioscopic catheter. Flushing to temporarily exclude the blood from the visual lights is accomplished through the thin-walled inner guiding catheter and a Y-connector.

ting. The angioscopic catheter is inserted very gently through this setting. The visual focus and lighting should be adjusted before insertion. The Y connector is used for flushing and preventing leakage of blood (Fig. 1-15). Following contrast arteriography through the outer guiding catheter to determine the exact site of occlusion, angioscopy is performed by manipulating the tip of the angioscopic catheter to a position just proximal to the occlusion. The observational target is brought into sight by using torque on the inner guiding catheter.

Flushing to Obtain Bloodless Visual Field

A flushing of 5% dextrose solution by hand injection or through the compression bag is made to obtain a bloodless field for the initial test visualization of the interior of the inner guiding catheter. A power injector can be applied for flushing at a rate of 1 to 3 ml per second for total amounts of 5 to 7 ml to achieve the transient bloodless visual field for several beats, depending on the rate and amounts of flow in the coronary system.

Angioscopy of the Intact Inner Wall, Atheroma Plaque, and Thrombus

Initially, the tip of the angioscopic catheter is located in the inner guiding catheter, thus the visual field is white. Then, as the scope is advanced to the distal end of the inner guiding catheter, the smooth surface of the intact wall of the coronary ostial or proximal area can be visualized.

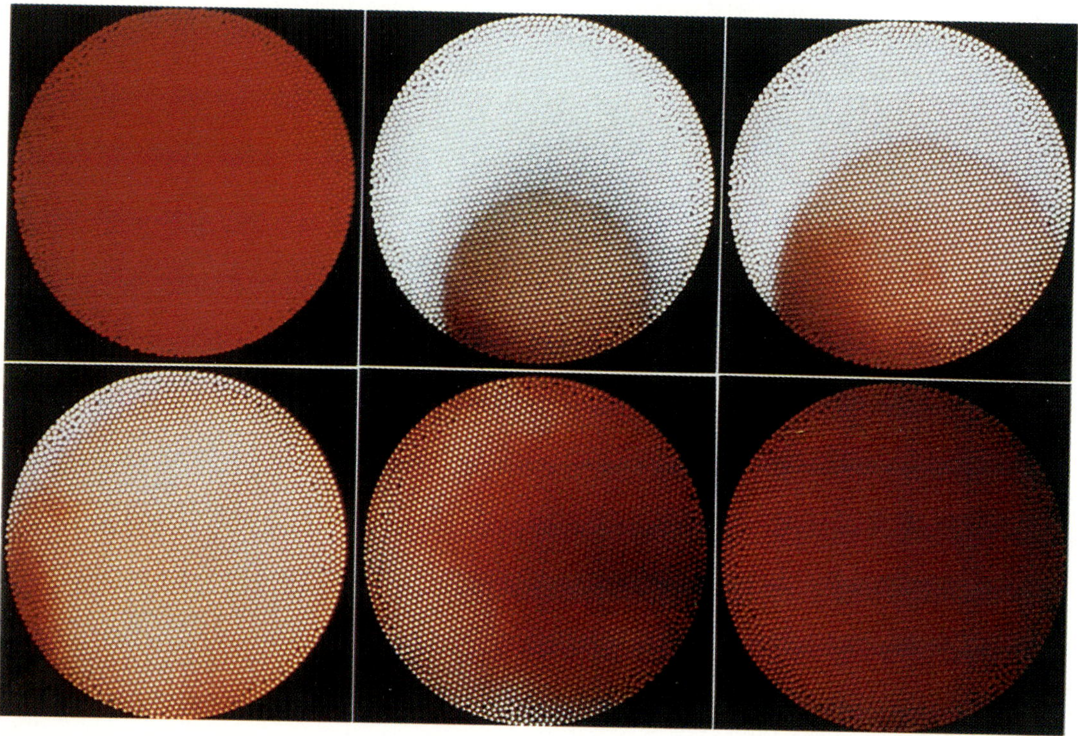

Fig. 1-16. Transient but clear visual images are obtained as seen in the top right two panels by flushing a warm, 5% dextrose solution at a rate of 0.3 to 3.0 ml per second, depending on the flow in the circulation.

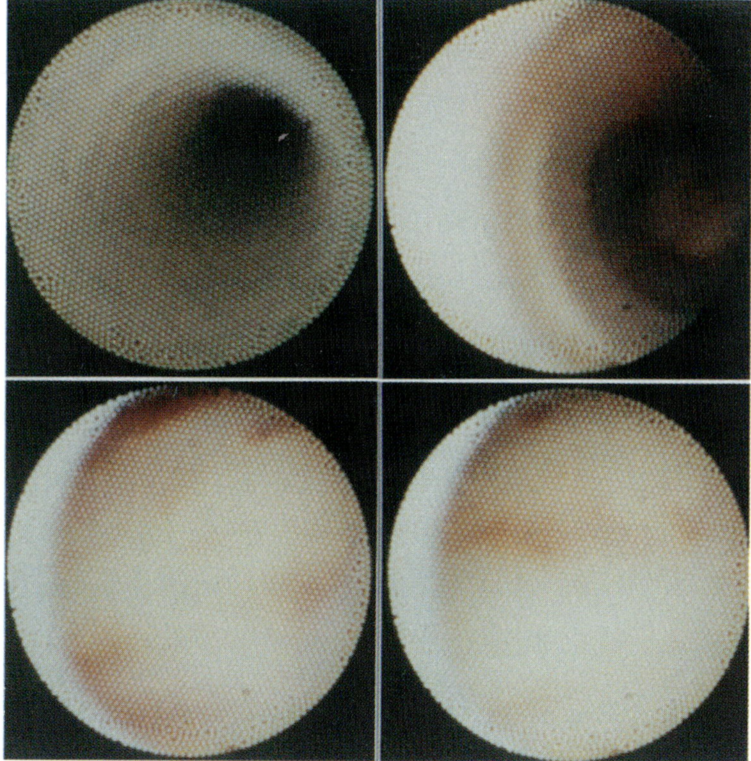

Fig. 1-17. Manipulation of the angioscopic catheter. *Top left,* The tip of the angioscopic catheter is initially positioned within the inner guiding catheter (IG), then advanced very gently toward the tip end of the IG and into the vascular lumen, as shown in the top left and bottom two panels.

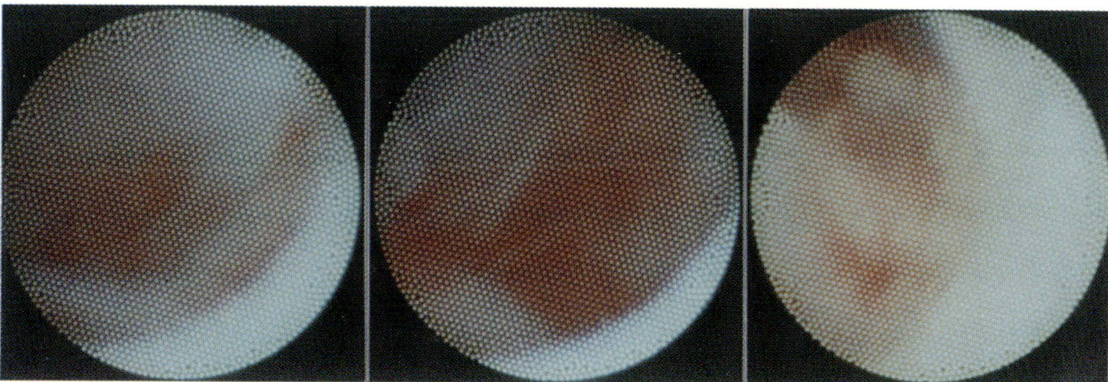

Fig. 1-18. Atheroma plaque in the proximal LAD artery. These images are taken following intracoronary thrombolysis, demonstrate a large atheroma plaque with residual thrombus, focal hemorrhage, and lipid-laden debris in its surface.

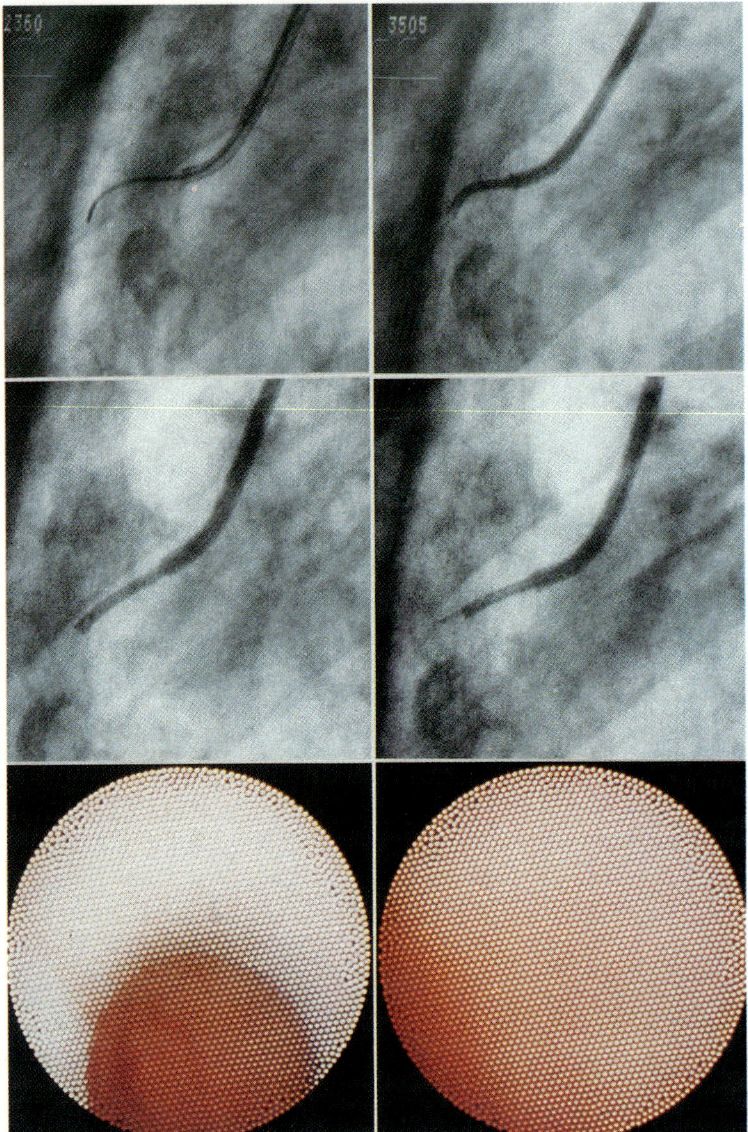

Fig. 1-19. Delivering the angioscopic catheter into the RCA. Initially a guidewire is inserted into the proximal RCA through an 8F PTCA guiding catheter *(top left panel)*, then the inner guiding catheter (IG) is inserted *(top middle panel* and *middle left panel)*, and the angioscopic catheter is advanced through the IG *(middle right panel)* into the lumen. The bottom left is the angioscopy of which tip-end is located within IG and then beyond the IG *(bottom right panel)*.

Flushing achieves a transient bloodless field as shown in the top two and bottom left panels in Fig. 1-16. As shown in Fig. 1-17, the tip of the angioscopic catheter was positioned initially within the inner guiding catheter, as in the top left panel, and advanced gently into the lumen, being careful not to damage the vascular wall and reducing the chance of intimal injury, as in top right and bottom two panels. In the bottom two panels you can see the large atheroma occupying the lumen of proximal LAD. Three photographs in Fig. 1-18 compare the different quality of images due to positioning of the tip of the angioscope. The left and middle panels are distant views of the atheroma of the proximal LAD, and the right panel is a close-up view detailing soft lipid laden debris.

Figure 1-19 shows the process of delivering the catheters into the right coronary artery (RCA). Through the PTCA guiding catheter as shown on the top left panel, the guide wire is advanced distally. With this, the inner guiding catheter is introduced into the proximal RCA as shown on the top right panel. The middle two panels demonstrate two different positions of the tip of the angioscopic catheter, and the bottom two panels are the angioscopic images taken at these catheter positions. The intraluminal images are seen through the guiding catheter as on the bottom left panel, while the entire image is of the wall itself when the tip is located beyond the distal end of the guiding catheter (bottom right panel). Figure 1-20 compares the radiographic silhouette of the RCA proximal ob-

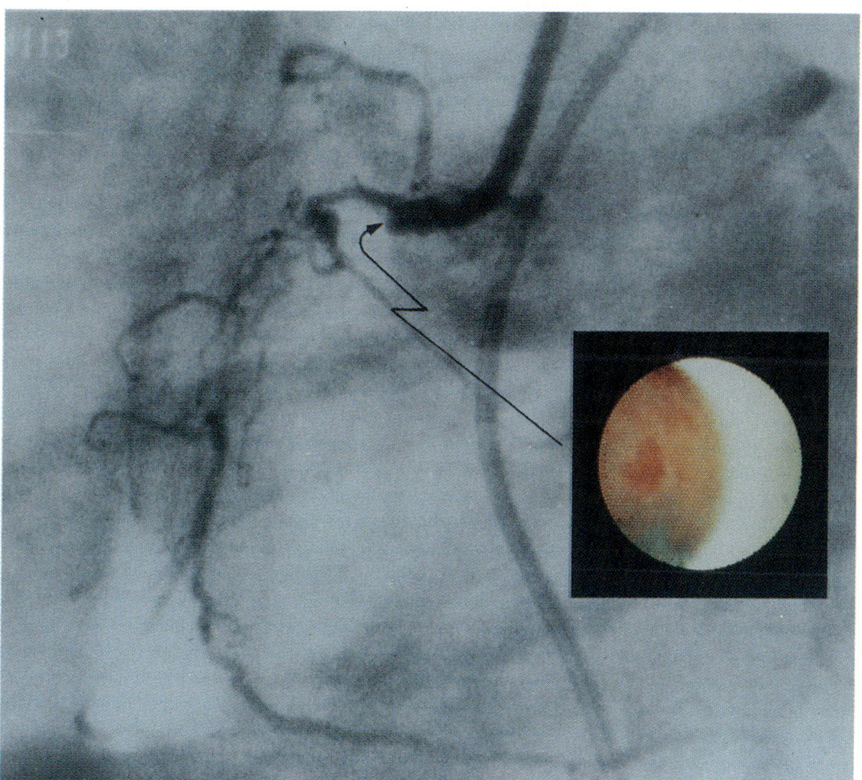

Fig. 1-20. Ulcer on the surface of a large occlusive atheromatous plaque in RCA No. 1 is visualized by lysing the proximal occlusive thrombi. This ulcer is not able to be seen by contrast anteriography.

struction to its inside view. The obstructed area was initially occupied by red thrombi, but by flushing, the large atheroma with its superficial debris or ulcer is visualized.

Angioscopy During PTCR and Emergency PTCA

To determine the intraluminal morphology before, and the immediate outcome of intracoronary thrombolysis (ICT), PTCA, using the above mentioned technique, was done in 15 patients during routine coronary arteriography. Table 1-1 shows a summary of the results.

In Fig. 1-21, the angioscopic images on the left show the proximal area of the complete occlusion of the LAD segment. The four right panels on this figure show the process of delivering the catheters into this area of LAD proximal obstruction. Following routine coronary artery guiding catheter placement, a guide wire, 0.28 mm in outer diameter, was introduced as shown in the second right panel. The tip of the guide wire was positioned proximal to the LAD occlusion as shown in the third right panel, and a soft tip inner guiding catheter insertion was made. Then the guide wire was removed, and the angioscopic catheter was gently inserted. The direction of viewing can be adjusted by manipulating both the inner guiding and angioscopic catheters. In the lower left three panels in Fig. 1-21, the white inside wall of the inner guiding catheter is seen, which indicates that the tip of the angioscope is positioned proximal to the distal end of the guiding catheter. With the tip of the angioscope located within the guiding catheter, images of the occlusive thrombi were seen, as in the upper panel. The left top angioscopic image is the occlusive thrombi. The left lower three panels are views of denudated plaque following intracoronary thrombolysis with urokinase infusion.

Figure 1-22 compares the angiograms and angioscopic images obtained in a 55-year-old male acute myocardial infarction (AMI) patient during PTCR and routine CAG. Both frames of the left and right panel were obtained at approximately the same time. As shown in the top panel, a totally occlusive thrombus was seen when the angiogram showed complete occlusion. Thrombus cracking and denudation were occurring at the same time as lengthening of the patent tract in the angiogram, as indicated in the second panel. The residual mixed thrombus and fibrin nettings coincided with the filling defects in the third panel. The recanalization and the residual stenosis were seen in the angiogram in the bottom right. Figure 1-23 compares conditions before and after the balloon angioplasty. As shown in the right panel, the cracking of thrombus and atheroma are created in an uneven fashion.

DISCUSSION

Current results indicate that the technique we developed for PTCA can be achieved safely during routine coronary arteriography by delivering the angioscopic catheter to a position just proximal to the observational target using the double guiding catheter system through the femoral artery. Although some transluminal techniques with limited utilities[9,10] and perioperative procedures[11,12] have been reported, the angioscopic determination of the morphologic aspects of coronary occlusion and the outcome of its recanalizing interventions possibly can be made for the first time by our method at the area where the F#5 guiding catheter can reach. In addition, the angioscopic catheter we developed and used in this series is extremely thin, disposable, and less expensive. These are obviously of advantage in combining this angioscopy technique with routine contrast arteriography during intracoronary thrombolysis and emergency PTCA in acute coronary event.

This combined method is promising in that it can provide an additional means to determine the composition of the occlusive lesions, assist in producing an effective recanalization,

Table 1-1. Results

1. Number of patients examined by angioscopy	15
2. Location of coronary occlusion-related AMI	LAD 9, LCX 2, RCA 4
3. Number of PTCR/PTCA	9/4
4. Size of guiding catheter being used	Outer: F#8.0/100 mm Inner: F#5.0/115 mm
5. Size of angioscopic catheter being used	0.7 mm/120 mm
6. Flushing volume of 5% dextrose solution	Rate: 0.5–3.0 ml/sec Total: 3.0–12.0 ml
7. Number of successful insertions of angioscopic catheter into proximal	LAD: 8/9 (89%) LCX: 1/2 (50%) RCA: 3/4 (75%)
8. Number of successful observations of occlusive lesion	LAD: 5/9 (56%) LCX: 0/2 (0%) RCA: 1/4 (25%)
9. Number of successful observations of the process of removing thrombus	LAD: 3/9 (30%) LCA: 0/2 (0%) RCA: 1/4 (25%)
10. Complication: Chest pain during catheterization	1/15(7%)

and characterize the atherosclerotic lesions lining the residual thrombus area and the residual thrombus.

Although the angioscopy by our technique can be made within the coronary area where the F#5 inner soft tip guiding catheter can reach, the principal barrier to achieve clear visual image is the flexibility of both inner guiding and CAS catheters. This obviously causes an inappropriate tip alignment, resulting in poor or narrow and fast-moving visual fields. In addition, the coupling in size of the catheters and vessel being examined can be responsible for obtaining unsatisfactory images. For example, relatively good images were obtained in midpath of LAD, LCX and RCA, while in larger vessels like proximal LAD, we had difficulties in visualizing the target lesion. On the other hand, a good fixation of the guiding catheter toward the target lesion in a nearly straight fashion can be attained in smaller vessels. Therefore, it can be difficult to maintain satisfactory tip alignment when manipulating the catheter during our technique because of both tortuosity of the artery and current lack of tip angulation mechanism.

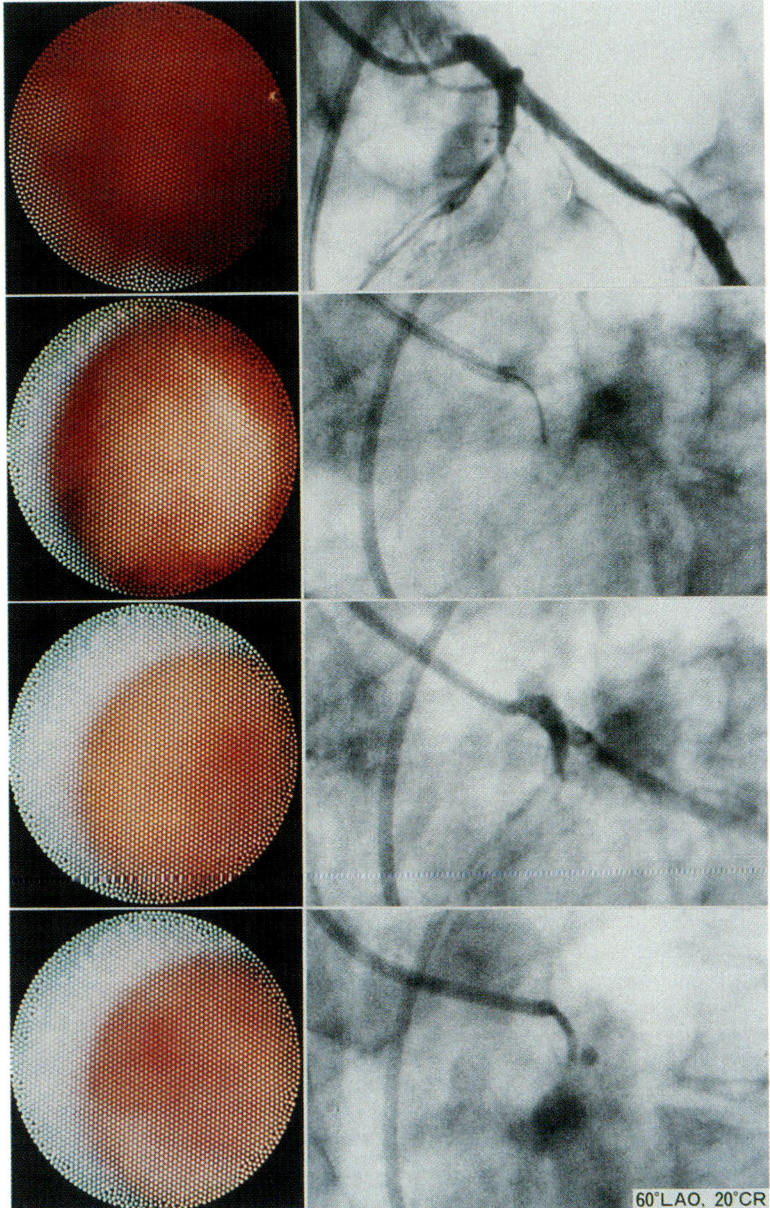

Fig. 1-21. Occlusive thrombus in the proximal LAD. Fluoroscopy shown in the right panel series demonstrates the process of delivering the angioscopic catheter into the LAD No. 6 occlusive lesion. The top left panel shows the proximal view of the thrombotic occlusion and the rest of the left panel shows the process of thrombolysis. The lumen is occupied by a large atheromatous plaque with abscess in the surface.

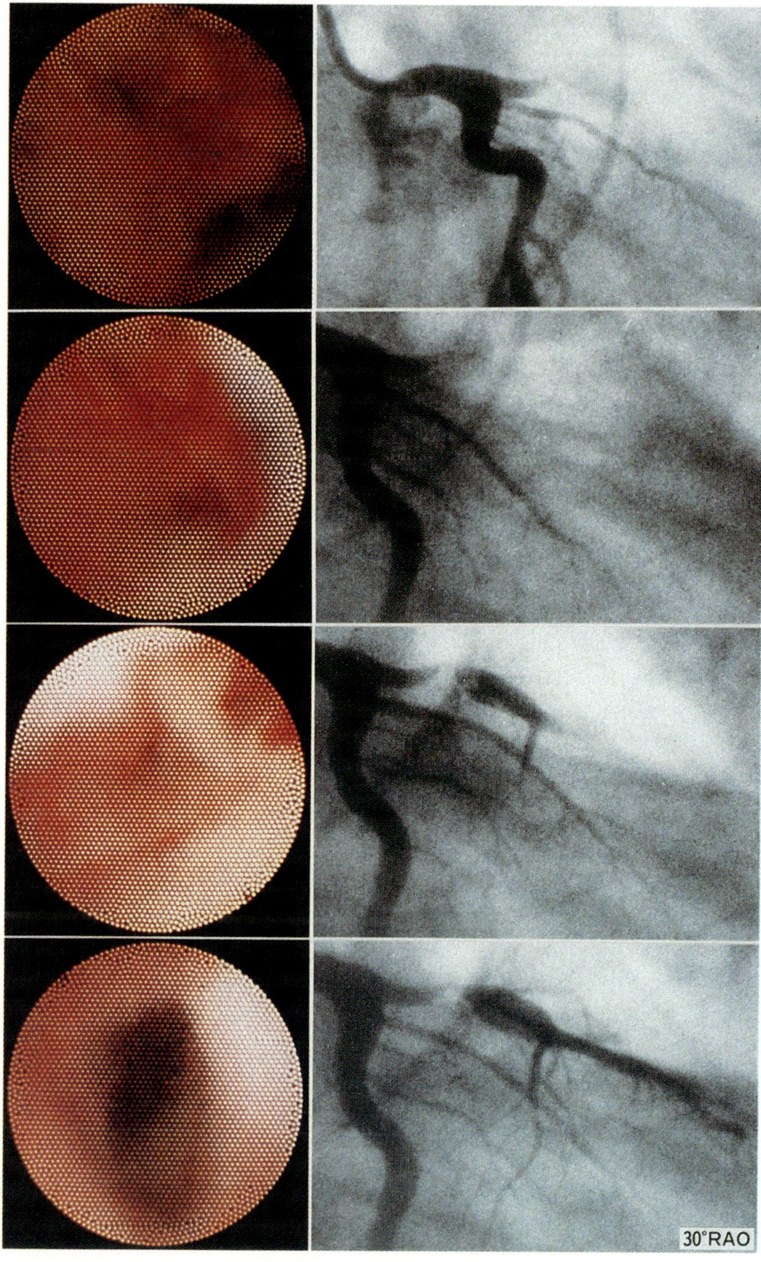

Fig. 1-22. Intracoronary thrombolysis. *Left,* Angioscopy demonstrates the process of thrombolysis; *right,* arteriography demonstrating the thrombolytic process.

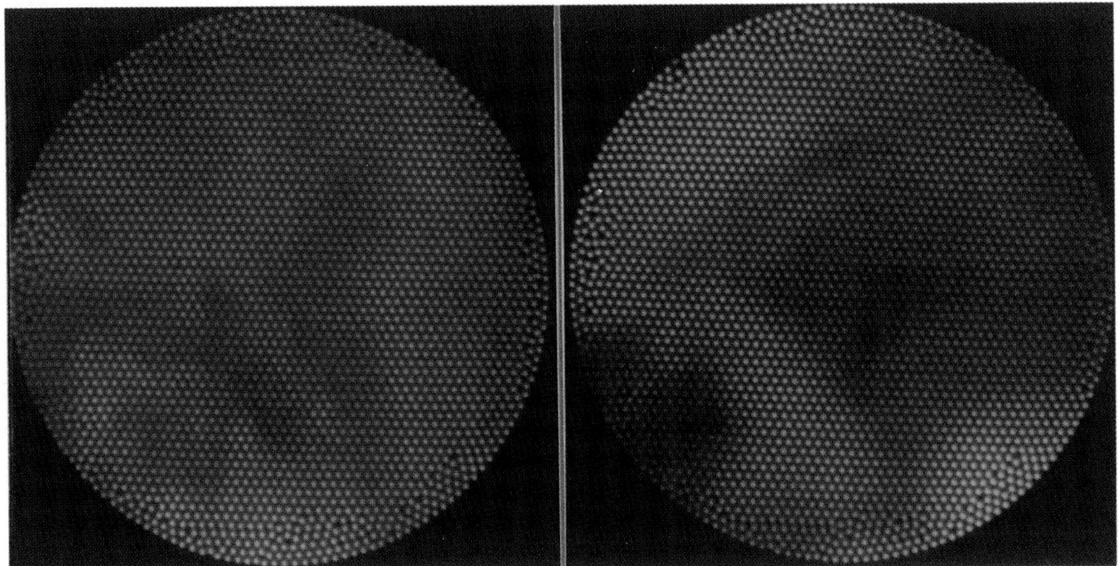

Fig. 1-23. Emergency balloon angioplasty. *Left,* Thrombotic occlusion is seen in the proximal LAD; *right,* the immediate outcome of PTCA is shown. Cracking of the mixed thrombi and atheromatous plaque, a flap, and focal hemorrhages are demonstrated.

However, this technique shows much potential for further technical advances, and we are currently continuing such efforts.

The angioscopically demonstrated plaques vary in both size and shape. They were xanthomatous in color, having focal hemorrhage or sometimes an abscess on the surface, which was partially or totally covered by red thrombi in AMI. Necrosis-ridden, mature coronary plaques, partially or totally covered by thrombi, seemed to be characterized by AMI. The cracking of these thrombi and plaques lysed residual thrombi and focal bleeding of the inner wall are likely to be the inner mechanisms of ICT and PTCA.

CONCLUSION

PTCA can be achieved by delivering the angioscopic catheter to a position just proximal to the observational target using the double guiding catheter technique through the femoral artery. This angioscopic visualization of the thrombotic and thrombolytic event possibly can be made at the area where a F#5 guiding catheter can reach. In addition, the angioscopic catheter used in this series is extremely thin and disposable.

Using this method during PTCR and PTCA during routine coronary arteriography is promising because it can

1. Determine the composition of the occlusive thrombus
2. Assist in producing an effective recanalization
3. Characterize the atherosclerotic lesions lining the residual thrombus area
4. Characterize the residual thrombus and the atherosclerotic lesions lining the wall

This technique shows much potential for further development in clinical and research applications, and we are continuing our efforts in this area.

REFERENCES

1. Davies, M.J., and Thomas A.C.: Plaque fissuring—the cause of acute myocardial infarction, sudden ischemic death, and crescendo angina, Br. Heart J. **53**:363, 1985.
2. Falk, E.: Unstable angina with fatal outcome: Dynamic coronary thrombosis leading to infarction and/or sudden death. Autopsy evidence of recurrent mural thrombosis with peripheral embolization culminating in total vascular occlusion, Circulation **71**:699, 1985.
3. Moise, A., Theroux, P., Taeymans, V., et al.: Unstable angina and progression of coronary atherosclerosis, N. Engl. J. Med. **309**:685, 1983.
4. Falk, E.: Plaque rupture with severe pre-existing stenosis precipitating coronary thrombosis: Characteristics of coronary atherosclerotic plaques underlying fatal occlusive thrombi, Br. Heart J. **50**:127, 1983.
5. Yusuf, S., Collins, R., Peto, R., et al.: Intravenous and intracoronary fibrinolytic therapy in acute myocardial infarction: overview of results on mortality, reinfarction and side-effects from 33 randomized controlled trials, Eur. Heart J. **6**:556, 1985.
6. Williams, D.O., Borer, J., Braunwald, E., et al.: Intravenous recombinant tissue-type plasminogen activator in patients with acute myocardial infarction: a report from the NHLBI thrombolysis in myocardial infarction trial, Circulation **73**:338, 1986.
7. O'Neill, W., Timmis, G., Bourdillon, P.D.V., et al.: A prospective randomized clinical trial of intracoronary streptokinase versus coronary angioplasty therapy for acute myocardial infarction, N. Engl. J. Med. **314**:812, 1986.
8. Topol, E.J., O'Neil, W.W., Langburd, A.B., et al.: A randomized, placebo-controlled trial of intravenous recombinant tissue-type plasminogen activator and emergency coronary angioplasty in patients with acute myocardial infarction, Circulation **75**:420, 1987.
9. Spears, J.R., Marais, H.J., Serur, J., et al.: In vivo coronary angioscopy, J.A.C.C. **1**:(5):1311, 1983.
10. Spears, J.R., Spokojny, A.M., and Marais, H.J.: Coronary angioscopy during cardiac catheterization, J.A.C.C. **6**:(1):93, 1985.
11. Sherman, C.T., Litvack, F., Grundfest, W.S., et al.: Demonstration of thrombus and complex atheroma by in vivo angioscopy in patients with unstable angina pectoris, N. Engl. J. Med. **315**:913, 1986.
12. Levin, D.C., and Gardiner, Jr., G.A.: Complex and simple coronary artery stenosis: a new way to interpret coronary angiograms based on morphologic features of lesions, Radiology **164**:675, 1987.
13. Inoue, K., Kuwaki, K., and Takahashi, M.: Transluminal cardioangioscopy, Circulation **68**(Suppl. III):7, 1983.
14. Inoue, K., Kuwaki, K., and Takahashi, M.: In vivo transluminal angioscopy, Circulation **70**(Suppl. II):622, 1984.
15. Inoue, K., and Kuwaki, K.: In vivo angioscopic demonstration of thrombus as a cause of cyclic flow variation in stenosed canine coronary artery, J.A.C.C. **7**:55, 1986.
16. Inoue, K., and Kuwaki, K.: Observation in vivo de al structure interieure des vaisseaux du chien utilisant un angioscope ultrafine fibre optique, La Lettre De Communication Medicale, May:14, 1986.
17. Inoue, K., Kuwaki, K., Ueda, K., et al.: Angioscopy guided coronary thrombolysis, J.A.C.C. **9**:62A, 1987.

Chapter **2**

Percutaneous Coronary Angioscopy

Raoul Bonan, MD, FACC

Percutaneous coronary angioscopy should permit a safe, nonsurgical, direct inspection of the coronary lumen and visualization of intracoronary lesions in order to improve diagnosis and allow future treatment.[1-8] This has been made possible with the development of ultrathin flexible fiberscopes; but to inspect distal coronary segments, especially those situated after coronary artery plaque, a safe "steerable" technique is necessary.

The purpose of this study was to evaluate the feasibility of angioscopic systems during cardiac catheterization before coronary angioplasty.

METHODS

Authorization was obtained from the Montreal Heart Institute Research and Ethical Committees to perform coronary angioscopy on patients undergoing percutaneous transluminal coronary angioplasty. Informed consent was obtained from each patient. The coronary angioscopy was made at the beginning of the procedure in the diseased vessel.

All human studies were made with an American Edwards Miniflex Angioscope (American Edwards Laboratories, Santa Ana, California), 1.0 mm in diameter and 150 cm in length. This flexible angioscope was made of 3000 fibers of 10 μm in diameter, with 12 concentrically arranged 0.1-mm illuminating fibers. It was first used in combination with a 5F "vector" catheter (Fig. 2-1A) and for the last patients, the tip of the angioscope was modified to accommodate a 0.014 guide wire on a 5- to 10-mm "guide rail" angioscope, and then it was used alone tracted on a 300-cm guide wire (Fig. 2-1B).

The angioscope was connected to an American Edwards Advanced Videoscopy System (AVS), which included an enhanced video camera, light source, and color monitor. The low-light sensitivity of the system makes the AVS "adaptable" to the intravascular condition.

Focus and lighting controls located on the camera head and console were easy to manipulate. Colors and focus (at 5 mm) were set before introduction, and light was monitored through the "camera operate control"; this angioscope resolved 0.3-mm pairs of lines at a lens-to-object distance of 5 mm. The color monitor was connected to a ¾-inch videotape recorder for continuous recording during pro-

A

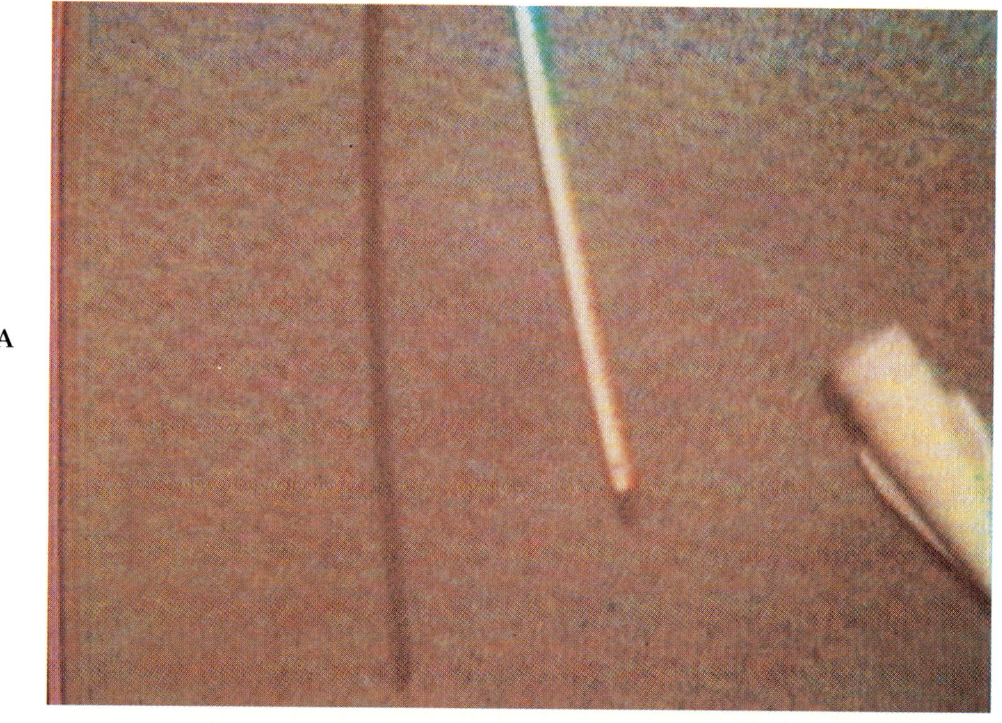

B

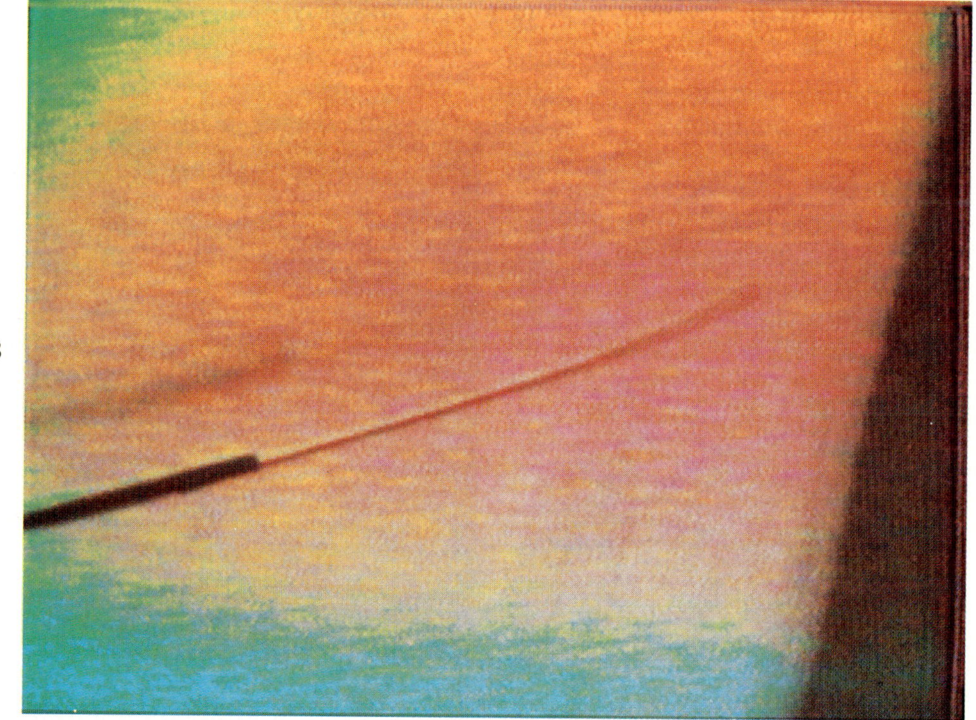

Fig. 2-1. A, A 5F vector catheter with black opaque tip and lateral holes. 1 mm angioscope of 3000 fibers of 10. **B,** "Guide rail" angioscope with 0.014-inch guidewire.

cedure, and photographs were secondarily obtained from the video.

A similar system was used experimentally on anesthetized sheep, percutaneously, obtaining visualization in the opposite femoral artery and coronary arteries. The angioscope used was bigger—an American Edwards Miniflex Angioscope, 1.3 mm in diameter, constructed of 6000 fibers.

Cardiac catheterization was performed from the right femoral artery in each patient using conventional 8F high-flow guiding catheters through an 8F introducer. After heparinization (5000 units) and repeat selective coronary arteriography, the 5F vector catheter through Y-connector was driven to the coronary stenosis on a conventional 0.014 guide wire. When the 5F catheter had reached the stenosis safely, the guide wire was withdrawn and replaced by the angioscope. The inner size of the 5F vector catheter's tip keeps the angioscope inside the catheter, preventing contact of the angioscope with the artery wall.

The two catheters were connected to a standard manifold for pressure monitoring and injection of either contrast medium or heparinized normal saline solution.

The visualization of the coronary lumen was then achieved by flushing heparinized normal saline solution under 300 mm Hg of pressure through the guiding catheter and the 5F "vector catheter"; supplement manual injection of the same solution was sometimes needed to achieve complete displacement of blood. It was necessary to withdraw the entire system in order to be coaxial for adequate visualization of the coronary artery lumen. After completion of the angioscopic attempt, the 5F catheter and the angioscope were removed, and a conventional coronary angioplasty was done.

When the "guide rail" angioscope was used, it was advanced to the coronary stenosis on a 300-cm 0.014 guide wire. With this kind of set-up, the guide wire crossed the stenosis only once and stayed in place during the entire procedure. For the angioplasty, the scope was exchanged for the balloon catheter; displacement of blood was then achieved from the guiding catheter. The guide wire helped the angioscope to stay coaxial with the arterial lumen.

RESULTS

Clear and typical images of the inside of the arteries were obtained in animal studies. The blood was displaced completely when the ratio between the diameter of the artery and the "vector catheter" was not out of proportion. It was possible to record images of bifurcation, branching of smaller arteries, platelet aggregation after wall traumatism by a guide wire, and circular and regular distal lumen of the artery (Figs. 2-2 through 2-4). Coronary artery visualization was more challenging than femoral artery visualization with complex and untreatable ventricular arrhythmia occurring after a few minutes of flushing.

Percutaneous coronary angioscopy was at-

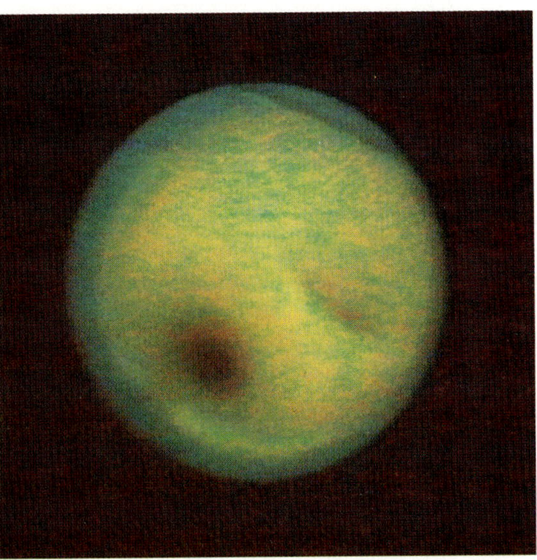

Fig. 2-2. Bifurcation in the sheep femoral artery visualized with the 1.3 mm angioscope of 6000 fibers.

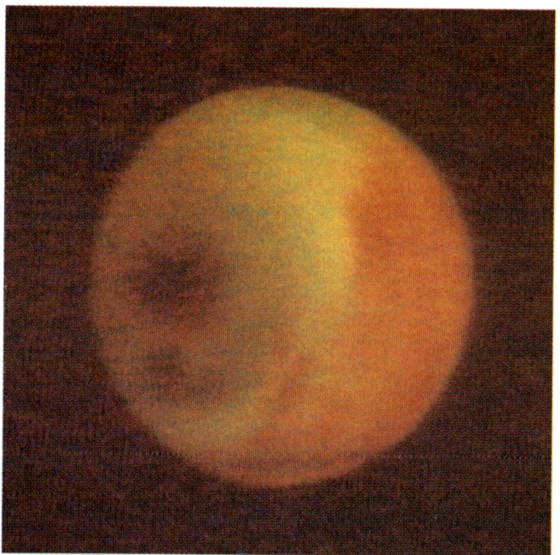

Fig. 2-3. Division of the sheep femoral artery observed with the 1.3 mm angioscope of 6000 fibers. Possible platelet aggregation on the left side of the artery wall after guidewire traumatism is seen. Note the regular circular aspect of the distal lumen.

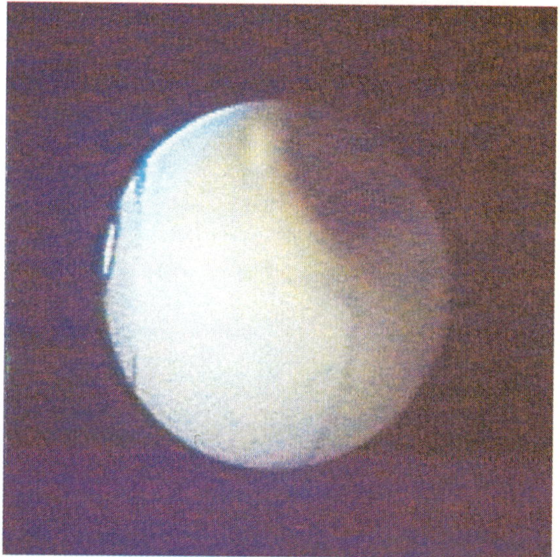

Fig. 2-4. Image of sheep coronary circumflex artery obtained with the 1.3 mm angioscope of 6000 fibers. Origin of a side branch is seen on the top.

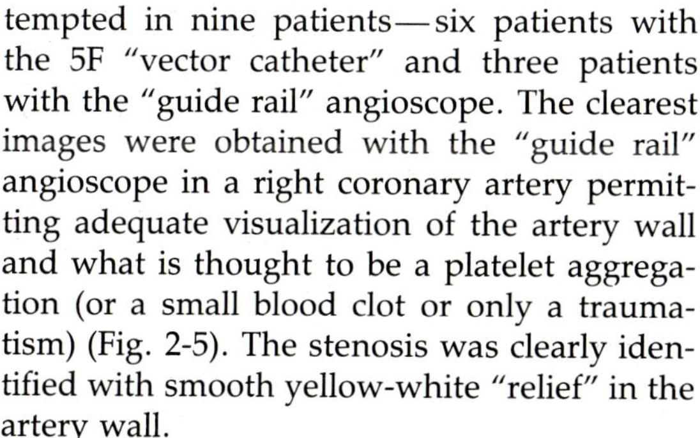

tempted in nine patients—six patients with the 5F "vector catheter" and three patients with the "guide rail" angioscope. The clearest images were obtained with the "guide rail" angioscope in a right coronary artery permitting adequate visualization of the artery wall and what is thought to be a platelet aggregation (or a small blood clot or only a traumatism) (Fig. 2-5). The stenosis was clearly identified with smooth yellow-white "relief" in the artery wall.

Adequate visualization of the lumen, dark inner regular circle (distal lumen) with reddish halo (wall) was obtained in six of eight catheterized arteries, until 6 cm from the ostium, with the 5F "vector catheter" and the angioscope (Fig. 2-6). In one case, even when the circumflex artery was deeply catheterized by the 5F catheter, it was impossible to manage the different curves with the angioscope and reach the tip of the catheter; in another case, a left anterior descending artery, the

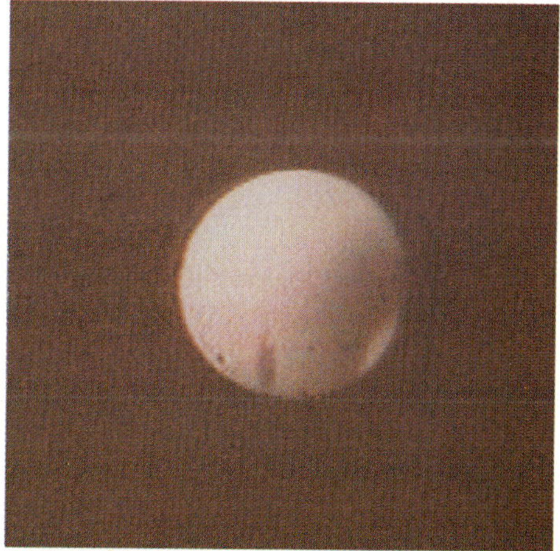

Fig. 2-5. Angioscopic image of a human right coronary artery obtained with the "guide rail" angioscope. The 0.014-inch guidewire is seen on the bottom right of the picture, on the arterial wall, along with the image of what is thought to be a platelet aggregation, a small blood clot, or only a traumatism.

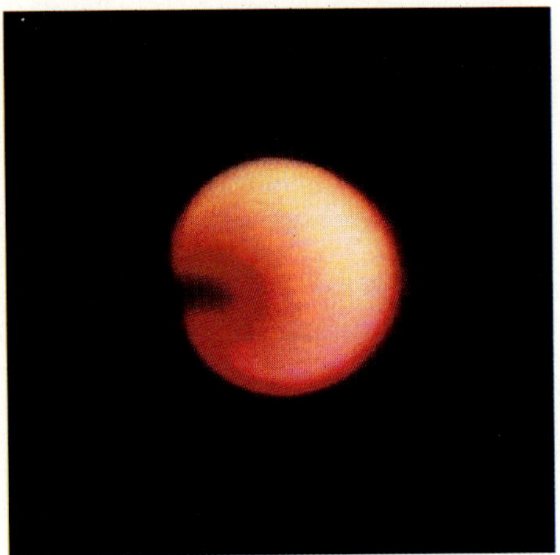

Fig. 2-6. Human percutaneous coronary angioscopic aspect of the lumen of a right coronary artery obtained with the 1 mm angioscope and the 5F vector catheter. Regular circular aspect of the distal lumen is seen.

flush was inadequate and no visualization was possible.

With the "guide rail" angioscope, only one attempt was successful—the right coronary artery. In a left anterior descending artery it was impossible to obtain enough flush to displace the blood, and in a bypass vein graft to a marginal circumflex artery, the patient developed chest pain as soon as the normal saline flush was started, forcing us to stop the angioscopy and proceed to the angioplasty.

On the eleven vessels studied, only seven lumens were visualized and from these, only four stenoses were recognized due to the necessity to be close (5 mm) and coaxial. Stenoses appeared as a dark crescent or a deformed dark circle (Fig. 2-7); a crescent shape stenosis was visualized even though it was not recognized on the coronary angiogram (Fig. 2-8).

Besides the chest pain already reported, a temporary complete heart block occurred during visualization (flushing) with the "guide rail" angioscope in a right coronary artery, necessitating temporary pacing support. T-wave inversion without symptom occurred during normal saline intracoronary flushing.

DISCUSSION

Percutaneous coronary angioscopy appears feasible and can be performed safely during cardiac catheterization before coronary angioplasty.[8] The real problem is to obtain enough flush to properly visualize the artery lumen. The development of new types of catheters or angioscopes, permitting such achievement is highly needed, working on displacement of anterograde or retrograde blood flow.

Image analysis is helped greatly by the use of a video system. The video system permits the recording of the entire procedure, which can be studied later, sequence by sequence, permitting the discovery of images obtained during transient displacement of blood (the use of video tapes makes it difficult to obtain good photographs).

The other difficulty is to keep a coaxial alignment of the angioscope within the lumen in order to visualize it. More often, the angioscope tip is directed toward the wall of the artery, especially after a curve. Then the reflection of the light dazzles the entire image. The withdrawal of the angioscopic system (5F vector catheter and the angioscope) permits coaxial positioning from time to time and then delivers an adequate image of the lumen, which is safer than readvancing the system without a guide wire.

The "guide rail" angioscope, even with its low rate of success in this series, seems more promising. Indeed, its conception offers steerability and the opportunity to stay coaxial or at least para-axial, and allows the deliverance of a fair amount of flush from the guiding catheter. More than that, it looks safer to use a 300-cm guide wire which crosses the stenosis only once and which will be used for the balloon angioplasty. The need for an opaque angioscope is imperative with this technique.

Percutaneous coronary angioscopy may

A

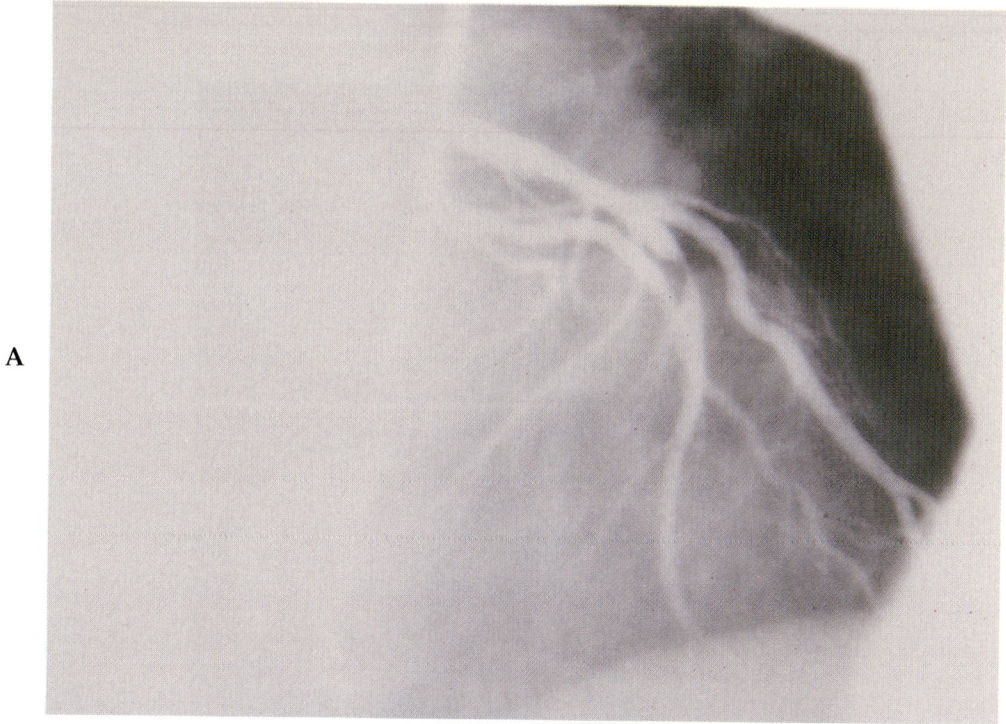

B

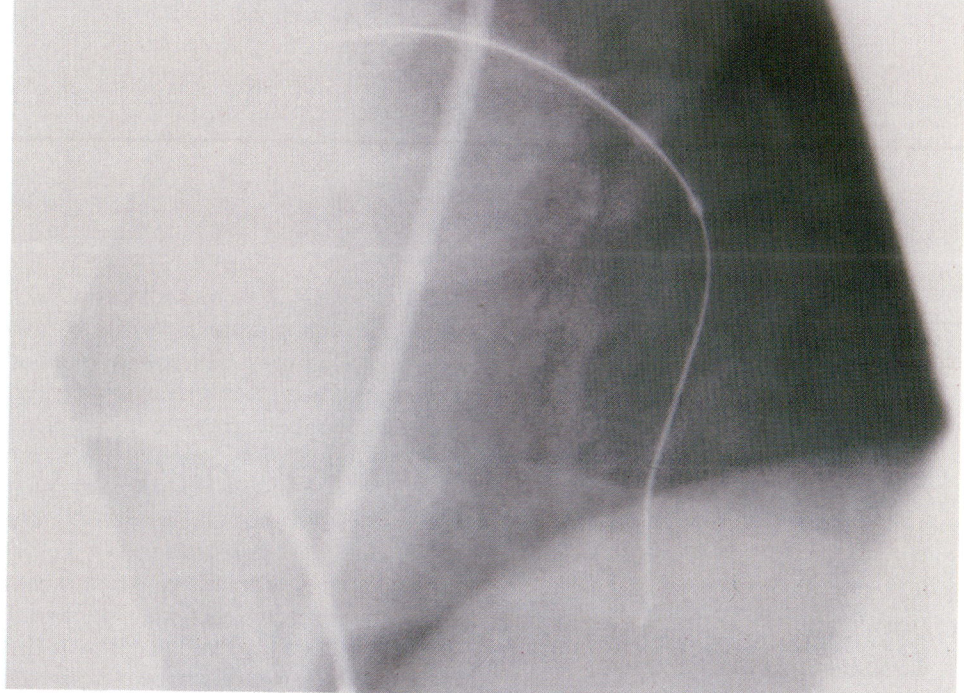

Fig. 2-7. A, Angiographic image of an LAD coronary artery stenosis. **B,** A 5F vector catheter is driven by a 0.014-inch guidewire to the stenosis.

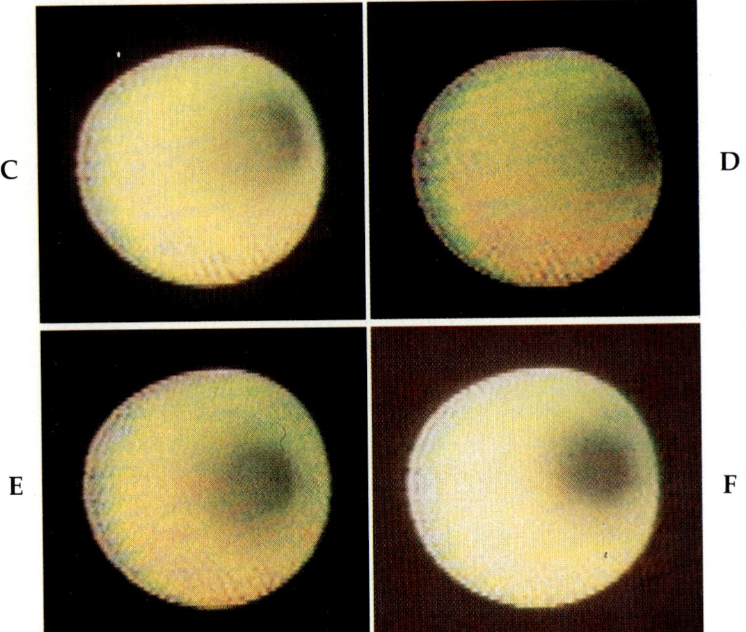

Fig. 2-7, Cont'd. C, D, E, F, Successive images obtained by withdrawing the angioscopic system (1 mm angioscope and 5F vector catheter). Small crescent-shape stenosis (between the one and three o'clock position) to a full circular lumen is seen.

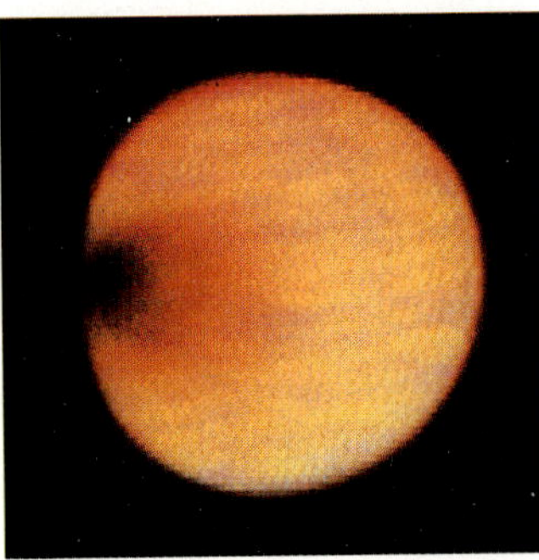

Fig. 2-8. Human percutaneous coronary angioscopy (1 mm angioscope and 5F vector catheter). Crescent-shape stenosis of an LAD artery is shown.

possibly identify and differentiate unactive atheromatous plaque (smooth surface) from active or "complex" plaque (irregular surface with intramural hemorrhage or intimal flap) and commands aggressive treatments.[6,7]

Quantitative assessment of a stenosis can be more accurate with angioscopy, particularly crescent-shaped stenosis, using the guide wire as size reference.[8]

The future of percutaneous coronary angioscopy will stand between the eventual risk of complication and the success of the visualization which needs to be improved by the development of new catheters and new video systems. It should contribute to future developments such as angioscopically guided laser or other angioplasty.

REFERENCES

1. Rhea, L., Walker, I.C., and Cutler, E.C.: The surgical treatment of mitral stenosis: experimental and clinical studies, Arch. Surg. **9**:689, 1924.
2. Greenstone, S.M., Shore, J.M., Heringman, E.C., et al.: Atrial endoscopy (arterioscopy), Arch. Surg. **93**:811, 1966.
3. Spears, J.R., Marais, H.J., Serur, J.M., et al.: In vivo coronary angioscopy, J.A.C.C. **1**:1311, 1983.
4. Cortis, B.S., Hussen, H., Chandra, S.K., et al.: Angioscopy in vivo, Cathet. Cardiovasc. Diagn. **10**:493, 1984.
5. Litwack, F., Grundfest, W.S., Lee, M.E., et al.: Angioscopy visualization of blood vessel interior in animals and humans, Clin. Cardiol. **8**:65, 1985.
6. Grundfest, W.S., Litwack, F., Sherman, T.C., et al.: Delineation of peripheral and coronary detail by intra operative angioscopy, Ann. Surg. **202**:394, 1985.
7. Sherman, T.C., Litwack, F., Grundfest, W., et al.: Coronary angioscopy in patients with unstable angina pectoris, N. Engl. J. Med. **315**:913, 1986.
8. Spears, J.R., Spokojny, A.M., and Marais, J.: Coronary angioscopy during cardiac catheterization, J.A.C.C. **6**:93, 1985.

Chapter 3

Coronary and Peripheral Vascular Angioscopy

James S. Forrester, MD, FACC
Andrew Jakubowski, MD
Ann Hickey, MD
Frank Litvack, MD
Warren S. Grundfest, MD

Angioscopy allows direct examination of the lumen and endothelial surface of blood vessels. Coronary arteries, bypass grafts, and peripheral vessels have been examined in the operating room, and percutaneous coronary angioscopy is being tested in the catheterization laboratory.[1] In this chapter, we will describe the history of angioscopy, how to perform the procedure, and how this information has led cardiologists to modify their views about the pathogenesis of coronary syndromes.

HISTORICAL PERSPECTIVE

The first use of angioscopy was probably in 1913 when Rhea and Walker used a rigid illuminated tube to visualize intracardiac structures at thoracotomy.[2] A decade later, Allen put a lens to the end of the scope, and reported good visualization of canine intracardiac structures.[3] It was the development of flexible fiberoptic bundles for the communication industry in the early 1960s, however, that led to use of fiberoptics in medicine. In 1966, Greenstone et al. used fiberoptics to visualize peripheral canine arteries using saline to displace the blood,[4] and a year later Gamble visualized cardiac chambers and large vessels through a fiberoptic placed within the balloon.[5] It was not until almost 20 years later that Spears first reported visualization of human coronary arteries.[1,6] In the same year our group began using angioscopes ranging from 0.85 mm to 2.8 mm in external diameter. We began by visualizing vessels in cadavers,[7] and ultimately developed the ability to perform routine studies in the cardiac and peripheral vascular operating room.[8] We are now attempting to develop the procedure for use in the cardiac catheterization laboratory.

METHODS

Angioscopic Equipment

Our angioscopes have an outer diameter of 0.7 to 2.8 mm. For small vessels, we use 0.70- to 1.5-mm outer diameter angioscopes (Advanced Interventional Systems, Costa Mesa, California and American Edwards Laboratories, Santa Ana, California) (Fig. 3-1). The devices contain 5000 to 8000 imaging fibers surrounded by a concentric ring of illumination fibers, and have a flexible plastic catheter housing. For larger vessels we use 1.4- to 1.8-mm angioscopes (Olympus Corporation of America, New Hyde Park, New York). These scopes also have a central imaging bundle with a surrounding concentric ring of illumination fibers sheathed in a polyvinyl chloride (PVC) jacket. Most of the angioscopes have line pair resolution exceeding 200 μm and approaching 64 μm at 5 mm. Minimum focus distance ranges from 2 to 6.5 mm. The longer focal length angioscopes are not usable in small tortuous vessels. We use a 1000-watt xenon light source (Storz, Los Angeles, CA) for illumination. The angioscopic images are relayed from the fiberoptic bundles through a video coupler to a light-sensitive (Sony DXC D1850) video camera. On-line images are viewed on a high-resolution (Sony PVM1960) video monitor. Permanent recordings are made using a ¾-inch (Sony 5800) video tape recorder.

Operative Technique

Peripheral bypass graft angioscopy is performed with control of blood flow by vascular tapes or clamps. Crystalloid irrigation solution, delivered through a coaxial angiocath connected to a 300-mm Hg pressurized bag, is used to flush away backflow. The volume of infusion depends on vessel size and the degree of occlusion. A patent vessel requires about 2 to 4 ml per second (total volume 200 to 400 ml) for 1.5 to 2 minutes of images. On the other hand, a completely occluded vessel needs only 2 ml per second for 10 to 15 minutes of images. We perform coronary artery and bypass graft imaging with the aorta cross-clamped after cardiac arrest. In coronary arteries, the angioscope is inserted through the distal arteriotomy; for vein grafts, the angioscope is passed through its proximal end before performing the aortic anastomosis.

Peripheral Vascular Surgical Procedures

We obtained good images in 85% of 60 patients who had angioscopy during peripheral vascular surgery.[9] The 15% failure rate was due primarily to inadequate clearance of retrograde or collateral blood flow. By angioscopy, we see misplaced sutures, redundancy of graft material, and intimal flaps incorporated into the anastomosis causing partial obstruction (Fig. 3-2). As a result, the changes in intraoperative management based on our angioscopic findings have been significant (Table 3-1).

We revised 3 of the 26 peripheral vascular anastomoses examined by angioscopy. Specifically, the anastomosis site was changed based on angioscopic detection of severe distal disease in one case. In another, an intimal flap that had been unknowingly incorporated into the distal infrageniculate anastomosis led to revision of the anastomosis. In the 23 anastomoses we did not revise, we often saw incorporation of atheromatous plaque into suture lines and small intimal fragments which did not appear to compromise flow. We have a follow-up program to determine whether these luminal irregularities cause long-term adverse effects.

We also have performed 48 femoral popliteal bypass procedures, of which 13 were in situ saphenous vein grafts. In 6 of the 13 (46%), we discovered competent valves which required repeat valvotomy.

In five cases we performed angioscopic inspection after graft thrombectomy. In four (80%) we found thrombus (Fig. 3-3) neointi-

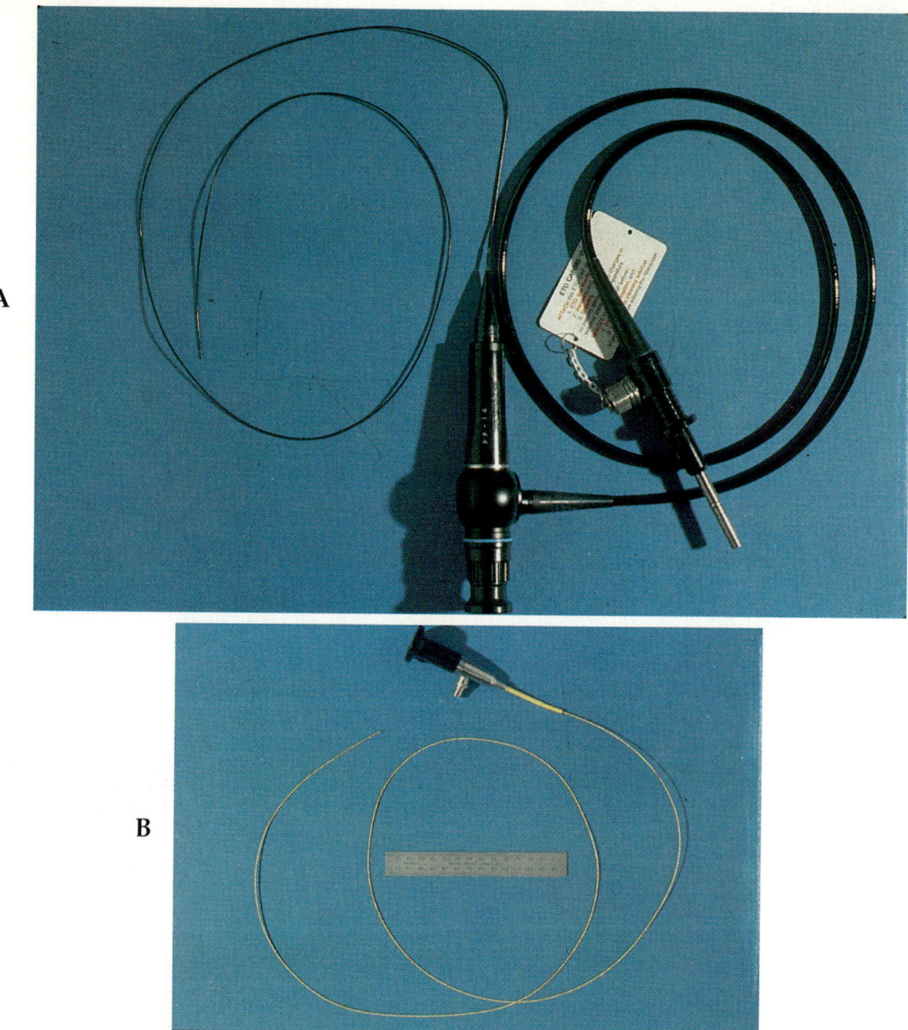

Fig. 3-1. American Edwards 0.85 mm (white) and Olympus 1.4 mm (black) angioscopes.

mal flaps, or atherosclerotic plaque, and performed repeat thrombectomy (Fig. 3-4).

Comparison of Angioscopy to Contrast Angiography

Coronary angioscopy has been compared to coronary angiography by several groups. Lee et al.[10] studied 11 stenoses at coronary artery bypass surgery. They reported that angioscopic cross-sectional measurements correlated well ($r = 0.90$, $p < 0.001$) with calculated angiographic stenosis. Our correlations have not been as good. We found that coronary angiography failed to detect three of four endothelial ulcerations and six of seven partially occlusive thrombi.[11] In three patients with acute percutaneous transluminal coronary angioscopy failure, angioscopy detected significant vessel dissection (two visible lumens) in

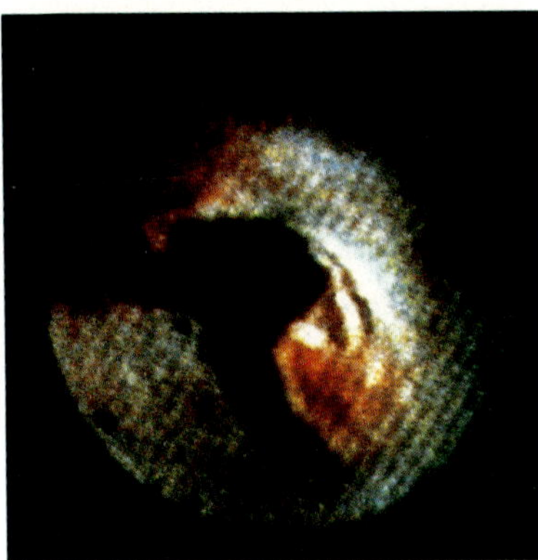

Fig. 3-2. This is the typical angioscopic image of a nonobstructive, free-floating intimal flap after thrombectomy. The clinical significance of this finding is not clear.

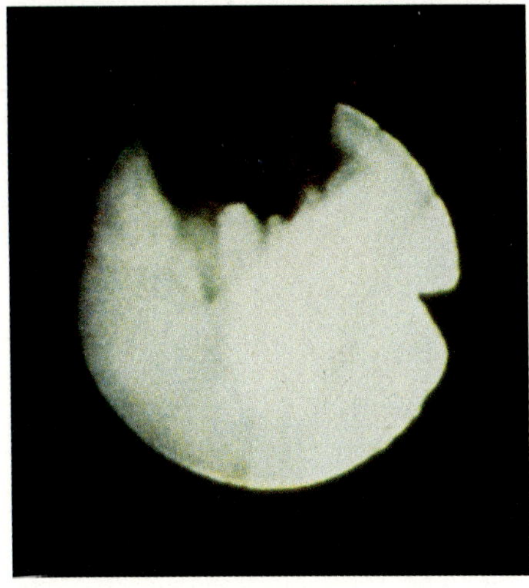

Fig. 3-3. Angioscopic view of a polytetrafluroethylene graft to the suprageniculate popliteal artery revealing retained thrombus. Balloon catheter is seen in the upper part of the image.

Table 3-1. Changes in Intraoperative Management in Peripheral Vascular Surgery Based on Angioscopic Findings

Change	*n*
Deletion of completion angiogram	3
Graft revision	2
Reexcision of venous valve	6
Revision of anastomosis	3
Repeat thrombectomy	4
	18

all of them, but only one patient was detected angiographically. Similar results have been obtained at peripheral vascular angiography by Van Steigman et al.[12] They found that arteriography failed to demonstrate one free floating clot, two endothelial ulcerations, and two intimal flaps. Ritchie et al.[13] found angioscopy to be superior to angiography for detection of intimal vascular details. These data indicate that angioscopy provides information not obtained by angiography. We believe that the study of the *entire* vascular tree is better performed by angiography, but that angioscopy shows the *details* of the intimal surface at one vascular site.

Establishing the Pathogenesis of Acute Coronary Syndromes

We have performed 87 angioscopic examinations in the first 60 patients studied during coronary artery bypass surgery. In five patients, images were obtained in a nonoffending artery (artery not held responsible for patient symptoms) and four had no intra-arterial images (graft inspection). Of the 51 patients with arterial examinations, diagnostic images were obtained in 38 (75%). The major cause of failure was insufficient irrigation. The left anterior artery was most easily accessible (46/87 studies), but other vessels were also examined (Table 3-2).

Coronary Atherosclerosis: A Modern Paradigm

Our experience with coronary angioscopy has led us to propose a paradigm of acute and

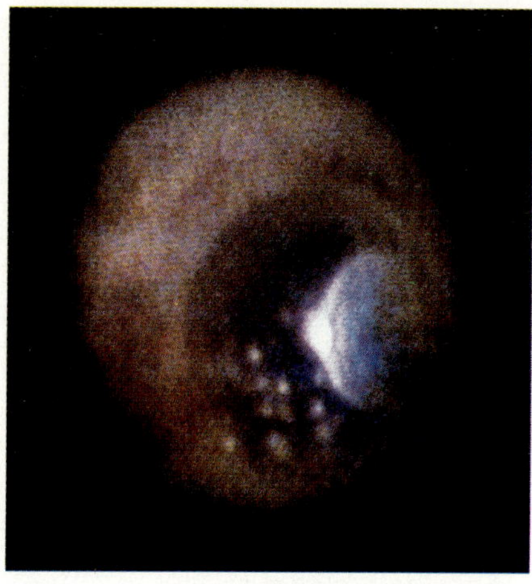

Fig. 3-4. The same graft as in Fig. 3-3 seen from below the obstruction with an inflated balloon.

Table 3-2. Arteries Inspected During Angioscopy in 60 Patients with Coronary Artery Disease

Artery	*Images*	*No. Images*	*Total No. of Inspections*
Left anterior descending	31	15	46
Diagonals	5	3	8
Left circumflex	17	9	26
Right coronary artery	3	3	6
Other branches	0	1	1
Total	56	31	87

chronic coronary disease.[14] We propose that coronary disease is a continually repeating cycle of clinical stability interrupted by acute syndromes. Our central idea is that this clinical cycle is driven by an unrecognized cycle at the endothelial surface, which determines the patient's specific symptom presentation (Fig. 3-5).

The first histopathologic cycle is stable atheroma-endothelial ulceration-platelet adhesion-ulcer healing. We believe that each of these states has a related clinical syndrome. The coronary arteries in stable angina have smooth, yellow-white atheroma on the endothelial surface. When the atheroma develops an endothelial ulceration, the clinical presentation becomes accelerated angina (increased frequency of angina without rest pain). If platelet aggregates that form on the ulceration embolize, either sudden death or ischemic cardiomyopathy result. When the ulcer heals there is rapid progression of the coronary stenosis at the site, but the clinical state returns to chronic stable angina.

The second cycle is endothelial ulceration-partial thrombosis-thrombus evolution-thrombus incorporation-stable atheroma. This cycle also has related clinical states. When a partially occlusive thrombosis develops on the endothelial ulceration, the patient experiences unstable angina. If the thrombosis proceeds to complete occlusion, acute myocardial infarction results. Coronary thrombi may lyse or may be incorporated into the vessel wall. When the thrombus is incorporated, it causes rapid progression of coronary stenosis. After lysis or incorporation, there is return to chronic stable angina. The cycles then repeat.

Events Preceding Coronary Thrombosis: Clinical-Histologic Features of the First Cycle

The basis of our paradigm is the correlation between symptoms and the details of endothelial surface we see in living patients. Because our angioscopic observations correspond directly to gross autopsy description, however, we also can infer the histologic appearance of these lesions. The first cycle consists of stable atheroma, endothelial ulceration, platelet adhesion, and healing with atheroma progression.

Stable atheroma. Figure 3-6 is an illustrative angioscopic image from the left circumflex coronary artery of a 65-year-old woman with a 2-year history of stable angina pectoris, 2.5-

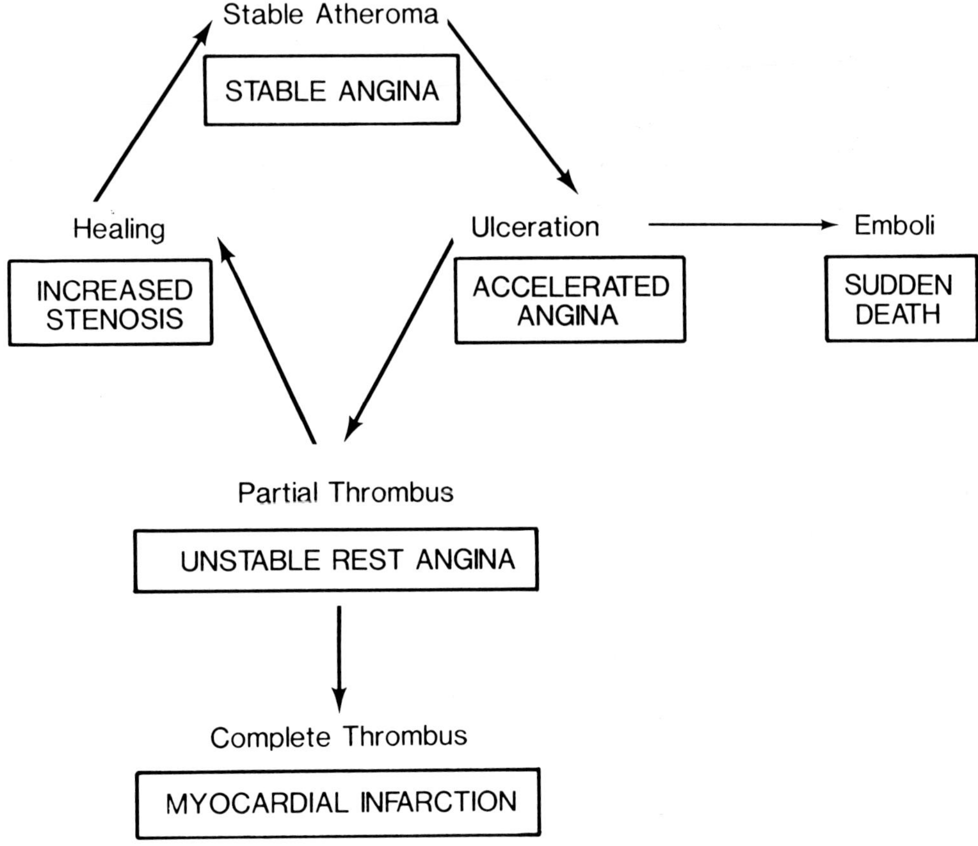

Fig. 3-5. The pathogenesis of acute coronary syndromes.

mm horizontal ST segment depression during exercise, a strongly positive thallium test consistent with multivessel disease, and greater than 90% stenosis in all three major coronary arteries. There is a smooth, crescent-shaped, yellow-white atheroma protruding into the coronary lumen. Angioscopy of the left anterior descending coronary artery revealed similar smooth atheroma.

Figure 3-7 shows a large, mature atheroma. The lumen has been markedly narrowed by a huge, fibrous plaque. To the right of the lumen, there is an area of necrosis. Although most of the necrotic core was lost in preparation, macrophages still line the wall of the abscess.

This lesion is typical of the atheroma we have seen by angioscopy in patients with stable atherosclerotic disease. The earliest nonobstructive lesions are oblong and oriented along the axis of flow; obstructive lesions have no regular shape and are usually eccentric. Histologically, these stable atheroma exhibit several stages of development which correspond to our angioscopic observations. The small nonocclusive oblong protrusions are fatty streaks, which are composed predominantly of lipid-laden macrophages. As the lesion enlarges and becomes partially obstructive, smooth muscle cells are found to have migrated from the media into the subendothelium, and the lipid-laden macrophages are covered by a fibrous cap. Thus, in stable, exercise-induced angina, the normal endothe-

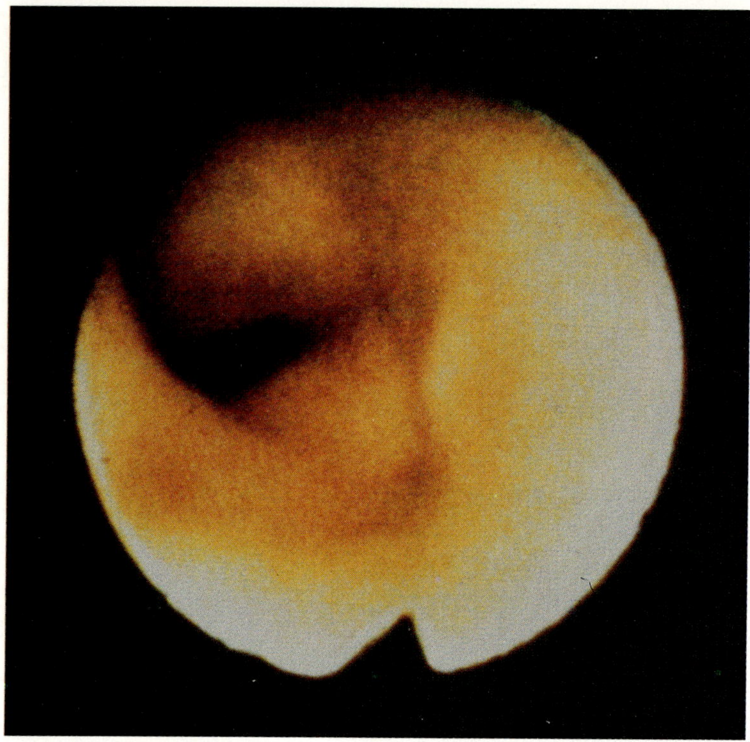

Fig. 3-6. Typical appearance of stable atheroma in a patient with stable coronary artery disease. The endothelial surface is smooth. No thrombus or plaque hemorrhage is apparent.

lial cells have been replaced by a heavier fibrous cap, but the endothelial surface itself remains intact. Although there is no doubt that the pathophysiologic basis of pain in stable angina is a transient increase in oxygen demand that exceeds the artery's capacity to deliver flow, we now believe that stable angina is the only syndrome in which this mechanism is the dominating factor.

Endothelial ulceration. In contrast to stable angina, when the clinical presentation is an unstable syndrome, we see changes in the endothelial surface. The least severe of the unstable coronary syndromes is accelerated angina (increasing frequency of angina without rest pain).

Figure 3-8 shows the endothelial surface of the left anterior descending coronary artery in a 75-year-old man with a 7-year history of stable angina and a 3-week period of accelerated angina pectoris. The accelerated syndrome was only partially responsive to nitrates and beta blockers. At angiography the patient was found to have an 80% to 90% stenosis in the left circumflex coronary artery. The endothelial surface is disrupted, and there is subintimal hemorrhage. There is, however, no thrombus attached to the endothelial surface. Microscopically, serial sections of ulcerations show progressive thinning of the fibrous cap as the point of rupture is approached.

The distinguishing feature between acute and stable coronary disease at angioscopy is this endothelial ulcer; thus far, all but one of our patients with accelerated angina have had endothelial disruption. Furthermore, the

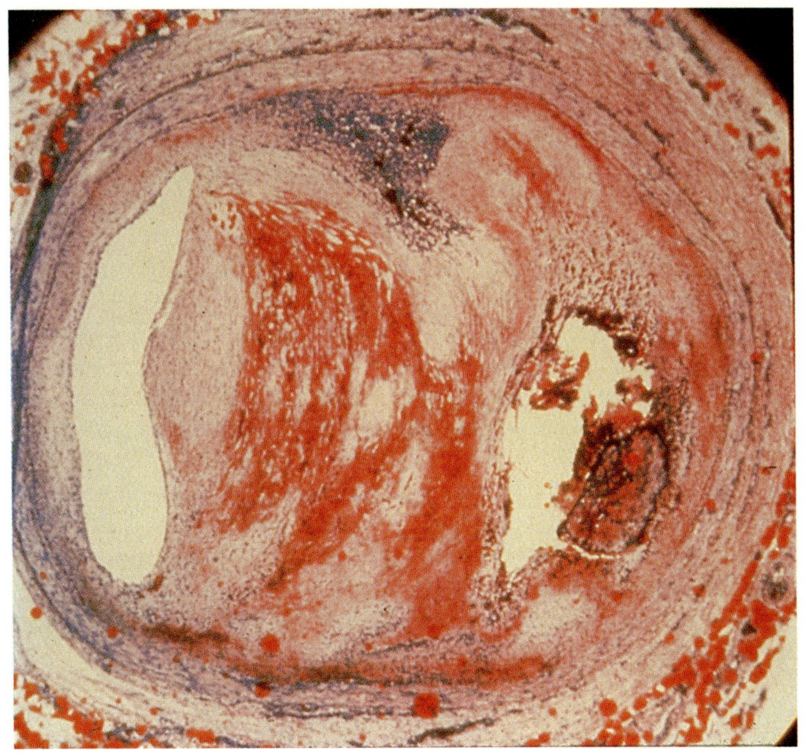

Fig. 3-7. An atheroma with a necrotic core covered by a fibrous cap (Reprinted with permission from Friedman, M. et al.: Am. J Pathol. **48:**19, 1986.)

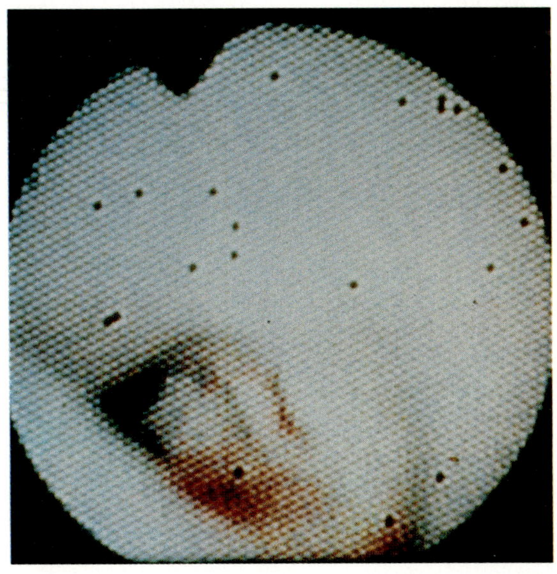

Fig. 3-8. An endothelial ulceration in the LAD coronary artery of a patient with accelerated angina.

acute lesion invariably lies in the coronary artery identified by electrocardiography as the one responsible for acute ischemic symptoms.[15] Although the cause of endothelial ulceration is not definitely established, a strong inferential case exists for erosion from within. Atheromas almost always lie beneath the ulceration, and the evolution of ulceration bears a histologic resemblance to rupture from within, induced by an inflammatory foreign body response. The mechanism by which ulceration causes angina may be through release of vasoconstrictive compounds such as thromboxane A_2 platelets which aggregate at the site.

Platelet aggregation. Despite the fact that endothelial disruption causes platelet aggregation, we do not always see a thrombus attached to the ulceration either at angioscopy or at autopsy. This suggests that platelet embolization, documented in the constricted canine coronary artery, also occurs in humans. Microemboli trigger fatal ventricular arrhythmias in humans. This is not to imply that sudden death is always caused by emboli, because people who die instantaneously (within 30 seconds) rarely have any type of acute coronary lesion.[16] The important point is that sudden death, like the other acute coronary syndromes, has more than one cause. Nevertheless, we believe that microemboli are an important cause of sudden ischemic cardiac death.

Coronary embolization is not necessarily fatal, and its frequency is probably much higher than we recognize. Because microemboli are not found in autopsies of patients with chronic coronary disease, they probably disappear by endogenous lysis. The alternative clinical outcome of endothelial ulceration with platelet microemboli, therefore, is another example of the chronic-acute-chronic cycle, in this case heart failure without history of infarction, in the presence of nonocclusive coronary disease. We believe that microemboli that lyse are an important cause of ischemic cardiomyopathy.

Healing with progression of stenosis. The ultimate evolution of endothelial ulceration is healing. Animal studies in our laboratory and others[17] demonstrate that experimentally induced endothelial disruption heals rapidly. After attachment of platelets, endothelial cells grow inward from the margins of the damaged surface, covering the platelet-fibrin mass. Simultaneously the platelets and fibrin are rapidly replaced by macrophages, smooth muscle cells, and fibrous tissue so that at 4 weeks the site of prior endothelial damage often is not readily identifiable. In humans, this is probably the most common outcome: Duncan et al.[18] found that 81% of 251 patients with new or worsening angina had returned to full-time work at 6 months; only 16% went on to have acute myocardial infarction. We believe that healing of the endothelial ulcer leads to stabilization of the acute coronary syndrome.

Reendothelialization of an ulceration over a ruptured atheroma, however, invokes an important permutation of the normal healing process. In the animal preparation, endothelial injury in the presence of hyperlipidemia results in accelerated development of atheroma.[19] We believe that precisely the same process occurs in human coronary disease, with or without clinical hyperlipidemia. This view conforms to clinical reality: 75% of patients with unstable angina exhibit rapid localized progression of stenosis when coronary angiography is performed soon after the acute episode.[20]

This pathogenetic mechanism, we believe, also occurs in stable angina. A critical insight from our angioscopic experience is that coronary endothelial ulceration can occur in the absence of a recognized change in symptom pattern; at coronary angiography, ulceration or thrombus also is reported in a small percentage of patients with stable angina.[21] Serial angiography clearly established the phenomenon of episodic localized progression. For instance, Singh[22] found that only 34 of 105 (33%) coronary stenoses exhibit progression at

4-year follow-up (7.8%/year). Rapid progression typically occurred with the abrupt development of new symptoms and frequently involved previously normal segments. We believe that endothelial ulceration without symptoms is the major (but unrecognized) cause of rapid localized atheroma progression in coronary heart disease.

The restenosis rate after percutaneous transluminal coronary angioplasty is 30%.[23] Our angioscopic experience in vivo has demonstrated that substantial endothelial disruption, undetectable by angiography, can be induced by balloon angioplasty in patients who are initially thought to have had a successful therapeutic procedure. We also believe that this same process—endothelial disruption, platelet aggregation, and accelerated fibroproliferative response—is the cause of restenosis after percutaneous transluminal coronary angioplasty.

In summary, the first cycle—ulceration, platelet aggregation, and healing—has several potential acute and chronic disease outcomes: accelerated angina, microembolization producing either sudden death or chronic heart failure, and healing with return to stable angina, often accompanied by accelerated progression of coronary stenosis.

When the Coronary Thrombus Forms: The Second Cycle

The second cycle consists of ulceration, partial thrombosis, thrombotic occlusion and lysis or incorporation with atheroma progression.

Partial coronary thrombosis. Figure 3-9 is from a 70-year-old man with new-onset, unstable rest angina (increasing frequency with rest pain). He had an inadequate in-hospital response to nitrates, beta blockers, calcium-channel blockers, and heparin. The electrocardiograms showed transient inverted T waves in the anteroseptal leads, but there was no creatine kinase elevation. His coronary angiogram revealed a 95% left anterior descending coronary stenosis. The angioscopic image was recorded just distal to the stenosis. There is a bright red partially occlusive thrombus just distal to the stenosis. The thrombus surface undulated during infusion of the clear viewing solution but was not dislodged from the endothelial surface by vigorous flushing.

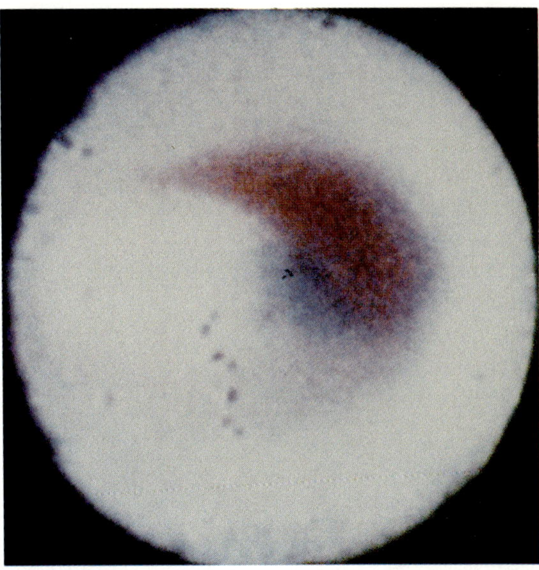

Fig. 3-9. A fresh partially occlusive coronary thrombus in a patient with unstable rest angina pectoris. (Courtesy Dr. Meyer Friedman.)

Figure 3-10 shows a coronary artery with a partially occlusive intraluminal thrombus. There is rupture of the fibrous cap that covered an atheroma cavity, and at the point of rupture there is thrombus formation. Beneath the point of rupture lies an atheroma, whose necrotic content has been partially removed during fixation.

Partially occlusive thrombus is typical of this clinical syndrome: 87% of our patients with unstable rest angina have had a thrombus; in contrast, we have not yet seen thrombus in stable coronary disease. Furthermore, when an intracoronary thrombus is removed at autopsy, it is attached to an ulcerated endothelial surface in over 90% of cases. We be-

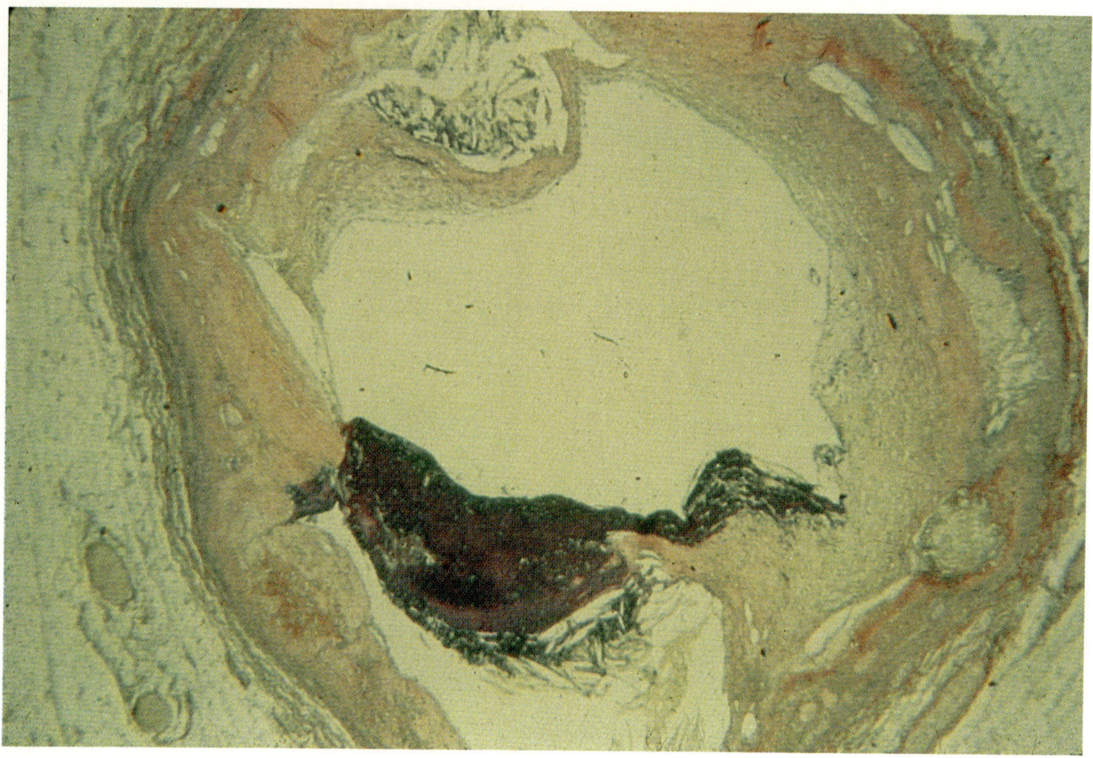

Fig. 3-10. A partially occlusive coronary thrombosis attached to an endothelial ulceration. (Courtesy Dr. Meyer Friedman.)

lieve that the continuum of clinical severity from accelerated angina to unstable rest angina has a pathologic parallel: that from endothelial ulceration to partially occlusive thrombosis.

Like the endothelial, the partially occlusive thrombus is also biologically unstable—its two short-term potential fates are lysis or progression to occlusion. The frequency of remission of unstable rest angina with supportive medical therapy[24] suggests that spontaneous lysis is common. The angiographic literature also suggests that endogenous lysis can occur fairly rapidly with supportive therapy. Rentrop et al.[25] found in patients with acute infarction a 90% prevalence of total obstruction in the first several hours, but after 14 days of conventional therapy it was only 33%. We believe that spontaneous lysis is a common outcome of both partial and totally occlusive coronary thrombosis.

Coronary occlusion. The alternative to lysis for the partially occlusive thrombus is progression to total occlusion, represented by the clinical syndrome of acute myocardial infarction. Both clinical and pathologic data support the hypothesis that partially occlusive thrombi can progress to occlusion over a period of days or weeks. In his review of the world literature, Fulton[26] found that 13% to 40% of patients with unstable angina progressed to myocardial infarction within 3 months, many within the first few days or weeks. Conversely, in patients with acute infarction, there was a prodrome of unstable angina in 30% to 65% of patients. Autopsy confirmation is provided by the identification of two or more thrombus layers, attributed to episodic growth over time, in 81% of thrombi from patients who die with unstable angina. We believe that some coronary thrombi progress slowly to occlusion and that acute myocardial infarction in this group should be almost entirely preventable.

Nonetheless, the more common presentation of myocardial infarction is sudden onset of chest pain, suggesting that in the majority of infarctions progression to total occlusion is rapid.

Figure 3-11 is from a 66-year-old man with a 1-year history of stable angina who had the sudden onset of severe chest pain that waxed and waned over several hours. During hospitalization, the pain recurred and an ECG revealed ST segment elevation in the inferior leads. He immediately received heparin and intravenous tissue-type plasminogen activator and experienced complete relief of pain within 30 minutes, but soon thereafter symptoms recurred. At angiography, he had total left circumflex coronary artery at the site of angiographic occlusion. There is a coronary thrombus obstructing approximately 90% of the lumen.

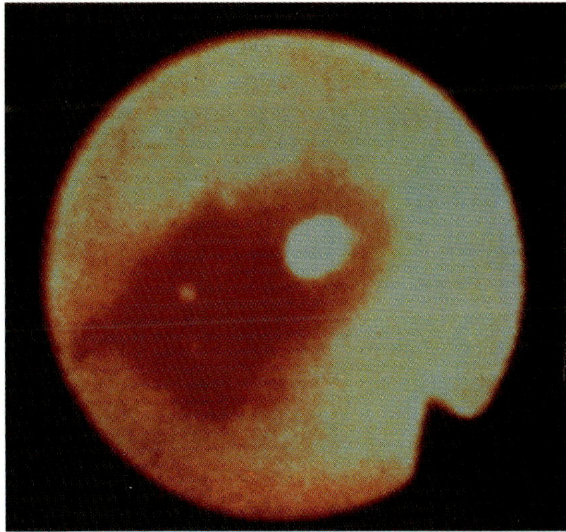

Fig. 3-11. A completely occlusive coronary thrombosis in the LAD coronary artery.

Figure 3-12 shows a portion of a thrombosed segment of the left anterior descending coronary artery of a patient who died 90 minutes after the onset of symptoms. A large atheroma cavity has ruptured into the lumen. The red-staining lipid content of the cavity, containing some cholesterol clefts *(arrows)*, constitutes the upper third of the thrombus, which occludes the lumen. The remaining two-thirds of the thrombus consists chiefly of platelets, with an outer fringe composed chiefly of erythrocytes. In the atheroma cavity, there are many cholesterol clefts, and an area of calcification lies in direct contact with the cavity.

In our paradigm, there are two competing forces which determine whether a thrombus completely obstructs the coronary artery: the mass of thrombus required to produce occlusion and the efficiency of endogenous lysis. Complete thrombotic occlusion is common (79%) when the preexisting stenosis is greater than 75% of the lumen, but uncommon (3%) when the preexisting stenosis is less than 75%.[27] Recurrence of occlusion after therapeutic thrombolysis is also clearly related to the magnitude of preexisting coronary stenosis. This principle also applies to balloon angioplasty, atherectomy, and laser angioplasty. It appears that even extensive endothelial disruption can heal without thrombotic occlusion when the residual stenosis is not severe. We believe that the magnitude of stenosis at the time of endothelial disruption determines whether the vessel remains patent or occludes.

Prognosis in stable coronary disease, therefore, is the product of two independent factors: percent stenosis and the phase of atheroma cycle. This explains the relative inaccuracy of prognostication based solely on "percent coronary stenosis" and "stress-induced ischemic abnormalities": one of the two fac-

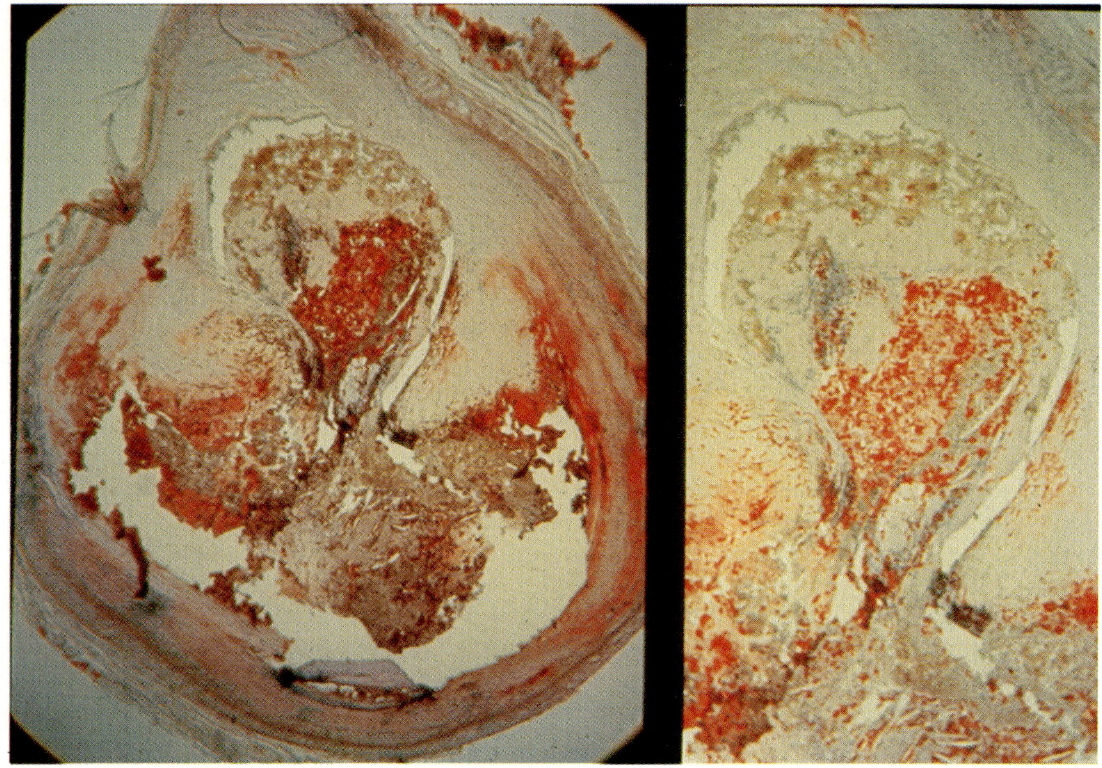

Fig. 3-12. A coronary thrombosis containing fragments of the endothelial surface and cholesterol clefts in a patient who died soon after the onset of an acute myocardial infarction. (Reprinted with permission from Friedman, M. et al.: Am. J. Pathol. **48:**19, 1966.)

tors determining prognosis is not assessed. Whether an ulceration and thrombus develop is determined by the atheroma cycle; the clinical outcome is determined by percent stenosis when this occurs. We believe that clinical prognosis is determined by both percent stenosis and the atheroma cycle; the unseen phase of the atheroma cycle is the "hidden factor" in coronary disease.

Thrombus incorporation. The thrombus cycle is completed by either endogenous lysis or incorporation of the thrombus into the vessel wall. By angioscopy, we often see no thrombus in vessels as early as 2 weeks after transluminal anterior myocardial infarction. Assuming that the transmural myocardial infarction was caused by an occlusive coronary thrombus, it has apparently undergone lysis. The endothelial surface is ulcerated, but there is no evidence of thrombus.

Figure 3-13 shows the alternative fate of coronary thrombus. The thrombus has been covered by a thin layer of endothelium, and the platelet-fibrin mass is being replaced by macrophages and fibrous tissue. In several more weeks, if the evolution of this thrombus parallels that in the animal, the lesion will be indistinguishable from the chronic stable atheroma. We believe that both thrombus incorporation and endothelial healing cause rapid progression of coronary stenosis. Like the first cycle, it also returns to the starting

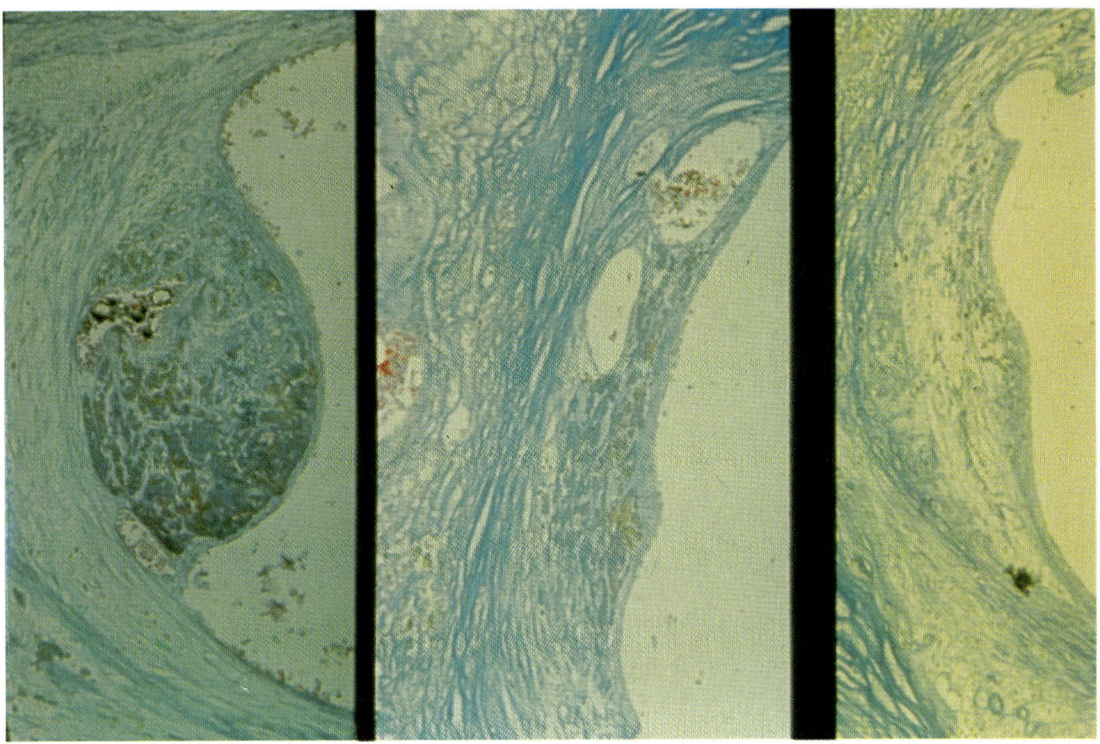

Fig. 3-13. Incorporation of thrombus into the wall of a coronary artery. The three sections are approximately 50 μm apart. The middle panel shows both thrombi infiltrated by connective tissue. The right panel shows the terminal portion of the thrombus incorporation. (Courtesy Dr. Meyer Friedman.)

point: a stable atheroma with stable angina pectoris.

The Coronary Artery Disease Paradigm and Its Therapeutic Implications

Our paradigm of coronary disease consists of linked histopathologic cycles based on endothelial ulceration and coronary thrombosis. Within each cycle there are specific endothelial conditions, each of which is responsible for the clinical syndromes we identify at the bedside. Our paradigm implies that between each transition there may be a brief opportunity for an intervention that can break the cycle. In principle, the intervention should be specific for the endothelial condition, and it can be inferred from the clinical presentation.

We need interventions that induce these four specific effects: prevent ulceration, inhibit platelet aggregation, lyse thrombus, and promote endothelial healing. We have no known interventions that cause the first or last effect. Ironically, these two classes of interventions are the most likely to interrupt the rapid progression of stable coronary atheroma. We suspect that erosion of the fibrous cap is caused by macrophages, which are known to cause both free radical formation and to produce enzymes capable of destroying collagen and elastin. Therefore, we believe that antioxidants[28] and anti-inflammatory agents[29] deserve immediate investigation as drugs that can impede atheroma rupture or promote ulcer healing.

In patients with endothelial ulceration, we need agents to inhibit platelet aggregation. If effective, these agents could reduce the rate of sudden death or development of ischemic cardiomyopathy from emboli and impede progression of thrombus to total occlusion and myocardial infarction. Some of these effects have been established by the Veterans Administration Cooperative Study of 1266 men with unstable angina who were randomly assigned to treatment with buffered aspirin or placebo. There was a 51% lower cardiac event rate at 3 months in the aspirin-treated group.[30] These results have been recently confirmed by a Canadian multicenter trial.[31] We believe additional antiplatelet agents (for example, prostaglandin derivatives) deserve trial in the full range of clinical disorders secondary to endothelial disruption (for example, after angioplasty).

In patients with unstable rest angina caused by partial thrombosis, arrest of progression to total occlusion by thrombolytic therapy requires investigation. As yet the data are limited. Lawrence et al.[32] found a large and statistically significant reduction in cardiac event rate at 3 months when patients with unstable angina received 24-hour treatment with intravenous streptokinase during hospitalization. We believe with attention to risk versus benefit, thrombolytic agents deserve trial in unstable rest angina; however, the rate of bleeding complications must be reduced well below that reported in acute infarction.

In summary, we see coronary disease as two interlocking cycles. The first consists of a stable atheroma that progresses to endothelial ulceration, platelet aggregation, and ulcer healing. The second cycle, which begins with the endothelial ulceration, progresses through partial thrombosis, complete occlusion, lysis, and thrombus incorporation. Each phase of the two cycles results in a clinical syndrome, and each may benefit from specific therapy. This paradigm links basic science to clinical practice, offers a testable hypothesis, and suggests that there is an opportunity for considerable advancement in the medical therapy of coronary heart disease.

If by this paradigm we can redirect the debate on coronary thrombus, it is because where others have seen resolution, we see lack of information. Although the new information from our first angioscopic explorations is limited, we believe that the missing link in our understanding of human coronary disease has been our inability to perceive its evolution. We know our paradigm may be "wrong": it is based on observations in selected patients, so ill that they required bypass surgery. But if it is in error, we will not mind being wrong. As Lewis Thomas says in *The Wonderful Mistake,*[33] "Biology needs a better word than 'error' for [its] driving force. . . . Or maybe error will do after all, when you remember that it came from an old root meaning to wander about, looking for something." Alternately, the thrombus may not progress to complete occlusion but rather stabilize and become incorporated into the atheroma, leading to *localized progression of coronary stenosis.* The typical clinical cycle of coronary disease—chronic stability punctuated by acute complications—is the result of this unrecognized cycle at the endothelial surface.

Evaluation of Coronary Artery Bypass Grafts

Examination of vein graft was easily accomplished. In particular, we were able to closely examine suture lines and the shape of the anastomosis. Based on angioscopic examination three anastomoses were revised due to misplaced sutures or unsuspected large intimal flaps. The frequency of change in the operative procedure due to angioscopy, however, is less than that at peripheral vascular surgery.

Limitations of Angioscopy

There are several technical problems with the first generation angioscopic devices that preclude widespread routine clinical use. A clinical angioscope must have a flushing channel and the ability to angulate its tip. The angioscope also must be made more flexible, because the first generation device is sufficiently stiff that in percutaneous use it could cause coronary artery spasm, dissection, or perforation.

Our intraoperative complication rate with angioscopy examination has been low. In two coronary patients, the angioscope tip raised small intimal tears that were of no recognizable clinical consequence. In two peripheral vascular patients, flaps were created. One flap occurred at a peripheral anastomotic site and led us to revise the anastomosis. We believe that the next generation of softer devices should further reduce this low complication rate.

CONCLUSIONS

Angioscopy offers a unique opportunity to visualize the abnormalities of the vascular endothelium that are responsible for the generation of clinical syndromes. Although angio scopy is still in its initial stage of development, the unique data it provides may become useful in several areas of research and clinical practice. In the surgical theater, angioscopic evaluation of the patency of anastomosis, particularly during peripheral vascular surgery, will probably become a complementary method to intraoperative angiography or surgical probes when the procedure can be completed in a few minutes. Angioscopy can also become an important surgical teaching tool because it allows direct inspection of suture lines.

The second major clinical application is percutaneous angioscopy. If we can develop percutaneous coronary angioscopy, we could assess the completeness of thrombolytic therapy. Perhaps most important, we also could inspect coronary artery stenoses before and after balloon dilatation, allowing us to define the pathophysiology of restenosis. We could then initiate additional therapy (for example, removal of intimal flaps) that could reduce the rate of restenosis. Even if these practical applications do not evolve, however, the images of coronary arteries in living humans, obtained during acute coronary syndromes, will forever alter our understanding of atherosclerotic disease.

ACKNOWLEDGMENTS

We wish to acknowledge the many vascular surgeons who have participated in the collection and analysis of angioscopic data: cardiac surgeons Myles Lee, M.D., Robert Kass, M.D., Aurelio Chaux, M.D., Carlos Blanche, M.D., Jack Matloff, M.D., and peripheral vascular surgeons: Robert Foran, M.D., Lewis Cohen, M.D., Philip Levin, M.D., David Cosman, M.D., Richard Treiman, M.D., and Robert Carrol, M.D. We are also grateful to Mr. Zev Lapin and Mr. Steven Meadow for their abiding interest and support of the research program. Part of this manuscript originally appeared in Circulation **75**:505-512, 1987. We also wish to acknowledge the generous contribution of the histologic illustrations by Dr. Meyer Friedman, whose research a quarter of a century ago has greatly influenced the ideas expressed herein.

REFERENCES

1. Spears, J.R., Spokojny, A.M., and Marais, H.J.: Coronary angioscopy during cardiac catheterization, J.A.C.C. **6**:93, 1985.
2. Rhea, L., and Walker, I.C., cited by Cutler, et al.: Arch Surg **9**:689, 1913.
3. Allen, D.S., and Graham, E.A.: Intracardiac surgery: A new method, J.A.M.A. **79**:1028, 1922.
4. Greenstone, S.M., Shore, J.M., Heringman, G.C., et al.: Arterial endoscopy (arterioscopy), Arch Surg **93**:811, 1966.
5. Gamble, W.J., and Irris, R.E.: Experimental intracardiac visualization, N. Engl. J. Med. **276**:1397, 1967.
6. Spears, J.R., Marais, H.J., Serur, J., et al.: In vivo coronary angioscopy, J.A.C.C. **1**:1311, 1983.
7. Litvack, F., Grundfest, W.S., Lee, M.E., et al.: Angioscopic visualization of blood vessels interior in animals and humans, Clin. Cardiol. **8**:65, 1985.
8. Grundfest, W.S., Litvack, F., Sherman, T., et al.: Delineation of peripheral and coronary detail by intraoperative angioscopy, Ann. Surg. **202**:394, 1985.
9. Grundfest, W.S., Litvack, F., Sherman, T., et al.: Definition of new pathophysiologic mechanisms and altered decisions: an outcome of intravascular angioscopy (abstract), J.A.C.C. **7**:153A, 1986.
10. Lee, G., Garcia, J.M., Corso, P.J., et al.: Correlation of coronary angioscopic to angiographic findings in coronary artery disease, Am. J. Cardiol. **57**:238, 1986.
11. Sherman, C.T., Litvack, F., Grundfest, W., et al.: Coronary angioscopy in patients with unstable angina pectoris, N. Engl. J. Med. **315**:913, 1986.
12. Van Steigman, G., Bartle, E.J., Pearce, W.H., et al.: Vascular endoscopy with a new laser capable angioscope, Lasers Surg. Med. **5**:170, 1985.

13. Ritchie, J.L., Nanses, D.D., Vracko, R., et al.: In vivo rotational thrombectomy—evaluation by angioscopy, Circulation **74**(II):457, 1986.
14. Forrester, J.S., Litvack, F., Grundfest, W., et al.: A perspective of coronary disease seen through the arteries of living man, Circulation **75:**505, 1987.
15. Sherman, C.T., Litvack, F., Grundfest, W., et al.: Demonstration of thrombus and complex atheroma by in-vivo angioscopy in patients with unstable angina pectoris, N. Engl. J. Med. **315:**913, 1986.
16. Friedman, M., Hanwaring, J.H., Rosenman, R.H., et al.: Instantaneous and sudden deaths: clinical and pathologic differentiation in coronary artery disease, J.A.M.A. **225:**1319, 1973.
17. van Aken, P.J., and Emeis, J.J.: Organization of experimentally induced arterial thrombosis in rats from two weeks until ten months: the development of an arteriosclerotic lesion and the occurrence of rethrombosis, Artery **11:**384, 1983.
18. Duncan, B., Fulton, M., Morrison, S.L., et al.: Prognosis of new and worsening angina pectoris, Br. J. Med. **1:**981, 1976.
19. Steele, P.M., Chesebro, J.H., Holmes, D.R., et al.: Balloon angioplasty in pigs: histologic wall injury as a determinant of platelet deposition and thrombus formation, Circ. Res. **57:**105, 1985.
20. Moise, A., Theroux, P., Taeymans, Y., et al.: Unstable angina and progression of coronary atherosclerosis, N. Engl. J. Med **309:**685, 1983.
21. Ambrose, J.A., Winters, S.L., Stern, A., et al.: Angiographic morphology and the pathogenesis of unstable angina pectoris, J. Am. Coll. Cardiol. **5:**609, 1985.
22. Singh, R.N.: Progression of coronary atherosclerosis: clues to pathogenesis from serial coronary arteriography, Br. Heart J. **52:**451, 1984.
23. Holmes, D.R., Vlietstra, R.E., Smith, H.C., et al.: Restenosis after percutaneous transluminal coronary angioplasty (PTCA): a report from the PTCA Registry of the National Heart, Lung and Blood Institute, Am. J. Cardiol. **53:**770, 1984.
24. Mulcahy, R., Daly, L., Graham, I., et al.: Unstable angina: natural history and determinants of prognosis. Am. J. Cardiol. **48:**525, 1981.
25. Rentrop, K.P., Frederick, F., Blanke, H., et al.: Effects of intracoronary streptokinase and intracoronary nitroglycerin infusion on coronary angiographic patterns and mortality in patients with acute myocardial infarction. N. Engl. J. Med. **311:**1456, 1984.
26. Fulton, W.F.M.: Pathogenesis of unstable angina preceding acute myocardial infarction. In Lichtlen, P.R., editor: Coronary angiography and angina pectoris, Stuttgart, George Thieme Verlag, 1976.
27. Falk, E.: Plaque rupture with severe preexisting stenosis precipitating coronary thrombosis: characteristics of coronary atherosclerotic plaques underlying fatal occlusive thrombi, Br. Heart J. **50:**127, 1983.
28. Lee, T.H., Hoover, R.L., Williams, J.D., et al.: Effect of dietary enrichment with eicosapentaenoic and docosahexaenoic acids on in vitro neutrophil and monocyte leukotriene generation and neutrophil function, N. Engl. J. Med. **32:**1217, 1985.
29. Lewis, D.H., Davis, J.W., Archibald, D.G., et al.: Protective effects of aspirin against acute myocardial infarction and death in men with unstable angina, N. Engl. J. Med. **309:**396, 1983.
30. Lewis, D.A.: Endogenous antiinflammatory factors. Biochem. Pharmacol. **33**(11):1705, 1984.
31. Cairns, J.A., Gent, M., Singer, J., et al.: Aspirin, sulfinpyrazone, or both in unstable angina: results of a Canadian multicenter trial, N. Engl. J. Med. **313:**1369, 1985.
32. Lawrence, J.R., Shepard, J.T., Bone, I., et al.: Fibrinolytic therapy in unstable angina pectoris: a controlled clinical trial, Thrombosis Res. **17:**767, 1980.
33. Thomas, L.: The wonderful mistake. In The medusa and the snail, New York, 1979, Viking Press.

Chapter 4

Considerations of Dosimetry for Laser-Tissue Ablation

Sipke Strikwerda, MD
John R. Kramer, MD
Firooz Partovi, PhD
Michael S. Feld, PhD

Balloon angioplasty (percutaneous transluminal coronary angioplasty—PTCA)[1] is currently a widely accepted procedure in the treatment of patients with obstructive coronary artery disease, but it is associated with a high recurrence rate. The tendency of restenosis of dilated vessels[2] may be due to the circumstance that the obstructing atherosclerotic plaque is remodeled but essentially left in place. Laser light is particularly promising because it may eliminate plaque tissue from the vessel lumen,[3-5] possibly leading to better long-term results. Preliminary experiments, however, using continuous wave (CW) laser radiation transmitted through guiding catheters incorporating optical fibers, were frequently complicated by vascular perforation or excessive coagulation injury.[5-7]

The objective of this work is to identify the relevant tissue and laser beam parameters in the interaction of laser radiation with biological tissue. Results are presented of a study undertaken to establish the relation between delivery parameters of CW argon ion laser light and the effect on atheromatous plaque. Finally, implications for laser catheter design and dosimetry for laser angiosurgery are discussed.

TISSUE AND LASER BEAM PARAMETERS

When laser radiation of low intensity is incident on a thin sample of biological tissue, a variety of optical phenomena may occur. The light may be partly reflected from the surface or transmitted through the sample. The other portion of the beam is attenuated by absorption and scattering as it penetrates the tissue. The thickness of the layer of tissue in which 63% (1-1/e) of the radiation entering the sample has been attenuated, is defined as the penetration depth.[8] The depth of penetration is a function of the wavelength-dependent absorption and scattering coefficients of the tissue. The penetration depth D is related to the absorption coefficient α and scattering coefficient β according to the equation

$$D = \frac{1}{\alpha+\beta}$$

When the absorption coefficient α (unit: cm^{-1}) is high, penetration depth is low, and laser radiation is confined to the most superficial layers of tissue. In case of a low absorption coefficient, the penetration depth is higher with scattering of light playing a more important role. Only absorption of laser radiation causes generation of heat. The interplay between laser wavelength and tissue properties, resulting in characteristic values of α and β, determines the distribution of light and, hence, the temperature profile in tissue.[9,10]

The wavelength of a CO_2-laser, at 10,600 nm in the far infrared (IR-C), is strongly absorbed by water and has a penetration depth in tissue of some nanometers to micrometers.[8,11] The ultraviolet (UV) wavelengths of an excimer laser (from 193 to 351 nm) also have very low penetration depths in biological tissue. They have been measured in cornea to be approximately 4 and 47 μm for wavelengths of 193 and 248 nm, respectively.[12] Because at the CO_2 and excimer laser wavelengths the deposition of laser energy is limited to the thinnest layer nearest the surface, these lasers are well suited for cutting and ablation of tissue. Because of the strong absorption, scattering of light beyond the top layer is minimal. The application of CO_2 and pulsed excimer laser radiation in atherosclerotic vascular disease, however, is limited by lack of a fiber optic delivery system to reliably transmit the optical energy to the treatment site.

The near infrared (IR-A) radiation of the CW Nd:YAG laser at 1,060 nm generally has a penetration depth in biological tissue in the order of millimeters. At this wavelength, heat is deposited in deeper layers, making it more suitable for tissue coagulation.[9,10]

Absorption of CW argon ion laser radiation (principal wavelengths: 488 and 514.5 nm) is strongly dependent on the presence of chromophores in the irradiated tissue, like melanin and hemoglobin. The penetration depth of argon ion laser light in atherosclerotic plaque has been reported to be about 300 μm.[13,14] Because of the intermediate depth of penetration in tissues that are not heavily vascularized or pigmented, the argon ion laser may be used for coagulation as well as ablative purposes. Whether exposure to argon ion laser light will primarily cause coagulation or tissue removal is dose dependent. Particularly at the argon ion laser wavelengths, where penetration strongly varies with the chemical and physical composition of the tissue involved, proper selection of delivery parameters is essential for a given surgical application.

Using CW laser radiation, heat is initially deposited in a "volume" of tissue, which is a function of penetration depth D and diameter d of the laser beam.[10,11] During the exposure, a temperature gradient develops to surrounding tissue, causing heat to flow out of the irradiated area. The rate at which heat diffusion takes place is a characteristic of tissue and can be expressed in terms of thermal conductivity (unit: W/cm °C) or thermal diffusivity (unit: cm^2/sec). Thermodynamic properties of vessel wall and plaque have been reported by Welch et al.[15] The effect of a laser procedure (that is, the absolute and relative extent of tissue ablation and coagulation) is ultimately determined by the *dosimetry* of the beam: the area of the light spot, the intensity (defined as incident power per unit area), the duration of the exposure, and the time interval between exposures.

DOSIMETRY STUDIES

A dose of laser light (or "photon dose") of given wavelength is fully described by the following *dosimetric parameters:*

1. Incident power (in watts)
2. Area of the beam (in mm^2)
3. Exposure time (in seconds)

To determine if removal of atherosclerotic plaque by CW argon ion laser radiation can be optimized while coagulation damage is minimized, we studied ablation of atheromatous tissue by laser exposures of varying dosimetry quantitatively and qualitatively.[16] For this purpose, we used 27 segments of human atheromatous aorta (each approximately 15 cm long) obtained at autopsy from 17 patients. The degree of atherosclerosis ranged from lightly diseased aortic wall containing fatty streaks to noncalcified, mild-to-moderate fibrous atherosclerotic plaque. The segments were rinsed and immersed in a bath of saline 0.9% at room temperature with the luminal surface facing upward.

Laser light was delivered to the tissue using an optically shielded laser catheter[17] in normal orientation to the plaque surface.[16-19] The transparent tip of the catheter, enclosing an optical fiber, was forced to be in contact with the plaque using a 35 gram mass (0.34 N). The diameter of the light spot at the tissue was controlled by choosing the appropriate distance between the output end of the optical fiber and the outer surface of the quartz shield.[17,19] We employed spot diameters of 1000, 750, 500, and 280 μm.

The input end of the optical fiber was aligned with the focused beam of a Coherent I-20 argon ion laser. Laser power was measured at the tip of the catheter and adjusted with a beam attenuator. A calibrated in-line power meter continuously monitored incident power. An electro-mechanical shutter placed in the laser beam path provided control of exposure time. Laser light was delivered to the plaque in many single exposures at a variety of fluence levels (Table 4-1). Fluence* was constructed from different combinations of power (1.5 to 10 watts), time (20 to 4000 msec), and spot diameter (280 to 1000 μm). At each combination of dosimetric parameters (spot size, power, exposure time), a minimum of six locations on the tissue sample were irradiated. A total of 914 exposures were made.

Table 4-1. Fluence Levels and Number of Exposures (Total: 914) for Each Spot Diameter in the Study

Spot Diameter (μm)	*Fluence (J/mm²)*						*No. of Exposures*
1000	—	1.3	2.6	5.1	7.6	—	247
750	0.8	1.4	2.3	4.5	6.8	9.1	342
500	1.0	1.8	3.2	5.1	—	10.2	253
280	—	—	3.2	5.7	—	10.2	72

After irradiating an aortic segment, the intima was inspected grossly and under a dissecting microscope. If a laser exposure had caused removal of tissue, the dimensions of the resultant crater were measured using a microscope with polarized surface illumination. Ablation depth was evaluated by focusing first on the bottom of the crater and then on the tissue surface, reading the travel of the microscope stage between the two planes from the calibrated focusing knob. Crater diameter was measured at the intimal surface using the eyepiece reticle of the microscope. After the measurements, all aortic segments were fixed and stored in 10% neutral buffered formalin for future histopathologic preparation. From representative specimens for each experiment, samples were chosen at random, embedded in paraffin, sectioned, and stained with hematoxylin-eosin.

EFFICIENCY OF TISSUE REMOVAL

Certain minimum levels of argon ion laser intensity and fluence have to be delivered to

**Fluence is defined as the product of incident power and exposure time divided by spot area, with units of joules per mm².[17,19] It follows from this definition that fluence is equivalent to the ratio of energy to spot area and, also, to the product of intensity and exposure time.*

atheromatous tissue before ablation starts.[20] When laser energy is converted to thermal energy in plaque, a spatial temperature distribution is present with heat diffusing radially outward to surrounding tissue.[10,21] The generation of heat at the target site should at least keep pace with thermal diffusion to cause a local temperature rise sufficient for tissue ablation. This explains the existence of a threshold value for intensity (in units of watts/mm^2 or joules/sec/mm^2). Intensity reflects the *rate* at which laser energy is delivered to a given area of tissue. A fluence threshold refers to a minimum amount of energy necessary to remove a certain tissue volume under that area. The "volume" of tissue being irradiated is a function of beam diameter and penetration depth of the light.[10,11] Obviously, only part of the energy deposited is used for ablation; the rest causes coagulation damage or reversible thermal effects.[15] We considered the lowest levels of intensity and fluence that produced tissue removal with *each* single laser exposure a *practical* ablation threshold. For each spot size, practical threshold values for intensity and fluence could be determined.[20,22]

Above intensity threshold, the depth of the ablation crater was found to be fairly uniform for different laser intensities at the same fluence level.[20,22] Figure 4-1 depicts ablation depth (mean ± SD) in atheromatous tissue versus fluence of CW argon ion laser light delivered in spots of 1000, 750, 500, and 280 μm diameter. Results are plotted against fluence only, with each fluence constructed from laser intensities above the practical threshold and exposure time. Measurements at different fluence levels in aortic segments originating from the same patient are interconnected. Below the practical fluence threshold, laser exposures do not or inconsistently produce tissue removal. The occurrence of ablation is consistently reproducible, however, using fluences at or above this threshold. Here, each data point (solid black dots) represents 26 ± 10 laser craters (mean ± SD). The standard deviations around the mean values of ablation depth include intrasample variability experimental variation, and depth variation between different intensity–time combinations that give rise to the same fluence. When more tissue segments were irradiated at a given fluence and spot diameter, sample-to-sample variability in mean ablation depth averaged 9% (range: 1% to 22%).

It is shown in Fig. 4-1A and 4-1B that, above the practical threshold, crater depth increases with fluence in a linear fashion for spot diameters of 1000 and 750 μm. The slope of these curves is an estimate for the incremental yield of the ablation process and has been calculated to approximate 0.14 and 0.11 mm^3/J for 1000- and 750-μm-diameter spots, respectively. The curve(s) in Fig. 4-1C for a 500-μm spot can be seen to taper off with increasing fluence. Because of the cylindrical geometry of the laser craters produced at this spot size, the volume of tissue removed by laser ablation was derived from crater depth and diameter. As a measure for efficiency, the ablation ratio or ablation yield, defined as volume removed per unit energy, was calculated for various fluences, and combinations of intensity and exposure time. At a 500 μm spot diameter, ablation ratio was maximal at a fluence of 5.1 J/mm^2 ranging from 0.08 ± 0.01 mm^3/J to 0.15 ± 0.02 mm^3/J (mean ± SD) for different tissue samples and laser intensities.[22] It follows that, using a fluence of 10.2 J/mm^2, the first half of the laser exposure attributes more to ablated tissue volme than the second half. This is most likely due to divergence of the beam as it exits the catheter, causing lower intensities at newly exposed layers of tissue as ablation progresses and the crater deepens, while the catheter tip remains on the tissue surface. Figure 4-2 illustrates the calculated decrease in intensity with increasing distance from the optical shield, for each of the four spot sizes used. The drop in intensity is steepest for an initial beam diameter of 280 μm, followed by 500, 750 and 1000 μm. Absorption and scattering of laser light by vaporous products and particulate debris pro-

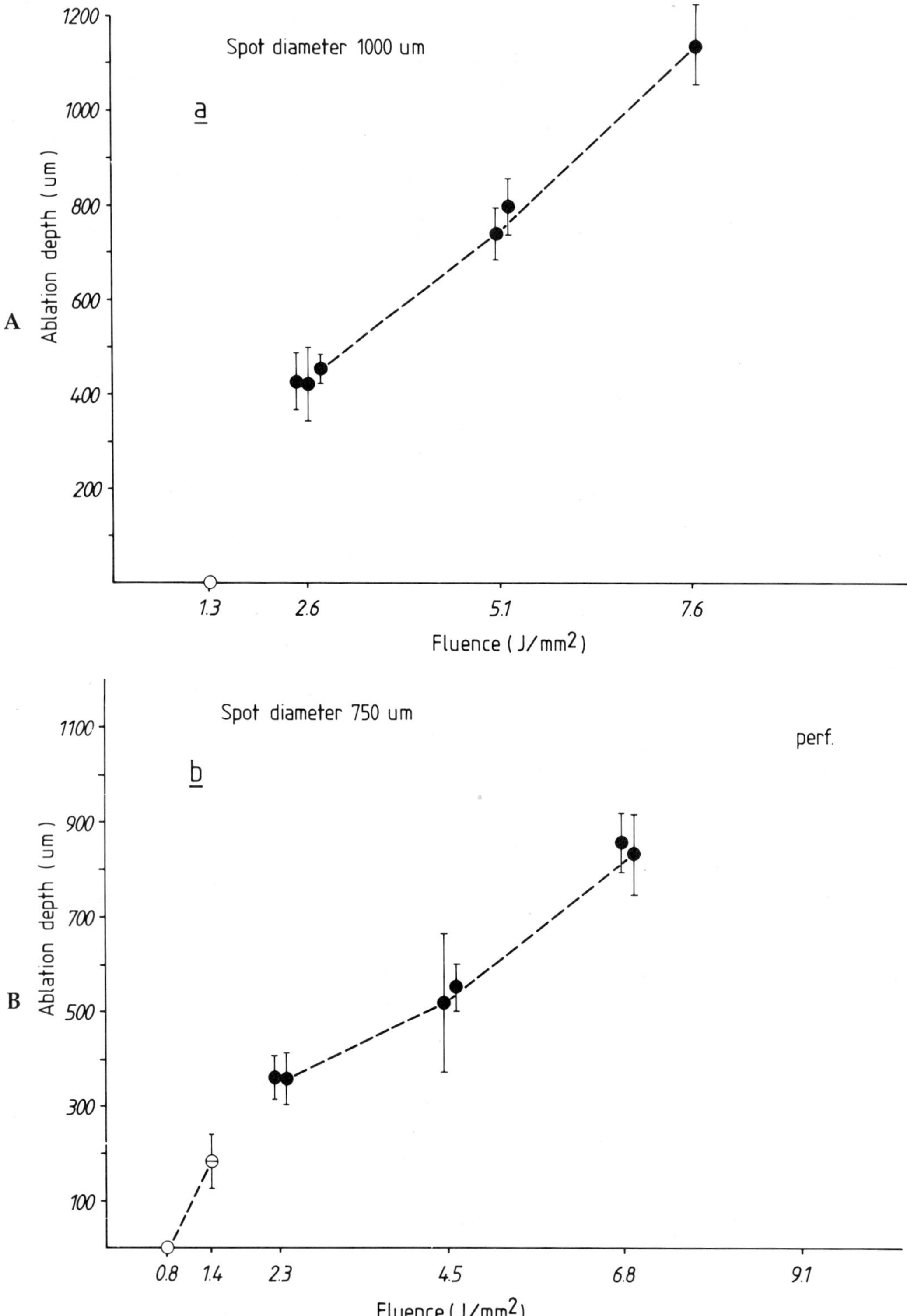

Fig. 4-1. For legend see opposite page.

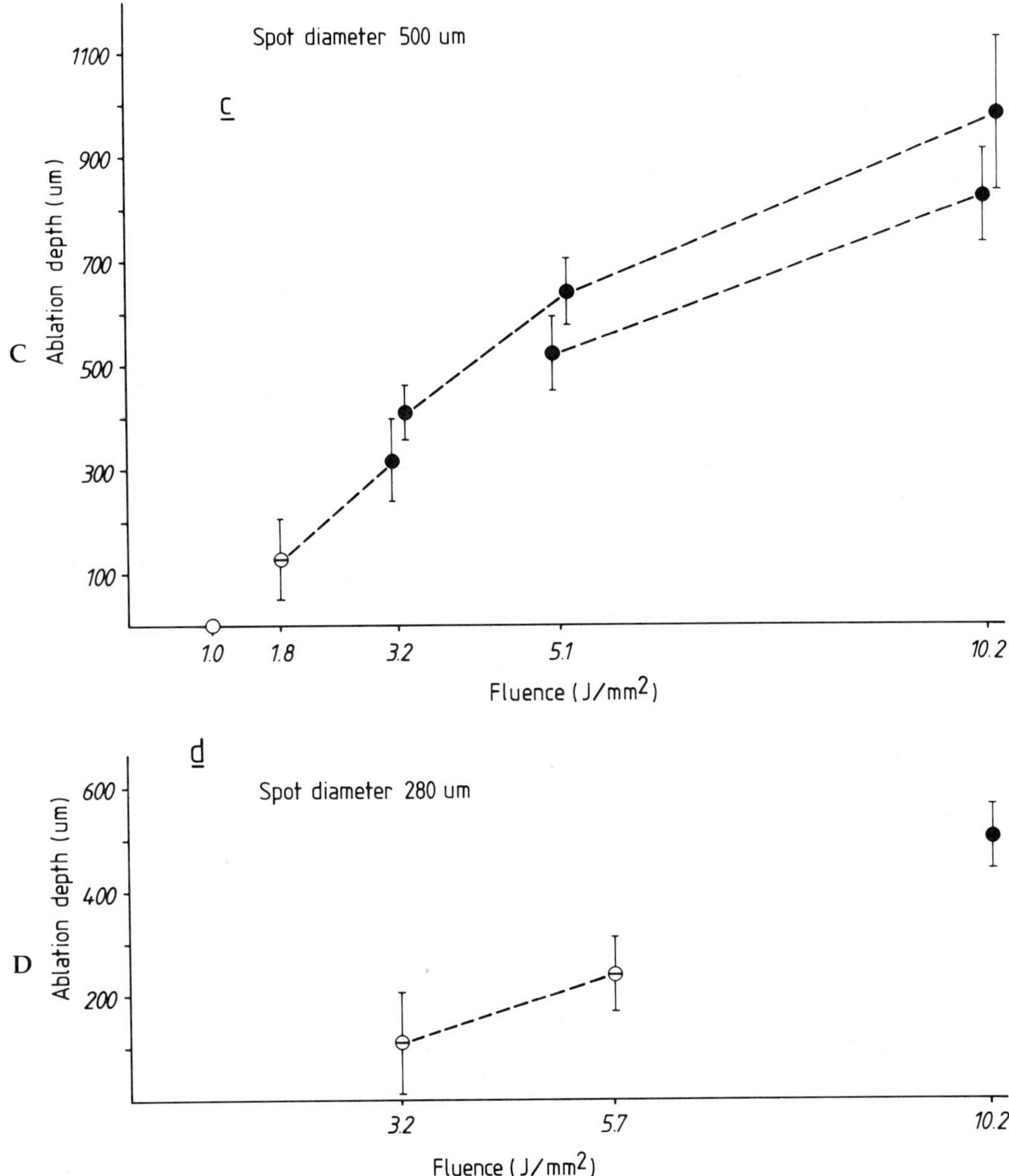

Fig. 4-1, con't. Ablation depth (mean ± SD) in atheromatous tissue versus fluence (J/mm^2) of cw argon ion laser light, delivered in spots of 1000 (**A**), 750 (**B**), 500 (**C**), and 280 (**D**) μm diameter. Measurements from tissue segments derived from the same patient are interconnected with a dashed line. A fluence of 9.1 J/mm^2 in a spot of 750 μm diameter consistently perforated (perf.) the approximately 1200-μm-thick aortic sample. (0, No ablation; θ, inconsistent ablation; ●, consistently reproducible ablation.)

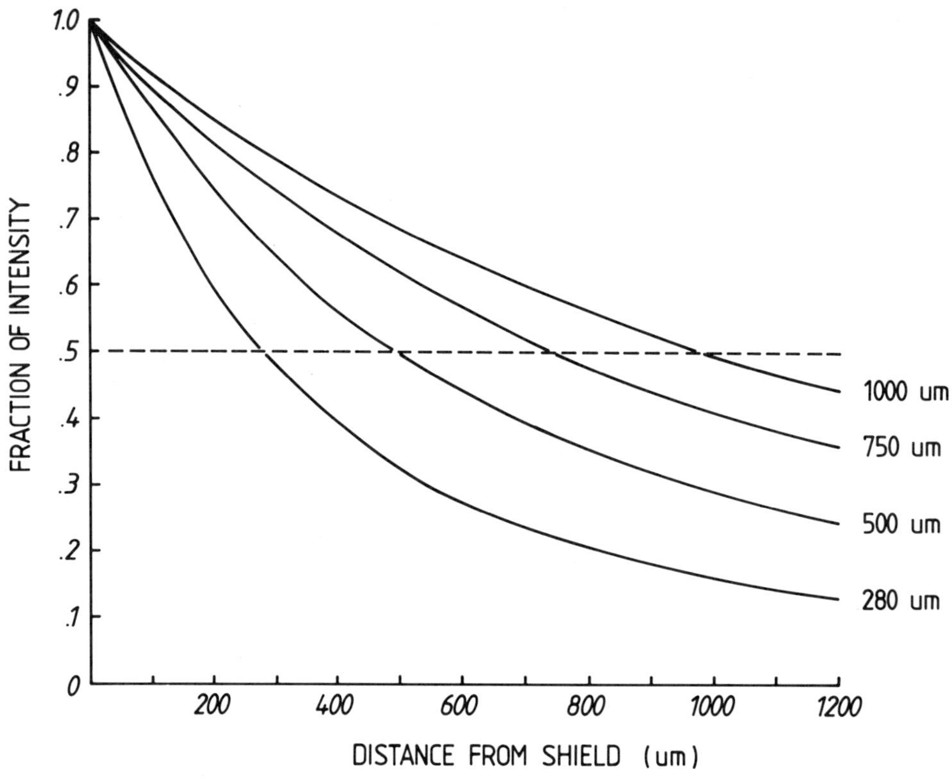

Fig. 4-2. The calculated decrease in intensity with increasing distance from the catheter tip for diverging laser beams (sine of the half angle = 0.21) in air with an initial diameter at the outside surface of the shield (i.e., spot diameter) of 1000, 750, 500, and 280 μm.

duced by tissue ablation, and thermal diffusion during a prolonged exposure may also cause a decrease in ablation efficiency.[22] The most inefficient ablation was observed using a spot diameter of 280 μm (Fig. 4-1D).

MORPHOLOGY

Gross and microscopic inspection of the exposed aortic segments revealed that, for a given spot diameter and fluence, carbonization was more evident when a low-intensity laser beam was used. High-intensity laser radiation appeared to produce relatively less char. Also, more carbonized remnants were present when large spot diameters were used, ablation of a greater amount of tissue naturally leaving more char behind.

A representative crater for each combination of spot size, fluence, and intensity was examined histologically. Figure 4-3 is a photomicrograph of a laser crater in aortic wall produced with a spot diameter of 280 μm and a fluence of 10.2 J/mm^2 of argon ion laser light. The duration of exposure was 210 msec, and the intensity was 48.7 W/mm^2 (power: 3 watts). The band of vacuolization (± 40 μm wide) lining the crater indicates extensive coagulation necrosis. Figure 4-4 is a photomicrograph of a laser crater produced with the same fluence and practically the same intensity (50.9 W/mm^2) and exposure time as the crater shown in Fig. 4-3. Here, however, spot

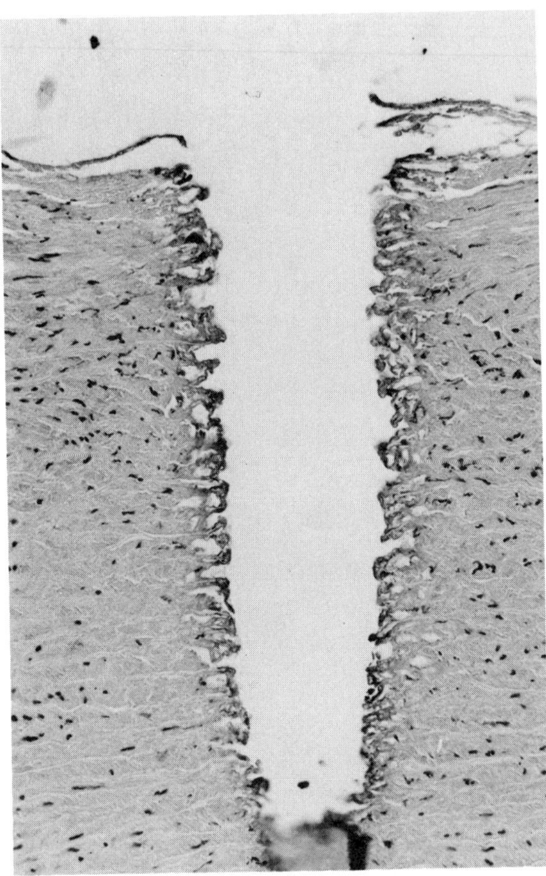

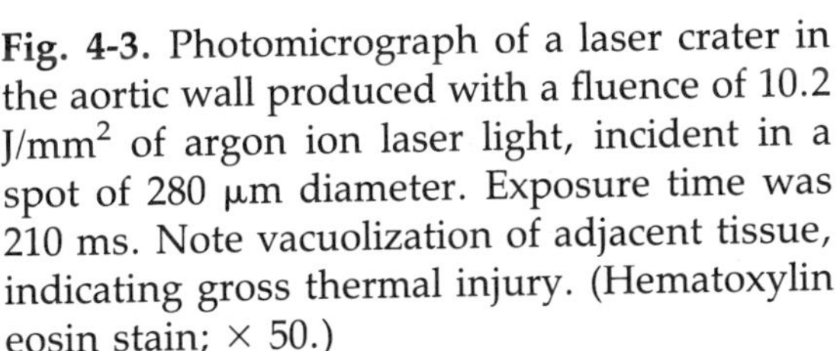

Fig. 4-3. Photomicrograph of a laser crater in the aortic wall produced with a fluence of 10.2 J/mm^2 of argon ion laser light, incident in a spot of 280 μm diameter. Exposure time was 210 ms. Note vacuolization of adjacent tissue, indicating gross thermal injury. (Hematoxylin eosin stain; × 50.)

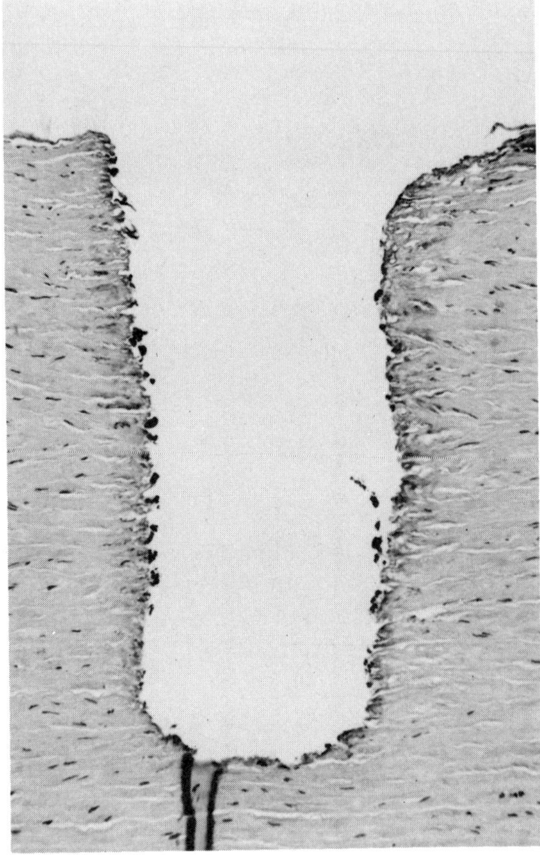

Fig. 4-4. Photomicrograph of a laser crater in the aortic wall after exposure to the same fluence as in Fig. 4-3, but delivered in a spot of 500 μm diameter. Exposure time was 200 ms. This crater is deeper with only mild hyperbasophilia and hypereosinophilia of adjacent tissue. (Hematoxylin eosin stain; × 31.)

diameter was 500 μm and beam power was 10 watts to compensate for the larger spot area. Mild hypereosinophilia and -basophilia of the perimeter and some carbon particles are visible with only slight evidence of coagulation, mostly toward the intimal surface. Overall thermal injury to remaining tissue at these laser parameters is considerably less than illustrated in Fig. 4-3. In Fig. 4-5, a crater in atheromatous tissue is shown after exposure to a fluence of 5.1 J/mm^2 of argon ion laser light delivered in a spot of 500 μm diameter. Exposure time was 333 msec, and the intensity was 15.3 W/mm^2. A cone-shaped area of vacuolization is evident with coagulation effects extending into the periphery of the crater, primarily near the intimal surface. Figure 4-6 illustrates a laser crater produced with the same fluence as in Fig. 4-5, but using a catheter with a spot diameter

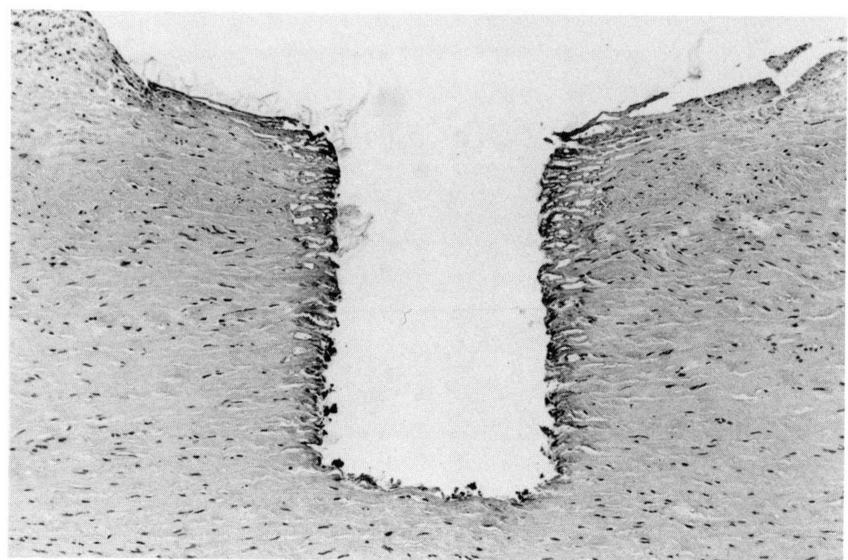

Fig. 4-5. Photomicrograph of a crater in an atheromatous plaque, irradiated with a fluence of 5.1 J/mm^2 in a spot of 500 μm diameter for a duration of 333 ms. Vacuolization and hypereosinophilia is evident and most extensive near the luminal surface. (Hematoxylin eosin stain; × 25.)

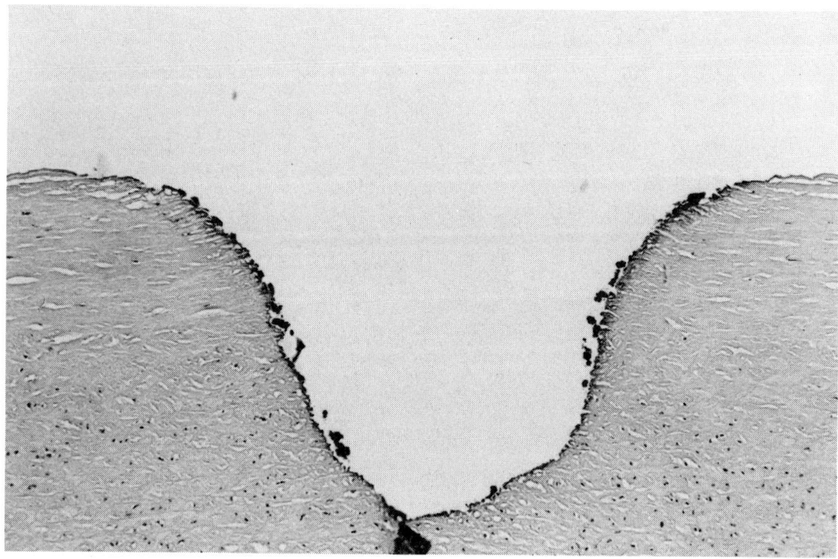

Fig. 4-6. Photomicrograph of a laser crater produced with the same fluence as used in Fig. 4-5. Here, however, spot diameter was 1000 μm and exposure time was 400 ms. Although carbonization seems more prominent, visible coagulation effects to the underlying vessel wall are considerably less. (Hematoxylin eosin stain; × 25.)

of 1000 μm. Here, exposure time was 400 msec, and the intensity was 12.7 W/mm^2. A thin rim of hyperbasophilia lines the ablation crater, and carbon particles are present. The fibrocellular structure of the remaining arterial wall is intact, and morphologic evidence of peripheral thermal injury is minimal.

The low efficiency observed when using a catheter with a 280 μm spot indicates that a substantial part of the incident fluence is not used for tissue ablation. Histopathologic examination of specimens with ablation craters produced at this spot size showed extensive coagulation damage at the periphery of the laser beam impact (Fig. 4-3). Two plausible explanations may exist for the favorable results seen when lesser radiation of the same fluence, and practically the same intensity and exposure time, is delivered in larger spot diameters. First, when laser radiation is incident in a small spot, internal scattering of light out of the beam[9,15] may cause heating and coagulation of surrounding tissue. Laser light delivered in a broader beam may be relatively less scattered. Second, heat being generated in a small volume may diffuse to the periphery earlier than heat present in a larger tissue volume[21] generated at the same rate. The thermal relaxation time γ* for a cylindrical Gaussian temperature distribution having a width equal to the spot diameter is proportional to the area of the spot under laser irradiation[21] and can be considered an estimate for the time delay after which significant heat diffusion takes place to boundary tissues. For a spot diameter of 280 μm, thermal diffusion may begin shortly after the start of the laser exposure leading to excessive coagulation damage and inefficient tissue removal. Heat, on the other hand, deposited in a volume under a larger diameter spot may be confined to this area for a relatively longer time period.

Thermal relaxation time is defined as the time required for the central temperature of a Gaussian temperature distribution with a width equal to the target's diameter to decrease by 50%.[21]

When both fluence ($\geq$ practical threshold) and spot diameter ($\geq$ 500 μm) were kept constant, short exposures of high-intensity laser light were found to result in efficient ablation and less coagulation injury in comparison with longer exposure times.[22] The rate of tissue heating and, therefore, the speed of the ablation process is determined by the intensity of the beam. High laser intensities allow a given fluence to be delivered in a short exposure. Because thermal diffusion out of a heated volume is a time-dependent phenomenon,[10,11,21] peripheral thermal injury due to heat diffusion is reduced when tissue is ablated rapidly using high laser intensities and short exposure times. The results of this study suggest that from the duration of the laser exposure relative to the thermal relaxation time of the irradiated tissue volume, a reasonable estimate can be derived from the presence and extent of secondary thermal damage adjacent to the ablated area. Peripheral thermal damage can be minimized using short exposures and the highest possible laser intensity in a spot of proper size.

IMPLICATIONS FOR LASER ANGIOSURGERY

Laser-mediated ablation of atherosclerotic obstructions may become a valuable clinical technique in the management of patients with coronary or peripheral artery disease. The transluminal application of laser light transmitted through optical fibers, however, has been associated with a high complication rate. Poor catheter design and inadequate understanding of laser light dosimetry may have been responsible for the high incidence of vascular perforation, coagulation necrosis, and aneurysm formation of normal vessel wall underlying the atherosclerotic plaque.[5-7] The optically shielded laser catheter[17] used in this study provides control of all three dosimetric parameters (spot size, power, exposure time) of argon ion laser light and allows reproducible delivery of predetermined "photon-doses" at a target site. In a dose-response investigation using atheromatous aortic wall, it was found that discrete portions of tissue may be removed with relatively little variation in the extent of ablation at a given laser dose.

One goal of the experiment was to define a range of dosimetric parameters that would yield a maximum ablation efficiency and a minimum of thermal injury to remaining tissue. Based on the results presented above, we recommend argon ion laser doses be employed, that are:

1. Emitted by catheters with a spot diameter of ≥ 500 μm
2. Of low fluence, at or just above the practial ablation threshold
3. Of high intensity to reduce exposure time

When a fluence is chosen at or just above threshold, one may expect removal of a *minimum* amount of tissue with *each* single exposure. At such dose, ablation is shallow (about 400 μm deep; see Fig. 4-1), thus reducing the risk of perforation. Another advantage of using low fluences is that (normal) tissue not in contact with the shield, some distance away from the catheter, receives a light dose below ablation threshold. Due to beam divergence (Fig. 4-2) and attenuation by blood elements, intensity and fluence decrease with distance from the shield. When low fluence doses are delivered to plaque in a relatively large spot using short exposures of high-intensity laser light, efficient tissue ablation occurs, and other thermal effects, at the periphery of the impact of the beam, are minimal.

Based on the concept of the optical shield, a laser catheter has been constructed incorporating multiple optical fibers.[23] The light spots of the individual fibers cover the entire surface of the shield allowing the catheter to be advanced into a composite crater after each fiber in the device has been "fired" once. Exposure conditions for ablation are restored once the shield is brought in contact with deeper layers of plaque, after which the firing sequence may be repeated. Between exposures, tissue is allowed to cool by means of a saline flush or by the bloodstream acting as a heat sink. Subsequent shallow "bites" in atherosclerotic plaque by a sequence of argon ion laser light exposures of proper dosimetry from a multifiber optically shielded catheter may remove obstructive lesions in atherosclerotic vascular disease with precision and control, and without excessive peripheral coagulation necrosis.

REFERENCES

1. Grüntzig, A.R., Senning, A., and Siegenthaler, W.E.: Nonoperative dilatation of coronary-artery stenosis: percutaneous transluminal coronary angioplasty, N. Engl. J. Med. **301**:61, 1979.
2. Holmes, D.R., Jr., Vlietstra, R.E., Smith, H.C., et al.: Restenosis after percutaneous transluminal coronary angioplasty (PTCA): a report from the PTCA registry of the National Heart, Lung and Blood Institute, Am. J. Cardiol. **53**:77C, 1984.
3. Lee, G., Ikeda, R.M., Kozina, J., et al.: Laser-dissolution of coronary atherosclerotic obstruction. Am. Heart J. **102**:1074, 1981.
4. Abela, G.S., Normann, S., Cohen, D., et al.: Effects of carbon dioxide, Nd-YAG, and argon laser radiation on coronary atheromatous plaques, Am. J. Cardiol. **50**:1199, 1982.
5. Abela, G.S., Normann, S.J., Cohen, D.M., et al.: Laser recanalization of occluded atherosclerotic arteries in vivo and in vitro, Circulation **71**:403, 1985.
6. Choy, D.S.J., Stertzer, S.H., Myler, R.K., et al.: Human coronary laser recanalization, Clin. Cardiol. **7**:377, 1984.
7. Lee, G., Ikeda, R.M., Chan, M.C., et al.: Limitations, risks and complications of laser recanalization: a cautious approach warranted, Am. J. Cardiol. **56**:181, 1985.
8. Sliney, D.H.: Laser-tissue interactions, Clin. Chest Med. **6**:203, 1985.
9. Halldórsson, T., and Langerholc, J.: Thermodynamic analysis of laser irradiation of biological tissue, Appl. Opt. **17**:3948, 1978.
10. Cummins, L., and Nauenberg, M.: Thermal effects of laser radiation in biological tissue, Biophys. J. **42**:99, 1983.
11. Wolbarsht, M.L.: Laser surgery: CO_2 or HF, IEEE J. Quantum Elect. **QE-20**:1427, 1984.
12. Puliafito, C.A., Steinert, R.F., Deutsch, T.F., et al.: Excimer laser ablation of the cornea and lens: experimental studies, Ophthalmology **92**:741, 1985.
13. Van Gemert, M.J.C., Verdaasdonk, R., Stassen, E.G., et al.: Optical properties of human blood vessel wall and plaque, Lasers Surg. Med. **5**:235, 1985.
14. Cothren, R.M., Kittrell, C., Willet, R.L., et al.: Controlled ablation of atherosclerotic plaque: experimental and theoretical dosimetry, J. Am. Coll. Cardiol. **7**:208A, 1986.
15. Welch, A.J., Valvano, J.W., Pearce, J.A., et al.: Effect of laser radiation on tissue during laser angioplasty, Lasers Surg. Med. **5**:251, 1985.
16. Strikwerda, S., Bott-Silverman, C., Ratliff, N.B., et al.: Dosimetry studies for argon ion laser light ablation of atheromatous plaque, Lasers Surg. Med. **6**:270, 1986.
17. Cothren, R.M., Kittrell, C., Hayes, G.B., et al.: Controlled light delivery for laser angiosurgery, IEEE J. Quantum Elect. **QE-22**:4, 1986.
18. Shelton, M.E., Hoxworth, B., Shelton, J.A., et al.: A new model to study quantitative effects of laser angioplasty on human atherosclerotic plaque, J. Am. Coll. Cardiol. **7**:909, 1986.
19. Strikwerda, S., Kittrell, C., Cothren, R.M., et al.: The evolving role of laser radiation in the treatment of atherosclerotic vascular disease, J. Med. Imaging, 1987. (In press.)
20. Strikwerda, S., Cothren, R.M., Partovi, F., et al.: Ablation thresholds of atheromatous tissue for argon ion laser light exposures. (To be published.)
21. Anderson, R.R., and Parrish, J.A.: Selective photothermolysis: precise microsurgery by se-

lective absorption of pulsed radiation, Science **220**:524, 1983.

22. Strikwerda, S., Bott-Silverman, C., Ratliff, N.B., et al.: The effects of varying argon ion laser intensity and exposure time on the ablation of atherosclerotic plaque, Lasers Surg. Med., 1987. (In press.)
23. Cothren, R.M., Hayes, G.B., Kramer, J.R., et al.: A multifiber catheter with an optical shield for laser angiosurgery, Lasers Life Sci. **1**:1, 1986.

Chapter 5

Thermal Ablation of Tissue by Laser Radiation

Firooz Partovi, PhD
Joseph A. Izatt, PhD
Carter W. Kittrell, PhD
Michael S. Feld, PhD
Sipke Strikwerda, MD
John R. Kramer, MD

The theoretical treatment of tissue ablation by laser radiation has been the subject of several investigations.[1-4] The importance of tissue ablation lies in its application to the surgical removal of unwanted tissue, particularly in percutaneous procedures such as the ablation of atheromas in arteries. It is crucial, in such applications, to have a way of determining the optimum laser wavelength and dosage parameters (power, spot diameter, exposure time) for removing a desired quantity of tissue. A prime factor in this optimization is the amount of energy transferred to the surrounding tissue, for this determines the extent of heating of that tissue and affects its subsequent healing and long-term recovery. When the treatment site is out of sight and the margin for error is small, the predictive power of a quantitative theory is of great value. A theoretical description of the process is useful not only as a framework for determining the optimal dosage and wavelength, but also as a guide for a better understanding of the process.

The purpose in developing a theory of ablation is to obtain quantitative relations governing the variables of interest in the ablation process. Armed with that knowledge, the surgeon can choose the proper photon dosage and be confident that, within statistical limits, the desired quantity of tissue will be removed and a predictable amount of energy will be deposited in the surrounding tissue.

However, it is in the nature of living matter to have variability, so that the tissue response in each individual case cannot be precisely predicted, whether by a theoretical approach or otherwise. There will be a statistical distribution of responses, as in any treatment. A knowledge of the average response and of the range of variation is extremely valuable to the clinician. A practical theory is expected to predict the average effect, and as such it does not need to be very sophisticated, although a sophisticated theory will generally lead to a better understanding of the basic phenomena. Experiments are needed to determine the range of variation, and the operating room procedures and devices should be designed so as to tolerate the variation. Careful monitoring and control by an experienced physician will be a permanent part of those procedures.

Naturally, a theory must be checked against experiment before it can be trusted, but one advantage of a sound theoretical formula is that it can also act as a guide to point out new domains of parameters that are likely to be useful and that need to be investigated. It is, therefore, fair to say that a satisfactory theory of ablation is a useful complement to empirical studies of the process.

The present work deals with a single laser beam applied during a single exposure. This is the necessary starting point for understanding more complex situations, in which the light is delivered by several beams[5] or in repeated exposures.[6,7] Additional variables, such as firing order, pulse duration, and repetition rate, would become part of the dosage specification in those situations. This chapter describes the ablation model and outlines the theory, and discusses the results and compares them to the experiments reported by Strikwerda.[8] (References made hereafter to experimental data are aimed at these experiments.)

THEORETICAL MODEL OF ABLATION

A detailed theory of thermal ablation with collimated laser light was published recently.[4] The heat diffusion equation and energy balance considerations were used in conjunction with a simple model of light distribution in tissue to derive the desired relationships. We will attempt in this analysis to present the most relevant features of those calculations plus a number of new features which have been added to make the theory applicable to the experiments cited above.

We begin with the simplest case. Suppose a uniform beam of laser light is incident at right angles onto the tissue, idealized to have a plane surface, homogeneous composition, and infinite depth (Fig. 5-1A). The beam is cylindrical with a well-defined *diameter*, d. It is composed of an enormous number of particles of light, or photons, all traveling on straight parallel paths until they enter the tissue. The optical properties of the tissue determine what happens next. As a photon passes through a little bit of tissue, three things can happen. The first is transmission: it passes through undisturbed. The second is scattering: the direction of travel is altered, but no energy is deposited. The third is absorption: the photon is absorbed by a chromophore (Greek for "colorbearing") within the tissue, and the optical energy is transferred to the tissue as thermal (or some other form of) energy. Photons may be scattered many times before being absorbed or leaving the tissue. Because of scattering, the beam of light will not be confined to the beam cylinder within the tissue but will spread to a broader region in a diffuse fashion. Absorption, on the other hand, will cause the light to be gradually extinguished as it moves farther from the point of incidence.

Ablation results depend on the dosage of light received by the tissue. Loosely speaking, "photon dosage" should mean the total light *energy*, E, delivered to the tissue. In general, however, the outcome of ablation will also depend on how fast a given quantity of energy is supplied and on how concentrated it is. Laser *power*, P, measures the energy delivered per unit time and therefore indicates how fast the energy is supplied. Laser *fluence*, ϕ, measures the energy incident on unit area of tissue and indicates how concentrated it is.

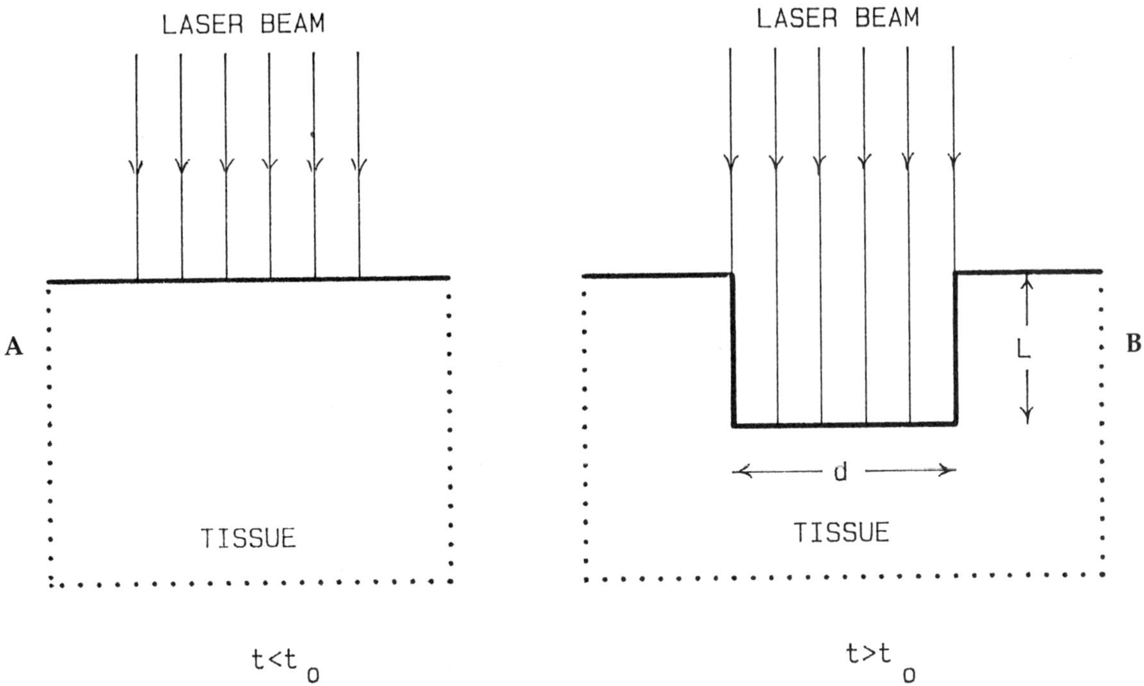

Fig. 5-1. Ablation with collimated laser beam. **A,** Before onset of ablation. **B,** After onset of ablation.

Beam *intensity*, I, measures both the rate and the concentration of the energy flow and is defined as energy incident on unit area per unit time. Relations among the various dosage parameters have been summarized in equation 2, in which A denotes the cross-sectional area $\pi d^2/4$ of the beam and t stands for the exposure time (during which the energy, E, is delivered). We shall use joule as the unit of energy, millimeter as the unit of length, and second as the unit of time. This gives watt (= joule per second) as the unit of power, joule per square millimeter as the unit of fluence, and watt per square millimeter as the unit of intensity.

Laser energy will heat each point of the tissue only to the extent that the light is absorbed there. A perfectly transparent or translucent medium is not heated by the passage of light. When the tissue beneath the laser beam acquires enough energy, it will undergo ablation, that is, disintegration and ejection of gas, liquid, and solid debris. Ablation creates a crater, which advances into the tissue along the beam cylinder at a constant rate until the beam is turned off. The diameter of the crater has been observed to be roughly equal to the beam diameter, d. Therefore d will denote the diameter of both the beam and the crater. The depth of the crater will be denoted by L (Fig. 5-1B). For ablation to actually occur, however, the light parameters must exceed certain thresholds, as explained in the following paragraphs.

The temperature rise in the illuminated parts of the tissue will set up heat conduction (heat diffusion) to the cooler parts, removing heat from the illuminated region. Some heat will also escape from the surface of the tissue through conduction or convection. When the beam intensity, I, is low, these heat losses will prevent the illuminated regions of the tissue from reaching high enough temperatures to be ablated. Therefore, for ablation to occur, the intensity must exceed a limiting value, I_0, called the *intensity threshold.*

With the intensity greater than threshold, it still takes some time, t_0, for the first layers of tissue to accumulate enough heat in order for ablation to begin. Accordingly, t_0 will be called the *time threshold.* If the beam intensity is only moderately higher than threshold, t_0 will be very long, allowing heat to reach deep into the peripheral tissue by means of conduction, and to cause significant damage. Therefore, intensities many times greater than threshold should be used for ablation of tissue. In fact, experiments have shown that even for intensities several times greater than threshold, ablation can still be quite erratic and unpredictable, unless the intensity exceeds what has been termed the "practical intensity threshold."[8]

We will assume in what follows that the beam intensity is much greater than threshold intensity. This is also a requirement to be met in practice, as argued above. At such high intensities, ablation will take place much faster than heat diffusion, so that the latter will no longer play a significant role. This eliminates the need for solving the heat diffusion equation, simplifying the analysis considerably. In this regime, intensity and exposure time enter the calculations as a product. In other words, if a given quantity of tissue is removed using a (high) intensity, I and the exposure time, t, the same quantity will be removed by using twice the intensity and half the time, so that the same value of the product (It) will yield the same result. (This is not true if ablation is carried out at an intensity near the threshold, I_0. In that case, a small decrease in intensity may increase the time substantially.) The product of intensity and exposure time is just the fluence, ϕ, defined earlier. Fluence measures the total energy falling on unit area of the tissue over the duration of ablation. The fluence delivered to the tissue during the time threshold, t_0, will accordingly be called the *fluence threshold*, ϕ_0. Ablation will begin only after the incident fluence ϕ has exceeded ϕ_0.

Using high intensities will suppress only the *conduction* of heat to the peripheral tissue. Energy can still escape the beam cylinder by means of light *scattering*. Speeding up the ablation process by an increase in intensity cannot reduce the amount of energy scattered to the periphery, because scattered energy escapes the beam cylinder at the speed of light. Tissue scatters light strongly, tending to spread it over a broad region and to reduce its effectiveness in ablation. However, the spread of light can be checked by absorption. The extent of light absorption changes dramatically with wavelength, and it is possible to control the spread of light by a suitable choice of the wavelength. Yellow and red light, for example, are not suitable for ablation, because they are only weakly absorbed by tissue. The blue-green light of argon ion laser is absorbed much more strongly, and with a penetration depth of a fraction of a millimeter, it affects only a moderate thickness of tissue beyond the beam cylinder. Other wavelengths in the mid-infrared or in the ultraviolet region have such short penetration depths that they leave virtually no heat in the tissue beyond a thin boundary layer. Clinical studies are needed to determine whether deposition of a certain amount of heat is beneficial or detrimental to the healing process.

Having looked at some of the concepts involved in ablation, we are now ready for the quantitative formulation. The object is to relate the depth, L, of the ablated crater to the total incident fluence, ϕ, and the beam diameter, d, with the intensity assumed to be much greater than the threshold intensity. We begin by the assumption that it takes a definite amount of energy to ablate a unit volume of tissue. This energy will be called the *heat of ablation*, h_{abl} and measured in joules per cubic millimeter. The volume of the crater (that is, of the removed tissue) therefore is equal to the available energy divided by h_{abl}.

Denoting the area of the crater by A and its depth by L, we may write,

$$\text{(volume of removed tissue)} = AL = \text{(available energy)} / h_{abl} \quad (1)$$

To calculate the available energy, we begin with the total incident energy and determine what fraction of it stays within the beam cylinder and is available for ablation. The total energy incident on the tissue during the ablation process is,

$$\text{(total energy, E)} = Pt = ItA = \phi A \quad (2)$$

The total energy must be corrected for various losses to arrive at the available energy.

First, a fraction, R, of the incident light is reflected at the surface of the tissue. (There are two kinds of reflection: specular reflection at the surface due to a mismatch in refractive index, and diffuse reflection due to backscattering within the tissue.) The net energy penetrating the tissue is therefore $(1 - R)$ times the total incident energy, or $(1 - R)\,\phi A$.

The next loss to consider is due to conduction and convection of energy outward from the surface of the tissue. Because we are assuming rapid ablation at high intensity, we may neglect this loss. (Reradiation of energy from the surface is also too small to be considered.) Similarly, heat conduction within the tissue away from the beam cylinder can be neglected, as can heat carried away by perfusion. As already pointed out, there simply is not enough time for slow processes such as conduction, convection, or perfusion to amount to anything when operating at high laser intensities.

Scattering of light within the tissue is an important cause of heat loss from the beam cylinder. We use the symbol f to denote the fraction of light energy that is *not* scattered out of the beam. Therefore the available energy is further reduced to $(1 - R)f\phi A$.

Finally, we must correct for the energy left in the tissue beneath the ablated surface after the beam is turned off. This tissue has been "preheated" by absorption of laser light passing through the ablating surface. The energy left there is the same as the energy delivered to the beam cylinder during the initial preheating period, t_0, before the onset of ablation. Thus we must subtract $(1 - R)f\phi_0 A$ from the above value to obtain an estimate of the energy available for ablation:

$$\begin{aligned}\text{(available energy)} &= (1 - R)f\phi A - (1 - R)f\phi_0 A \\ &= (1 - R)f(\phi - \phi_0)A \quad (3)\end{aligned}$$

Substituting this equation in equation 1, we obtain the desired relation:

$$\text{(volume of removed tissue)} = LA = (1 - R)f(\phi - \phi_0)A/h_{abl} \quad (4)$$

or

$$L = (1 - R)f(\phi - \phi_0)/h_{abl} \quad (5)$$

This equation relates the crater depth, L, to the laser fluence, ϕ, delivered to the tissue. It explicitly exhibits the fact that no ablation will take place unless the fluence, ϕ, exceeds the threshold fluence, ϕ_0. Of course, it has been assumed implicitly that the intensity, I, is much greater than threshold intensity, I_0. The beam diameter, d, enters the equation through the definition of ϕ, equation 2, and —as we shall see—through the factor f.

It is convenient to define two new quantities that characterize the ablation process. The *ablation yield*, Y, is defined as the volume of tissue removed per unit incident energy, and the *ablation efficiency*, η, is defined as the ratio, energy available for ablation divided by net energy penetrating the tissue. To calculate Y, we simply divide equation 4 by equation 2:

$$Y = [(1 - R)f(\phi - \phi_0)A/h_{abl}]/\phi A$$

or

$$Y = (1 - R)f(1 - \phi_0/\phi)/h_{abl} \quad (mm^3/J) \quad (6)$$

To calculate η, we first multiply equation 2 by $(1 - R)$ to get the net energy penetrating the tissue, and then divide the result into equation 3, the available energy:

$$\eta = [(1 - R)f(\phi - \phi_0)A] / [(1 - R)\phi A]$$

or

$$\eta = f(1 - \phi_0/\phi) \qquad (7)$$

Notice that in the definition of efficiency, the available energy is compared to the energy *penetrating* the tissue, not the energy incident on it. That is why the reflectance, R, has no effect on efficiency as defined here. The advantage of defining efficiency in this way is that it will indicate the heat loss to the remaining tissue only and not to the medium outside the tissue. After all, we are not worried about wasting energy so much as we are concerned about losing it to the tissue we intend to save.

The parameters R, h_{abl}, f, and ϕ_0 need to be determined before the results of equations 5, 6, and 7 can be used. Each of these in turn depends on one or more parameters characterizing the tissue and the laser beam. Values of most of these parameters are subject to sizable uncertainties arising from biological variations, variations with temperature, and lack of reliable measurements. Reported measurements are generally carried out at room temperature, whereas some tissue properties, such as absorption coefficient and reflectance, are expected to be quite different when the tissue is undergoing ablation. For these reasons, we have allowed some flexibility in assigning values to the parameters of interest so as to optimize the agreement between theory and experiment. The (in vitro) ablation experiments used for comparison in the next section employ the blue-green light of argon ion laser on segments of human atheromatous aorta,[8] and the values quoted below are appropriate for that case.

The *reflectance,* R, at the tissue surface can, in principle, be calculated if the optical properties of the tissue are known.[3,9] However, it is in any case advisable to measure this parameter in the laboratory, perferably under the conditions of ablation. We will use a value of 0.20, somewhat lower than but consistent with preliminary measurements on mild atherosclerotic plaque carried out at room temperature.[10] (See also van Gemert et al.[3,9], whose measurements yield a value of $R \simeq 0.28$.)

The heat of ablation, h_{abl}, will depend on tissue composition and ablation mechanism. Different laser wavelengths and power levels will favor different ablation mechanisms. Continuous wave (CW) lasers in the visible or infrared range are expected to induce predominantly thermal evaporation of water in soft tissues. In this mode, vaporized tissue water escapes in an explosive manner, carrying with it microscopic fragments of other material that make up the tissue. We shall use this as our model for estimating the heat of ablation. The value h_{abl} will first be calculated for pure water and then multiplied by the volume percentage of water in tissue. The heat used by other tissue components will be neglected.

Heat of ablation for water consists of two parts: the heat, h_0, necessary to raise the temperature of water from its ambient value in the tissue to the boiling point, and the *latent heat of vaporization,* h_v, to turn water into steam:

$$h_{abl} = h_0 + h_v \quad \text{(water)} \qquad (8)$$

The values h_0, h_v, and h_{abl} are measured in joules per cubic millimeter. Denoting the needed temperature rise by T_0 (degrees Celsius), we have

$$h_0 = \rho c T_0 \qquad (9)$$

where ρ is the *density* (grams per cubic millimeter), and c is the *specific heat* (joules per gram per degree Celsius) of water. It is suspected that the tissue water is superheated before it is vaporized. If this occurs, T_0 will be higher, increasing h_0, but a corresponding decrease in h_v will compensate for it, leaving

h_{abl} practically unchanged. For in vitro experiments, the ambient tissue temperature is about 20°C, resulting in a T_0 of 100 − 20 = 80°C. This, combined with a density of $\rho = 10^{-3}$ g/mm^3 and specific heat of c = 4.18 J/g°C, will yield a value of about 0.33 J/mm^3 for h_0. The latent heat, h_v, for water is about 2.25 J/mm^3, so that h_{abl} for pure water is about 2.58 J/mm^3. Assuming water makes up 70% of the tissue volume and neglecting the contribution of the other 30%, we find $h_{abl} \simeq 1.8$ J/mm^3 for soft tissue. For high-peak-power pulsed lasers and for hard tissue, which is more effectively removed with such lasers, other processes in addition to the thermal evaporation of water are likely to play dominant roles, so that the above estimate of h_{abl} will not necessarily hold for those cases.

To calculate the fraction, f, of the laser energy that is not scattered out of the beam, one must first determine the scattering and absorption properties of the tissue and then solve the radiative transfer equation[11] to find the light distribution within the tissue. The transfer equation is a formidable integro-differential equation for a function of five variables. Various approximations to the solution, such as the Kubelka-Munk and the diffusion approximations[11] and the 7-flux model[12] have been proposed. Rather than attempting to solve this equation, we have assumed a crude, but physically plausible picture of light energy distribution within tissue. A similar approximation was used in a previous publication.[4] The assumption is that the light energy density decreases exponentially within the tissue both in the forward direction along the beam and laterally away from the beam. The characteristic length for the exponential decay is the distance over which the energy density decreases by a factor (1/e), where e ≃ 2.7. In the forward direction, this will be called the penetration depth, D. In the earlier work, D was also used for the decay length in the lateral direction exterior to the beam. This resulted in f = d/(d + 4D). With only one parameter, D, to characterize the light distribution in the tissue, this model cannot account for the known anisotropy of light scattering in the tissue, which is predominantly forward directed. To account for that, we may assume the lateral decay length to be some fraction of D, say μD. A value of (1/2)D will be used for the present calculations, yielding

$$f = d/(d + 2D) \tag{10}$$

As expected, for beam diameters large compared to the penetration depth, f approaches unity; for d small compared to D, it approaches zero. D has been measured for the blue-green argon ion laser light in atherosclerotic plaque by Cothren et al.,[13] who quote a value of 0.38 mm. Taking D to be the reciprocal of the attenuation coefficient μ measured by van Gemert et al.,[3,9] we arrive at 0.315 mm. A value of D ≃ 0.3 mm will be used in this work.

Fluence threshold, as defined earlier, is the laser fluence (that is, energy per unit area) that must fall on the tissue before ablation begins. Clearly, ablation can begin only when the top layer of tissue has absorbed an energy equal to h_{abl} per unit volume. Now, for the assumed model of light distribution in tissue, the absorption coefficient is f/D[4], and since only a fraction (1 − R) of the incident fluence penetrates the top layer of the tissue, we must have

$$h_{abl} = (1 - R)(f/D)\phi_0$$

or

$$\phi_0 = Dh_{abl} / [(1 - R)f] \tag{11}$$

Substitution of ϕ_0 from this equation into the results of equations 5, 6, and 7, followed by some manipulation, changes them to the following forms:

$$L = (1 - R)f\phi / h_{abl} - D \tag{12}$$
$$Y = (1 - R)fL / [(L + D)h_{abl}] \tag{13}$$
$$\eta = fL / (L + D) \tag{14}$$

These results have been derived for a collimated laser beam. In applications inside the arteries, the laser light would be delivered by an optical fiber housed in a catheter, and the output light would not be collimated. Instead, a diverging cone of light with the half angle Θ would emerge from the tip of the fiber (Fig. 5-2). The sine of this angle is referred to as the numerical aperture of the fiber and was found to be about 0.21 in experiments performed with argon ion laser light.[8]

As the beam diverges, its diameter increases, and its intensity decreases in inverse proportion to the square of the diameter, so that the laser beam no longer has a unique diameter, or intensity. These and other quantities that vary along the diverging beam must be defined at some fixed distance from the tip of the fiber to make them unambiguous. We will therefore agree to define and measure these quantities at the surface of the tissue, assuming, of course, that the fiber tip stays fixed during the ablation. Accordingly, we will henceforth use the term "spot diameter" (rather than beam diameter) for d, alluding to the spot of light formed on the tissue surface before the onset of ablation. The new definitions, which apply to d, I, I_0, ϕ, ϕ_0, and any function of these quantities, are identical to the old definitions when $\Theta = 0$. In spite of the beam divergence, the experimental craters were observed to be roughly cylindrical with a diameter approximately equal to the spot diameter, d (Fig. 5-2). This allows us to continue to use the symbol d to denote both the spot diameter and the crater diameter.

Beam divergence complicates the calculation of crater depth, but the dominant effect is the loss of energy to the sides of the crater (see Fig. 5-2). To take this factor into account, we need to go back and correct the available energy, equation 3. Unlike the other factors that reduce the available energy, this one depends on the depth of the crater. When the crater depth is zero, all the light falls on the spot to be ablated, but as the crater grows deeper, less light is available at its bottom for ablation, the crater advances more slowly, and the ablation yield and efficiency go down. At an instant when the crater depth is L, the ratio of the laser power incident on the crater floor to the total laser power incident on the tissue can be calculated from the geometry of Fig. 5-2. The result is approximately $1/(1 + \epsilon)^2$, where,

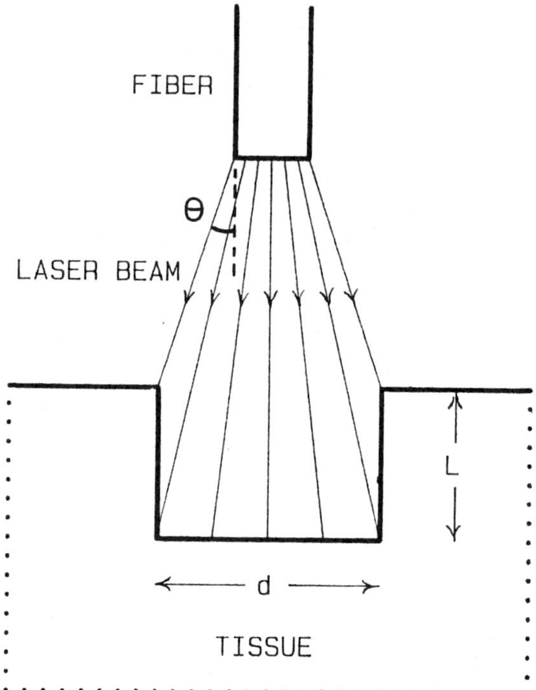

Fig. 5-2. Ablation with a diverging laser beam. Some of the light falls on the crater wall, resulting in lower intensity at the bottom.

$$\epsilon = (2L/d)\tan(\Theta) \qquad (15)$$

The factor $1/(1 + \epsilon)^2$ is equal to unity when ablation begins ($L = 0$) and reaches its smallest value when ablation ends. Therefore, the overall factor affecting the available energy is an average of $1/(1 + \epsilon)^2$, taken over the duration of ablation. That average turns out to be 1/b, where,

$$b = 1 + \epsilon + (1/3)\epsilon^2 \qquad (16)$$

Therefore, the energy available for ablation is given by

$$(\text{available energy}) = (1 - R)f(\phi - \phi_0)A/b$$

which replaces equation 3. The rest of the calculation proceeds as before, and we simply state the results: The right hand sides of equations 4, 5, 6, and 7 are divided by b, as was done for equation 3. Equations 12, 13, and 14 are replaced by

$$bL + D = (1 - R)f\phi/h_{abl} \quad (17)$$
$$Y = (1 - R)fL / [(bL + D)h_{abl}] \quad (18)$$
$$\eta = fL / (bL + D) \quad (19)$$

The rest of the equations and definitions are unchanged. Notice that if the beam is collimated, Θ is zero, making b equal to one, and the new equations become identical with the old, as they should.

An important effect of beam divergence is to decrease the efficiency η of ablation as evidenced by the additional factor b in the denominator of equation 19. Therefore, even a short-wavelength excimer laser, with its strong absorption in tissue, would cause some peripheral heating if administered through a fiber.

DISCUSSION OF THE RESULTS

Equations 17, 18, and 19 are the desired theoretical results. Equations 10, 15, and 16 serve to define the parameters f and b appearing in the results. The easiest way to use the results is to choose values for the dimensions of the crater (diameter d and depth L) and to use equation 17 to calculate the fluence ϕ needed to realize those dimensions. Equations 18 and 19 will then give the ablation yield Y and efficiency η for the desired crater size. The crater diameter is taken to be the same as the spot diameter.

Once the fluence ϕ is determined, it must be translated into incident power and exposure time with the help of equation 2. This can be done in three steps: (1) choose an intensity value much higher than the threshold intensity for the given spot size; (2) divide the intensity into ϕ to get the exposure time; (3) multiply intensity by the spot area $\eta d^2/4$ to get the incident power. The threshold intensity is given by the following expression[4] (note, however, that the equation in the reference may seem different, because it is expressed in terms of thermal diffusivity, κ, rather than the thermal conductivity, K. Also, the factor $(1 - R)$ is absent there, because intensity and fluence values are assumed to have been corrected for reflection):

$$I_0 \simeq 2KT_0/[fd(1 - R)] \quad (20)$$

Here K, the thermal conductivity of the tissue, is estimated to be 4.2×10^{-4} W/mm°C,[14] resulting in threshold values that range from 0.94 W/mm^2 for a spot diameter of d = 0.28 mm to 0.14 W/mm^2 for d = 1 mm.

Of course, equations 17, 18, and 19 are valid only when the right hand side of equation 17 is positive. This means the fluence, ϕ, must be larger than threshold fluence, ϕ_0, given by equation 11. Notice that when the divergence angle is zero (parallel beam), then b = 1 and ϕ is a linear function of L, whereas in general, it is a cubic function (see Fig. 5-3). Accordingly, the ablation yield, Y, and efficiency, η, continue to increase with increasing L when the beam is parallel, but for a diverging beam, they decrease after reaching a maximum (see Fig. 5-4). Another source of inefficiency that would cause a similar trend in Y is the attenuation of the intensity caused by the masking effect of the escaping steam and debris, but this is neglected in our analysis.

The constants going into the theoretical formulas are not accurately known, particularly under conditions of ablation and, in any case, are subject to a considerable degree of biological variability. This prompted us to adjust some of the constants so as to obtain the best

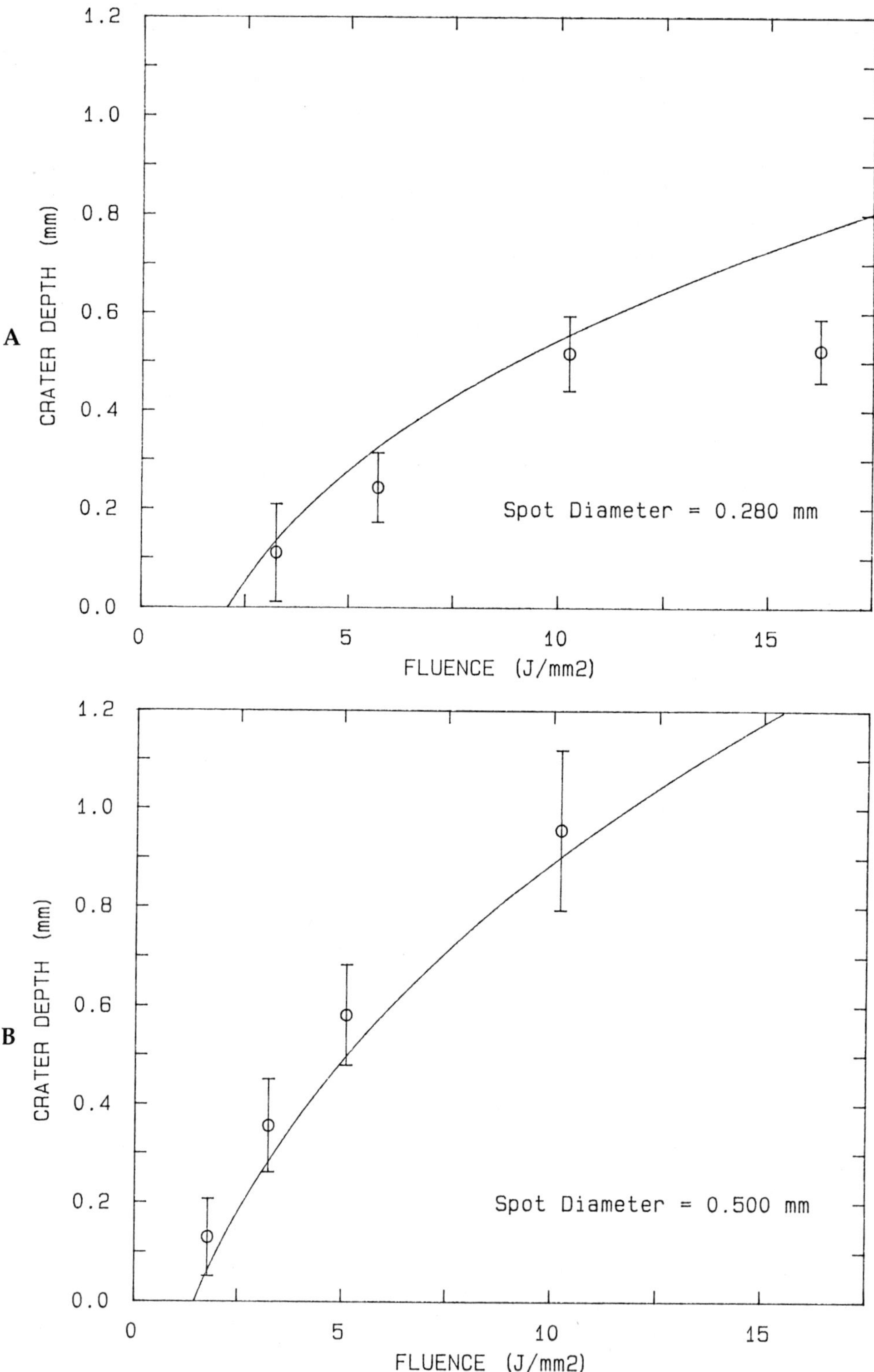

Fig. 5-3. Crater depth as a function of fluence. **A,** Spot diameter d = 0.280 mm; **B,** d = 0.500 mm; **C,** d = 0.750 mm; **D,** d = 1.000 mm.

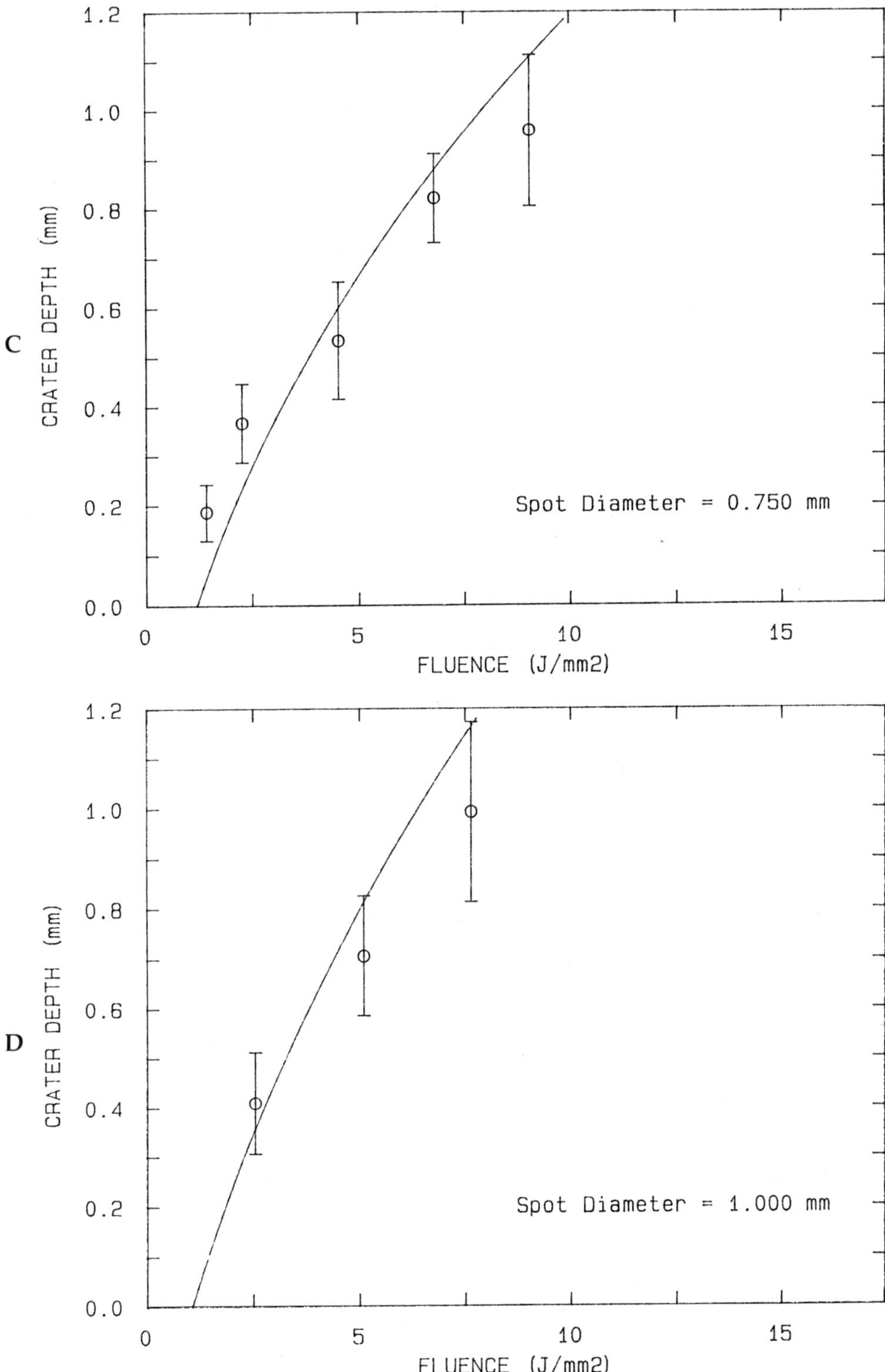

Fig. 5-3, cont'd. For legend see opposite page.

fit to the experimental data. The encouraging result was that the adjusted constants remained close to their measured values. The complete set of constants used in numerical calculations are as follows:

$$R = 0.2$$
$$D = 0.3 \text{ mm}$$
$$h_{abl} = 1.8 \text{ J/mm}^3$$
$$\sin(\Theta) = .21$$

Figure 5-3 shows crater depth, L, plotted versus fluence, ϕ, for four different spot diameters. The curves represent the theoretical result of equation 17, while the experimental points represent some 1000 ablation runs, reported by Strikwerda.[8] Each experimental point on the graph represents the average of a large number of in vitro ablation runs with the blue-green light of the argon ion laser on segments of human atheromatous aorta. Many runs were made at each combination of intensity, I, and exposure time, t, and there were several combinations of I and t for each fluence level, ϕ = It. Often, data from different samples are averaged to obtain the same data point. The error bars represent standard deviations.

Those runs that failed to produce a crater or that perforated the artery wall have not been used because a one-to-one correlation does not exist between ϕ and L for these cases. In other words, *any* fluence less than ϕ_0 will fail to produce a crater, and *any* fluence greater than a certain level will result in perforation. Experimentally, the runs that failed to create craters did not always fall below the fluence threshold, even after allowing for the usual statistical uncertainty. This makes ablation near fluence threshold somewhat unpredictable and calls for setting higher "practical" threshold levels.[8]

The ϕ-intercepts in Fig. 5-3 are the theoretical fluence thresholds given by equation 11. Values range between 1 and 2 J/mm^2 for the four spot diameters, decreasing with increasing spot size.

Figure 5-4 shows the calculated efficiency, η, as a function of crater depth, L, for four spot diameters. The same curves can be read as plots of ablation yield, Y, versus crater depth, provided the vertical scale on the right is used. The graphs show that the efficiency is very small for very small crater depths. This is because an amount of energy, $A\phi_0$, must be given to the tissue before ablation can begin. At the other extreme, when the crater is very deep, a large fraction of the light falls on the crater wall as a result of the beam divergence, and the efficiency goes down again. Somewhere between the two extremes is the "optimum" crater depth, which corresponds to maximum efficiency. Hence, to maintain efficiency, deep holes should be made in several steps, with the catheter moved closer at each step. Notice also that the efficiency is greater for larger spot sizes, as is the optimum crater depth.

Efficiency is an important indicator because it provides information on the amount of heat retained by the tissue. For example, an efficiency of 0.3 means 70% of the energy is left in the tissue and 30% is ejected with the ablated material. (This is not true for the inefficiency caused by beam attenuation from debris mentioned above. In that case the lost energy heats the blocking debris, not the tissue.)

Figure 5-5 shows the relative discrepancy between experiment and theory. Each circle on this graph represents one ablation run. Missing are some 250 trials that failed to produce a crater and about 25 that perforated the tissue. Points that fall on the same vertical line correspond to runs repeated under the same power, spot diameter, and exposure time on one or more samples. Runs differing in some of these parameters are set off horizontally from each other. The horizontal ordering is as follows: All runs with a lower spot diameter, d, are to the left of those with a higher d, so that the horizontal axis is divided (unequally) into four regions corresponding to d = 0.28, 0.50, 0.75, and 1.0 mm. Within each spot size, lower intensity runs

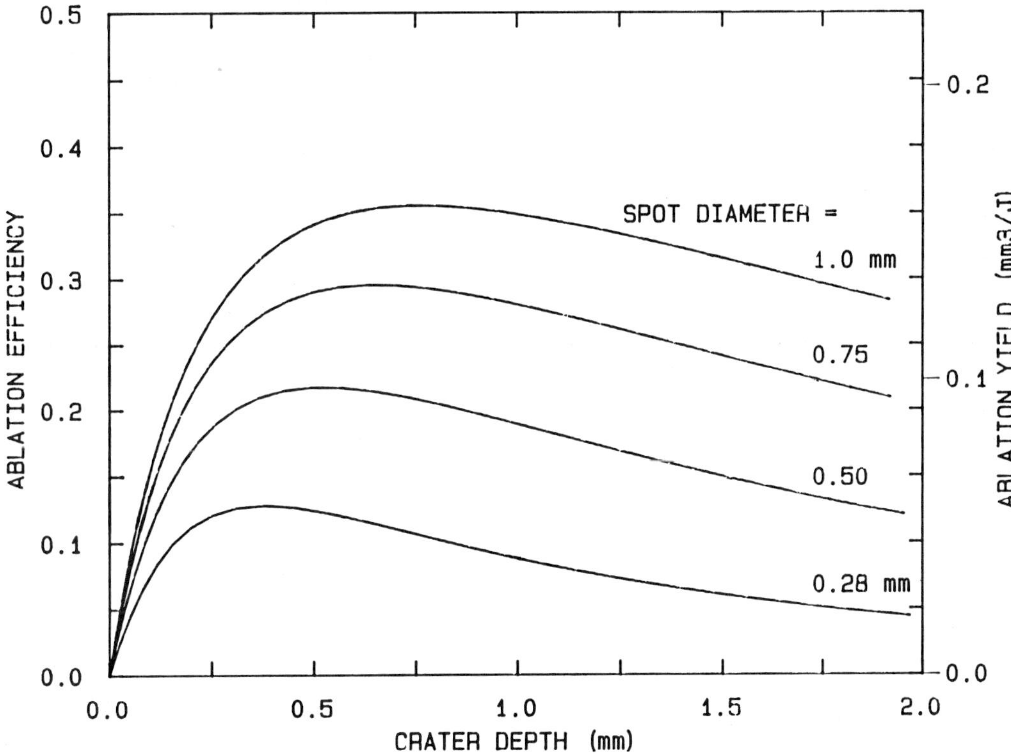

Fig. 5-4. Ablation efficiency and yield as a function of crater depth for four spot diameters. The left vertical scale is used for efficiency, and the right scale is used for yield.

take precedence, and within each spot size and intensity, lower exposure times come first. We chose to plot every run rather than statistical averages to exhibit the extent of variation from run to run and also to highlight the size of the whole project.

The discrepancy between experiment and theory is calculated as follows:

$$\text{(relative discrepancy)} = \frac{\text{theoret. fluence} - \text{exp. fluence}}{(\text{theoret. fluence} + \text{exp. fluence})/2}$$

The theoretical fluence is calculated by substituting the experimental values of L and d into equation 17 and solving for ϕ. Experimental fluence is just the product of incident power and exposure time divided by the area of spot, all taken from experiment. The numbers on the vertical axis of Fig. 5-5, however, do not represent the above quantity exactly, except near 0. Instead, "40%" means that experimental fluence is 40% lower than the theoretical fluence, and "−40% means that the theoretical fluence is 40% lower than experiment. If there were complete agreement between theory and experiment, all the points would line up on the horizontal line, labeled "0". The constants R and D have been adjusted to give a least-square fit to this line. The graph shows that most of the experiments agree with theory to within 40%. It also shows that the experiments performed with the same dosage parameters (points lying on the same vertical line) vary among themselves to a comparable degree. Hence, one can say that

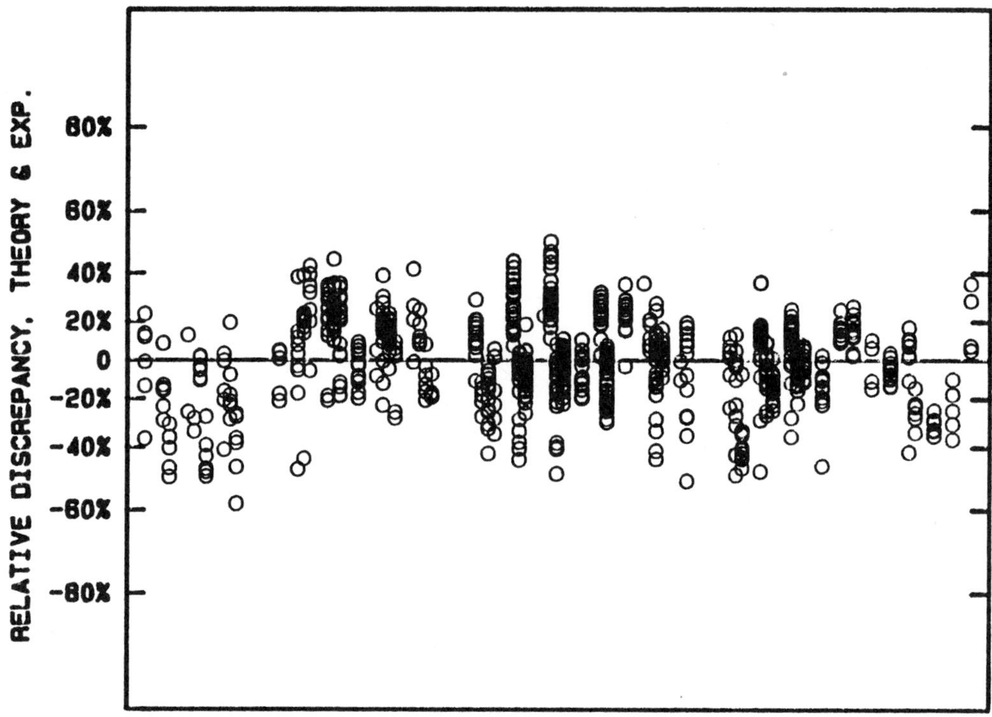

Fig. 5-5. Relative discrepancy between theory and experiment. The horizontal axis indicates a particular ordering of the data; see text for details.

the agreement between theory and experiment is good. Figure 5-5 illustrates the statistical spread and the limits of predictability expected of most biological systems—a situation familiar to clinicians and one they have learned to cope with.

CONCLUSIONS

The simple theory presented here shows that ablation can be quantified. Furthermore, it agrees with experiment within the uncertainties inherent in the latter. In addition, it lays the groundwork for systematic studies of ablation and is a step toward establishing dosimetry for the process. Finally, it can be considered a starting point for studying multifiber and/or pulsed ablation and ablation of other tissue types, particularly hard calcified plaque.

Predictions of the theory correspond to the average response and are not intended to provide a precise photon dosage for each individual case. Therefore, the methods and devices used in the operating room must be so disigned as to allow for statistical variation, perhaps with a system of continuous monitoring. Nonetheless, if the range of variation is known, a theory that predicts the average response is a powerful tool; it is much better than "shooting in the dark."

The theory has been developed with the assumption that the laser intensity must be much higher than threshold, if undue heating of peripheral tissue is to be avoided. (See Partovi et al. for the case of arbitrary intensity.[4]) Other factors that affect ablation efficiency are: (1) a beam divergence reduces efficiency; (2) larger spot sizes are more efficient; (3) crater depth is optimum when it is roughly equal to the spot diameter (see Fig. 5-4); and (4) laser wavelengths that are absorbed more strongly result in higher efficiency.

To further our understanding of ablation we need a better model of light distribution in tissue, theoretical and experimental studies of temperature distribution in the peripheral tissue and measurement of the optical and thermal properties of tissue, particularly under conditions of ablation.

ACKNOWLEDGMENTS

Useful discussions with other members of the Lester Wolfe Laser Angiosurgery group at the Cleveland Clinic Foundation, American Hospital Supply Corporation, and MIT are gratefully acknowledged. Part of this work was performed at the MIT Laser Research Center.

REFERENCES

1. Langerholc, J.: Moving phase transitions in laser-irradiated biological tissue, Appl. Opt. **18**:2286, 1979.
2. Laufer, G.: Primary and secondary damage to biological tissue induced by laser radiation, Appl. Opt. **22**:676, 1983.
3. van Gemert, M.J.C., Schets, G.A.C.M., Stassen, E.G., et al.: Modeling of (coronary) laser-angioplasty, Lasers Surg. Med. **5**:219, 1985.
4. Partovi, F., Izatt, J.A., Cothren, R.M., et al.: A model for thermal ablation of biological tissue using laser radiation, Lasers Surg. Med. **7**:141, 1987.
5. Cothren, R.M., Hayes, G.B., Kramer, J.R., et al.: A multifiber catheter with an optical shield for laser angiosurgery, Lasers Life Sci. **1**:1, 1986.
6. Bellinger, R., Shi, De-Xiu, Gomes, E., et al.: Radiation of human atherosclerotic plaque with midinfrared (3 μm) and CO_2 (10.6 μm) lasers: a histologic comparison, Lasers Surg. Med. (abstract) **7**:80, 1987.
7. Sartori, M., Henry, P.D., Sauerbrey, R., et al.: Tissue interactions and measurement of ablation rates with ultraviolet and visible lasers in canine and human arteries, Lasers Surg. Med. **7**:300, 1987.
8. Strikwerda, S., Bott-Silverman, C., Ratliff, N.B., et al.: The effects of varying argon ion laser intensity and exposure time on the ablation of atherosclerotic plaque, Lasers Surg. Med. 1987. (In press.)
9. van Gemert, M.J.C., Verdaasdonk, R., Stassen, E.G., et al.: Optical properties of human blood vessel wall and plaque, Lasers Surg. Med. **5**:235, 1985.
10. Baraga, J., personal communication.
11. Ishimaru, A.: Wave propagation and scattering in random media, New York, 1978, Academic Press.
12. Welch, A.J., Yoon, G., and van Gemert, M.J.C.: Practical models for light distribution in laser-irradiated tissue, Lasers Surg. Med. **6**:488, 1987.
13. Cothren, R.M., Kittrell, C., Willett, R.L., et al.: Controlled ablation of atherosclerotic plaque: experimental and theoretical dosimetry, J. Am. Coll. Cardiol. **7**:208A, 1986.
14. Chato, B.T., editor: Advanced heat transfer, p. 395, Chicago, 1969, University of Illinois Press.

Chapter 6

Peripheral Laser and Mechanical Angioplasty: 1987
The Stanford Experience

Robert Ginsburg, MD

In January 1987, we established a new unit called the Center for Interventional Vascular Therapies (CIVT) at Stanford University Hospital. The impetus for its creation was the rapidly expanding number of devices being developed for the treatment of occlusive vascular disease. We believed that in order to provide objective and scientific perspectives to this ever-growing and frenzied area of medicine that a new approach was needed.

The goal of the CIVT is to focus on the artery as an organ regardless of the end-organ it ultimately supplies, and this approach is different from traditional medical teachings. The CIVT is composed of cardiologists, interventional radiologists, and vascular surgeons as well as cardiac surgeons engaged in a coordinated effort to care for patients. Moreover, the unit strives to offer the patient "one-stop shopping" for their vascular problems, and encourages second opinions and "failure analysis" of previous vascular interventions. Additionally, a full complement of diagnostic and therapeutic modalities is offered to the patient including risk-factor modification, drug therapy, angioplasty, and surgery.

As part of our angioplasty program, we are presently evaluating the following devices: 1-mm angioscope (Machida), the Kensey catheter (Cordis), Rotablator (Biophysics International), and Laserprobe (Trimedyne). It is in context of this brief overview of our program that our experience with these new devices is presented.

ANGIOSCOPE

The device we are presently evaluating is a 1-mm flexible angioscope (Machida, Orangeburg, New York). The scope is ethylene oxide sterilized and reusable. It requires a xenon light source and a video camera, monitor, and tape recorder.

The scope is used for viewing both the peripheral and the coronary arteries. A guiding catheter (5F to 8F) is first inserted to the most distal site of the area to be examined using standard guidewires. Once in place, the scope is inserted through the guiding catheter to its most distal end. The guiding catheter is then flushed with saline. The flow rate is not fixed and depends on the volume and the rate of flow of blood in the vessel being examined.

Usually 100 to 200 ml are infused during an examination. As with other nonvascular scoping procedures, a much better view is obtained when the catheter and angioscope together are withdrawn (retrograde) through the vessel. If the scope is advanced alone, there is the risk of perforation or dissection, but more importantly, the scope has the tendency not to remain coaxial and only the wall is visualized.

As the angioscope technology advances, so does our enthusiasm for this device. We believe its indications will be primarily for diagnosis and in therapeutic decision making. As we are all acutely aware, an angiogram shows only shadows and can suggest but not prove underlying pathophysiology. On the other hand, the scope can rapidly and precisely determine what is occluding the lumen of the vessel. This new, readily obtainable information has altered our approach to treating patients. We can now carefully choose the appropriate device or agent depending on the visually observed disease state.

The limitations of the scope is its expense, especially the "start-up" costs needed for the video equipment and camera. The scopes are fragile and need care during use and sterilization. Most importantly, steering or guiding systems still need to be designed to permit full potential use of the angioscope.

ROTATING-TIP (KENSEY) CATHETER

We are presently participating in clinical trials using the Kensey catheter for the treatment of total occlusions of both the peripheral and coronary arteries. This device is described in detail in another chapter, but, in brief, the catheter has a small rotating "cam"-like tip that spins at 45 to 90K rpm and is perfused with saline or dilute contrast at 20 to 30 ml/min. This device is designed primarily for totally occluded vessels. It does not have a guidewire system and must be advanced carefully under fluoroscopic guidance. Because the tip is a fixed size, for most vessels, balloon angioplasty is needed to further improve the luminal diameter.

This catheter is most effective on vessels occluded with thrombus or a semisolid "gruel"-like material. The device does not work well in areas of fibrous capped lesions where there is the tendency to seek the path of least resistance most commonly the subintimal plane.

A unique feature of the device is that contrast is ejected from the distal tip at high velocity. The contrast penetrates the wall of the vessel and can even extravasate. Not infrequently, during a procedure it appears that the device has perforated the vessel when in reality the contrast has extravasated along the subintimal plane within the boundaries of the vessel giving the inexperienced operator a degree of anxiety.

Overall, this device is "user friendly," and the equipment needed to operate it is not complex and is physically small. The device requires patience and, unlike the Laserprobe, it is advanced very slowly and in most cases advances forward on its own power. The risk of perforation is small unless it is manually pushed out of the vessel. Although excellent for total occlusions, it probably will not be useful to enlarge mildly stenotic vessels.

We have used the 8F device in 30 peripheral arteries and the 5F device in 3 coronary arteries. Problems that need to be resolved are flexibility and steerability. To cross tortuous vessels, these characteristics need to be improved. If this can be accomplished, then the device will find its place in the cath lab.

ROTABLATOR

The Rotablator is a diamond-studded tip that spins at 140,000 rpm over a coaxial wire to "sand" or smooth the lumen of stenotic vessels. This device is intended for vessels with diffuse disease but not total occlusions. The advantages of this device over others are

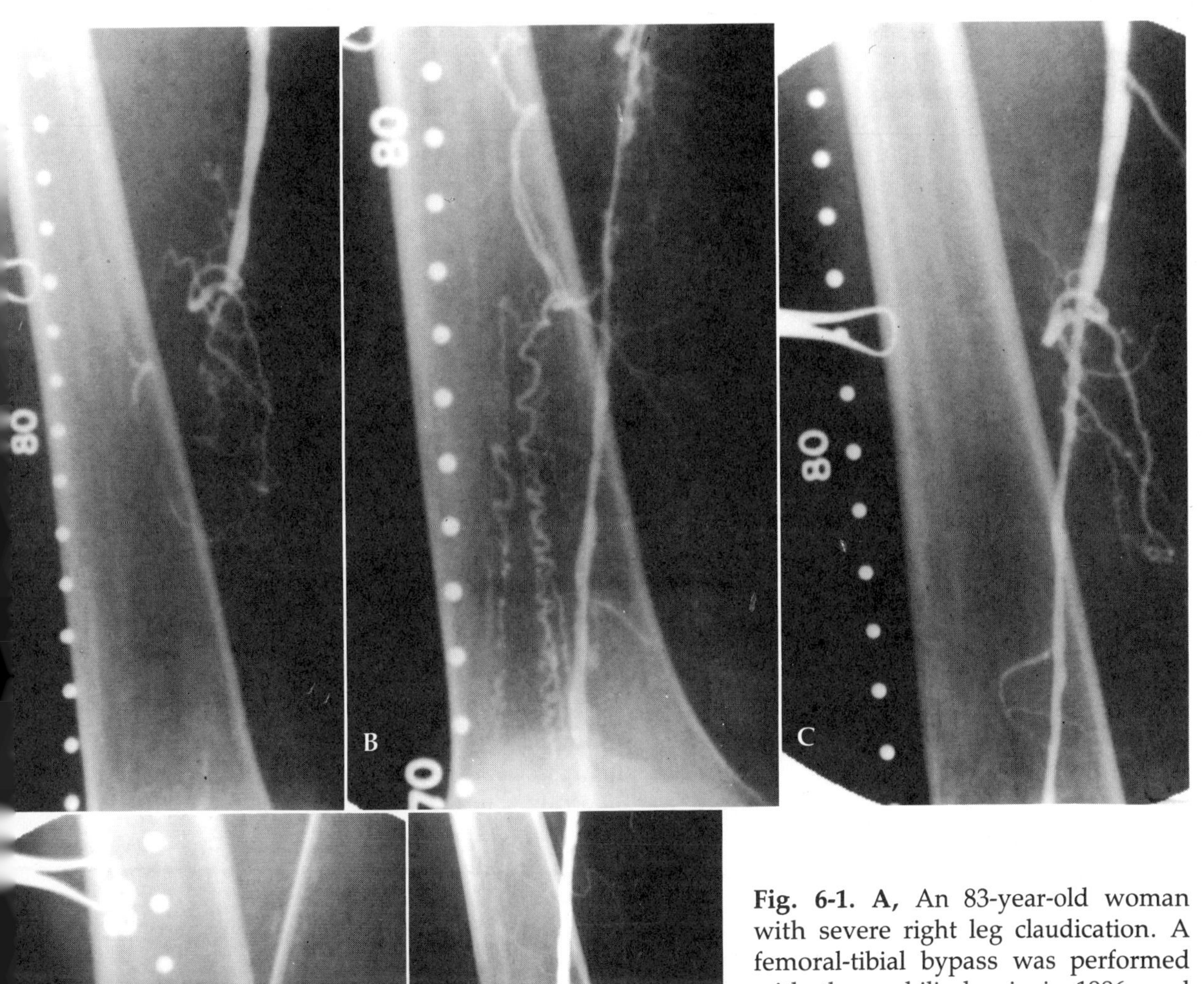

Fig. 6-1. A, An 83-year-old woman with severe right leg claudication. A femoral-tibial bypass was performed with the umbilical vein in 1986, and failed shortly after surgery. Occlusion is seen in adductor canal. Standard guidewire would not cross obstruction and a hot laserprobe (10 W, 8 seconds) was used to pass through blockage. **B,** After laserprobe a small channel was opened (No. 80). **C,** Rotablator (145,000 rpm) was used to enlarge the luminal diameter. Tip of Rotablator is seen at No. 76. **D,** Balloon angioplasty was performed subsequent to 1c to increase functional cross-sectional area. **E,** Final result. Patient was heparinized overnight and discharged the following day on aspirin with good popliteal pulse.

that it passes coaxially over a 0.009'' guidewire, is very flexible, is available in a variety of sizes, and the catheter is air-driven.

To date we have used the device percutaneously to treat three patients with diffuse peripheral vascular disease. The device is easy to use and is quite effective. The largest tip we have used is 2.5 mm, which will fit through an 8F Hemaquet arterial sheath.

Emboli have not as yet been a clinical problem although carefully looked for angiographically. However, spasm, especially in the smaller trifurcation vessels, has occurred. This is not treatable with either nitrates or calcium blockers. Time (usually 30 to 45 minutes) is the best treatment. Whether or not this vasospasm will be a clinical problem remains to be determined. The issue of restenosis, although now a major limiting factor of balloon angioplasty, was not appreciated 10 years ago, and its prevention was not a primary goal of lasers.

The basic question many ask is why use lasers in the first place. For the majority of physicians, their first experience with lasers was not dissimilar from that of the lay public. In the late 1970s, lasers became larger than life on the cinema screen, and these backlot fantasies were soon extrapolated into clinical medicine, particularly into cardiovascular medicine. However, anyone who was tempted to work in this area soon realized the many difficult technological hurdles to be overcome.

Laser energy, as described in other chapters in this book, can be delivered through fiberoptic transmission cables. The flexibility and size of these glass fibers permit their use through guiding catheters and, therefore, access to arterial vessels of almost any size and location. One of the major problems still facing us today is, however, the delivery of this energy from a small-diameter fiber to a large target site. Many ingenious and creative engineering designs and models have been developed over the years and implemented clinically, but as yet none solves all the problems faced in the treatment of vascular disease. Some of the limiting factors include the size of the device that can be safely inserted into an artery (usually no greater than 9F or 0.118 inch), flexibility of the fiber, thermal injury to nontarget tissue, and perforation through the wall of the vessel.

A critical problem in the design and testing of laser devices has been the lack of a suitable model of human atherosclerosis. Most animals do not spontaneously develop atherosclerosis. One of the most available animal models for vascular disease is the high-cholesterol-fed rabbit in whom the vessels are first mechanically debrided of their endothelial cells with a balloon. These vessels can appear angiographically to be similar to humans', but histologically the vessels are not comparable because they are primarily comprised of foam cells and very soft noncalcified material. Moreover, other animals such as the pig or monkey can similarly develop disease, but these animals are not easy nor inexpensive to use for scientific study. Because of these less than ideal animal models, many of these new devices had to be tested directly in humans, to determine their efficacy. It became generally accepted to use the peripheral leg arteries for testing, because the arteries were in a less hazardous position compared to carotid or coronary arteries. The peripheral arteries have now become a standard site for the development of new therapies.

MORE THAN A TEST BED?

In the United States, the treatment of peripheral vascular disease has primarily been under the purview of the vascular surgeon. Specialists in internal medicine generally had less of an interest in this clinical problem, possibly because there was little to offer therapeutically other than surgery, and, therefore, most were of the persuasion that this

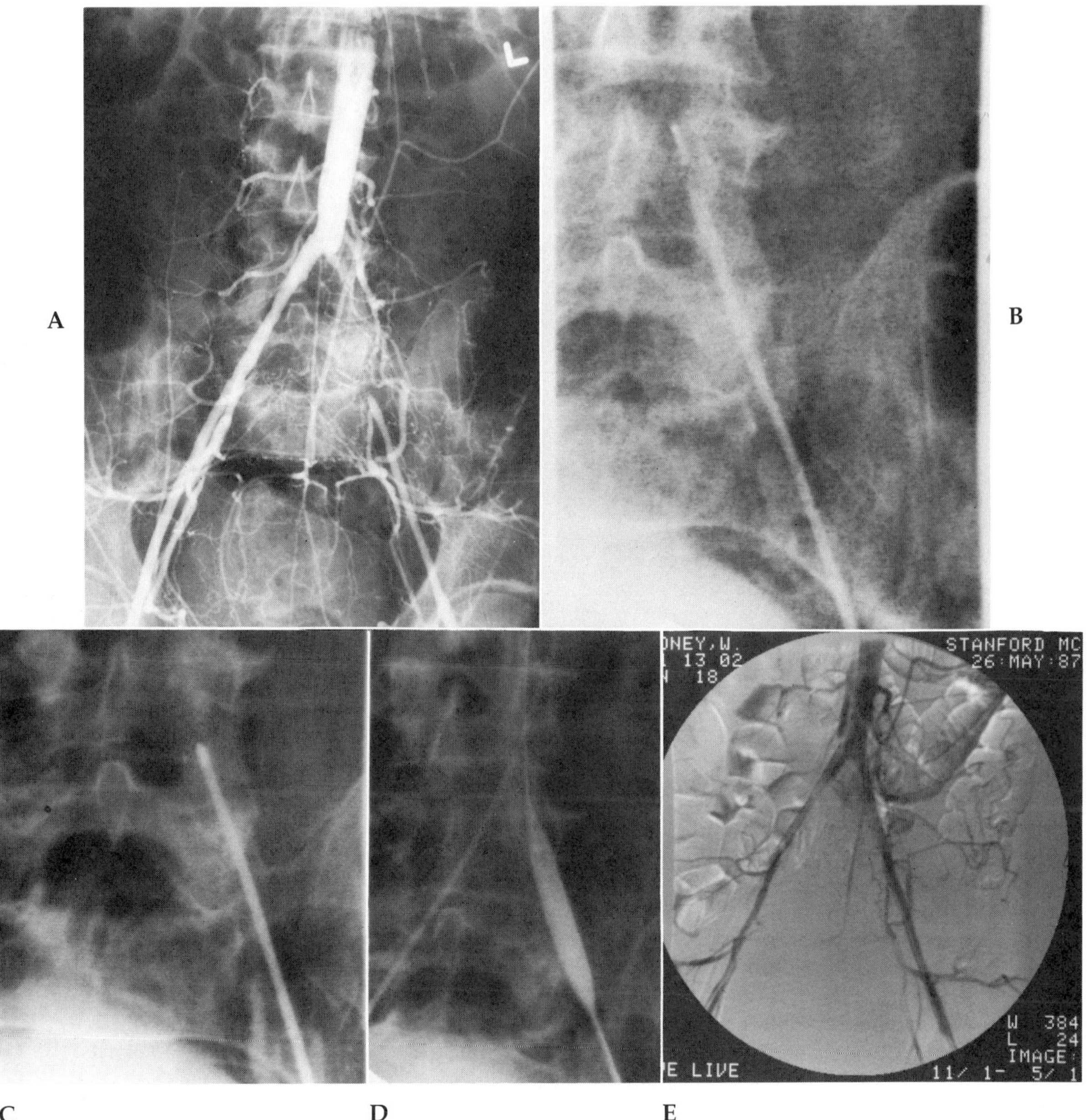

Fig. 6-2. **A,** A 61-year-old man with occluded left common iliac artery. **B,** Laserprobe was unable to pass retrogradely (subintimal). **C,** Kensey catheter was unable to pass retrogradely (subintimal). **D,** Wire was passed around the bifurcation and antegradely through the left lesion. The wire was retrieved from the left common femoral artery by a basket, and a balloon was passed retrogradely over the wire through the obstruction. **E,** Postprocedure angiogram.

was almost solely a surgical problem. More recently, with better understanding of the pathophysiology of vascular disease, balloon angioplasty, and the limited long-term viability of bypass grafts, there has been renewed interest in alternative methods in the treatment of peripheral vascular disease.

At Stanford, our initial clinical studies with percutaneous laser angioplasty were done in the peripheral (leg) vessels of patients with severe end-stage vascular disease. We chose this route because the peripheral vessels offered us relatively straight arteries, variable complexity of lesions, accessibility to external compression in case of perforation, relatively safe environment in case of distal emboli, and, most importantly, they were amenable and accessible to surgical bailout should it be required. This was our original rationale in using this cohort of patients.

In September 1985, we reported our initial experience with percutaneous transluminal laser angioplasty (Radiology **156**(3):619, 1985). We made the following observations: First, laser energy could be passed successfully through silica fiber bundles and delivered into an arterial vessel. Second, the glass fiber could be passed in many but not all cases through atherosclerotic lesions in similar fashion to a guidewire. Third, the procedure was painful if there was insufficient cooling by blood saline or contrast around the fiber tip to protect normal vessel wall. Fourth, if the vessel was severely diseased, the fiber could go subintimal and perforate in similar fashion to, but more easily than a guidewire.

One of the goals in the early development of laser angioplasty was to use the laser to debulk significant amounts of atheromatous material from the lumen of the vessel to improve hemodynamic flow. Also, it was desired that this procedure would replace and not be an adjunct to balloon angioplasty. Also, it became obvious to us that peripheral vascular disease was complex and unpredictable. Our goal was to use the peripheral vessels as a testing ground without the expectation that the then state of the art was sufficient realistically to be a definitive treatment solution for this disease.

DO LASERS HAVE A ROLE IN THE TREATMENT OF PERIPHERAL VASCULAR DISEASE?

The answer to this question, based on the technology available in 1987, is a qualified maybe. We are witnessing two disciplines—angioplasty and peripheral vascular disease treatment—undergoing rapid maturation and change. As previously pointed out, the disease process in the leg arteries is complex. How to determine the pathophysiology of the artery from a shadow seen angiographically is as yet undefined. Moreover, the approach in the health-care system toward diagnosing and treating peripheral vascular disease is changing from a purely surgical disease to more of a medical problem. Many physicians are just becoming aware of the options available to treat their patients.

Patients with claudication need to be evaluated carefully to determine if this is due to ischemia and whether this is a result of inflow or distal disease. Patients with iliac, common femoral, or profunda disease need to be treated aggressively because limb loss can occur. However, the most commonly diseased vessel in the leg, the superficial femoral artery, rarely needs to be reopened if the other major vessels are open. A superficial femoral artery occlusion usually can be treated best by an exercise program, medication, and having the patient stop smoking. The SFA usually first occludes Hunter's canal and then occludes retrograde. Even if it is reopened, long-term potency is not spectacular. This vessel is, however, long and straight and is ideal for devices such as the hot-tip probe.

Overall, lasers in their present configuration can help but are of limited usefulness in the overall therapy of peripheral vascular disease.

CLINICAL EXPERIENCE WITH LASERPROBE

The Laserprobe (Trimedyne, Inc., Santa Ana, California) is the only laser-driven cardiovascular device clinically approved for general use by the FDA (as of late 1987). The approval indications were the use of this device for the treatment of otherwise impossible cases of peripheral vascular disease. It was believed that the device would be useful in cases in which standard "Dotter" or balloon procedures were determined to be unsatisfactory. Several other laser angioplasty devices are in early clinical trials.

In practice, the hot-tip probe is primarily an assist device to be used in conjunction with balloon angioplasty. The above-knee peripheral vessels are quite large, ranging from 5 to 8 mm in diameter. This discrepancy in size almost mandates for most cases that balloon angioplasty be used along with the device. However, the peripheral vessels below the knee become quite small, down to 1.0 mm in size, and in these vessels the mismatch in size is less apparent and at least theoretically the hot-tip probe alone could be the primary angioplasty device.

The hot-tip probe is believed to be most useful in totally occluded vessels. In the peripheral vessel, total occlusions are most common in the superficial femoral, popliteal, and tibioperoneal trunk, respectively. Atherosclerotic lesions develop in the adductor canal where the vessel crosses through interosseous membranes. The plaque becomes hemodynamically critical and totally occludes, and the thrombus begins to propagate in retrograde fashion. The overall composition of the totally obstructed vessel depends in part on the duration of the obstruction and the extent of involution that occurs along with calcium and fibrous tissue deposition.

Once heated, the hot-tip probe travels along the path of least resistance. In vessels with a relatively soft thrombus core, the probe works well and has little opportunity to perforate or cause thermal injury to normal vessel wall. However, in the rock-hard, old, solid atherosclerotic lesions, there is a much greater chance for the probe as well as guidewires to enter into and traverse the endarterectomy or subintimal plane. If the probe can find its way back into the true lumen more distally, then this is not a major concern, but in most cases it remains subintimal. The subintimal path is hazardous, and the risk of perforation or severe thermal injury is high. Therefore, the limitations of the probe are not necessarily the technology itself but the variable complex nature of the vascular disease.

The Laserprobe has several configurations. One useful one is the "monorail" probe which has a small hole on the side of the head to permit use of a 0.018" or smaller guidewire system. Although the wire system doesn't help in total occlusion, sometimes there are tandem lesions with a right proximal lesion and a total distal lesion. The ability to use the probe with a steerable guidewire is a great help to deliver the probe past tortuous nonoccluded lesions to the target site. However, the "monorail" system is presently only available on the 2.0-mm tip, limiting the guiding catheters that can accommodate it.

Technically there is a significant learning curve in the use of the probe, not dissimilar to that in the use of balloon angioplasty. The fiber-optic cable itself is relatively flimsy and not easy to steer or direct. In peripheral vessels, we have developed a preference for the 1.5-mm probe. Using the Seldinger technique, we usually insert a 8F Hemaquet sheath with check valve into the artery. Although one could insert the probe directly into the sheath, there is usually a tremendous amount of leakage around the small fiber cable at the

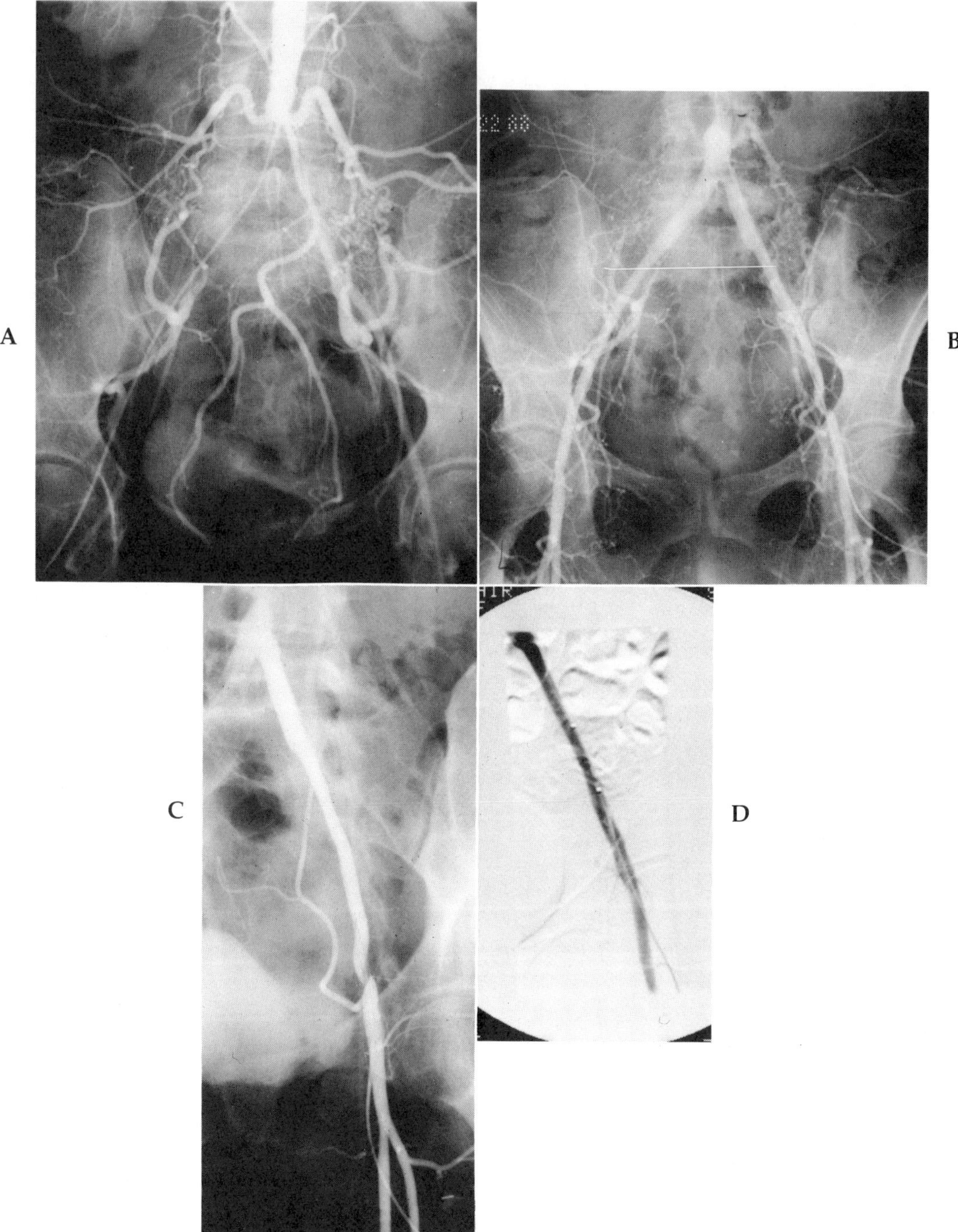

Fig. 6-3. A, A 50-year-old woman with severe bilateral claudication. She refused aorto femoral bypass surgery. **B,** Both iliac arteries were approached retrogradely using new hydrophilic glidewire (Meditech/Terumo). Balloons were used to perform bilateral angioplasty. **C,** Postprocedure angiogram shows widely patent vessels, but left external iliac/common femoral junction shows an area of stenosis, probably trauma from the arterial sheath). **D,** Three months after the procedure stenosis of 3c successfully dilated with balloon.

check valve. Therefore, we prefer to insert through the sheath a multipurpose coronary guiding catheter and at its proximal end to connect a Y connector with an adjustable O ring valve. This prevents back leakage, but permits control and manipulation of the fiber cable. In practice, the guiding catheter is advanced to the target site. A saline or dilute contrast solution is infused through one arm of the Y connector and then is advanced through the distal end of the guiding catheter. The laser is activated, and the hot tip is advanced. The direction of the probe can be controlled in part by torquing the guiding catheter. The smaller 1.5-mm probe heats up quite rapidly and does not need a long warm-up time (usually only a few seconds). We have found that intermittently pulsing the probe gives better thermal control of the tip because it is an "unforgiving" instrument. Once a tract is made, the probe commits itself to continuing to follow the path it creates. Not infrequently, this is an undesirable subintimal path. If the probe is successfully advanced through the lesion, the operator may not want to lose the lumen which could occur if the probe is withdrawn. Therefore, the proximal end of the fiber can be cut, and the fiber cable can be used as a guidewire, being careful to realize that the distal tip cannot be pulled back through the balloon catheter because of its size. Balloon angioplasty can now be performed and when completed the combined systems can be removed.

POTENTIAL PROBLEMS WITH THE PROBE

Clinical experience with the probe is not extensive, although it is now available for general clinical use in the therapy of peripheral disease. Therefore, questions such as long-term potency and untoward effects of thermal injury are unanswered. However, preliminary experience suggests that this is not much of a concern.

The primary difficulty in using the probe or any other device in totally occluded vessels is in guiding the instrument down the true lumen of the vessel. In patients with extensive and old disease, there is a high likelihood of the instrument entering the subintimal or endarterectomy plane. When this occurs rarely can satisfactory long-term result be obtained. One disadvantage with the probe is that if it tracts subintimally, there is a greater risk of thermal injury to surrounding normal wall as well as perforation.

Another potential problem is in smaller distal vessels of the peripheral. When the vessel diameter approaches the diameter of the probe itself there is a greater risk of thermal injury. This occurs because there is less blood flow cooling the surrounding tissue. Also more of the probe is in contact with the total surface of the vessel, and, therefore, there is greater dissipation of the thermal energy to potentially normal vessel wall. Whether or not this will become a significant clinical problem is unknown.

WHAT'S HOT, WHAT'S NOT

Due to unexplained electronic problems with our laser, it was not always operational when we were about to advance the Laserprobe. Therefore, we discovered by chance during one of these power failures that the probe works well even when cold. The "football" shape of the Laserprobe evidently permits the probe to "snowplow" through the soft core of an obstructed vessel, and in many instances this is the true lumen.

Because of this early observation, we have randomized our patients to use of the hot or cold probe. To date we have found that the probes work well unheated, but that there are specific situations when thermal energy is needed.

SUMMARY

The results of our comparative trial of the Laserprobe, Kensey, and balloon for peripheral angioplasty are shown in Table 6-1. The comparative characteristics of these devices are listed in Table 6-2.

From February to August 1987, 61 patients were entered into the study. All lesions were first approached with standard guidewires and catheters. If a wire could be passed, then primary balloon angioplasty was performed. If this was not successful, then either the Laserprobe or the Kensey catheter was used.

The data to date suggest that a successful procedure is directly related to the extent of the disease present. In the "impossible" lesions, the new devices are successful about 20% of the time.

Table 6-1. Center for Interventional Vascular Therapies, February to August 1987

	Laserprobe Hot/Cold	*Balloon*	*Kensey*	*Total*
Iliac	5/1	5	4	15
SFA/TRI	8/5	16	17	46
Total	13/6	21	21	61
Success	16/26%	95%	19%	52%

CONCLUSION

Many new technologies are being developed for the treatment of occlusive vascular disease. At present, no one device is ideal for all clinical situations. The process of atherosclerotic vascular disease is complex, and much still needs to be understood. These new devices all complement one another and are needed for the high-volume complex angioplasty laboratory. However, because they are useful in only limited cases, we would not recommend them for general use until more studies are completed.

Table 6-2. Comparative Characteristics of Angioplasty Devices

	Laserprobe	*Rotablator*	*Kensey*	*Atherocath*
Indications:				
Total obstructions	Yes	No	Yes	No
Diffuse disease	Yes	Yes	Yes	No
Focal disease	N/A	Yes	Yes	Yes
FDA approval:				
Peripheral artery	Yes	No	Pending	Yes
Coronary arteries	No	No	No	No
Need balloon angioplasty	Yes for >2.5-mm vessel	Yes for >2.5-mm vessel	Yes for >2.5-mm vessel	No
Unit cost: (approximate)				
Drive source	$92,000	$5,000	$10,000	$ 90.00
Delivery system	$ 390	$ 600	$ 500	$600.00
Perforation risk	Yes	No	Yes	No

Chapter 7

Laser Angiosurgery:
A Biomedical System Using Photons to Diagnose and Treat Atherosclerosis

Michael S. Feld, PhD
John R. Kramer, MD

Laser angiosurgery[1-3] is an overall term used by colleagues at the Cleveland Clinic Foundation and the Massachusetts Institute of Technology to describe a large, ongoing research project aimed at the development of intraoperative and percutaneous catheters that can recognize and ablate intra-arterial atherosclerotic obstructions with a precisely controlled and aimed photon beam. Because the power of the beam is immense, and because the arterial wall is thin and easily damaged by heat, there is little room for error, necessitating a sophisticated and complex delivery system.[4] This chapter describes our approach to the use of laser light in the vascular system, that is, laser angiosurgery (LAS).

LASER CATHETER DESIGN

The LAS catheter is based on a multifiber approach, in which the distal tip is formed of an array of optical fibers encased in a protective, transparent shield[5,6] (Fig. 7-1). As the lesion is contacted, blood is displaced, providing the light exiting the fibers with a clear path to the target. Each fiber produces a small light spot at the tip of the shield, irradiating a correspondingly small "field" of tissue. The fibers are arranged inside the shield so that the spots all overlap, providing coverage of the entire distal tip of the device. Tissue fields are irradiated sequentially. Thus, with a series of small spots (typically 0.5 mm in diameter), a large diameter arterial lumen (typically 2 to 3 mm in diameter) can be recanalized.

There are two distinct aspects of the LAS removal process: target recognition and target ablation. Each tissue field is treated individually. A given field is first diagnosed, and then it is ablated or spared, as indicated. The objective is to remove the diseased tissue causing the stenosis, leaving healthy tissue and blood intact. The functions of recognition and ablation are best discussed separately.

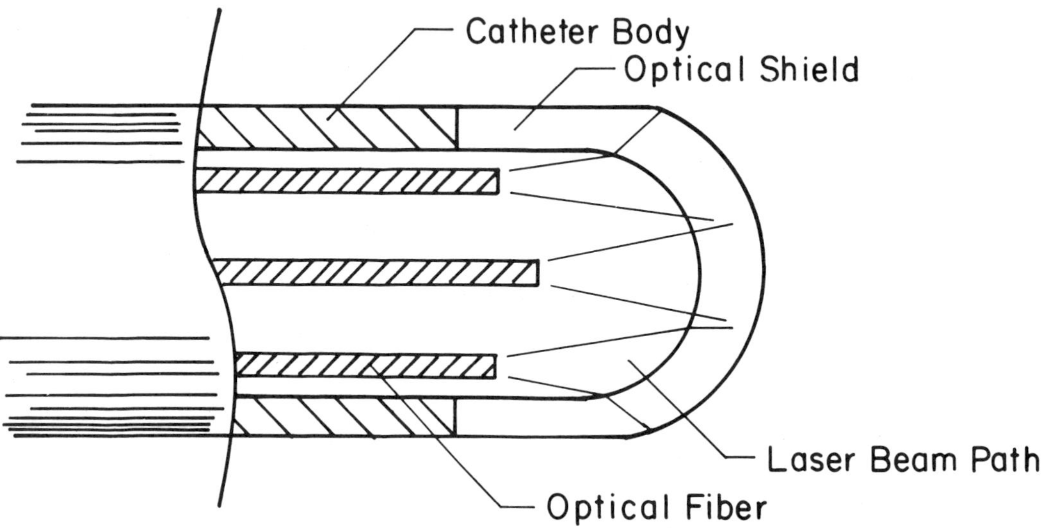

Fig. 7-1. Cross-sectional diagram of a multifiber laser catheter with an optical shield. Three fibers are shown, along with the laser beam path of each. Note that the beams must be arranged so that light covers the entire surface of the shield.

TARGET RECOGNITION

The purpose of target recognition is to determine the identity of a given tissue field. The field may be normal or diseased, or it may be filled with blood. The LAS recognition scheme is based on a process called "spectral diagnosis."[7] In the specific spectral diagnostic technique used at present, called laser-induced fluorescence, blue-green argon ion laser light at 476 nm emitted from a fiber impinges on a given tissue field, causing emission at longer wavelengths (500 to 650 nm). Some of this fluorescence is collected by the fiber and carried back to the proximal end of the catheter, where it is analyzed with a spectrometer. The spectral pattern of this light is distinct for normal and diseased tissue, enabling a diagnosis to be made[8] (Fig. 7-2). As blood does not fluoresce, its presence can also be determined.

This process of spectral diagnosis can be performed rapidly, tissue field by tissue field, under computer control. It uses low-intensity exciting light, sufficiently weak to ensure that the tissue is not damaged and its spectral response is not altered. Once target determination is accomplished, high-intensity light from the same laser source can be used to ablate the tissue.

TARGET ABLATION

Strikwerda et al.[5,9] have demonstrated that relatively char-free craters can be consistently produced in atherosclerotic plaque if the appropriate light intensity and exposure time are used. Once over a practical threshold (intensity $\simeq$ 25.5 watts/mm^2, fluence $\simeq$ 3.2 J/mm^2), ablation depths are predictable even when aortic segments exhibit varying stages of disease and come from different patients.

By analyzing Strikwerda's data, Partovi et al.[10] have been able to theoretically model the ablation process and mathematically predict

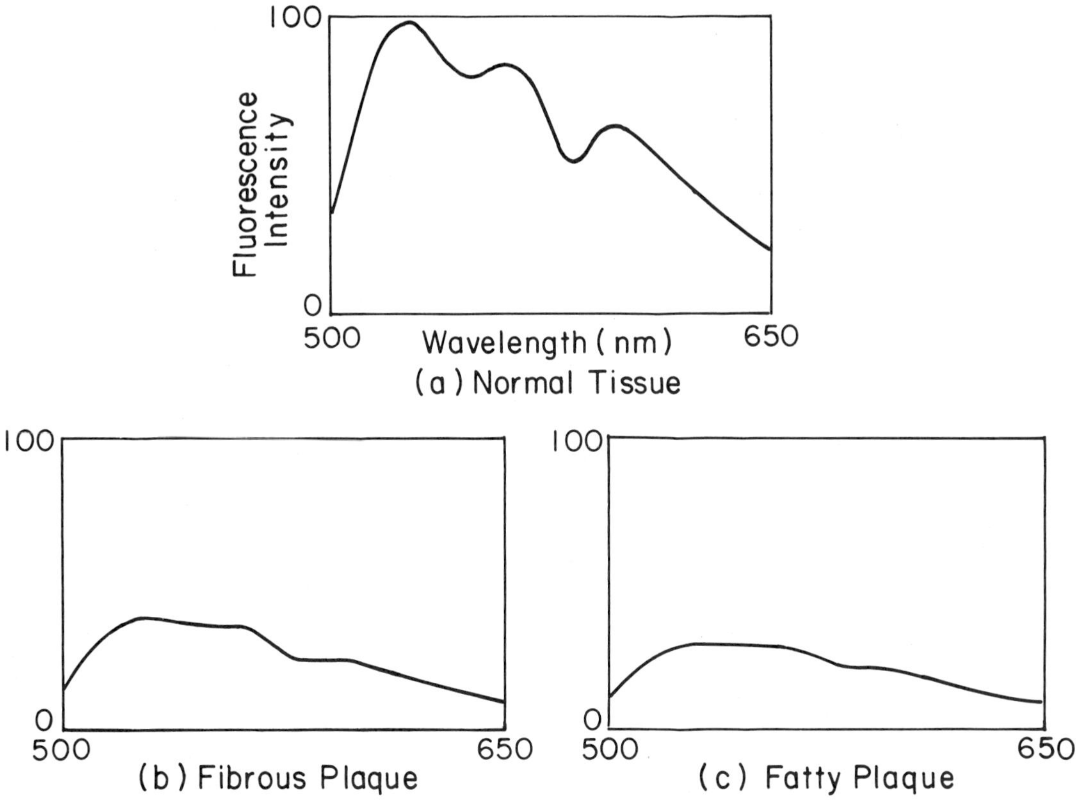

Fig. 7-2. Typical fluorescence spectra for **A**, normal tissue, **B**, fibrous plaque, and **C**, fatty plaque. Fluorescence intensities are given in arbitrary units.

crater depth in relation to the photon dose delivered:

$$l \simeq v(t - t_0) = [f(x)/h_{abl}] \cdot (I - I_0) \cdot (t - t_0) \quad (1)$$

where

- l = crater depth
- v = ablation velocity
- t = exposure time
- t_0 = threshold time
- $f(x)$ = fraction of light absorbed in the cylinder of tissue being removed
- x = d/D, with d the diameter of the light spot and D the penetration depth of light in the tissue
- I = laser intensity (power/unit area)
- I_0 = threshold intensity
- h_{ab1} = amount of heat needed to reach water-steam phase transition temperature and then evaporate a unit volume of tissue

The parameters D and f(x) characterize the interplay of scattering and absorption and are determined by the tissue properties and the wavelength of light used. Similarly, h_{abl} depends on the composition of the target tissue. However, the factors I, t, and d can be controlled by the delivery system itself. This provides the basis for precise photon dosimetry.

Experiments with samples of fresh cadaver arterial wall have established the laser light parameters required for a useful working range. To obtain reproducible tissue craters, the intensity, I, should be much larger than the threshold intensity, I_0. In this limit equation 1 reduces to

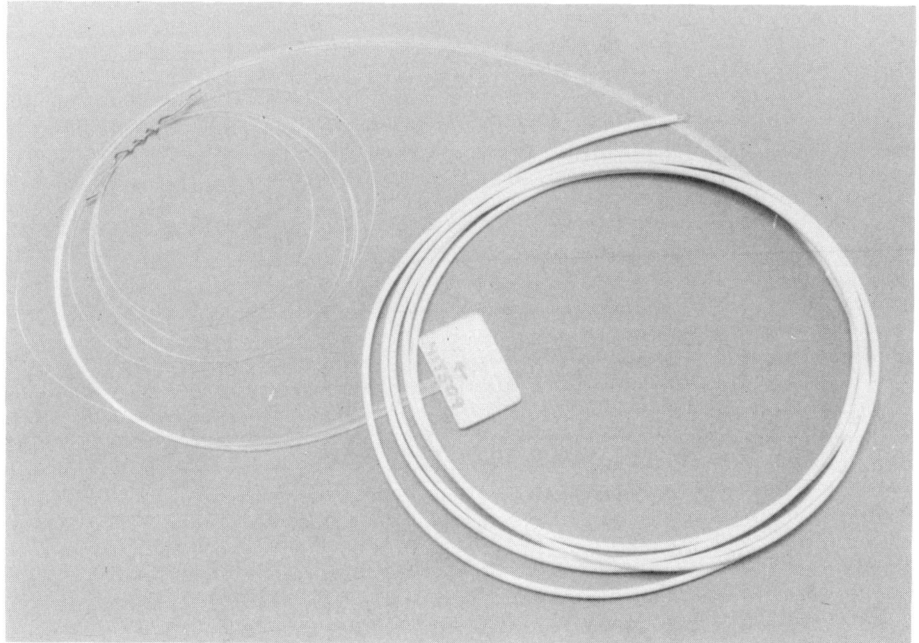

Fig. 7-3. An 8F, 20 fiber optically shielded laser angiosurgery catheter. Nineteen fibers are contained within the optical shield, while 1 fiber is separate from the catheter, allowing power measurements.

$$\begin{aligned} l &= [f(x)/h_{ab1}] \cdot (\Phi - \Phi_0) \\ &= D(\Phi/\Phi_0 - 1) \end{aligned} \qquad (2)$$

with Φ = It the fluence (J/mm^2) of the impinging light beam, and $\Phi_0 = h_{ab1} \cdot D/f(x)$, the threshold fluence. In this regime the independent values of intensity and exposure time are not important, but only their product.

The laser angiosurgery system has been designed to allow physicians to control the delivery of a predetermined photon dose, Φ:

$$\begin{aligned} \Phi &= [\text{power (watts)} \times \text{time (seconds)}] \\ &\quad \div \text{spot area (mm}^2\text{)} \end{aligned} \qquad (3)$$

OVERALL SYSTEM CONSIDERATIONS

The laser angiosurgery catheter (Fig. 7-3) is designed to control beam intensity by predetermining spot diameter. Interfacing of the catheter and the delivery system, therefore, allows control of dosimetry (power, exposure time, and spot diameter). The delivery scheme is shown in Fig. 7-4.

Additionally, the LAS catheter protects the optical fibers with an optical shield and is capable of producing a large new lumen using an array of optical fibers with overlapping spots which can be fired sequentially (one round) and in series (many rounds, one after the other).[11,12] Because target recognition is feasible, not all fibers need be fired when in contact with an eccentric lesion.[7]

A new interventional operating room incorporating a laser angiosurgery system has recently been constructed at the Cleveland Clinic Foundation (Fig. 7-5). A Coherent Innova 100 argon ion laser is housed in a closet outside the operating room so that surgeons are isolated from the noise of the power supply and cooling water. Light is transmitted to the operating room by a 50-micron fiber-optic

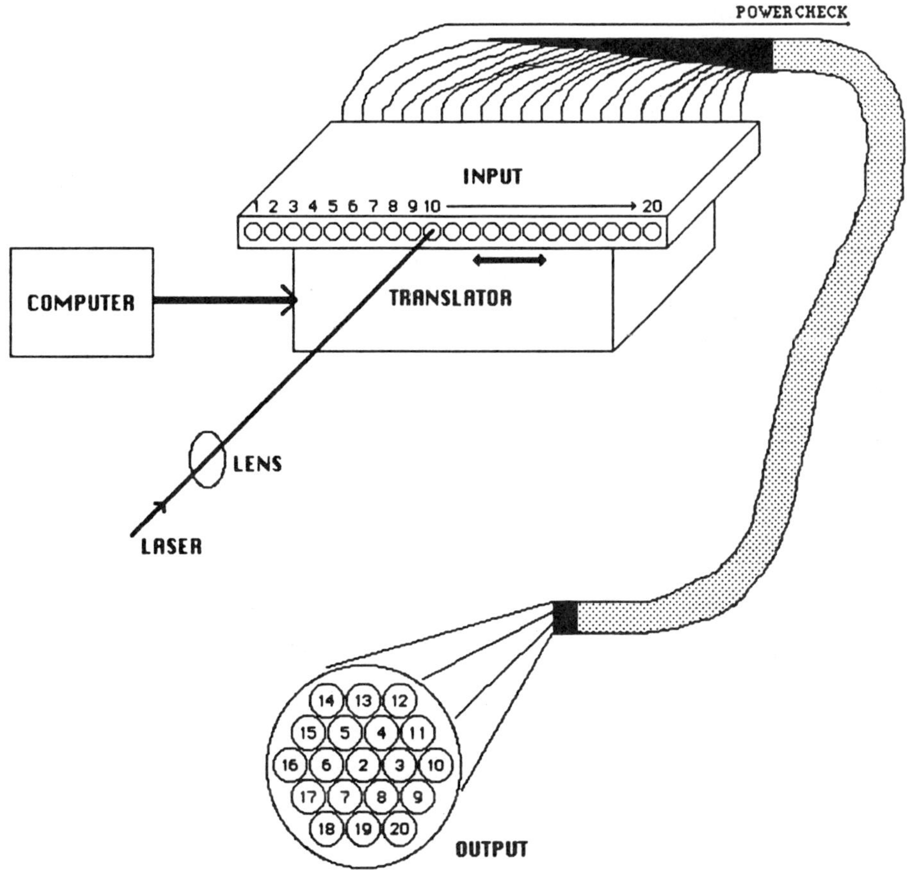

Fig. 7-4. Laser angiosurgery system.

cable strung through the ceiling. In the operating room the fiber-optic cable is connected to a small optical bench which sits near the patient and contains the hardware for timing exposures and focusing the beam into the LAS catheter. A foot pedal allows the surgeon to control beam entry into the operating room. A computer controls laser power and exposure time.

The system has been tested extensively in vitro[13] in cadaver arteries, both normal and with fibrous plaque. The catheter removes 0.16 mm^3 of tissue for each joule of energy delivered. This ablation yield varies by less than 10% over a wide range of operating parameters and does not change with repeated firing despite the accumulation of small amounts of char on the optical shield.

Kjellstrom et al., using a canine model, have shown in vivo that the system allows removal of local, fibrotic obstructions without vascular perforation.[14] Histologic evaluation of arterial segments from animals followed for up to 60 days after laser angiosurgery showed

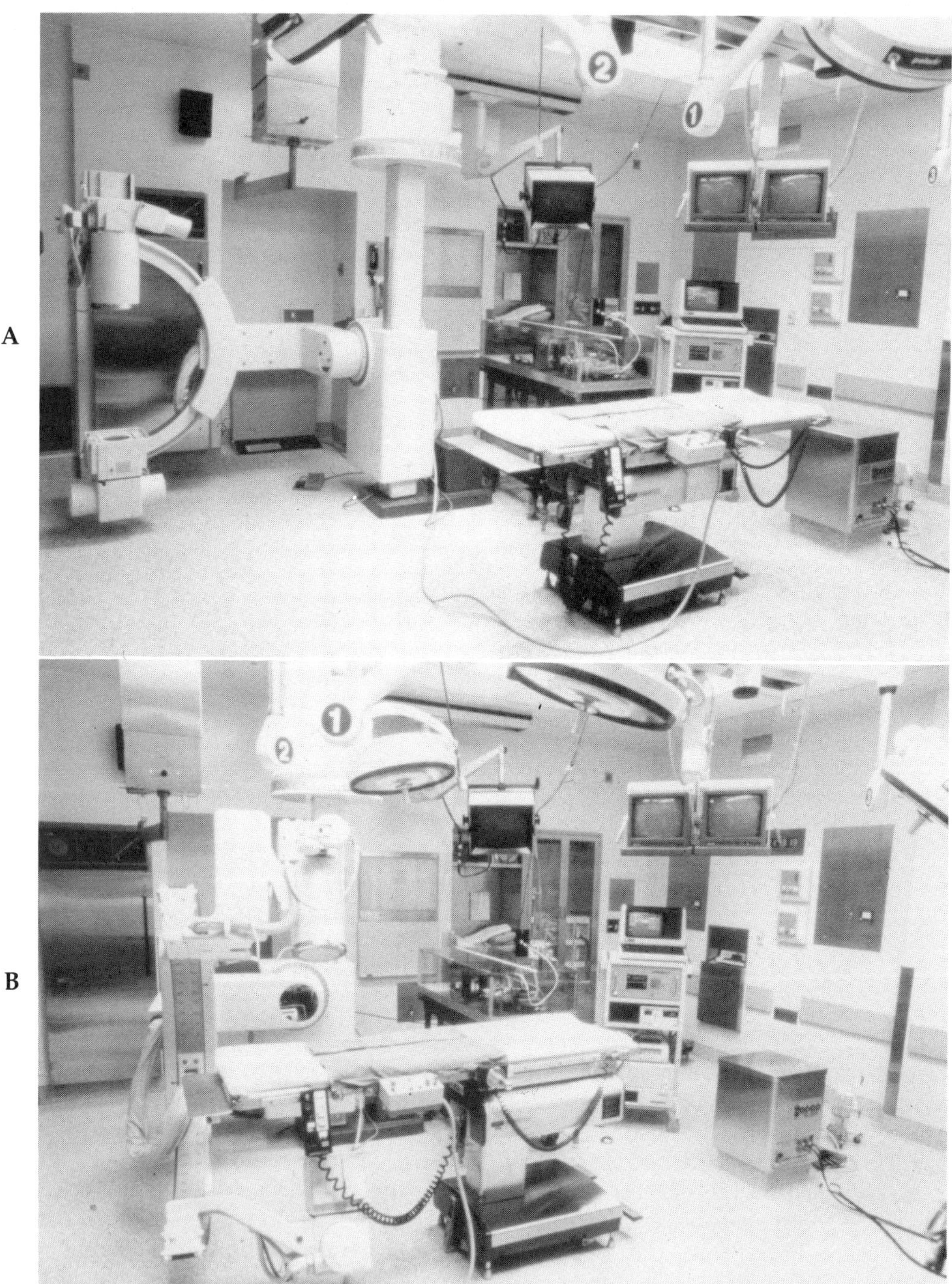

Fig. 7-5. Laser angiosurgery operating room. **A,** "Operating room" configuration for intraoperative experiments, and **B,** "catheterization laboratory" configuration for percutaneous experiments.

reendothelialization of the treated area within 30 days, confirming the earlier work of Gerrity et al. in which a different wavelength (one that could not be transmitted through a fiber) was used.[15]

FUTURE DIRECTIONS

The LAS system has a sound scientific basis. Several additional steps are now planned. Clinical ablation studies are presently in progress. Focal atherosclerotic obstructions in the proximal left anterior descending coronary artery are being removed with the LAS catheter passed retrograde through an arteriotomy prior to anastomosing the left internal mammary artery to the treated vessel. While the bypass introduces competitive flow, it protects the patient in the event of acute thrombosis at the treatment site. Preliminary results in patients undergoing recatheterization 6 weeks after surgery indicate treated segments remain patent. If this is a consistent finding, future protocols will involve the removal of distal lesions, beyond the protection of a bypass graft. This study does not use the spectroscopic guidance system, which has been tested independently in the operating room, and needs now to be incorporated in the full system. Another area of interest is the use of new ablation strategies. Because argon ion laser light does not effectively remove calcified materials, research is in progress on alternate ablation strategies capable of removing hard tissue. Finally, research is ongoing on alternate spectral diagnostic schemes capable of sensing various disease entities in arteries and, perhaps, elsewhere in the body.

REFERENCES

1. Kittrell, C.: Strategic plaque initiative, The Spectrograph **6**:1, 1987.
2. Goth, P.R., Kramer, J.R., Kittrell, C., et al.: Multifiber optically shielded catheter for laser angiosurgery, In Katzir, A., editor: Optical fibers in medicine II, Proc. SPIE **713**:58, 1987.
3. Kjellstrom, B.T., Cothren, R.M., and Kramer, J.R.: The use of lasers in vascular and cardiac surgery, Acta. Chir. Scand. (In press.)
4. Kramer, J.R., Strikwerda, S., Kittrell, C., et al.: Laser angiosurgery: a brief overview of tissue micromachining with spectral diagnostics, In Bruschke, A.V.G., Spaan, J.A.E., and Gittenberger, A.C., editors: Coronary circulation, from basic mechanisms to clinical implications, Boston, Martinus Nijhoff, 1987.
5. Cothren, R.M., Kittrell, C., Hayes, G.B., et al.: Controlled light delivery for laser angiosurgery, IEEE, J. Quantum Electron. **22**:4, 1986.
6. Cothren, R.M., Hayes, G.B., Kramer, J.R., et al.: A multifiber catheter with an optical shield for laser angiosurgery, Lasers Life Sci. **1**:1, 1986.
7. Hoyt, C.C., Richards-Kortum, R.R., Costello, B., et al.: Remote biomedical spectroscopic imaging of human artery wall, Science. (Submitted for publication.)
8. Kittrell, C., Willett, R.L., de Los Santos-Pacheo, C., et al.: Diagnosis of fibrous arterial atherosclerosis using fluorescence, Applied Optics **24**:2280, 1985.
9. Strikwerda, S., Bott-Silverman, C., Ratliff, N.B., et al.: The effects of varying argon ion laser intensity and exposure time on the ablation of atherosclerotic plaque, Lasers Surg. Med. (In press.)
10. Partovi, F., Izatt, J.A., Cothren, R.M., et al.: A model for thermal ablation of biological tissue using laser radiation, Lasers Surg. Med. **7**:141, 1987.
11. Cothren, R.M., Kramer, J.R., Hayes, G.B., et al.: Engineering of a multifiber catheter with an optical shield for laser angiosurgery, IEEE Engineering in Medicine and Biology. (In press.)
12. Kramer, J.R., Bott-Silverman, C., Ratliff, N.B., et al.: Removal of atherosclerotic plaque using multiple short exposures of argon ion laser light, Am. Heart J. **113**:1038, 1987.
13. Cothren, R.M., Costello, B., Hoyt, C., et al.: Tissue removal using an 8F multifiber shielded laser angiosurgery catheter, Lasers Life Sci. (Submitted for publication.)
14. Kjellstrom, B.T., Bylock, A.L., Bott Silverman, C., et al.: Removal of surgically induced fibrous arterial plaques by argon laser angiosurgery using a multifiber delivery system: an experimental study in the dog, J. Thorac. Cardiovasc. Surg. (Submitted for publication.)
15. Gerrity, R.G., Loop, F.D., Golding, L.A.R., et al.: Arterial response to laser operation for removal of atherosclerotic plaques, J. Thorac. Cardiovasc. Surg. **85**:409, 1983.

Chapter 8

New Sources for Laser Angioplasty:
Er:YAG, Excimer Lasers, and Nonlaser Hot-Tip Catheters

Robert F. Bonner, PhD
Paul D. Smith, PhD
Louis D. Prevosti, MD
Martin B. Leon, MD

With the rapid implementation of percutaneous transluminal balloon angioplasty over the last decade, interventional cardiologists have sought the next generation of catheter-based techniques which might exhibit greater clinical efficacy in a wider patient population. The concept of laser angioplasty has generated enormous expectations of precise, high-technology remodeling of diseased arteries through microsurgical ablation of obstructions. The potential of laser pulses to vaporize an obstruction, rather than merely reform it, appears the key to the prospects of this new technology. The first generation laser angioplasty devices have rapidly gone from simple designs using available technology (argon lasers and commercial silica optical fibers) to clinical trials. From the limitations of these first attempts have come both minor modifications using existing technology (hot-tip and sapphire-tipped systems), alterations in catheter delivery systems (including multifiber over-the-wire designs), and a search for newer laser systems capable of greater precision and predictability and the ability to ablate calcified as well as soft tissue obstructions.

The overly aggressive and premature clinical use of poorly characterized laser angioplasty systems seems to be fueled by exaggerated expectations for laser angioplasty and a limited understanding of laser microsurgery. The enthusiasm for techniques of ablating atheroma with a laser must be tempered by the possible complications: acute arterial wall perforation, particulate embolization, thrombus formation, and long-term adverse effects of thermal and photochemical damage to the vessel wall. Acute perforations have been a major problem with current laser angioplasty systems. In our opinion, new systems are required which provide precise, predictable ablation of variable composition atherosclerotic obstructions with effective guidance to prevent transmural perforation. The clinical utility of laser angioplasty rests on a convincing demonstration that, compared to balloon angioplasty, it can reestablish flow safely with lower risk, with lower incidence of restenosis, or in a wider range of potential patients.

There are three critical elements for laser microsurgery through a catheter: (1) the precision and predictability of the ablation process in diseased vessels, (2) the short- and long-term biological response to the ablated surface, and (3) guidance control of the ablation in order to prevent perforation. The implementation of these three elements in a durable but highly flexible catheter capable of percutaneous access of the human coronaries is a formidable engineering task.[1] From a practical standpoint, the compatibility of any system design with routine clinical use requires a reliability and operational simplicity which may be the ultimate test of any system engineered for efficient ablation of all obstructive lesions without perforation.

Using a laser to perform microsurgical ablation of arterial obstructions requires a design concept meticulously executed in a laser and delivery catheter. The ultimate objective of almost all efforts has been the ablation of atheroma by a percutaneous catheter. The laser system should be able to ablate fatty, fibrous, and calcified plaque (1) with a high energy efficiency, (2) with minimal damage to the remaining vessel wall, (3) while creating an ablated surface amenable to rapid healing and reendothelialization without augmented thrombogenicity, (4) while creating particulate debris of the smallest possible size that is minimally thrombogenic and cytotoxic, and (5) with minimal risk of optical fiber damage while providing the most flexible of fiber delivery systems. If the effects of a given laser are highly variable and crude with thrombogenic surfaces and thermal or acoustic damage to the entire vessel wall, the most elaborate of feedback controls will be unable to provide the interventional cardiologist with an efficacious tool.

PHYSICAL CONCEPTS OF LASER VAPORIZATION OF TISSUE

Our objective is to develop a pulsed laser system transmitted through flexible fiber optics that is capable of precise, predictable ablation of targeted tissue with minimal damage to the remaining tissue. CW argon and Nd:YAG angioplasty systems inherently cause a large zone of thermal injury and are unable to ablate calcified atheroma. Thus, the physical effects of laser beams on tissues and optical fibers must be the starting point for the analysis of the various laser angioplasty systems. Laser light when absorbed by a targeted tissue is generally converted into thermal energy. In certain cases, it may result in coagulation of tissue (denaturation of structural proteins), melting of fatty deposits or other structures (solid or gel to liquid phase transitions), direct breakage of chemical bonds by high-energy photons, tissue combustion, or ablation by vaporization. If sufficient laser energy is delivered, the local deposition of heat can build until the tissue reaches the vapor point, leading to vaporization of the tissue (Fig. 8-1). Unless the power density within the tissue is extremely large (leading by nonlinear mechanisms to plasma formation, breaking of chemical bonds, and acoustic wave generation), the deposition of energy within the tissue will be initially determined by its effective absorption coefficient for the wavelength used, a′(l).

Scattering of light by tissue can alter its local absorption from that predicted by Beer's law (that is, e^{-ax} where a is the linear absorption coefficient). If isotropic scattering of a photon typically occurs before it is absorbed, the volume in which the photons are absorbed will be wider than the direct laser beam and shallower than predicted by Beer's law (the effective absorption coefficient $a' > a$ as in Fig. 8-2A). On the other hand, if most photons are absorbed before they have been

Thermal Vaporization of Tissue

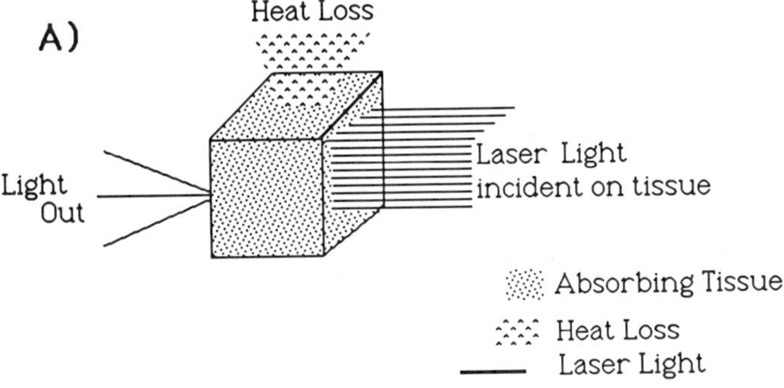

Energy Absorbed = Light Incident − Light Out − Heat Loss

B)

To Vaporize tissue (2/3 water) requires:	0.26 Joules to heat from 37 C to 100 C
	1.50 Joules to boil water
	1.76 Joules per cubic mm

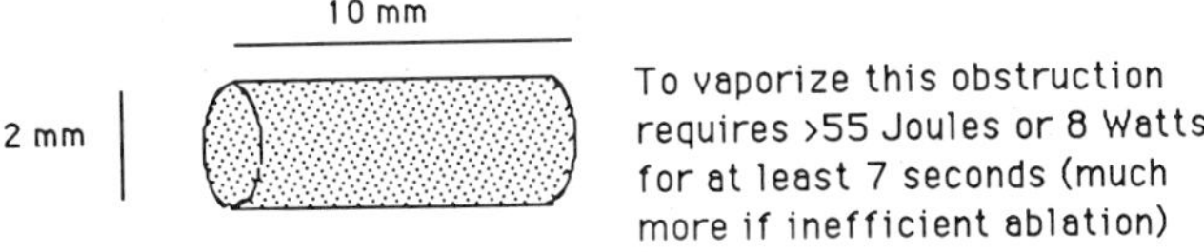

Fig. 8-1. Laser-induced thermal vaporization of tissue occurs when the net energy absorbed by a surface volume of tissue indicated in **A** exceeds the energy required to vaporize the water in the tissue as shown in **B.**

significantly scattered ($a >> \sigma_{sc}$, the isotropic scattering coefficient), the beam will be absorbed as predicted by Beer's law directly below the surface spot (as in Fig. 8-2B). For atheroma and normal artery wall, a is on the order of 10 to 30 cm^{-1} and σ_{sc} is 10 to 20 cm^{-1} for most visible wavelengths where Fig. 8-2A applies. With decreasing wavelength in the ultraviolet, a increases rapidly (~200 cm^{-1} at 308 nm and ~500 cm^{-1} at 275 nm) due largely to strong protein and nucleic acid absorption. In the infrared, water absorption peaks also result in very strong absorption (a ~ 90, 650, and 8000 cm^{-1} at 1950 nm, 10600 nm, and 2900 nm, respectively) for all tissue in vivo. Thus the energy of the incident laser pulse will be initially absorbed with an exponential distribution into the tissue (as in Fig. 8-2B) such that 63% of the energy will be deposited within a distance of 1/a of the surface.

Throughout the laser pulse, this absorbed light energy can provide the thermal energy

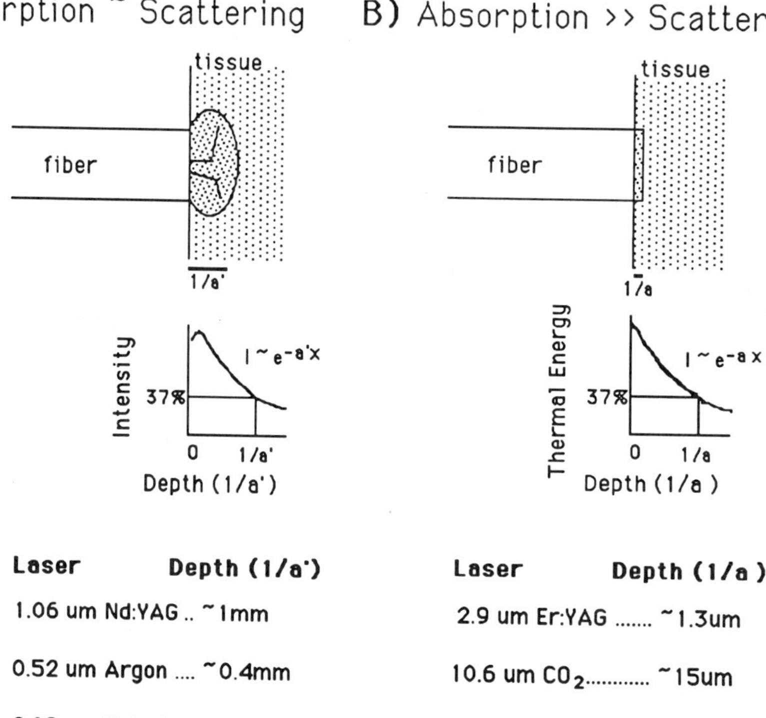

Fig. 8-2. Absorption of light in tissue is dependent on both the absorption coefficient, a, and the scattering coefficient σ_{sc} both of which varies with wavelength of the light. **A,** For many visible and near-infrared wavelengths $\sigma_{sc} \sim a$ and the light incident on the tissue is diffusely scattered before being absorbed within the tissue. The absorption depth is ~1/a′ where a′ > a owing to the effects of light scattering. **B,** For wavelengths with strong protein or water absorption light is absorbed near the surface (within ~1/a) before being scattered.

to vaporize the surface layers (Fig. 8-3A). During the pulse the heat can diffuse deeper into the tissue (Fig. 8-3B). At threshold for thermal ablation, the heat of vaporization of the tissue is deposited by the end of the pulse in a thin surface layer (for example, duration 3 in Fig. 8-3A and ~4.5 in Fig. 8-3B). For efficient ablation, most of the absorbed energy in each pulse should be used in vaporizing the tissue (durations >6 in Fig. 8-3). Thus the zone vaporized per pulse should be >1/a (where 1/a is the absorption space constant). If convective losses are negligible and vaporization of a surface layer can occur almost instantaneously after the heat of vaporization is deposited in this surface layer, we can predict laser pulse parameters for efficient ablation: (1) pulse duration T(sec) < $900/a'^2$ and (2) pulse fluence of ~6000/a′ J/cm^2 (roughly 2000 J/cm^3, at a depth of x > 1/a′). Under these conditions, the laser pulse can be expected to vaporize a soft tissue layer of a depth of ~x with a transient temperature rise of >60° C above ambient, lasting ~T sec, at a distance

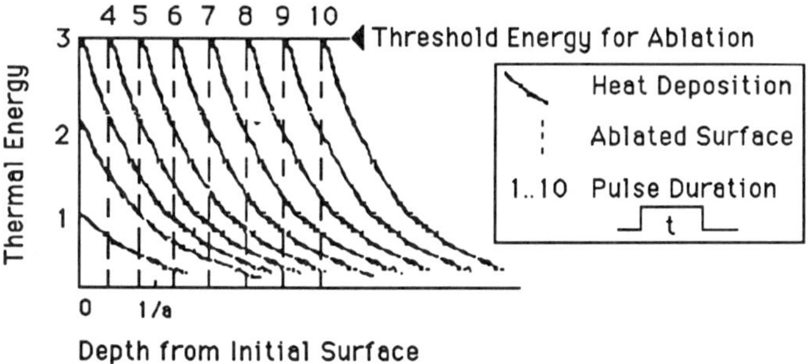

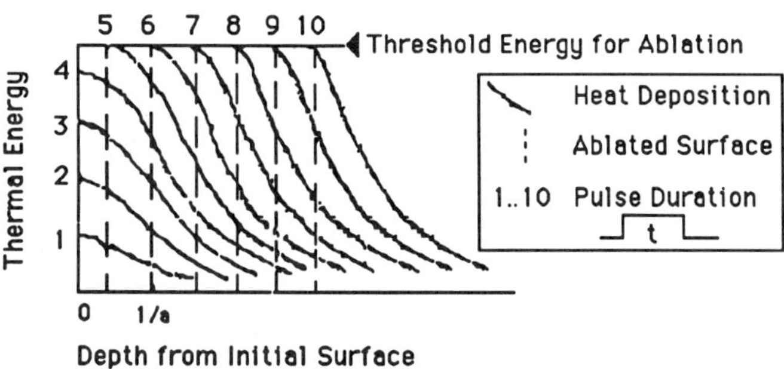

Fig. 8-3. Efficient thermal ablation occurs when most of the absorbed light energy is used to vaporize the surface layers rather than heat the surrounding tissue that remains. **A,** If the laser energy is supplied rapidly enough, sequential ablation of absorbing layers occurs before appreciable thermal diffusion. **B,** For slightly lower power laser pulses, thermal diffusion may increase the ablation threshold and reduce efficiency for near threshold pulses while having little effect on the efficiency of pulse lengths that remove a layer >>1/a.

of ~2/a′ into the wall of the crater. Thus, thermal ablation in tissue can be performed more precisely with more localized thermal damage to the remaining tissue for those wavelengths with a greater effective absorption coefficient a′.

Using these approximations, we can use the measured average atheroma absorption coefficients to generate approximate values for pulse duration, pulse energy and power density, and depth of ablation step for reasonably efficient thermal ablation of tissue as a function of wavelength (Table 8-1). Many conditions may modify this basic approximation for thermal ablation by lasers: (1) convective currents may increase thermal loss from a target, particularly in a wet field for longer pulse durations or repetitive pulses,[2] (2) for hard tissues such as bone or calcified plaque, thermal ablation may be a less efficient or

Table 8-1. Theoretical Parameters for Efficient Thermal Ablation of Atheroma Using Different Wavelengths

λ	α'	*1/e Depth (μm)*	*$\Delta\tau$ (ms)*	*Fluence (J/cm^2)*	*Thermal Damage ($2/\alpha'$) (μm)*
275 nm	500	20	3.6	12	40 μm
308 nm	200	50	22	30	100
500 nm	30	330	900	200	660
1.92 μm	100	100	90	60	200
2.9 μm	8000	1.3	0.1	1	3
10.6 μm	650	15	2.5	9	30

even ineffective means of tissue removal if the force generated by vaporization of tissue water is not able to disrupt the calcified structures, (3) the effects of shock waves generated by short, high power pulses and large tissue absorption coefficients may increase ablation efficiency,[3] and (4) multiple photon absorption may introduce nonlinear, powerdependent absorption and ablation associated with intramolecular bond breakage.[4]

For a given pulse duration, the efficiency of thermal ablation at a given wavelength usually increases with increasing pulse energy, particularly when operating near the ablation threshold. This will be so only as long as the ablative vaporization in a layer provided the heat of vaporization occurs without a significant delay (compared to the time necessary to provide the surface tissue layer with 2 J/mm^3). For thermal ablation to be efficient, we want to provide energy rapidly to the tissue avoiding thermal diffusion losses, but not so rapidly that the ablative process cannot keep up with the energy deposition at the surface (leading to superheating of the surface layer) or that large shock waves are created (which may increase efficiency at the expense of creating irregular surfaces, large tissue fragments, and deep fissures within the vessel wall). Furthermore if we decrease the pulse duration to much below a reasonably efficient pulse duration (that is, to $<< 900/a'^2$), the power density in the transmitting fiber is unnecessarily increased. At high power densities, fiber damage becomes increasingly likely for constant pulse energy (that is, tissue ablation). Thus by delivering a constant pulse energy in a decreasing pulse duration (from Dt $>> 900/a'^2$ to Dt $<< 900/a'^2$), one can go from no ablation with thermal damage, to efficient ablation with minimal thermal damage, to less efficient ablation (superheating) or erratic ablation (shock wave damage) and rapid fiber damage.

Clearly, one must carefully choose laser wavelength, pulse duration, pulse energy, and compatible optical fibers for optimizing microsurgical ablation of tissue by a catheter (Table 8-1). With these physical principles in mind, we have evaluated a number of different laser and thermal angioplasty systems.

CW LASER AND HOT-TIP ANGIOPLASTY

Continuous heating of a tissue surface can lead to efficient ablation of soft tissue if (1) the rate of heat delivery is rapid enough to overcome thermal losses (diffusion and convection) and (2) the fiber is continuously advanced to keep up with the ablation. In a wet field, convective losses can be large. These losses can be minimized and efficiency can be optimized by keeping direct contact of the probe on the tissue. Such an optimized system requires > 7 W/mm^2 (probe cross-sectional area) with probe velocity ~2 mm/sec. The early use of continuous Ar laser light delivered through bare fibers or metal-tipped fibers[5,6] approximated these conditions with the addition of significant mechanical force necessary to propel the probe through the lesions in the vessels (typically ~30 g/mm^2 or 3 atmospheres pressure). In reports where significantly less thermal energy than ~3 J/mm^3 is delivered per volume of vessel recanalized, thermal ablation does not account for the observed results. Rather the effects may arise from mechanical displacement and remodeling (similar to balloon angioplasty) and thermal coagulation or melting of atheroma. For example, a 1.5-mm catheter delivering 12 W can at best vaporize 2 cm of uncalcified obstruction in an artery in no less than ~8 seconds.

The disadvantages of such systems for coronary angioplasty are (1) the high velocity of ablation which must be maintained in order to prevent excessive local thermal damage of the vessel wall, (2) the high risk of perforation and excessive thermal damage to the artery wall, and (3) the inability of such low peak power thermal systems to ablate calcified atheroma. Although intuitively we felt that these systems would not in the long-term prove efficacious, it was clear that they were being widely used in clinical studies which might show some unpredicted advantages of a large zone of thermal injury to the vessel wall due to favorable long-term biologic responses. When such systems made with relatively stiff fiber optic catheters are advanced with significant force, the effects on atheroma might be similar to those proposed for laser coagulation through an inflated balloon catheter.[7] These hot-tip systems do not, however, require a laser. The only technological reason for using a laser in such systems is the ease of transmitting 8 to 12 W of laser power through a small, rugged optical fiber. Lu and Bowman[8] of our group at the NIH have demonstrated the feasibility of using electrical and chemical reaction "hot-tip" catheters in vivo to recanalize obstructions (Fig. 8-4). Such systems offer potential advantages of (1) reduced cost, (2) portability, (3) improved reliability and easier maintenance in a clinical environment, and (4) providing surface temperature sensing and feedback control to optimize the thermal process. At the NIH, animal experiments with flexible, nonlaser thermal catheters suggest that recanalization of soft fatty atheroma produced by diet and balloon barotrauma is much easier than thermal recanalization of implanted dense human xe-

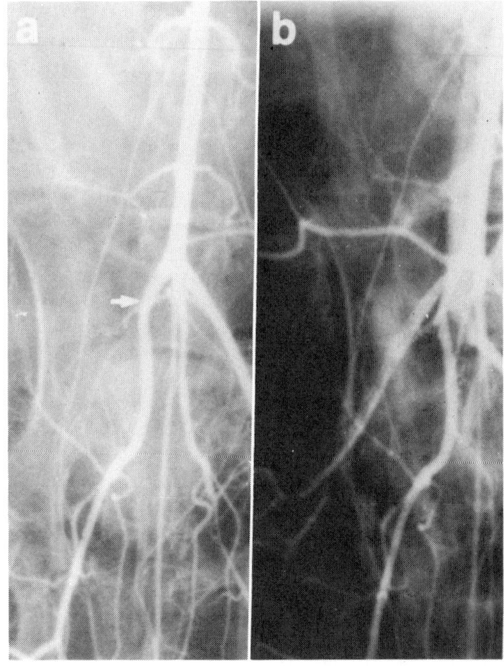

Fig. 8-4. Electrical hot-tip catheters have successfully recanalized atherosclerotic rabbits with occluded femoral arteries. Typical angiograms taken before **(A)** and **(B)** after the procedure are shown. Arrow in **A** indicates totally obstructed vessel recanalized in **B.**

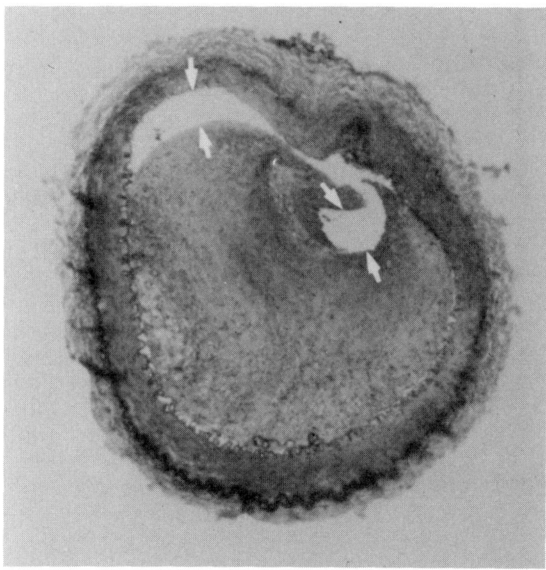

Fig. 8-5. Rabbit vessels recanalized with a hot-tip catheter typically show a new luminal surface formed by coagulation and compression and with significant intraluminal plaque remaining.

nografts of more variable and stiffer composition including calcification. As shown in Fig. 8-5, the thermal remodeling of the obstructing lesion may be associated with compression, dehydration, and coagulation of tissue rather than its fragmentation by vaporization. Furthermore, we suspect that much of the success reported in clinical trials of the laser hot-tip systems is due to the mechanical force applied to the lesion as the catheterizer forces the stiff probe through lesions rather than thermal ablation. The necessity of applying large mechanical forces in order to advance the catheter may also explain the persistent problems with perforations with laser hot-tip systems.

SELECTIVE ABLATION OF ATHEROMA

It may be of practical advantage for the ablative laser angioplasty catheter to preferentially remove atheroma by exhibiting lower thresholds or greater efficiency for the removal of atheroma. If atheroma has a higher effective absorption coefficient than that of the surrounding normal tissue at a given laser wavelength, then the threshold pulse fluence for ablation will be proportionally lower and at pulse fluences near this threshold the ablation efficiency may be significantly higher. Prince et al.[9] demonstrated such selective ablation using a flash-lamp pumped dye laser at 480 nm. This selectivity is the result of the yellow pigment in fatty lesions, which increases the absorption coefficient of this tissue for blue light by almost twofold. Thus for a given pulse of energy, twice as much energy is absorbed in any thin layer near the surface. This surface layer heats to the vapor point more rapidly and thus reaches the threshold for ablation at lower values of total energy delivered to the tissue (or lower average surface irradiance). We have demonstrated this selectivity of ablation using both a repetitively pulsed dye laser at 480 nm and a cw Argon laser at 488 nm (Fig. 8-6). Selectivity between tissue types is conferred at average tissue irradiances which are above threshold for soft, pigmented atheroma but not for unpigmented normal tissue (2 to 6 W/mm^2). This same selectivity has been observed for normal tissue impregnated with hemoglobin which also absorbs strongly at these wavelengths. For atheroma without pigmentation, such preferential ablation is not observed. At any wavelength for which the effective absorption coefficient for atheroma is higher than for normal wall, such preferential effects can be observed when operating at or below the threshold for ablating normal tissue. With increasing irradiance, ablation efficiency for unpigmented soft tissue increases and this selectivity for pigmented tissues diminishes rapidly. Therefore, in order to use this selectivity, it is necessary to maintain tissue laser dosimetry very accurately, direct probe-tissue contact, and avoid blood absorption.

It is possible that such selective effects could also arise from the increase in tissue turbidity (decrease in mean distance before scattering) associated with atheroma. In such a case the apparent absorption coefficient increases merely because light diffuses back and forth before it travels the 1/e distance for absorption (Fig. 8-2A). Thus the path that light travels to a given depth is longer; and light is more superficially absorbed. Such an effect can only be significant when the absorption coefficient is rather weak (that is, scattering coefficient ≥ absorption coefficient as shown in Fig. 8-2A).

By quantitating the ablation on human necropsy aorta under saline, we conclude that the cumulative effects of subthreshold 2-μsec dye laser pulses (< 0.42 J/mm^2 each at five to seven pulses per second) and CW argon laser (at 2.5 to 5 W/mm^2) are roughly equivalent in their ability to ablate soft yellow atheroma or hemorrhagic tissue while not ablating either normal or atheromatous tissue which is unpigmented (Fig. 8-6). This effect might be used to provide limited selectivity for soft, pigmented obstructions, if dosimetry is precisely controlled and the probe is held in contact with the tissue. Because hemoglobin strongly absorbs 480-nm light, laser angioplasty with a thin layer of blood between the target tissue and the probe might be efficient at slightly lower fluences than predicted in Table 8-1. In this case, however, selectivity would be lost.

HOLMIUM: YAG/YLF LASERS IN THE INFRARED

The holmium solid-state lasers in various crystal substrates (YAG, YLF, and YSSG) operate at 2.1 μm (2.088 and 2.106) which is near a water absorption peak at 1.93 μm. Although this water absorption peak has an absorption coefficient of 140 cm^{-1} at 1.93 μm[10] (tissue absorption ~100 cm^{-1}), the absorption of water falls off to 30 cm^{-1} by 2.09 to 2.11 μm, the wavelengths of the holmium lasers. Thus for this laser, tissue absorption coefficient a is~21 cm^{-1} (a′ slightly more) which is approximately the value for Ar laser lines (488 and 516 nm). Tissue effects would not be expected to be much different from high power Ar laser systems presently in use. Currently available holmium lasers give 200-μsec pulses of up to 1 J which are easily transmitted by 100- to 200-μm flexible silica fibers selected for high infrared transmittance. Our preliminary results with wet field ablation of diseased arteries (both soft and calcified atheroma) through these fibers show tissue histology rather similar to argon laser ablation (200-μm zone of thermal damage) but with some signs of mechanical disruption of the tissue often associated with shock waves (Fig. 8-7). Additionally, calcified tissue is ablated, although with very low efficiency (~50 J/mm^3) and high thresholds (~6.3 J/mm^2). Both of these effects probably arise from the short pulse and high peak powers of the laser relative to the Ar laser. The holmium laser is a relatively small reliable solid-state laser with very high peak powers (~5000 W). Although it may be easier to maintain and more portable than a high power (10 to 20 W) argon laser, it does not appear to provide fundamental ablative advantages over the argon laser systems already extensively examined. Because it relies on water absorption of approximately equal magnitude for all normal and diseased arteries, the ablation would not be selective when operating near threshold (as are Ar and pulsed dye lasers operating near the hemoglobin and flavin absorption peaks) unless the apparent absorption coefficient in atheroma is significantly greater due to its consistently higher scattering coefficient σ_{sc}.

PULSED LASERS WITH STRONG TISSUE ABSORPTION: A COMPARISON OF EXCIMER AND Er:YAG LASERS

Favorable early reports on excimer laser in vitro ablation of atheroma[11,12] have led to re-

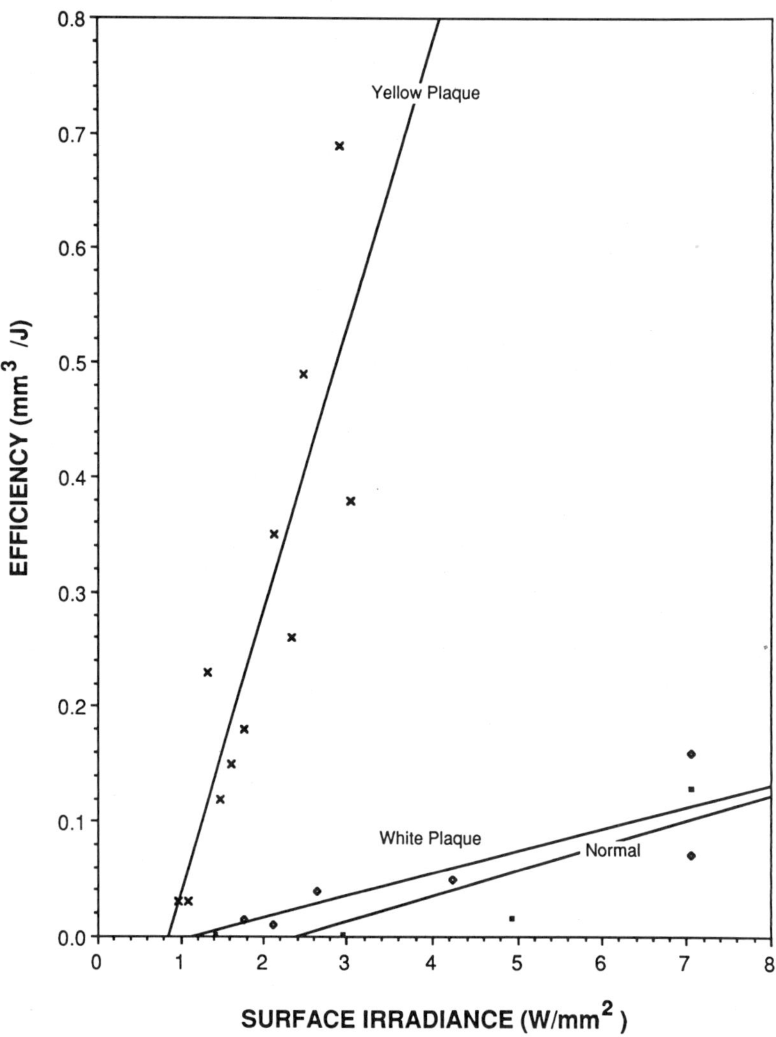

Fig. 8-6. The dependence of ablation efficiency on surface irradiance with an argon laser at 488 nm for pigmented and unpigmented atheroma and normal artery from human necropsy are compared. At surface irradiance values near threshold (1.5 to 3.0 W/mm^2) the pigmented atheroma can be selectively ablated.

cent attempts to develop prototype excimer laser angioplasty systems, most of which use XeCl excimer lasers at 308 nm or XeF at 351 nm. In vitro studies have shown that the 308-nm excimer laser (with pulse lengths between 10 and 200 nsec) gives precise and efficient ablation of both soft and calcified tissues (the latter with higher thresholds and lower efficiencies) at pulse fluences capable of being delivered in silica fibers (<13 J/cm^2). Beginning 2 years ago, we collaborated with laser and optical fiber specialists at the Naval Re-

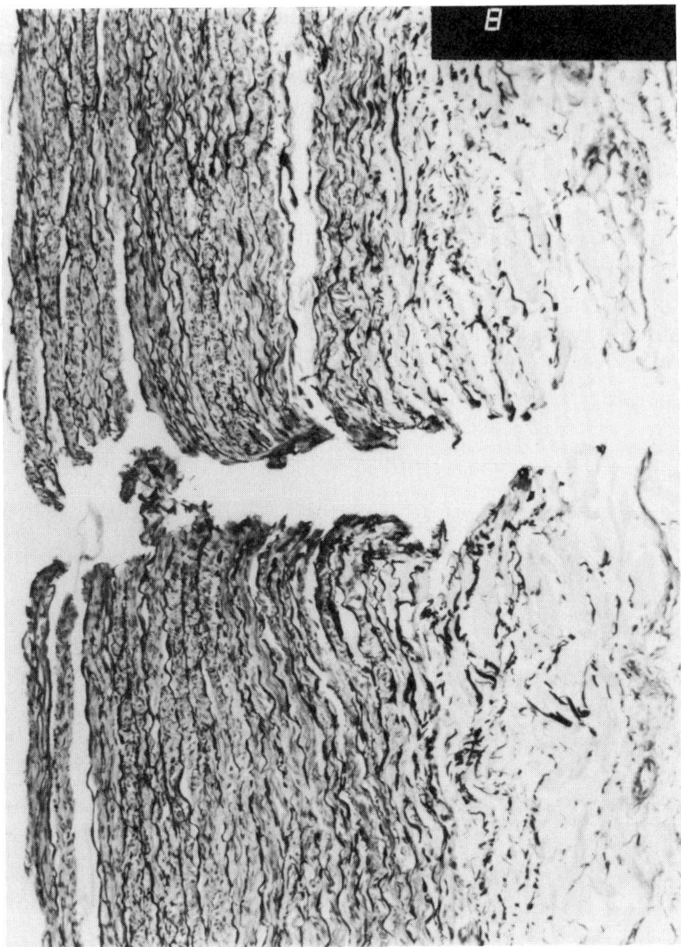

Fig. 8-7. Histology of ablation craters created in human necropsy arterial specimens with the holmium:YAG laser at 2.09 μm (200/μsec pulse length, 300 to 800 mJ) delivered through low hydroxyl silica fibers in a wet field typically shows little thermal damage but severe acoustic damage in the form of fissures and surface irregularities.

search Lab (NRL) to demonstrate equivalent results using 70-μsec pulses from a small Er: YAG laser at 2.9 μm transmitted through zirconium fluoride glass fibers.[13-15] The combination of the precise surface remodeling without thermal damage and the ability to ablate calcified atheroma make both these lasers attractive candidates for a new generation of laser angioplasty systems.

In order to evaluate which of these lasers might be a better technology to refine for clinical use, we have compared the ablation parameters and mechanisms, fiber optic damage and possible catheter designs for these two very different laser sources.[15] We delivered both erbium and XeCl laser pulses in air and through optical fibers onto the surface of tissue. The lasers were repetitively pulsed at 1 to 5 pps (at low pulse rate to minimize cumulative thermal effects of previous pulses). We determined the surface fluence (energy per unit area per pulse) on the target, the total number of pulses delivered and quantified the histological effects on the tissue by microscopy (including the dimensions of the ablated crater and the damage to the surrounding tissue). With the pulsed erbium lasers, delivered both through air (direct gaussian beam) and in a saline field through zirconium fluoride optical fibers, the craters were precise with minimal damage to the remaining tissue for both normal artery wall, all forms of human atheroma, and bone (Fig. 8-8). Tissue ablation using either Er:YAG or excimer (KrF at 248 nm and XeCl at 308 nm) lasers in air and through fibers in a wet field gave comparable efficiencies and thresholds (Figs. 8-9 and 8-10). For all tissues, ablation with these lasers show histologically precise craters without coagulation necrosis or adjacent thermal injury. For noncalcified tissue, ablation threshold for erbium lasers (with 70-μsec pulses) was 6 mJ/mm^2 which was comparable to the KrF laser (5 mJ/mm^2) and lower than for XeCl (18 mJ/mm^2). The ablation

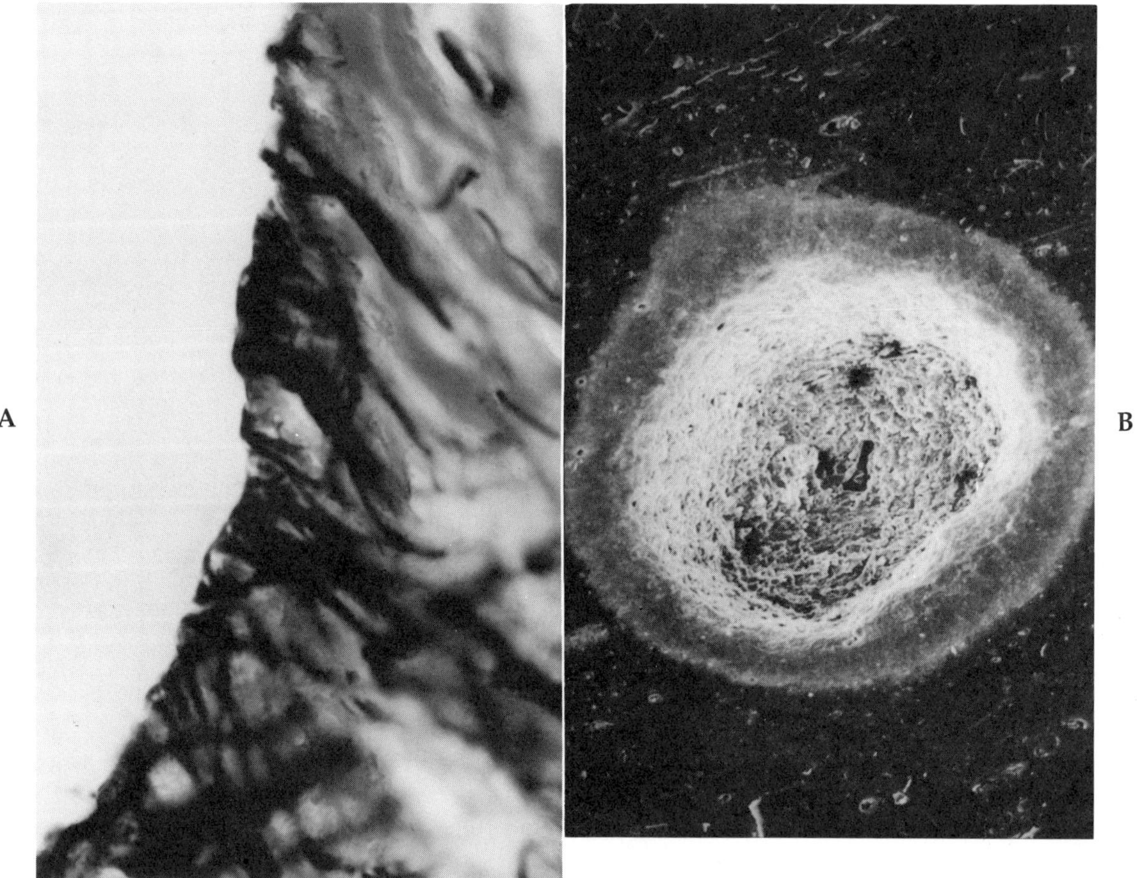

Fig. 8-8. Histology of the craters created with the Er:YAG laser by **A,** wet field ablation of arterial wall using optical fibers and **B,** heavily calcified tissue show smooth surfaces (within 5 μm) and little thermal damage (~5/μm).

thresholds and efficiencies in air and in a wet field were essentially the same.

Er:YAG ABLATION

The Er:YAG laser gives efficient ablation at the parameters predicted in Table 8-1 (100-μsec pulses at fluence of 10 mJ/mm^2) for thermal vaporization. It is important that we observed the same efficiency in a wet field, even though a very thin layer of water will totally absorb the laser pulse. This high efficiency, of course, requires probe–tissue contact. Surprisingly, the ablation appears linear up to pulse fluences ~1000 mJ/mm^2 and ablation depths of ~1 mm (which is ~700 1/e depths) without evidence of shock wave disruption of the tissue. This suggests that the laser heats a thin surface laser to the vaporization point. This layer is then rapidly ejected in a time less than 200 nsec (<<200 μsec/700), during which very little additional energy is deposited in this surface layer. This process continues throughout the 200-μsec laser pulse resulting in an efficient continual etching of the surface to a depth proportional to the pulse fluence. To verify this mechanism, we compared the ablation depth per pulse for normal Er:YAG (200 μsec) and Q-switched Er:YAG (300 nsec) pulses at the same fluence (~2400 mJ/mm^2). For the longer pulse the ablation depth was >1000 μm, whereas it was only 60 μm for the Q-switched pulse. For the shorter pulse, the efficiency drops dramatically because the surface layer (~1.3 μm) is superheated and remains in the beam for ~6 nsec. Thus during a 300 (that is, 50 × 6) nsec pulse, one can only ablate ~50 1/e depths (60 μm). By using the longer pulse Er:YAG, one can maintain high efficiencies of ablation (~0.6 mm^3/J) without fiber damage for pulse fluences >3000 mJ/mm^2, because 6 nsec is a negligible fraction of 200 μsec. This sequential

Er:YAG Laser through Fiber Optics on Aorta

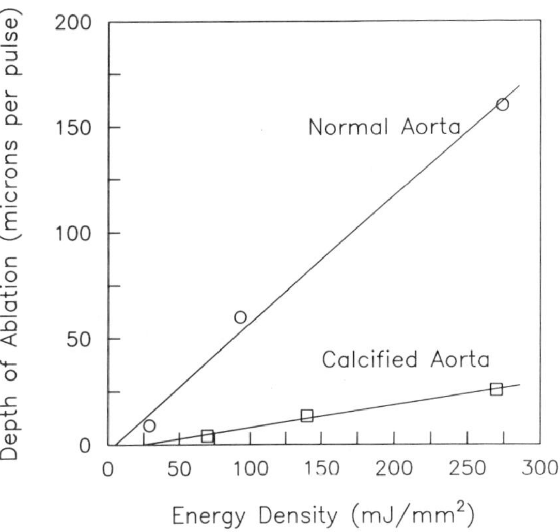

Fig. 8-9. The dependence of ablation depth on pulse fluence for wet field ablation of human necropsy specimens with the Er:YAG laser at 2.9 μm delivered through zirconium fluoride glass fibers shows a low threshold and high efficiency for both soft arterial tissues and heavily calcified atheroma.

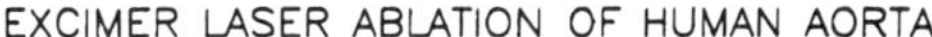

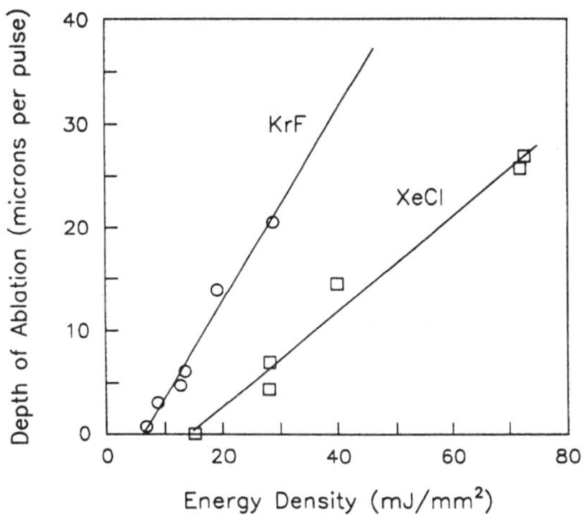

Fig. 8-10. The dependence of ablation depth on pulse fluence for ablation of soft tissues with excimer lasers at 248 nm and 308 nm is comparable to that for Er:YAG lasers for pulse fluences below 100 mJ/mm^2.

etching during a pulse also minimizes shock waves and due to the very local surface absorption allows efficient ablation of heavily calcified tissue. At the end of each pulse only ~10 mJ/mm^2 remains in a superficial ~2-μm layer of tissue at the base of the crater (as shown for time #10 in Fig. 8-4) which decays to ambient over several hundred μsec. Thus, the zone of thermal injury is confined to ~5 μm.

XeCl EXCIMER ABLATION

The 40-nsec pulses of XeCl excimer laser at 308 nm show very similar ablation and efficiency to that of the Er:YAG over the range of 20 to 100 mJ/mm^2. This is not predicted by the values in Table 8-1, which assume linear absorption of ~200 cm^{-1} at 308 nm (compared to 8000 cm^{-1} at 2.9 μm) leading to thermal vaporization. Additionally, infrared video thermography of the surface temperature of tissue exposed to pulses at the ablation threshold for the XeCl laser shows a temperature elevation of only ~20° C (energy deposition of ~60 mJ/mm^3), which is also inconsistent with thermal vaporization. All these measurements were performed at low pulse rates (1 pps). At higher pulse rates (~50 pps), thermal vaporization may be more important. There have been a number of suggestions[4,12] that the excimer laser ablation is the direct result of bond breakage by high-energy UV photons. Recently we have demonstrated power-dependent (that is, nonlinear) peptide bond breakage in blood cells and plasma for peak irradiances >1 MW/cm^2 (pulse fluences of 0.5 mJ/mm^2 for our 40-nsec pulses), which are presumably the result of the sequential absorption of two photons by the same protein molecule within the laser pulse.[16] The sum of the energy in these two photons is great enough to break peptide bonds. Such molecular fragmentation may play a significant role in the precise tissue ablation with the excimer at low pulse rates. The clean edges of ablation may be the boundary at which a significant fraction of macromolecules are fragmented. A concern for the long-term biological response of artery wall exposed to this radiation is the high likelihood of point damage to DNA and proteins. Complete DNA inactivation[16] occurs at cumulative doses of ~10–50 mJ/mm^2. Point DNA defects might occur many space constants (1/a ~50 μm) from the fiber. "Two-photon" ablation would be expected to show a decrease in efficiency as the pulse length increases from 40 nsec (in contrast to thermal vaporization mechanism which would be pulse length independent for pulses up to 1 msec long as shown in Table 8-1). Thus, if this molecular fragmentation mechanism is necessary for the precise ablation observed with this laser, increasing the pulse length in order to decrease fiber damage will be accompanied by some loss in ablation efficiency.

As one increases the XeCl laser pulse energy to >100 mJ/mm^2, fiber damage becomes a critical factor due to nonlinear mechanism within the silica fiber. Working at these higher fluences without a fiber, we have seen plasma formation at the tissue surface which (1) decreases ablation efficiency and (2) creates shock waves which create fissures in the underlying muscle wall.

If one uses an excimer at low pulse energies (which are easier to transmit through flexible optical fibers) and high repetition rates (for example, 308 nm at 50 pps and 10 mJ/mm^2), then thermal ablation may become the predominant ablative mechanism. In this case, the ablation efficiency will increase with pulse rate (or average power). The thermal damage to the artery wall would increase dramatically (>100 μm in Table 8-1) from that observed with the more efficient high-energy pulses (Fig. 8-9). Similarly when using the XeF excimer at 351 nm where tissue exhibits a weaker absorption (1/a ~100 μm), low-energy pulses at high repetition rates will create significant thermal damage due to the higher average powers and the inefficiency of the ablative process.

FIBER-OPTIC TRANSMISSION 308 nm AND 2.9 μM

A critical component of laser angioplasty is a flexible, catheter-based fiber-optic delivery system. The cw argon laser transmitted through silica fibers was already in medical use when the first attempts of laser angioplasty were made. It was an easy choice on the basis of available technology. The pulsed CO_2 laser might be a good choice due to its ablation precision and laser efficiency and medical compatibility, if only a good flexible fiber were available. The laser–fiber-optic catheter system must be highly flexible and durable while transmitting pulses resulting in efficient tissue ablation. The larger the fiber diameter, d, the more energy it may carry without internal damage (pulse energy ~d^2), but the stiffer it becomes (as d^4). Thus, a small flexible fiber optic compatible with a coronary catheter must have a very high damage threshold (laser pulse energy per unit cross-sectional area of the fiber core) for the laser used. A flexible coronary catheter requires the use of fibers ~100 to 200 μm in diameter with a bend radius of ~5 mm (Fig. 8-11). To ablate tissue efficiently with either XeCl or Er:YAG lasers, one must supply ~30 to 40 mJ through a fiber to a 1-mm^2 surface.

The excimer lasers have inherently very short pulses (5 to 200 nsec). Therefore, very high peak powers (0.4 gigawatt/cm^2 for a 40-nsec, 40-mJ pulse carried in 600-μm diameter fiber) result when this pulse is focused onto a small fiber. All optical materials start to exhibit damage at peak irradiances near this level at 308 nm due to nonlinear field strength dependent processes. Using commercial silica fibers, 0.4 gigawatts/cm^2 is the maximum level that we have transmitted before catastrophic damage to the fiber (or 4 mJ in a 200-μm fiber). Taylor[17] has characterized a variety of commercial silica fibers for their transmission and damage thresholds at excimer wavelength and showed that, as theoretically predicted, the damage threshold increases as ~the square root of the pulse duration (that is, only a factor of 2 in going from 40 nsec to 200 nsec). It will be very difficult to increase significantly either the damage threshold (peak power) of silica fibers or the pulse length of the excimer (beyond 200 nsec). Thus, although it is easy to ablate atheroma in vitro through a 600-μm commercial silica fiber in contact with tissue and transmitting 8 to 15 mJ pulses (fluence ~30 to 60 mJ/mm^2), one has severe constraints when trying to design a flexible and reliable catheter for use with the XeCl laser. We have made a prototype flexible multiple fiber bundle (seven 200-μm silica fibers as diagrammed in Fig. 8-11A) for use with the excimer laser, but have serious doubts about the reliability of such a design. As one attempts to design a versatile, durable catheter for the XeCl excimer laser source, many restrictions on the design arise because the fiber damage threshold is not much higher than necessary for the ablation atheroma, particularly that which is calcified.

Our early work at the NRL with prototype Er:YAG laser and zirconium fluoride glass fiber demonstrated the feasibility and some practical advantages of this technology for laser angioplasty. It must, however, be stressed that at that time there was no commercial source for either the laser or fiber. Recently, the flash-lamp Er:YAG laser emitting up to 1 J per pulse at 2.9 μm at repetition rates of up to 5 to 10 pps has become commercially available. From our experience, this laser appears to be ideally suited to its use in medical environments for microsurgery due to its size, reliability, and ablative effects. Silica fiber absorbs this wavelength too strongly to be useful for 1- to 2-m long catheters. The zirconium fluoride glass fiber can be manufactured by the same methods as conventional silica fiber and has the potential for being nearly as strong and durable. The refinement of the technology for large-scale production of zirconium fluoride glass with the reproducible strength and high damage thresholds neces-

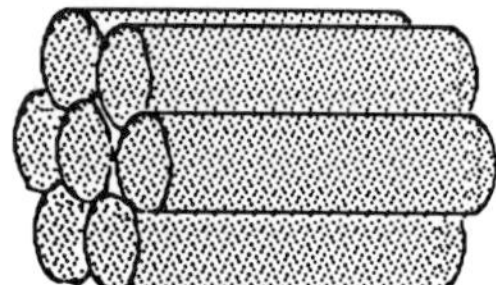

A) Flexible Densely-packed Multiple Fiber Probe

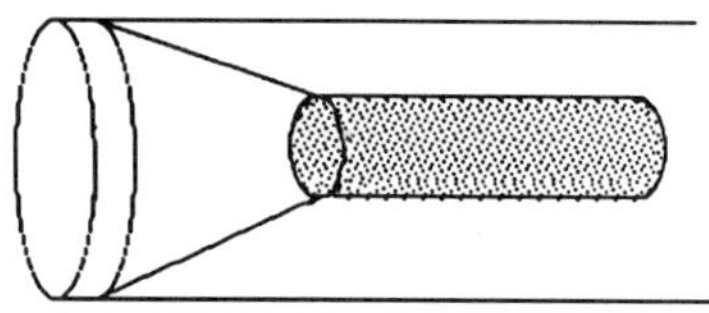

B) Windowed Catheter with Flexible Single Fiber

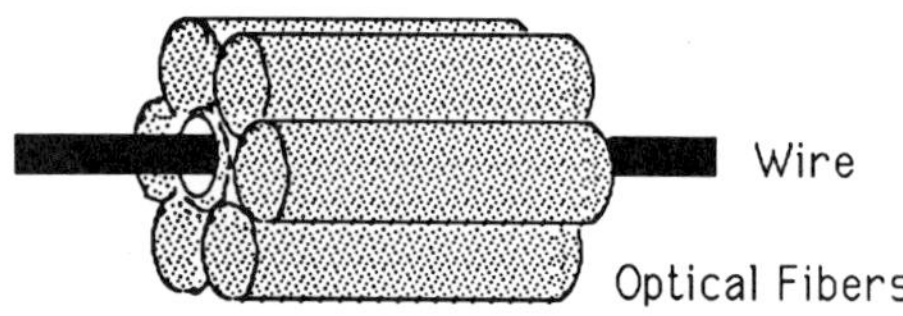

C) Flexible Densely-packed Multiple Fiber Probe with over-the-wire Guidance

Laser Catheter Design Concepts

Fig. 8-11. Flexible laser catheter design concepts require the use of small, flexible glass optical fibers. **A,** and **C,** Dense packed arrays of small fibers increase flexibility over larger single fibers. **B,** Windowed catheters using a small single fiber require that the damage threshold of the fiber is greater than the tissue ablation threshold.

sary for laser angioplasty requires additional commercial effort. We have, however, seen dramatic improvement in the strength of this fiber to where it is typically nearly as strong (tensile strength ~ 80 kpsi) as silica fiber and in selected samples can transmit >300-mJ pulses (200-μsec duration) through a 200-μm core. Thus, in contrast to the excimer laser systems, the Er:YAG laser appears to be physically compatible with a variety of flexible catheter designs while operating at highly efficient pulse energies (Fig. 8-11).

GUIDANCE

Second generation laser angioplasty systems using Er:YAG or XeCl lasers might approach the ideal of precise, localized ablation of all forms of atheroma. When operating at low pulse rates (~5 pulses per second), ablation velocities of 0.2 to 0.5 mm/sec with minimal damage to the underlying artery wall might be achieved while using a flexible catheter and minimal force. Such a tool without effective guidance might perforate the wall of tortuous vessels, such as the coronaries. There have been a variety of guidance systems employed in existing prototype laser angioplasty systems using other lasers. Over-the-wire systems (with either concentric or eccentric wires), concentric balloon catheters, or optical sensing catheters (probe-and-fire), all attempt to minimize perforation risk. The success of any of these guidance systems will depend on the flexibility and durability of the catheter and the details of its design as well as the ablative precision of the laser system. For this reason, we feel it is of critical importance that the intrinsic damage thresholds for 100- to 200-μm fibers be greater than the laser pulse energies needed to ablate a 1-mm^2 surface. This may be a critical factor limiting the applicability of excimer lasers at pulse energies needed for precise ablation. On the other hand, the prototype commercial zirconium fluoride fibers exhibit very high damage thresholds relative to energies needed for efficient ablation of ~1-mm^2 surface of atheroma in a wet field.

CONCLUSIONS

There have been a large number of laser/fiber-optic systems developed for clinical microsurgery at a variety of accessible anatomical sites. The first argon laser angioplasty systems were quite similar to systems used for endoscopic photocautery and opening of airway obstructions. Percutaneous coronary laser angioplasty requires a much greater flexibility and precision than any other endoscopic laser systems presently in clinical use. Currently available cw laser angioplasty systems and "hot-tip" catheters may be acceptable in large, straight peripheral arteries, but are too crude for efficacious use in small, tortuous, "unforgiving" coronary arteries. If techniques using such hot-tip laser angioplasty systems are proven efficacious, they will likely be supplanted by nonlaser hot-tip catheters using electrical or chemical production of heat.

Our focus has been to develop a pulsed laser system transmitted through flexible fiber optics which is capable of precise, predictable ablation of targeted tissue with minimal damage to the remaining tissue. The flash lamp-driven Er:YAG laser provides laser pulses at nearly optimal pulse durations for highly efficient tissue ablation with the greatest possible precision for a thermal process using ubiquitous tissue absorption. The laser pulses can be delivered to the surface of a tissue in a wet field by zirconium fluoride optical fibers at an intrafiber fluence in excess of 9000 mJ/mm^2 as compared with efficient tissue ablation of 50 microns per pulse at 90 mJ/mm^2. This technology appears to provide a means of performing precise laser microsurgery to many heretofore inaccessible sites within the body. It is appropriate for calcified as well as soft tissue ablation. The competing technology of excimer laser angioplasty appears to be less promising due to the complexity of the laser and its use in a clinical environment and the limitations on catheter design due to optical fiber damage at the high peak powers necessary for efficient ablation of atheroma.

REFERENCES

1. Leon, M.B., Smith, P.D., and Bonner, R.F.: Laser angioplasty delivery systems: design considerations. In White, R.A., and Grundfest, W.S., editors: Lasers in Cardiovascular Disease, 1987, pp. 44–63.
2. Meyers, S.M., Bonner, R.F., Rodrigues, M.M., et al.: Phototransection of vitreal membranes with the carbon dioxide laser in rabbits, Ophthalmology **90:**563, 1983.
3. Bonner, R.F., Meyers, S.M., and Gaasterland, D.E.: Threshold for retinal damage associated with the use of high-power neodymium:YAG lasers in the vitreous, Am. J. Ophthalmol. **96:**153, 1983.
4. Srinivasan, R., and Leigh, W.J.: Ablative photodecomposition action of far ultraviolet (193 nm) laser radiation on polyethylene/terephthalate films, J. Am. Chem. Soc. **150:**220, 1985.
5. Abela, G.S., Normann, S.J., Cohen, D.M., et al.: Laser recanalization of occluded atherosclerotic arteries in vivo and in vitro, Circulation **71:**403, 1985.
6. Ginsburg, R., Wexler, L., Mitchell, R.S., et al.: Percutaneous transluminal laser angioplasty for treatment of peripheral vascular disease: clinical response with 16 patients, Radiology **156:**619, 1985.
7. Spears, J.R.: PTCA restenosis: potential prevention with laser balloon angioplasty (LBA), Am. J. Cardiol. 1987. (In press.)
8. Lu, D.Y., Leon, M.B., and Bowman, R.L.: Electrical thermal angioplasty: catheter design features, in vitro tissue ablation studies, and in vivo experimental findings, Am. J. Cardiol. 1987. (In press.)
9. Prince, M.R., Deutsch, T.F., Matthews-Roth, M.M., et al.: Preferential light absorption in atheromas in vitro: implications for laser angioplasty, J. Clin. Invest. **78:**295, 1986.
10. Hale, G.M., and Querry, M.R.: Optical constants of water in the 200 nm to 200 μm wavelength region, Applied Optics **12:**555, 1973.
11. Grundfest, W.S., Litvack, F., Forrester, J.S., et al.: Laser ablation of human atherosclerotic plaque without adjacent tissue injury, J. Am. Coll. Cardiol. **5:**929, 1985.
12. Srinivasan, R.: Ablation of polymers and biological tissues by ultraviolet lasers, Science **234:**559, 1986.
13. Esterowitz, L., Hoffman, C.A., Tran, D.C., et al.: Angioplasty with a laser and fiber optics at 2.94 μm, SPIE **622:**1986.
14. Bonner, R.F., Smith, P.D., Leon, M.B., et al.: Quantification of tissue effects due to a pulsed Er:YAG laser at 2.9 μm with beam delivery in a wet field via zirconium fluoride fibers. In Optical fibers in medicine II, ed. by A. Katzir. SPIE **713:**2, 1986.
15. Bonner, R.F., Smith, P.D., Leon, M.B., et al.: A new erbium laser and infrared fiber system for laser angioplasty (abstract). Circulation **74**(suppl 2):361, 1986.
16. Prodouz, K.N., Fratantoni, J.C., and Bonner, R.F.: Use of laser-UV for inactivation of virus in blood products, Blood **70:**589, 1987.
17. Taylor, R.S., Leopold, K.E., and Singleton, D.: Fiber optics for high power excimer lasers. CLEO Annual Meeting Baltimore, 1987.

Chapter 9

Laser Angioplasty of Peripheral Arteries with a Sapphire-Tip Catheter

Jean L. Fourrier, MD
Jean M. Brunetaud, MD
Phillipe Marache, PhD
Serge Mordon, PhD
Jean M. Lablanche, MD
Michel E. Bertrand, MD

The cardiovascular applications of laser angioplasty are receiving growing attention, and several reports have demonstrated that totally occluded peripheral vessels can be recanalized with percutaneous transluminal laser angioplasty. The laser delivery in blood vessels can be achieved by three different methods.

1. Laser angioplasty can be performed with a bare optic fiber coupled to different laser sources (Nd-YAG and argon).[1-5] However, there are several practical limitations to this technique: (a) the vaporization creates a narrowed tunnel, (b) the direct contact with the blood results in back burning of the distal tip of the optical fiber, and (c) the sharp edge of the fiber can cause wall injury and even perforations.[6-8]
2. Laser angioplasty has been performed with modified bare fiber characterized by a metallic protection of the distal tip. This could be achieved with the hot-tip system allowing thermal angioplasty.[9-12]

   A combination of free laser vaporization and thermal effects was obtained with the hybrid system of Abela.[13]
3. Finally, the distal tip of the optical fiber can be protected by a synthetic sapphire and lensed balls.[14-16] In this study

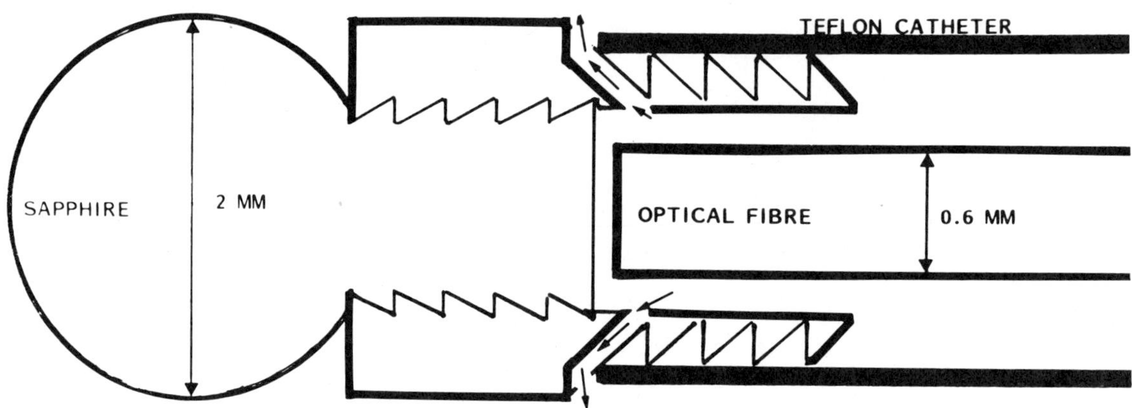

Fig. 9-1. Laser angioplasty catheter with the sapphire connected to the catheter.

we report the preliminary results obtained with sapphire-tip laser angioplasty.

METHODS

We designed an optically modified laser catheter with the following characteristics (Fig. 9-1):

1. We used a synthetic round sapphire, 2.2 mm in diameter (Laser Sonics, Santa Clara, California). This anisotropic and birefringent crystal has a high melting point (2020° C) and combined with a Nd-YAG laser source, its refractive index is 1.7545 for 1064 nm. The sapphire has a focusing effect with a focal length located 2 mm beyond the tip of the probe.
2. The optical fiber is a quartz optic fiber, 600 microns in diameter.
3. This fiber was introduced into a Teflon catheter (7F). Figure 9-1 shows that the sapphire was screwed onto a metallic universal connector attached to the Teflon catheter. The distal tip of the fiber is very close to but not in contact with the proximal part of the sapphire. The Teflon catheter was continuously washed by a saline solution. This infusion allows a permanent cleaning of the interface between sapphire and the optical fiber to prevent the back burning of the latter.

   The circulation of this infusion (20 ml/min) from the proximal part of the catheter to the two side holes cools the sapphire, the metallic connector, and the vessel wall during laser emission. Finally, the two side holes allow injection of contrast medium to verify the position of the catheter in the vessel.
4. The laser source was a Nd-YAG with a wavelength of 1020 nm (Cilas, France), a power range from 5 to 45

watts, and a possibility of exposure time from 0.2 to 10 seconds.

POPULATION STUDY

This study included 20 patients (17 men, 3 women) ranging in age from 42 to 73 years (mean 55). All had severe symptoms and were candidates for surgery. Eight patients had severe intermittent claudication. Seven patients had additional rest pain, and five had skin ulcerations. The lesions were located on the superficial femoral artery in 16 and on the popliteal artery in 4 patients. Angiography detected a narrowing in 2 patients and a total obstruction in 18 patients. The length of the occlusion ranged from 5 to 45 cm.

All the patients gave their informed consent. They received nifedipine (60 mg) and aspirin (500 mg/day) before the procedure. A premedication was obtained with an IV injection of 50 mg of chlorazepate.

PROCEDURE

A 8F sheath was introduced into the femoral artery under local anesthesia. After IV injection of 10,000 units of heparin, the tip of the catheter, with its metallic connector clearly visible under fluoroscopy, was placed closed to the occlusion which was detected by small injections of contrast medium.

With the probe placed at 2 mm of the occlusion (focal length of the sapphire), the laser emission was started. Most often, several shots at 40 J were able to open a new tunnel in which the probe was introduced. Additional laser shots at 15 J were done while the probe was gently and slightly advanced into the atherosclerotic segment. The progression of the catheter was repeatedly checked by injection of contrast medium. As a result of laser vaporization, small bubbles could be seen around the sapphire. When the occlusion was crossed, the catheter was pulled back and the new tunnel was opacified. Most often the procedure was completed by a balloon angioplasty.

EVALUATION OF THE IMMEDIATE RESULTS

The luminal diameter along the tunnel created by laser angioplasty was carefully measured with a calibration factor calculated from the size of the metallic connector (2 mm). Sapphire laser angioplasty was considered successful if a channel 2 mm in diameter was obtained without complications (perforation or embolization).

RESULTS

The procedure was successful in 17 patients; this result was obtained with laser angioplasty alone in 3 patients; most often (13 cases) the new channel had a small diameter (2 to 2.5 mm), and the procedure was completed by balloon angioplasty.

Figure 9-2 shows a typical example of a patient with a total occlusion of the lower part of the superficial femoral artery. After laser angioplasty a new channel, 2 mm in diameter, was obtained, and balloon angioplasty obtained a marked enlargement of the vessel and a satisfactory result. A similar result is observed in another patient (Fig. 9-3).

In these series, there was one case of wall entry and two perforations. In these patients, the intermittent opacification of the recanalized channel showed an extravasation of the contrast medium. Laser delivery was stopped, and these perforations were without clinical consequence.

After the procedure, the patients were studied clinically with doppler velocimetry, and a second angiographic study was performed 2 months later. Reocclusion occurred in three patients within the first week of the

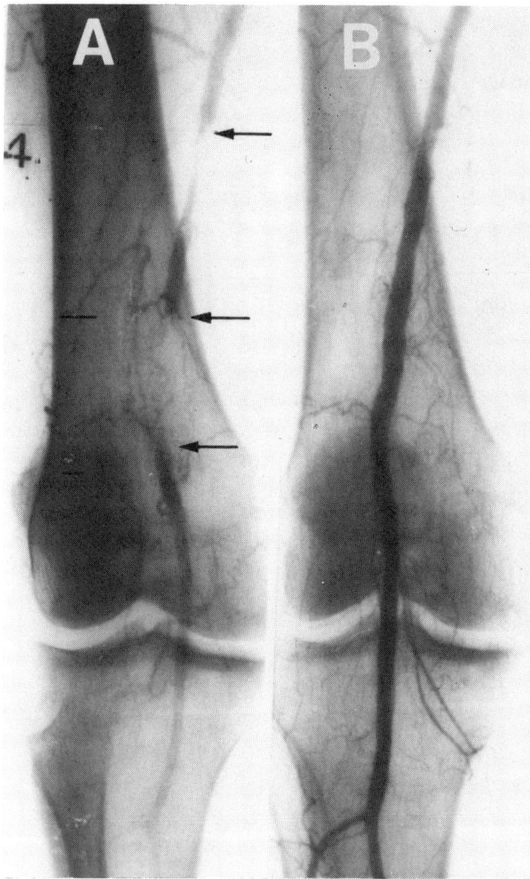

Fig. 9-2. A, Total occlusion of the lower part of the superficial femoral artery. Occlusion is preceded by a long narrowing. **B,** Final result after laser recanalization completed by balloon dilatation.

procedure. Two months later, angiography showed three additional reclosures. The ten remaining patients had a marked improvement of their clinical conditions. Five patients had a sustained good result 1 year after the procedure, and one of them still shows excellent results 18 months after laser angioplasty.

The results are summarized in Table 9-1: there were 16 technical successes; early reclosure was observed in 3 patients and late reclosures were detected by angiography at 2 months in 3 other patients. The rate of current patency was 50%.

DISCUSSION

Over the past 5 years, several studies have reported the results of in vivo or in vitro experimental studies concerning the effects of laser on blood vessels. However, there are few clinical reports concerning laser angioplasty of peripheral vessels in humans. The first attempts were done with optical bare fibers. However, some limitations rapidly occurred with this technique: the sharp edge of the tip of the optical fiber could induce wall injury and even perforation. Moreover, some charred particles could occur at the tip of the fiber as a result of the back burning due to the high-power energy delivered through the blood. Finally, the laser-created channel was narrowed, and this could explain the high rate of reclosure observed with this technique.

Different authors have proposed to protect the optical fiber with a metal cap: thus, thermal angioplasty with the hot tip system was currently applied by Sanborn and Cumberland. With these probes the diameter of the channel was increased, but, in most cases, the technique required a complementary balloon angioplasty.

In 1986, a new optically modified probe was developed with a sapphire located at the tip of the catheter.

The sapphire offers several advantages: First, the sapphire protects the bare optic fiber, and, because the interface between these two parts is continuously washed with saline, the detrimental back burning effect of the distal fiber tip is avoided. Second, the round sapphire tip of the catheter is less aggressive to the arterial wall. Third, the sapphire probe is able to focus the laser beam; thus, the depth of vaporization is more limited than with conventional bare fibers; moreover, the thermal inertia is rather short and this could

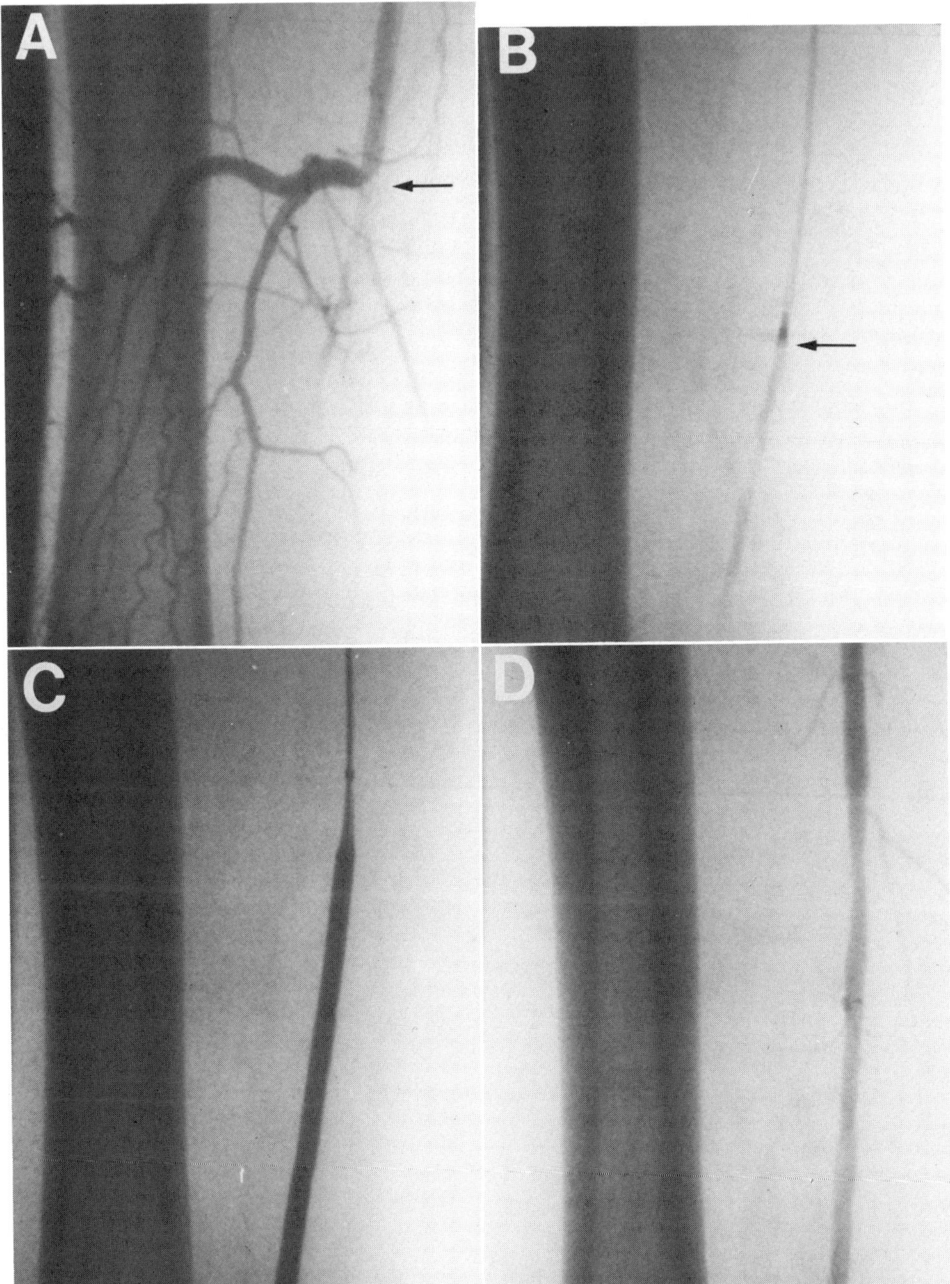

Fig. 9-3. A, Total occlusion of the femoral artery with an important collateral circulation. **B,** New channel obtained by laser recanalization. One can clearly distinguish the tip of the catheter with the metallic connector. **C,** Balloon dilatation. **D,** Final result. Note the disappearance of the collateral circulation.

Table 9-1. Overall Outcome

Number of patients	20
Number of procedures	20
Technical success	16 (80%)
Technical failure	4 (20%)
Early reclosure	3
Late reclosure	3
Sustained good result	10 (50%)

limit the thermal damages along the arterial wall. Finally, from several experimental studies we performed in vitro and in vivo, we concluded that a sapphire laser probe can induce a wider crater than that obtained with a bare fiber tip. These results were recently confirmed by Geschwind et al.[17]

Experimental studies performed in our laboratory showed that a sapphire probe connected to an Nd-YAG laser source was able to vaporize safely atherosclerotic plaques, even with calcifications. Therefore in a second stage, sapphire laser angioplasty was applied to the recanalization of occluded peripheral arteries. The preliminary results reported in this study are already encouraging, but a certain number of problems are still unsolved. The first problem concerns the flexibility of the catheter which should be improved to facilitate the vessel selection; this could be solved with the use of very thin (but possibly more fragile) optical fibers. The second issue concerns the necessity of a steerable system. However, it is not so easy to design a catheter with a coaxial lumen for an optical fiber and a steerable guide wire. These technical improvements are needed to increase the safety and the quality of the procedures.

In conclusion, preliminary results suggest that laser angioplasty with a sapphire-tip catheter may recanalize total occlusion of peripheral vessels, but long-term follow-up studies are required to determine the exact impact of this laser treatment.

REFERENCES

1. Geschwind, H., Boussignac, G., Teisseire, B., et al.: Recanalization of human arteries using Nd-YAG laser carried by optical fiber, J. Biomed. Eng. **6**:281, 1984.
2. Ginsburg, R., Kim, D.S., Guthamer, D., et al.: Salvage of an ischemic limb by laser angioplasty: description of a new technique, Clin. Cardiol. **7**:54, 1984.
3. Choy, D.S.J., Stertzer, S., Myler, R.K., et al.: Human coronary laser recanalization, Clin. Cardiol. **7**:377, 1984.
4. Geschwind, H., Boussignac, G., Teisseire, B., et al.: Percutaneous transluminal laser angioplasty in man, Lancet **1**:844, 1984.
5. Geschwind, H., Boussignac, G., Teisseire, B., et al.: Conditions for effective Nd-YAG laser angioplasty, Br. Heart J. **52**:484, 1984.
6. Isner, J.M., Donaldson, R.F., Funai, J.T., et al.: Factors contributing to perforations resulting from laser coronary angioplasty: observations in an intact human post-mortem preparation of intraoperative laser coronary angioplasty, Circulation **72**:(suppl II):II-191, 1985.
7. Crea, F., Abela, G.S., Fenech, A., et al.: Transluminal laser irradiation of coronary arteries in live dogs: an angiographic and morphologic study of acute effects, Am. J. Cardiol. **57**:171, 1986.
8. Ben Sachar, G., Spector, M.L., Morse, D.E., et al.: Hazardous byproducts of laser irradiation: a qualitative and quantitative study (abstract), J. Am. Coll. Cardiol. **7**:46A, 1986.
9. Sanborn, T.A., Faxon, D.P., Haudenschild, C.C., et al.: Experimental angioplasty: circumferential distribution of laser thermal energy with a laser probe, J. Am. Coll. Cardiol. **5**:934, 1985.
10. Cumberland, D.C., Sanborn, T.A., Tayler, D.I., et al.: Percutaneous laser thermal angioplasty: clinical experience in peripheral artery occlusions (abstract), J. Am. Coll. Cardiol. **7**:211A, 1986.
11. Sanborn, T.A., Cumberland, D.C., Tayler, D.I., et al.: Human peripheral percutaneous laser assisted balloon angioplasty (abstract), Am. Soc. Laser Med. Surg. **6**:40, 1986.
12. Cumberland, D.C., Tayler, D.I., Welch, C.L., et al.: Percutaneous laser thermal angioplasty: initial clinical results with a laser probe in total peripheral artery occlusions, Lancet **1**:1457, 1986.
13. Abela, G.S., Normann, S.J., Cohen, D.M., et al.: Laser recanalization of occluded atherosclerotic arteries in vivo and in vitro, Circulation **71(2)**: 403, 1985.
14. Fourrier, J.L., Lablanche, J.M., Brunetaud, J.M., et al.: Angioplasty by contact sapphire: in vitro study (abstract), Lasers Surg. Med. **6**:177, 1986.
15. Fourrier, J.L., Marache, Ph., Brunetaud, J.M., et al.: Laser recanalization of peripheral arteries by contact sapphire in man (abstract), Circulation **74**:II-204, 1986.
16. Fourrier, J.L., Brunetaud, J.M., Prat, A., et al.: Percutaneous laser angioplasty with sapphire tip (letter), Lancet **I**:105, 1987.
17. Geschwind, H.J., Kern, M.J., Vandormael, M., Efficiency and safety of optically modified fiber tips for laser angioplasty, J. Am. Coll. Cardiol. **10**:655, 1987.

Chapter 10

Observations on Intraoperative Laser Coronary Angioplasty

James J. Livesay, MD, FACC

Recent studies have explored the use of lasers for relief of atherosclerotic obstruction. High-intensity light energy from a variety of laser sources is capable of plaque ablation by a unique process called photovaporization. Using proper laser dosimetry, plaque removal can be accomplished with microscopic precision. Innovative delivery systems have been designed to transmit laser energy to remote intravascular targets. Experimental studies have shown that arterial healing occurs rapidly within 2 to 3 weeks after laser ablation through migration of endothelial cells. Further refinements in laser delivery systems have stimulated clinical investigation of the role of laser angioplasty for catheter-directed and intraoperative application in peripheral and coronary artery disease.

Nearly 20% of coronary patients presenting for surgical revascularization have significant atherosclerotic disease involving the distal coronary tributaries. The presence of distal disease may limit the effectiveness of bypass surgery by compromising myocardial perfusion and by diminishing long-term graft patency. The finding of distal coronary disease influences the selection of patients for treatment and alters the procedure recommended for revascularization. In the past, a variety of techniques has been employed for treatment of distal disease; however, limitations of each have stimulated interest in developing alternate methods for revascularization. In 1984, a prospective clinical trial was organized at the Texas Heart Institute to assess the effectiveness of laser angioplasty as an adjunct for coronary revascularization in patients with distal atherosclerotic disease.

HISTORY OF LASER DEVELOPMENT

The origin of laser theory can be traced to Albert Einstein in 1917.[1] In 1960, the first laser was constructed by Theodore Maiman using a synthetic ruby crystal.[2] Almost immediately, the laser's potential for relief of atherosclerotic plaque was recognized by McGuff.[3] Interest in laser angioplasty was renewed in 1978 after advances occurred in the technology of lasers and optical fibers. Early work by Macruz,[4] Choy,[5] Lee,[6] and coworkers demonstrated the potential for plaque ablation using the argon laser transmitted by tiny optical fibers. As other laser wavelengths were investigated, the operational parameters necessary for precise control were identified and undesirable thermal damage to the arterial wall was avoided.[7-11] Histologic studies revealed remarkably clean incisions in atheromatous plaque using a variety of lasers.[8-13]

Initial clinical investigations with laser catheters by Ginsburg[14,15] in 1984 and others[16-18] demonstrated relief of arterial stenosis in femoral and popliteal arteries. The concept of intraoperative laser angioplasty for use as an adjunct for coronary revascularization was proposed in 1983.[19,20] The first clinical experience with laser angioplasty in the coronary arteries was reported by Choy in 1984. Working in Toulouse, France, these investigators performed intraoperative laser angioplasty in eight patients for relief of proximal stenosis prior to distal bypass grafting.[21] Although their initial results indicated relief of stenosis in seven of eight patients, subsequent angiograms demonstrated early occlusion of all laser-treated segments, presumably due to thrombosis from competitive flow.[22] In 1985, Livesay et al. reported preliminary results of the first FDA-approved clinical trial of laser angioplasty. "Laser endarterectomy" was used for intraoperative revascularization in patients with distal coronary disease.[20,23,24] Successful relief of stenosis was achieved by laser technique in 15 of 16 coronary arteries in 8 patients. Angiographic patency was demonstrated in 75% of arteries after the procedure.[23,24] In subsequent reports in 1986, Sanborn,[25] Cumberland,[26] and Crea[27] have described percutaneous techniques for laser angioplasty in combination with balloon angioplasty to relieve proximal coronary stenosis during cardiac catheterization.

INDICATIONS

Intraoperative laser angioplasty may be used to enhance the potential for revascularization in patients with difficult anatomical obstruction who require coronary bypass surgery.[20] Patients are selected for bypass surgery based on the usual clinical and anatomical criteria after consideration of their symptomatic status and angiographic findings. The indications for intraoperative laser angioplasty include the finding of severe atherosclerosis in one or more distal coronary vessels. Distal disease can be categorized as tandem stenosis, discrete distal stenosis, multiple stenosis in a series, long diffuse stenosis, or total occlusion. Infrequent problems such as distal coronary artery dissection or plaque disruption at the site of a distal anastomosis also may be corrected by laser technique. Intraoperative laser angioplasty also can be used for localized debridement of plaque at the arteriotomy in preparation for anastomosis or for relief of ostial stenosis at the origin of major tributaries. Relative contraindications to the laser procedure include heavily calcified arteries, small tributaries (less than 1.5 mm in outer diameter), and vessels with anticipated low flow rates due to prior infarction or poor runoff.

PATIENTS AND METHODS

Between January 1985 and June 1987, 25 patients underwent intraoperative laser angioplasty as an adjunct to coronary bypass grafting for treatment of a variety of coronary lesions. The patients (22 men and 3 women) ranged in age from 38 to 73 years. Multiple risk factors for atherosclerosis were present in this group of patients, including diabetes, hyperlipidemia, and cigarette smoking in the 6 youngest patients whose ages ranged from 38 to 49 years. Peripheral vascular disease was present in one third of the patients. Three patients had undergone a prior coronary bypass procedure 3 to 10 years earlier and presented with progression of atherosclerosis and graft closure. Of the 25 patients, 22 had triple vessel disease, and all had significant distal coronary disease. Two patients had diffuse involvement of a single coronary artery. One patient also had a tight ostial stenosis (95%) of the left main coronary artery.

The operative techniques employed for coronary revascularization in this patient group are similar to those reported at our institution in 30,646 patients.[28] During the operative procedure, moderate hypothermia perfusion and cold cardioplegia arrest provide the ideal environment for microscopic repair of complex coronary disease. Aortic cross clamping and continuous suction of the ascending aorta are used to remove blood, vapor, or debris during the procedure.[29] Distal plaque is identified by palpation and inspection. A distal arteriotomy is placed at a site preselected for bypass anastomosis. Intraluminal probes are used to confirm the location of the distal stenosis and to assess the internal diameter of critical stenoses before and after treatment.

A specially designed CO_2 laser is prepared for use with a small hollow wave-guide (1.5 mm in diameter) attached for intracoronary transmission. The wave-guide is introduced through the arteriotomy and advanced until it abuts the obstructive plaque[20] (Fig. 10-1). After the laser is aligned visually for coaxial passage, a series of laser pulses is used until the plaque is completely removed. Calibrated probes are used to reassess luminal size and relief of stenosis. Angioscopic inspection can be used to evaluate the results. Additional cardioplegic infusion or saline irrigation is helpful in removing any carbonized residue or potential debris. After laser angioplasty, the complementary distal bypass is completed with either saphenous vein graft or internal mammary artery.

CLINICAL AND ANGIOGRAPHIC RESULTS

The therapeutic objective of the combined laser–bypass procedure was to provide complete revascularization in patients with distal atherosclerotic disease. An average of 3.75 bypass grafts were placed in each patient. In addition to bypass grafting, laser angioplasty was used to remove obstructive lesions in 46 coronary artery segments. Other techniques were employed as well including manual coronary endarterectomy in four arteries, balloon dilatation in five arteries, vein patch angioplasty in five arteries. The CO_2 laser was effective in removing obstructive plaque under direct vision at the arteriotomy and in remote intraluminal locations 6 to 40 mm away. Successful ablation of plaque was observed in 42 of 46 lesions (91%). The laser was used in virtually all coronary artery locations, both epicardial and intramyocardial. An ostial lesion of the left main coronary artery was relieved using an approach through the aortic root. The laser procedure was effective in removing distal obstructions, relieving ostial stenosis, reopening total occlusions, correcting localized dissections, and debriding diffuse atheromatous lesions. Despite the presence of intramural calcium in nearly half the distal arteries treated, the laser was successful in removing plaque in all but two instances in which manual endarterectomy was required. Perforation occurred in one artery when the laser was misaligned.

The clinical course of this patient group has not differed from other similar patients undergoing coronary revascularization. There have been no early or late deaths. Two patients sustained perioperative myocardial infarctions: one due to a protamine reaction and the second in an area of previous infarction supplied by a small diseased artery. An antiplatelet regimen was used in all patients.[30] One patient required reoperation for postoperative tamponade and subsequently developed complications requiring prolonged hospitalization before recovery.

Postoperative coronary angiography has been performed in 18 patients within 3 months of surgery. The angiographic appearance of the laser-treated arteries revealed satisfactory relief of stenosis in localized distal

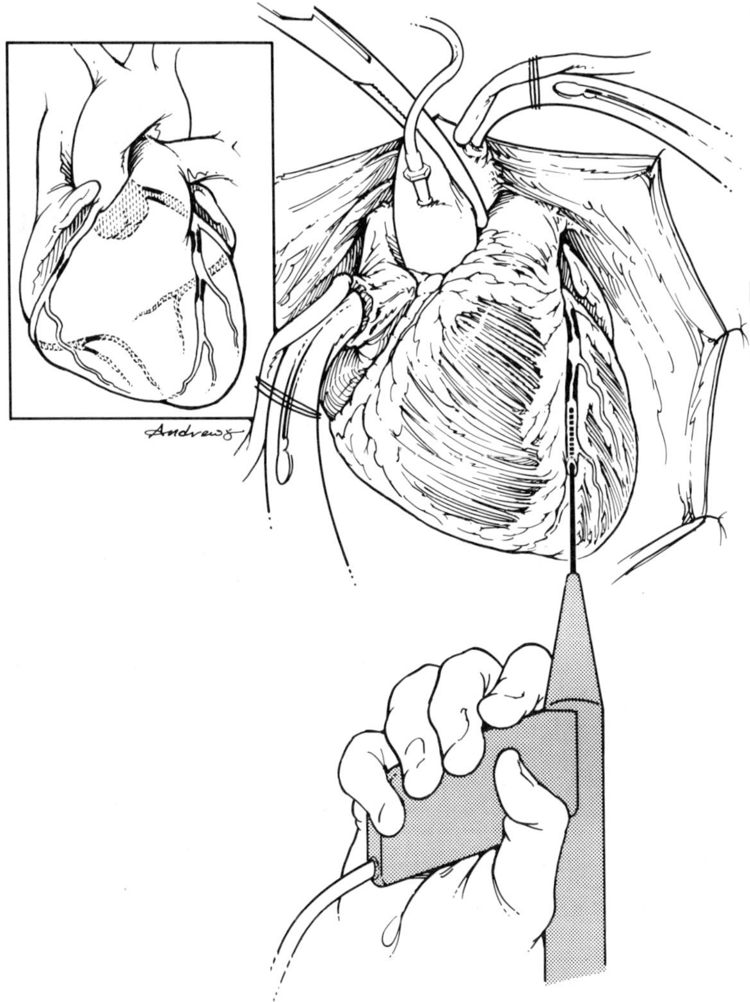

Fig. 10-1. Operative technique of laser endarterectomy for relief of distal coronary disease. A hand-held CO_2 laser is used to remove critical coronary stenosis of the distal artery. A small, hollow laserprobe is inserted through the distal arteriotomy. After relief of distal stenosis, a bypass graft is used to complete revascularization.

stenosis, long diffuse lesions, total occlusions, and multi-segment stenoses (Fig. 10-2). Early patency was observed in 47 of 52 bypass grafts (90%) and in 35 of 37 (95%) bypassed coronary arteries in the absence of distal disease. The angiographic patency of diseased distal arteries after laser angioplasty was somewhat lower (76%—29 of 38 arterial segments). Early thrombosis, which occurred in nine laser-treated arteries, was due to a combination of factors including small arterial size, low flow rates, endothelial ablation, and

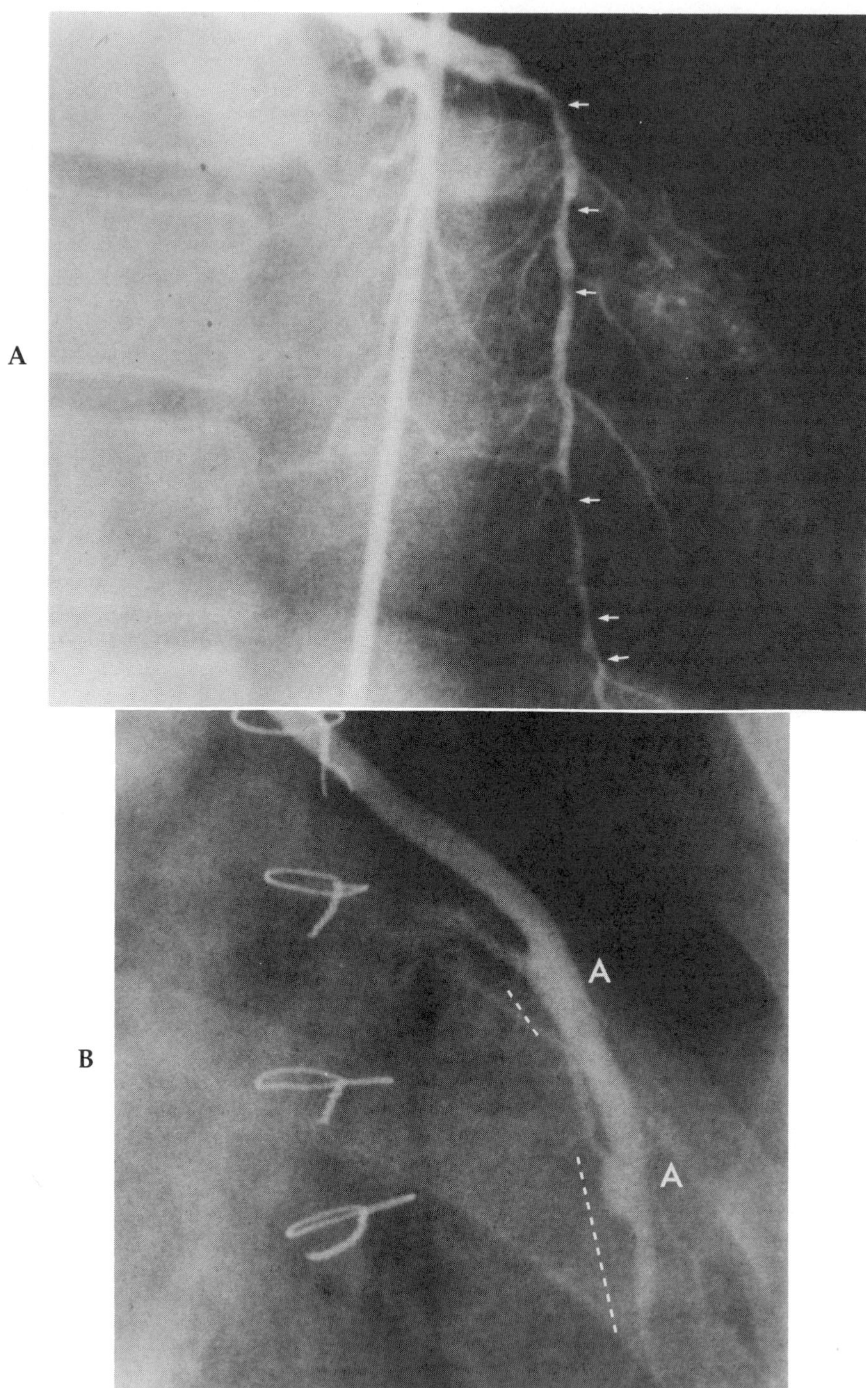

Fig. 10-2. For legend see opposite page.

unrelieved distal obstruction. The early patency rates after laser angioplasty in diseased distal coronary arteries was comparable to the results achieved by manual coronary endarterectomy.[31]

COMMENTS

Intraoperative laser angioplasty has proven to be a useful adjunct to conventional techniques for coronary revascularization. Laser technique offers several advantages, particularly in those patients with distal coronary disease. It affords a unique method of plaque ablation which can be used to relieve stenosis at some distance from the arteriotomy or to enable plaque sculpturing and repair of dissections under direct vision. Plaque removal can be accomplished without the need for the extensive dissection of the artery required by manual endarterectomy; and it avoids the problem of intimal flaps. Nevertheless, both procedures accomplish plaque removal by endothelial ablation, and therefore carry an increased risk of thrombosis especially in small arteries or in low flow situations. While satisfactory relief of stenosis can be achieved by laser angioplasty in a high percentage (91%) of diseased arteries, angiographic patency is demonstrated in a somewhat lower percentage (76%) due to the problem of early thrombosis. Anticoagulant regimens may play a role by enhancing early and late arterial patency rates. Surgical strategies are needed to enhance revascularization in patients with complex coronary disease and to ensure selection of the optimal technique for each anatomical problem. The future development of laser angioplasty affords great promise for new clinical tools that likely will augment present techniques for catheter-directed and intraoperative revascularization.[32]

Fig. 10-2. A, Preoperative left coronary angiogram illustrates diffuse, multisegment stenosis of the LAD coronary artery. Arrows designate multiple sites of stenosis in the proximal, middle, and distal vessel. Note the multiple small diagonal and septal tributaries arising from the midportion of the LAD. **B,** Postoperative angiogram demonstrates a patent saphenous vein graft with anastomosis (*A* label) to the mid and distal LAD. The dashed lines indicate arterial segments treated by laser endarterectomy. Note the improved angiographic appearance of the vessel and prompt filling of tributaries after multisegment laser endarterectomy.

REFERENCES

1. Boraiko, A.A: Lasers, "a splendid light," National Geographic March, 1984.
2. Maiman, T.H.: Stimulated optical radiation in ruby, Nature **187:**493, 1960.
3. McGuff, P.E., Bushnell, D., Soroff, H.S., et al.: Studies of the surgical applications of laser (light amplification by stimulated emission of radiation), Surg. Forum **14:**143, 1963
4. Macruz, R., Martins, J.R.M., Tupinamba, A., et al.: Therapeutic possibilities of laser beams in atheromas, Arq. Bras. Cardiol. **34:**9, 1980.
5. Choy, D.S.J., Stertzer, S.H., Rotterdam, H.Z., et al.: Laser coronary angioplasty: experience with 9 cadaver hearts, Am. J. Cardiol. **50:**1209, 1982.
6. Lee, G., Ikeda, R.M., Kozina, J., et al.: Laser dissolution of coronary atherosclerotic obstruction, Am. Heart J. **102:**1074, 1981.
7. Abela, G.S., Normann, S., Cohen, D., et al.: Effects of carbon dioxide, Nd-YAG, and argon laser radiation on coronary atheromatous plaques, Am. J. Cardiol. **50:**1199, 1982.
8. Grundfest, W.S., Litvack, F., Forrester, J.S., et al.: Laser ablation of human atherosclerotic plaque without adjacent tissue injury, J. Am. Coll. Cardiol. **5:**929, 1985.
9. Kramer, J.R., Bott-Silverman, C., Ratliff, N.E., et al.: Removal of atherosclerotic plaque using multiple short exposures of argon ion laser light. (Submitted for publication.)
10. Livesay, J.J., Johansen, W.E., Sutter, L.V., et al.: Experimental technique of laser coronary endarterectomy and its immediate effects on atherosclerotic plaques in cadaver hearts, Tex. Heart Inst. J. **11:**280, 1984.
11. Livesay, J.J., and Johansen, W.E.: Prevention of arterial wall damage during laser endarterectomy. Proceedings of the ICLAEO '84. Laser Institute of America, 1984.
12. Deckelbaum, L.I, Isner, J.M., Donaldson, R.F., et al.: Use of pulsed energy delivery to minimize tissue injury resulting from carbon dioxide laser irradiation of cardiovascular tissues, J.A.C.C. **7**(4):898, 1986.
13. Geschwind, H., Fabre, M., Chaitman, B.R., et al.: Histopathology after Nd-YAG laser percutaneous transluminal angioplasty of peripheral arteries, J.A.C.C. **8**(5):1089, 1986.
14. Ginsburg, R., Kim, D.S., Guthaner, D., et al.: Salvage of an ischemic limb by laser angioplasty: description of a new technique, Clin. Cardiol. **7:**54, 1984.
15. Ginsburg, R., Wexler, L., Mitchell, R.S., et al.: Percutaneous transluminal laser angioplasty for the treatment of peripheral vascular disease: clinical experience in sixteen patients, Radiology **156:**619, 1984.
16. Abela, G.S., Seeger, J.H., Barbieri, E., et al.: Laser angioplasty with angioscopic guidance in humans, J.A.C.C. **8:**184, 1986.
17. Cumberland, D.C., Sanborn, T.A., Taylor, D.I., et al.: Percutaneous laser thermal angioplasty: initial clinical results with a laser probe in total peripheral artery occlusions, Lancet **I:**1457, 1986.
18. Geschwind, H., Boussignac, G., Teisseire, B., et al.: Percutaneous transluminal laser angioplasty in man, Lancet **1:**844, 1984.
19. Livesay, J.J., Johansen, W.E., Sutter, L.V., et al.: Can laser endarterectomy extend the limits of coronary revascularization? Lasers Surg. Med. **3**(2):173, 1983.
20. Livesay, J.J., and Cooley, D.A.: Laser coronary endarterectomy: proposed treatment for dif-

fuse coronary atherosclerosis, Tex. Heart Inst. J. **11**:276, 1984.
21. Choy, D.S.J., Stertzer, S.H., Myler, R.K., et al.: Human coronary laser recanalization, Clin. Cardiol. **7**:377, 1984.
22. Choy, D.S.J.: Laser applications in cardiovascular disease, Semin. Intervent. Radiol. **3**:1, 1986.
23. Livesay, J.J., Hogan, P.J., and McAllister, H.A.: The development of laser angioplasty, H.E.R.Z. **10**:343, 1985.
24. Livesay, J.J., Leachman, D.R., Hogan, P.J., et al.: Preliminary report on laser coronary endarterectomy in patients, Circulation **72**(III):302, 1985.
25. Sanborn, T.A., Faxon D.P., and Kellett, M.A.: Percutaneous coronary laser thermal angioplasty, J.A.C.C. **8**(6):1437, 1986.
26. Cumberland, D.C., Starkey, I.R., Oakley, G.D.G., et al.: Percutaneous laser-assisted coronary angioplasty, Lancet **1**:214, 1986.
27. Crea, F., Davies, G., McKenna, W., et al.: Percutaneous laser recanalization of coronary arteries, Lancet **2**:214, 1986.
28. Livesay, J.J., Cooley, D.A., Hallman, G.L., et al.: Early and late results of coronary endarterectomy: analysis of 3,369 patients, J. Thorac. Cardiovasc. Surg. **92**(4): 649, 1986.
29. Isner, J.M., Clarke, R.H., Donaldson, R.F., et al.: Identification of photoproducts liberated by in vitro argon laser irradiation of atherosclerotic plaque, calcified cardiac valves and myocardium, Am. J. Cardiol. **55**:1192, 1985.
30. Cheseboro, J.H.: Effect of dipyridamole and aspirin on late vein-graft patency after coronary bypass operations, N. Engl. J. Med. **310**:209, 1984.
31. Keon, W.J., Akyurekli, Y., Bedared, P., et al.: Coronary endarterectomy: an adjunct to coronary artery bypass grafting, Surgery **86**:859, 1979.
32. Livesay, J.J.: Laser angioplasty: exploring a new frontier, Tex. Heart Inst. J. **14**:1, 1987.

Chapter 11

Early Results of Peripheral Laser Angioplasty and Preliminary Experimental Work on Coronary Laser Angioplasty

Leonard A. Nordstrom, MD

In the last decade, percutaneous transluminal angioplasty (PTA) has evolved from treatment of peripheral vascular lesions to treatment of progressively more complex coronary lesions. Despite this impressive progress, angioplasty remains limited to those lesions that can be traversed mechanically with a guidewire and catheter,[1] by the risk of subintimal dissection and subsequent reclosure of the artery,[2] and by a relatively high rate of restenosis[3] requiring either a repeat procedure or bypass-graft surgery. Common to each of these limitations is the mechanism of PTA's therapeutic action—dependence on mechanical probing and compressive remodeling,[4] rather than actual removal of plaque material. Although the intravascular use of lasers is still considered experimental, lasers possess unique optical properties that may complement angioplasty. Because laser light is coherent, it can be transmitted over a distance through optical fibers and guided to an obstructed site by a catheter. The collimated beam can be focused intensely to permit precise removal of tissue and thus create a new channel. Furthermore, because laser light is monochromatic, the characteristic wavelength emitted may be selectively absorbed by target tissues.

Integrating laser, fiber-optic, and PTA technologies requires a laser–catheter delivery system specifically designed for intravascular use.[5] This delivery system must include mechanisms to generate, transmit, and control laser energy within the arterial lumen. More specifically, a delivery system must address the following practical considerations:

1. The ability to adapt to a clinical environment: The laser must be suited for use in the catheterization laboratory; it must be safe, reliable, and user friendly.
2. Absorption characteristics of plaque and artery tissues: To utilize the monochromatic nature of laser light, the "ideal" wavelength should match wavelength of peak absorption by plaque tissue. Wave-

lengths absorbed less efficiently require greater incidental energy to elicit tissue response. If the absorption characteristics of plaque differ from those of artery wall tissue at any wavelength, selective ablation of plaque tissue must be possible.

3. Energy characteristics: Laser energy may be delivered in either of two forms—continuous wave or pulsed. The tissue removal pattern associated with each mode differs. Short intervals of pulsed energy yield minimal thermal conduction to surrounding tissue, because heat conduction is a time-dependent process.[6] Consequently, less charring and coagulation occur in pulse-irradiated tissues. However, transmitting the high peak power of pulsed energy through optical fibers is difficult, whereas continuous wave energy is easily transmitted using available fiber-optic technology.

4. Suitability of fiber optics: To preserve a percutaneous approach, the delivery fiber must be flexible, biocompatible, and small enough to be inserted into a catheter lumen.

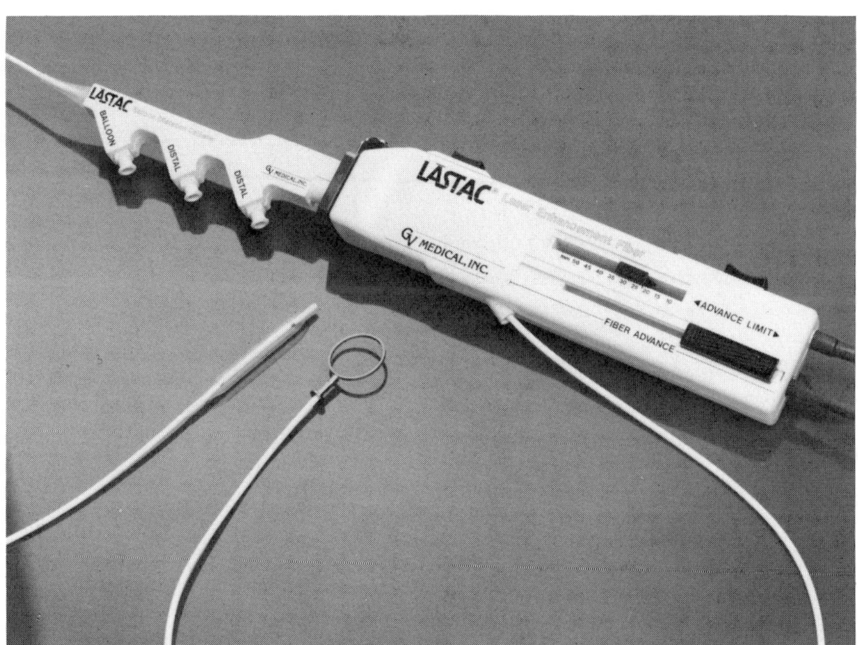

Fig. 11-1. Laser energy is transmitted to the vascular lesion through an optical fiber inserted into the lumen of the balloon dilatation catheter. A 200 μm fiber is housed in the laser-enhancement fiber (LEF) control handle that connects to the balloon catheter handle. The LEF control handle provides a mechanism to position the fiber in the artery lumen (fiber advance slide) and activate the laser.

5. Transmission through fluid field: Intravascular laser delivery requires the transmission of laser energy through blood, or through a field where saline has replaced blood. For wavelengths absorbed by both blood and saline, a contact probe is necessary; however, the size of recanalized channel will be restricted to the probe's diameter, which in turn has size limitations as described above.

Recognizing each of these delivery system requirements, a laser-enhanced angioplasty system (LASTAC ® System, GV Medical Inc., Plymouth, Minnesota) was developed. An argon-laser power source generates laser energy which is transmitted through an integrated laser catheter (Fig. 11-1).

Thrombus, a major constituent of vascular lesions, readily absorbs the blue-green light of argon laser energy. Argon laser light can be transmitted through water, and, therefore, saline is perfused during lasing to clear blood from the lasing field. Although plaque poorly absorbs argon laser light, emerging evidence suggests that plaque may absorb argon wavelengths more efficiently than normal artery wall tissue, thereby minimizing the risk of thermal injury to surrounding healthy tissue.[7-10]

The light beam is controlled through the centering characteristics of the balloon catheter and an altered laser beam profile. The optically engineered fiber tip delivers a light beam diverged from 10° to 40°, as measured in saline. Beam divergence accomplishes three objectives: It brings the therapeutic, power-dense area of light closer to the fiber tip, where beam direction can be managed (Fig. 11-2). Divergence maximizes tissue removal by presenting a wider beam profile to target tissues within the artery; also, divergence geometrically dissipates laser energy as distance increases, according to the inverse square law (Table 11-1). Further control of the laser beam is achieved by coaxial alignment of the fiber tip, upon inflation of a centering balloon dilatation catheter.

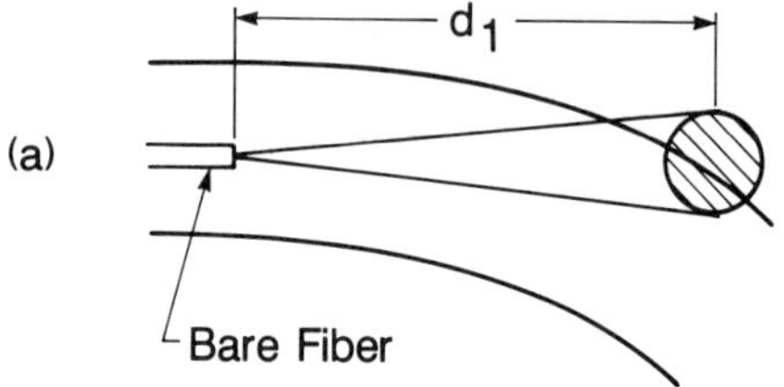

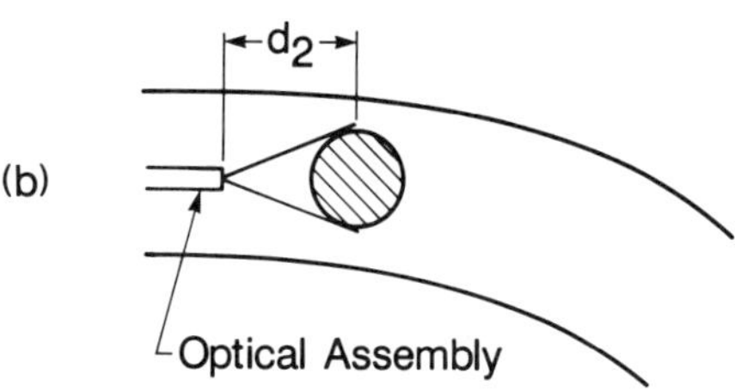

Fig. 11-2. A, A bare optical fiber (cone angle of 10 degrees) projects a light spot of therapeutic size at greater than 10 mm (d_1) from the fiber tip. **B,** The optical assembly diverges the light beam to a 40-degree cone angle. By comparison, the optical assembly reduces this distance (d_2) to 3 mm, where beam direction can be controlled.

The following presents preclinical and early clinical evaluations of the safety and effectiveness of this concept.

IN VITRO EXPERIMENTS

The effects of increased laser beam divergence have been evaluated in an in vitro bench tissue experiment,[11] in which tissue removal, using bare optical fiber, was compared to that using a fiber with an optical assembly mounted on the distal tip. The bare fiber produced a light cone of 10°, while the optical assembly diverged the light cone to 40° (both as

Table 11-1. Power Density for a Cone Angle of 40° at Varying Fiber Tip-to-Tissue Distances

Distance from Tissue Surface (mm)	*Power Density* at 10 Watts (Watts/mm²)*
1	23.8
2	6.0
3	2.7
4	1.5
5	1.0

$$\text{*Power Density} = \frac{10 \text{ watts}}{\text{Area of Spot}}$$

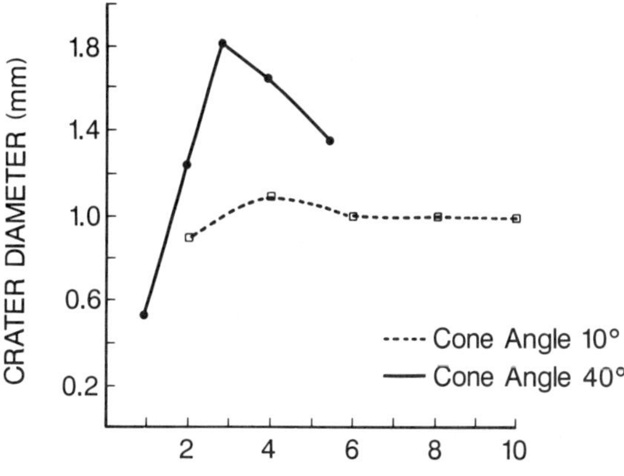

Fig. 11-3. Light intensity, from a diverged beam, rapidly decreases below the threshold necessary for consistent tissue destruction, beyond 3 mm from the fiber tip. Consequently, the diamteter of the resulting crater of tissue removed is also decreased.

measured in saline). The target was atherosclerotic aorta tissue mounted in a petri dish and immersed in 37° C saline. Both fibers were adjusted to deliver laser energy at a 90° angle incident to the tissue, and positioned to within 2 mm of the tissue surface. Laser energy was delivered at 10 watts for 10 seconds, while saline was infused at 10 ml/min. Distance was increased incrementally to 10 mm, with tissue ablation quantitated for each exposure.

The optical assembly significantly increased mean crater diameter ($P < 0.001$) at shorter distances: at 3 mm from the fiber tip the mean crater diameter was 1.81 mm. Beyond 3 mm, light intensity from the diverged beam rapidly decreased below the required threshold for consistent tissue response. By contrast, tissue ablation was relatively constant up to 10 mm from the bare fiber tip, with no appreciable increase in mean crater diameter noted at any distance (Fig. 11-3). Thus, by diverging the beam with an optical assembly, a larger, therapeutic, power-dense light spot is brought closer to the fiber tip to improve control.

The area of tissue ablation, resulting from argon laser exposure using a diverged beam, typically is surrounded by a thin zone of coagulative necrosis and carbonization, together measuring 0.2 to 0.5 mm in depth without thermal changes in adjacent muscularis (Fig. 11-4).

IN VIVO EXPERIMENTS

Two experiments were performed to evaluate control of laser exposure in situ through coaxial alignment of the fiber. In the first animal model,[12] thc abdominal aortas of New Zealand white rabbits were irradiated; in the second model, occluded and nonoccluded femoral arteries of mongrel dogs were experimentally treated.[11]

Atherosclerotic Rabbits

Three groups of rabbits received treatments of either balloon angioplasty (11 rabbits); laser

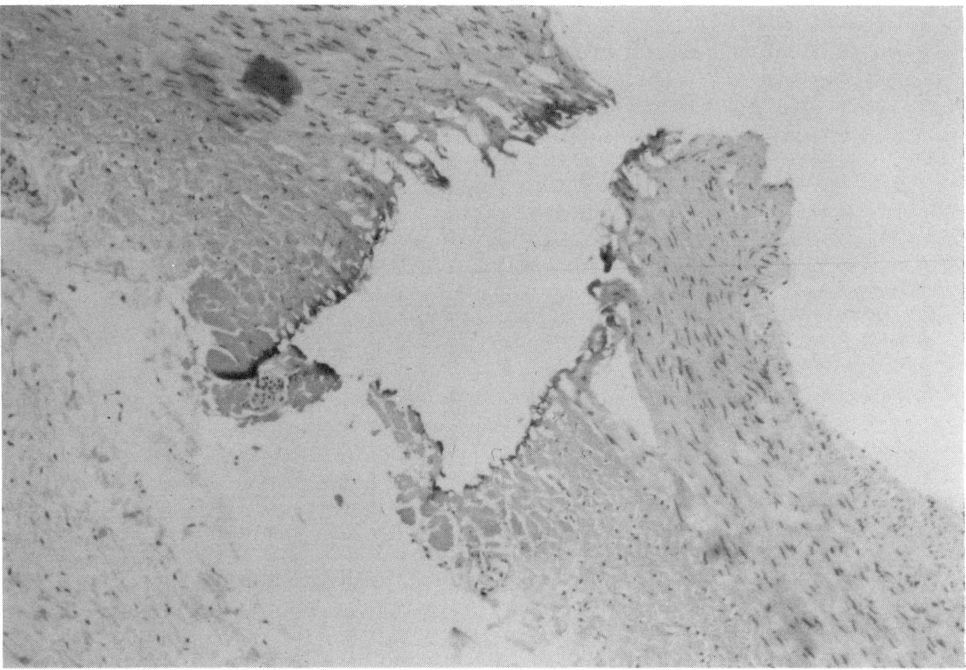

Fig. 11-4. Histology of tissue ablation resulting from argon laser exposure using a diverged beam in an arterial segment in vitro.

exposure, with the beam coaxially aligned via a centering balloon (14 rabbits); or a combined treatment of laser exposure with balloon angioplasty (13 rabbits). The control group (9 rabbits) was catheterized but received no treatment. The initial rationale for this experiment was to induce high-grade stenoses of the abdominal aorta, and then to compare the efficacy of the three treatments in subsequent recanalization. The stenoses were produced by a combination of endothelial abrasion and a high-cholesterol diet. However, the average stenosis, as revealed by angiography, was less than 33% with few high-grade obstructions noted. Recanalization, therefore, was quite variable, and no conclusions could be drawn from any of the treatment groups. Regardless, we noted significant results, in that no vessel perforations occurred in any of the 27 laser-treated rabbits. Neither the laser treatment nor the combined laser-with-balloon angioplasty treatment caused any histological evidence of charring, vacuolization, or coagulation. Similar studies[13,14] have reported a high incidence of laser-induced injury with even lower exposures, using this same experimental model. This study demonstrated that correct coaxial positioning of the fiber tip afforded control of the laser light beam.

Canine Model

Due to the problems encountered with atherosclerotic rabbits, a canine model was developed to further evaluate the coaxially aligned/diverged beam concept of laser control. Using the mongrel dog as a model, a total of 16 femoral arteries were occluded in an acute preparation. Human atherosclerotic plaque tissue (3 to 5 mm long) was mounted to an aluminum stent and stationed within the arterial lumen by surgical ligation. Additionally, three unoccluded arteries were exposed to high doses of laser to study potential thermal effects.

The laser catheter was introduced through a carotid cutdown and advanced distally to the obstruction site, where 800 J of laser energy were delivered. In 12 lasing attempts, no vessel perforations occurred and no gross or histologic evidence of thermal injury was observed. Even when relatively high doses (2400 J) were delivered in the unoccluded arteries, thermal injury was not evident in macro- and microscopic examinations. In the occluded artery series, two lasing attempts were aborted because coaxial position of the catheter could not be demonstrated fluoroscopically. Two vessel perforations did occur early in the series and were felt to be secondary to inadequate coaxial positioning of the fiber tip.

This series of experiments successfully demonstrated that high levels of laser energy could be delivered safely in situ, through coaxial placement of the fiber tip and divergence of the light beam.

Early Clinical Experience

This integrated system is being applied clinically in the treatment of human peripheral vascular disease (PVD). Patient selection follows an approved Food and Drug Administration (FDA) investigational protocol; all patients give informed consent prior to participation.

The procedure calls for removing as much plaque as possible with the laser and remodeling residual plaque by balloon dilatation. Twenty-eight procedures have been performed in the superficial femoral artery and two in the iliac artery. Total occlusions, averaging 9.0 cm in length (range: 1 to 37 cm), constituted 70% of the lesions treated.

Using standard PTA approach, the balloon catheter is advanced distally to the obstruction site over a 0.018-inch guidewire, and the patient is given 4000 to 5000 units of heparin intravenously. After documenting the obstruction's proximity by angiography, the guidewire is removed, and an optical fiber is introduced into the catheter lumen. With the fiber tip positioned 2 mm from the target and coaxially aligned by balloon inflation, 10 watts of laser energy are delivered for 2 to 10 seconds. A control system synchronizes perfusion of saline (10 to 30 ml/min) initiated 5 seconds prior to and continued during lasing, which flushes blood from the lasing field and cools the artery wall. The amount of energy used in these procedures varied between 60 and 2,730 J; the mean exposure was 954 J per case.

The sequence described is repeated as the laser catheter is advanced to allow tissue removal and, at the same time, balloon angioplasty. Tissue removal is verified periodically through fluoroscopy. Once the lesion is traversed, angiography is repeated, usually revealing uneven and incomplete tissue removal. Consequently, in longer lesions, a 10-cm balloon was inserted, and additional dilatations were performed. Figures 11-5 and 11-6 show the angiographic results pre- and postprocedure for laser-treated superficial femoral and iliac lesions, respectively.

Laser-enhanced angioplasty was successful in 28 of 30 procedures (93%). Two unsuccessful attempts occurred early in the series, in patients with 8- and 10-cm total occlusions—both of these technical failures were attributed to intimal dissection. Three lesions reclosed within 24 hours; these were presumed to be thrombotic occlusion. The remaining early reclosure was secondary to emboli that resulted from recanalizing a synthetic graft, which had been occluded over its entire segment. After several failed surgical interventions on this patient, an amputation was necessary. No other significant complications have occurred; there was one clinically insignificant perforation.

At follow-up examinations averaging 3 months (range: 1 to 14 months), 20 arteries remain patent based on the alleviation of symptoms and improved ankle/brachial indices, yielding a follow-up patency rate of 71%. This series is further described in Table 11-2.

Work in Progress

The primary challenge and ultimate goal for percutaneous transluminal laser angioplasty is, of course, to provide a safe, more effective, and less invasive alternative for treating coronary vascular disease. The encouraging success in treating human PVD has led to the initial experiments in vivo, using canine coronary models. Safe delivery of PTLA within coronary vasculature compels one to recognize two additional considerations:

1. Coronary arteries are smaller

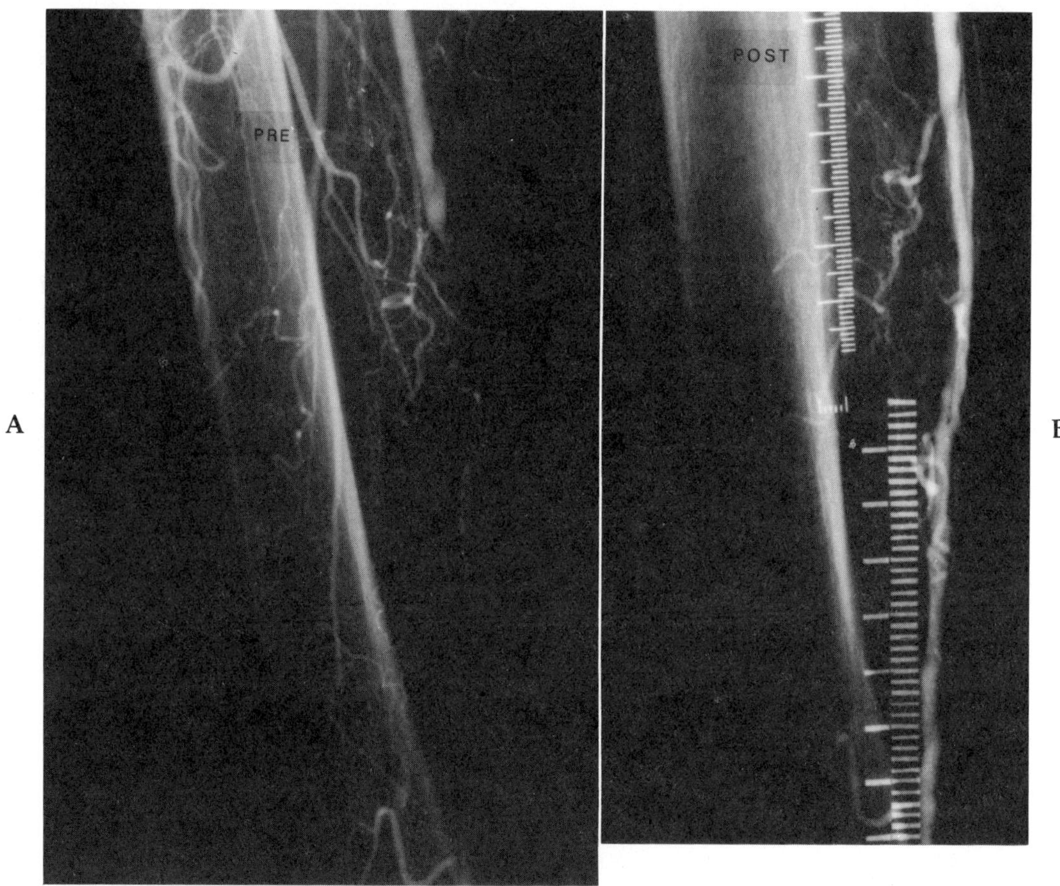

Fig. 11-5. A, A 7 cm total occlusion in a 75-year-old woman with life-style-limiting claudication of 24 months' duration. **B,** Result after 20 exposures, totaling 800 J, followed by three dilatations at 3 atm for 60 seconds. Ankle/brachial index was increased from 0.54 (preprocedure) to 0.98 (postprocedure).

Fig. 11-6. A, A 6 cm total occlusion of the left common iliac artery. **B,** Result following 32 exposures at 10 W for 2 seconds (500 J), and four dilatations at 6 to 14 atm for 90 to 180 seconds. Ankle/brachial index was increased from 0.58 (preprocedure) to 0.75 (postprocedure).

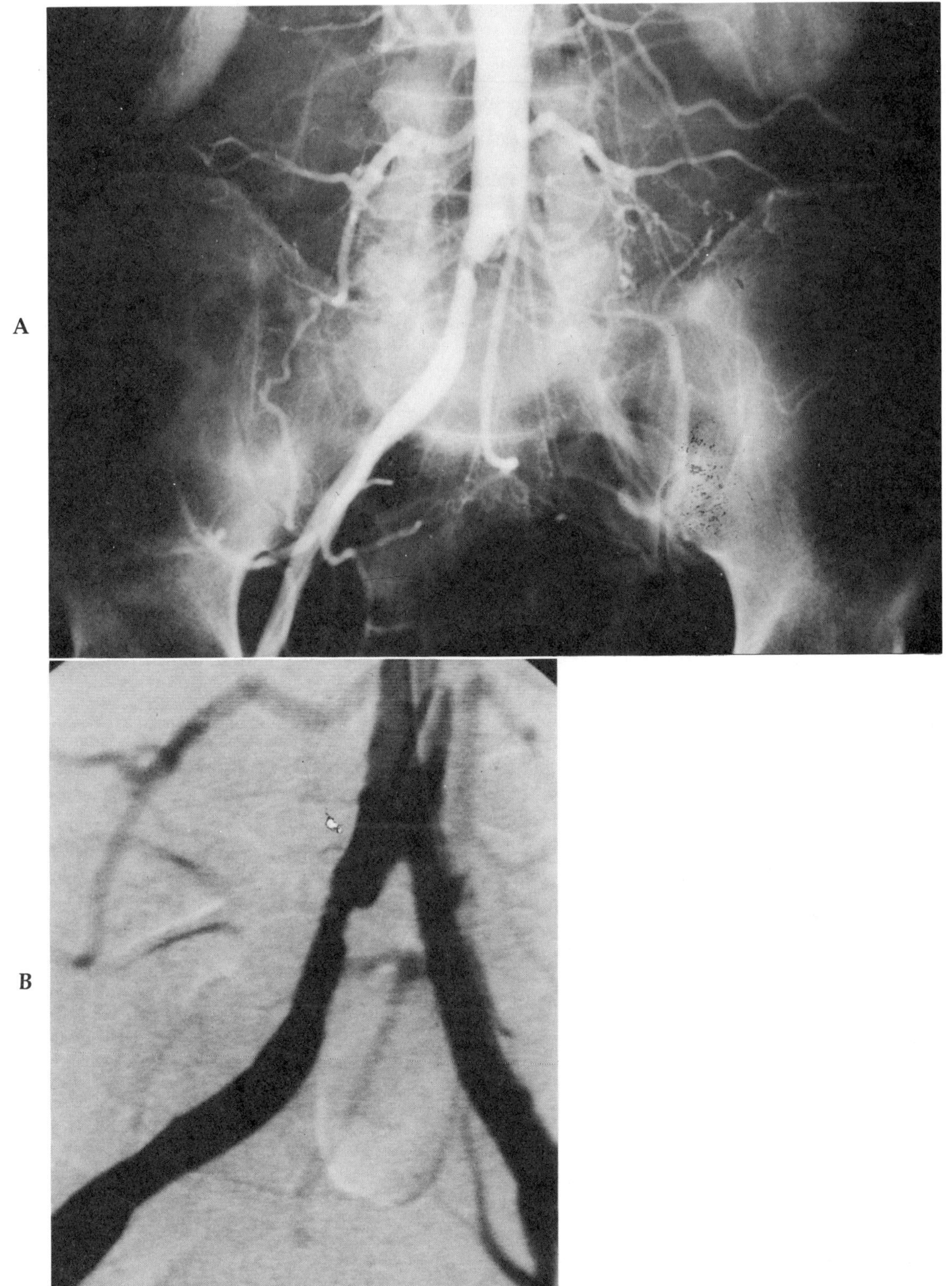

Fig. 11-6. For legend see opposite page.

Table 11-2. Subgroup Analyses

	Patent	*Technical Failures*	*Reclosure Early*	*Reclosure Late*
N	20	2	4	4
Lesion type				
Stenoses	9	0	0	0
Total occlusions	11	2	4	4
Lesion length (cm)	$\bar{x}$ = 7.5	$\bar{x}$ = 10	$\bar{x}$ =17	$\bar{x}$ = 5.0
(Range)	(2-15)	(9.5-10)	(3-37)	(1-7)
Average Joules:	780	1540	1553	489
ABI Post-Treatment	+0.24	−0.04	+0.18	+0.22
X Pre	0.61	0.72	0.64	0.62
X Post	0.85	0.68	0.82	0.84
Time to Restenoses				
Mean	—	—	24 hr.	3 mo.
Range	—	—	—	1-5 mo.

and more tortuous than peripheral arteries.

2. The heart is a dynamic environment; arteries are not only moving with each heartbeat, but are changing in curvature and diameter between systole and diastole.

Coaxial placement is essential for effective laser control, as supported by preclinical and early clinical experience, and it becomes a critical concern when working in the heart. The initial results in dogs, using the balloon configuration designed for peripheral use, proved disappointing. Two prototype balloon configurations were specially adapted for coronary use as a result of these initial failures. The safety of these prototype balloons as evaluated, as measured by angiography, hemodynamic measurements, and histopathology in a series of three canine coronary models.

In the three series of dogs, the femoral artery was entered using standard percutaneous approach. A multipurpose guiding catheter was passed into the ascending aorta, subsequently catheterizing the left coronary artery (LCA). The specially designed coronary catheter then was passed into the LCA through the guiding catheter, over a 0.014-inch guidewire. The optical fiber successfully negotiated the acute bends of left anterior descending (LAD) or circumflex (LCx) coronary arteries; no mechanical perforations occurred. Thoracotomy made a number of observations of the canine coronary vasculature possible, and so was performed in each treatment. With the coronary vasculature exposed, it was possible to observe coaxial alignment of the fiber by activating a low power beam of argon light (0.1 to 0.25 watts) down the artery lumen. A diffused beam following the linear displacement of the artery indicated coaxial alignment; an intense spot of light on the vessel wall indicated a misdirected fiber. By opening the dogs' chests, the immediate effects of lasing could be evaluated while lasing was performed.

Both balloon prototypes were used to deliver 68 laser exposures to 22 target sites in the LAD or LCx. Laser exposures consisted of 5 to 10 watts of energy delivered for 0.5 to 8.5 seconds: the mean exposure was 77 J/site (± 19 J). All specimens were subsequently examined histologically for laser effects.

A total of 20 of the 22 sites were irradiated without perforation; two LAD perforations were observed angiographically during the procedure and were confirmed by histology. Five additional perforations (four occurring in the LAD; one in the LCx) that presented periarterial hematomas were noted histologically, but none of these microscopic perforations resulted in hemodynamic effects. The periarterial hematomas were tolerated by each of the animals, all of which survived until sacrifice. Histological examinations of the remaining treatment sites further determined that thermal injury was either absent or slight. Using considerably lower power levels, equal or higher perforation rates have been reported in the literature of in vivo coronary laser studies.[15]

Several factors may have contributed to the LAD perforations. Proper positioning of the fiber tip may not have been achieved, because the fiber tip could not be observed perpendicular to the long-plane axis of the artery, using single-plane fluoroscopy. This was not true in the LCx. Second, due to the small diameter, the LAD may have been more intolerant of the thermal effects of lasing. Third, the smaller radius of curvature and tortuosity of the LAD made it difficult to place the catheter tip precisely.

A second series of dog experiments examined possible thrombogenicity following coronary laser exposures. Sites in the LAD or LCx were treated (respectively) with laser energy concomitant with balloon dilatation, or with balloon dilatation alone. From the partial results available, no histological evidence of thrombogenesis was observed, nor were any vessel wall perforations noted. However, full histological findings are pending for this series at this time.

In our most recent series of dog experiments, we have attempted lasing through an obstructed coronary artery. An induced chronic occlusion of the LAD has been attempted by denuding a segment of the artery's endothelium, isolating that segment by ligatures and introducing topical thrombin and canine blood. The resultant clot is permitted to adhere for 1 to 2 hours before the ligatures are released. After a 3- to 14-day convalescence to permit further fibrosis and aging of the lesion, obstructions were evaluated by angiography.

Successfully occluding the coronary vessels of dogs has proved difficult; to date, only two experiments have been prepared satisfactorily. In both of these animals, coronary approach with the fiberoptic catheter system was successful, and some thrombotic material was removed. Histological results were not available at this time. Further investigation of this model's suitability for the experimental treatment described is needed before significant results may be reported.

CONCLUSION

Laser-enhanced angioplasty is a useful adjunct to balloon angioplasty for treating PVD. Early clinical results mentioned were successful in 93% of the patients treated; more long-term studies are needed, however, to examine the impact of restenosis in laser-treated arteries.

Initial experimentation in canine coronary models suggests that high-energy laser can be successfully delivered and controlled in coronary arteries, but first, coaxial alignment of the optical fiber must be achieved by employing a specially designed coronary balloon catheter.

REFERENCES

1. Anderson, H.V., Roubin, G.S., and Lkeimgruber, P.P.: Primary angiographic success rates of PTCA, Am. J. Cardiol. **56:**712, 1985.
2. Cowley, M.J., Dorros, G., Kelsey, S.F., et al.: Acute coronary events associated with percutaneous transluminal coronary angioplasty, Am. J. Cardiol. **53:**12C, 1984.
3. Kent, K.M., Bentivoglio, L.G., Block, P.C., et al.: Long-term efficacy of percutaneous transluminal coronary angioplasty (PTCA): report from the National Heart, Lung, and Blood Institute PTCA registry, Am. J. Cardiol. **53:**27C, 1984.
4. Castaneda-Zuniga, W.R., Gormanek, A., Tadavarthy, M., et al.: The mechanism of balloon angioplasty, Radiology **135:**565, 1980.
5. Isner, J.M., and Clarke, R.H.: Laser angioplasty: unraveling the Gordian knot, J.A.C.C. **7**(3):705, 1986.
6. Welch, A.J.: The thermal response of laser irradiated tissue, IEEE J. Quantum Electron. **20**(12):1471, 1984.
7. Prince, M.R., Deutsch, T.F., Mathews-Roth, M.M., et al.: Preferential light absorption in atheromas in vitro, J. Clin. Invest. **78:**295, 1986.
8. Van Gemert, M.J.C., Verdaasdonk, R., Stassen, E.G., et al.: Optical properties of human blood vessel wall and plaque, Lasers Surg. Med. **5:**235, 1985.
9. Bowker, T.J., Edwards, P., Hall, T.A., et al.: Optical transmission of normal and atheromatous arterial wall: a spectral analysis, Cardiovasc. Res. **20:**393, 1986.
10. Prince, M.R., Deutsch, T.F., Sharpiro, A.H., et al.: Selective ablation of atheromas using a flashlamp-excited dye laser at 465 nm, Proc. Natl. Acad. Sci. U.S.A. **83:**7064, 1986.
11. Nordstrom, L.A., Castaneda-Zuniga, W.R., Lindeke, C.L., et al.: Laser angioplasty: controlled delivery of argon laser energy. (In press.)
12. Nordstrom, L.A., Castaneda-Zuniga, W.R., Grewe, D.D., et al.: Laser-enhanced transluminal angioplasty: the role of coaxial fiber placement, Semin. Intervent. Radiol. **3**(1):47, 1986.
13. Abela, G.S., Normann, S.J., Cohen, D.M., et al.: Laser recanalization of occluded atherosclerotic arteries in vivo and in vitro, Circulation **71**(2):403, 1985.
14. Lee, G., Ikeda, R.M., Theis, J.H., et al.: Acute and chronic complication of laser angioplasty: vascular wall damage and formation of aneurysms in the atherosclerotic rabbit. Am. J. Cardiol. **53:**290, 1984.
15. Anderson, H.V., Zaatari, G.S., Roubin, G.S., et al.: Coaxial laser energy delivery using a steerable catheter in canine coronary arteries, Am. Heart J. **113:**37, 1987.

Chapter **12**

Observations on Laser Thermal Angioplasty

Timothy A. Sanborn, MD

By partially removing obstructing atheroma or thrombus through vaporization of tissue rather than merely stretching or fracturing plaque as in conventional balloon angioplasty,[1] laser angioplasty or laser recanalization has the potential to serve as an aid or alternative to balloon angioplasty by:

1. increasing the initial success rate for lesions that are difficult or impossible to treat by conventional means
2. decreasing the incidence of restenosis after angioplasty

However, in initial experimental studies and early clinical trials with bare argon laser fiberoptics, the technique was limited by inadequate delivery systems resulting in an unacceptable high perforation rate[2-6] and the creation of small recanalized channels that resulted in poor long-term patency.[4] The key limitation in these early trials of laser angioplasty was the lack of an adequate catheter system for safe and effective intravascular delivery of laser energy. The first, but certainly not the last, laser fiberoptic catheter system that shows promise in preliminary animal and clinical trials is a laser-heated metallic-capped device on a laser probe.[7]

LASER THERMAL ANGIOPLASTY: EXPERIMENTAL RESULTS

In the last few years a novel fiberoptic laser delivery system has been developed (Trimedyne, Inc., Santa Ana, Calif.) in which argon laser energy is converted to heat in a rounded metallic cap at the end of a fiberoptic probe (Fig. 12-1). With this device, temperatures of over 400° C can be generated at the metallic cap.[7]

Initial studies in experimental atherosclerotic animals compared angiographic and histologic results using this new laser device with those of a bare fiberoptic probe.[2,8] In a series of in-vivo experiments involving the iliac arteries of 24 atherosclerotic rabbits, improved safety and efficacy of laser thermal angioplasty using this modified fiber was demonstrated compared with a conventional bare fiberoptic probe.[2] The results of angiography indicated that widening of luminal stenosis was seen in only 2 of 12 animals treated with the standard fiberoptic system compared with 8 of 12 animals treated with laser thermal angioplasty ($p < 0.01$). In these eight animals, the mean percent stenosis was 68% before

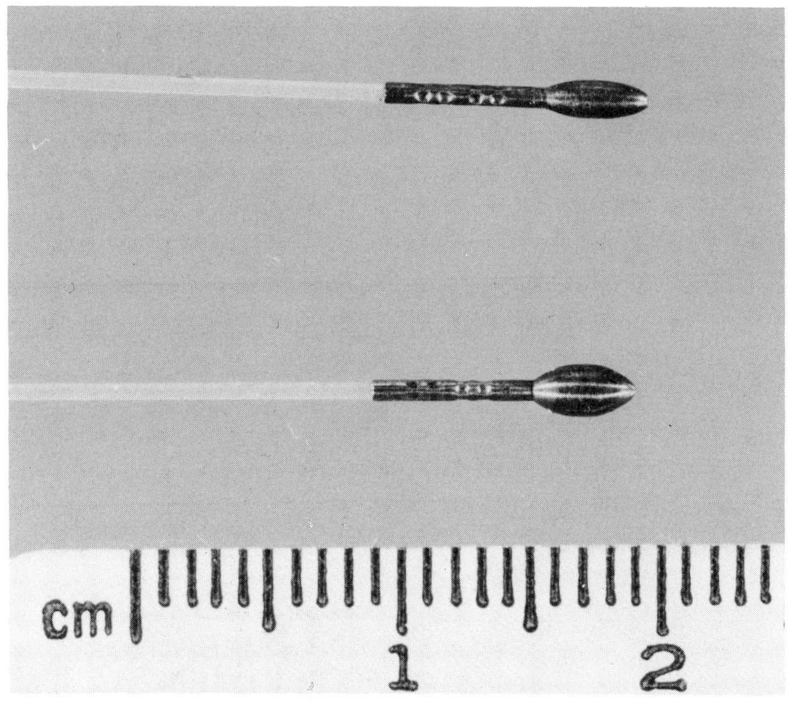

Fig. 12-1. A 1.5 mm laserprobe *(top)* and a 2 mm laserprobe *(bottom)*. (Reproduced with permission of Sanborn, T.A., et al: J. Vasc. Surg. **5**:83-90, 1987.)

treatment and was reduced to 13% after treatment. An angiographic example of laser thermal angioplasty is shown in Fig. 12-2. More importantly, perforation of the vessel wall occurred frequently with the fiberoptic fiber (9 of 12 animals) as opposed to only one mechanical perforation in 12 animals treated with the laser probe ($p < 0.001$). With the use of smaller, more flexible fiberoptics (less than 300 μm core diameter) mechanical perforation was eliminated entirely.

In histologic examination 30 minutes after laser angioplasty, strikingly different results were obtained with the two fiber systems (Fig. 12-3). With direct laser radiation from the bare fiberoptic, a deep but localized laser defect with near perforation of the vessel wall was noted along one side of the artery. There was associated charring, a gradient of thermal

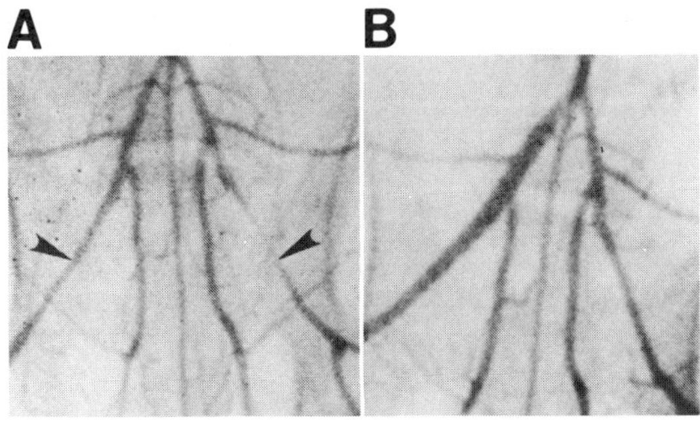

Fig. 12-2. Angiographic example of laserprobe results demonstrating **A** diffuse right iliac disease and more discrete higher grade left iliac lesion that were both successfully treated with good angiographic improvement **B.** (Reproduced with permission of Sanborn, T.A., et al.: Circulation **75**:1281-1286, 1987, and the American Heart Association.)

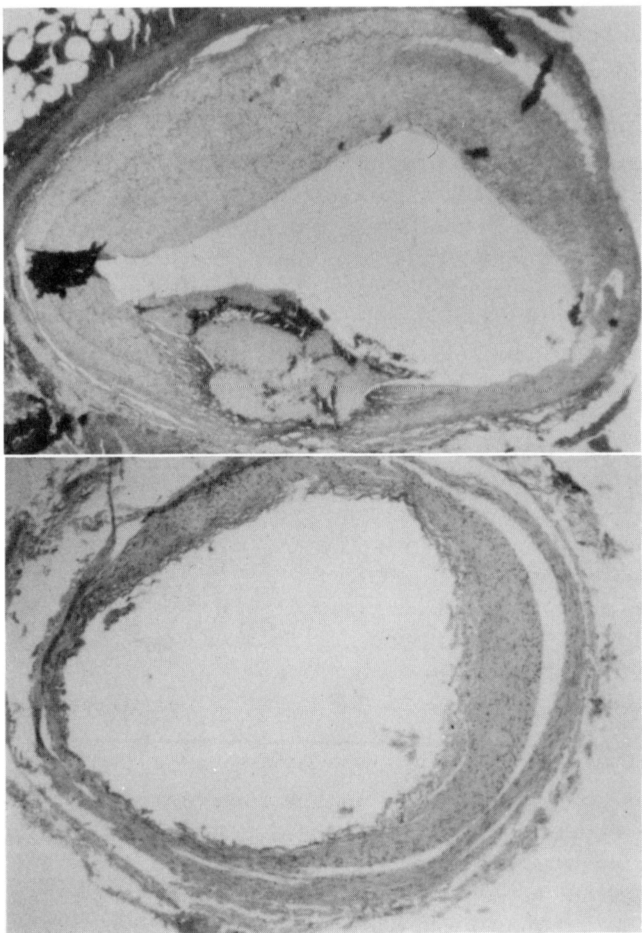

Fig. 12-3. Histologic specimens of iliac artery. *Top,* Example of direct argon laser radiation resulting in a localized laser defect along one side of the vessel wall that extends through the neointima into the media. A gradient of thermal injury characterized by cell swelling and tissue edema is also noted. In addition, considerable thrombus is present that fills the newly formed laser defect. *Bottom,* Example of circumference. (Hematoxylin eosin stain; × 80.) (Reproduced with permission of Sanborn, T.A., et al.: J. Am. Coll. Cardiol. **5**:934-938, 1985, and the American College of Cardiology.)

injury, and considerable thrombus formation. As is seen in Fig. 12-3 *(top)*, the major part of this eccentric lesion was not affected by the laser energy, thus indicating the problem of aiming the laser beam. In contrast, those vessels treated with the laser-heated metal probe showed histologic evidence of thermal injury distributed evenly around the entire luminal circumference. This thermal effect was associated with minimal charring, a gradient of thermal injury, and thinner, flatter thrombus formation. These histologic data suggest that circumferential rather than localized distribution of energy is a factor in these improved experimental results.

These results are confirmed in a series of postmortem human coronary artery xenografts transplanted into the canine femoral artery.[8] Angiography demonstrated recanalization in all five arteries treated with the laser-heated probe and three of five arteries treated with the bare fiberoptic. Only one perforation occurred with the metallic-capped fiber compared with three perforations using the bare fiberoptic. Interestingly, a larger 1.5 mm laser-heated probe was capable of creating a larger channel in the occluded arterial segment.

Recent follow-up angiographic and histologic studies in atherosclerotic rabbits demonstrated good long-term patency with minimal thrombogenesis and a very mild proliferative response to laser thermal angioplasty with a 1.5 to 2.0 mm laser-heated probe.[9] On histology, reendothelization of the luminal surface was noted as early as 2 weeks after laser thermal angioplasty. At 4 weeks the neointima was thin with a fibrous cap and minimal fibrocellular proliferation.

In a recent comparative study, laser thermal angioplasty was found to have less restenosis with a significantly larger luminal diameter (1.6 $\pm$ 0.5 mm vs. 1.0 $\pm$ 0.4 mm) when angiography was repeated 4 weeks after angioplasty.[10] At that time histologic examination revealed less fibrocellular proliferation after laser thermal angioplasty, whereas those vessels treated with balloon angioplasty demonstrated evidence of prior fracture and dissection of the vessel wall with more of a fibrocellular proliferative response (Fig. 12-4). Morphometer analysis of histologic cross-sections of these pressure-perfused arteries confirmed a significantly large luminal area after laser thermal angioplasty compared with balloon angioplasty (1.24 $\pm$ 0.62 mm^2 vs. 0.6 $\pm$ 0.45 mm^2; $p < 0.05$). Thus in rabbit iliac stenoses, laser thermal angioplasty was associated with less restenosis and produced a significantly larger mean luminal diameter and mean luminal area than conventional balloon angioplasty. These results may be due to the different pathophysiologic mechanisms involved in these two techniques.

LASER-ASSISTED BALLOON ANGIOPLASTY IN PERIPHERAL VESSELS

After demonstrating the safety and efficacy of this device in experimental animals,[2,8-10] a collaborative clinical trial was initiated at Boston University Medical Center and Northern General Hospital, Sheffield, England, to first determine the safety and efficacy of this laser-heated probe in performing percutaneous laser thermal angioplasty to recanalize lesions before using conventional balloon angioplasty.[11-13]

Patient Population

All patients had severe peripheral vascular disease and suffered from either limiting claudication or rest pain, gangrene, and threatened limb loss. Initial evaluation included a history and physical examination as well as a Doppler ankle-arm index (AAI), which was also used for follow-up after angioplasty. Patients were pretreated with oral aspirin (75 or 325 mg once a day).

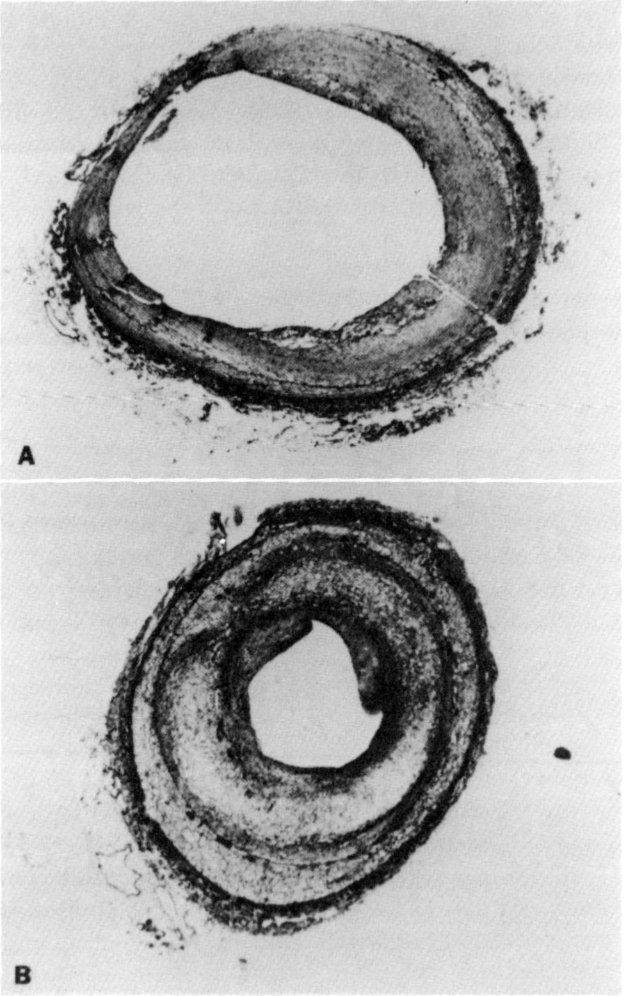

Fig. 12-4. A, Cross-section of a patent rabbit iliac vessel 4 weeks after laser thermal angioplasty, demonstrating minimal fibrocellular proliferative response and a thin, condensed fibrous cap. **B,** Histologic section 4 weeks after balloon angioplasty, revealing moderate fibrocellular proliferation caused by the dilatation, which partially fills the lumen and obliterates the prior dissection planes between the neointimal flaps and the media (Verhoff–van Gieson elastin stains; × 40.) (Reproduced with permission of Sanborn, T.A., et al.: Circulation **75:**1281-1286, 1987, and the American Heart Association.)

Laser Equipment

The laser system at Boston University consisted of a 14 W argon laser system (Optilase, Model 900, Trimedyne, Inc., Santa Ana, Calif.) coupled to a sterile disposable laser-heated metallic-capped fiberoptic, which consisted of a 300 μm diameter core fiberoptic fiber with a 1.0 to 2.5 mm metallic cap at the distal end of the fiber (Laserprobe-PLR, Trimedyne, Inc., Santa Ana, Calif.). At Northern General Hospital, the laser-heated probe was coupled to an argon laser generator from Heraeus Cooper Laser Sonics, Santa Clara, CA.[13]

Percutaneous Procedure

The majority of the procedures were performed by percutaneous arterial puncture of the ipsilateral femoral artery under local anesthesia. The equipment required (catheters, wires, other equipment) was identical to that utilized in conventional arterial catheterization. After cannulation of the superficial femoral artery, 5000 units of heparin was administered intraarterially and initial angiography was performed to document the lesion. To introduce the laser probe into the artery, an introducer sheath with good sealing around the laser fiberoptic and guidewire (0.04-inch "plus" wire) was necessary. We found the arterial sheath with the best prevention of backbleeding to be one manufactured by Cook (Model VCF–8.5–38, Cook, Inc., Bloomington, Ind.). The laser-heated probe was inserted into this introducer sheath and advanced under fluoroscopic guidance to the proximal origin of the lesion until contact was made between the probe tip and the lesion as verified by angiography and tactile feedback. Five to ten second pulses of 8 to 13 W of argon laser energy were then delivered from the laser generator to the probe. After the initial warm-up period of 2 to 3 seconds while maintaining gentle pressure on the probe in order to initiate advancement, the probe was then advanced through the lesion with a continuous motion. Care was taken to keep the tip moving as it cooled down after laser pulse delivery to avoid adherence to the arterial wall. If adherence was noted on gentle withdrawal of the probe, a repeat laser pulse was delivered to free the probe and a continuous motion was applied to the tip during the subsequent cooling period. Progress of the probe through the lesion was monitored fluoroscopically with several injections of 3 to 5 ml of contrast solution given through the arterial sheath to confirm the position of the device. After the lesions were crossed with the laser-heated probe, one final pulse was delivered on slow withdrawal of the probe through the lesion to maximize the luminal diameter. When the probe tip reached the proximal end of the lesion, laser power was discontinued and the probe moved back and forth for 5 seconds during cooling. The laser probe was then removed and an angiogram performed to document the luminal diameter produced by the procedure.

Because the luminal diameter produced by laser thermal angioplasty with the current 1.0 to 2.5 mm diameter device was considered inadequate in these large 4 to 5 mm peripheral vessels, the laser procedure was followed in all cases by conventional balloon angioplasty to obtain a definitive lumen that was documented by a final angiogram. The arterial sheath was subsequently removed and systemic heparin was administered for 24 hours unless a hematoma was present. The patients were discharged within 24 to 48 hours on 75 or 325 mg of aspirin a day.

Local Femoral Cutdown Procedure

Rarely, either marked obesity or high-grade proximal superficial femoral artery disease precluded a safe percutaneous approach. In these cases, under local anesthesia and mild sedation, a small cutdown was made to expose the common femoral artery for direct arterial puncture and subsequent laser and balloon angioplasty through an 8.5F sheath.[12]

Initial Results

In this initial series, laser recanalization was successful in 39 of 41 vessels for a 93% angiographic success rate with minimal complications and no vessel perforation.[11,12] In this study, the most commonly used laser probe size was the 2 mm diameter metal tip. The average laser wattage was 10 W (range 4 to 13 W). Representative angiograms are shown in Figs. 12-5 and 12-6.

Probe Detachment

Early in this clinical trial, probe tip detachment from the fiberoptic occurred in two patients; one of these probes could be retrieved and removed. Subsequent to this early experience, a safety (anchor) wire was incorporated into the device to add stability to the joint between the fiberoptic and the metal tip and to prevent further probe detachment. In addition, by keeping the probe moving constantly during laser delivery and the cooling period, it was found that adherence to the vessel wall, one of the potential causes of probe detachment, was significantly reduced.

Use in Total Occlusion

Once the safety and efficacy of laser thermal angioplasty was demonstrated in peripheral vessels, the next step was to demonstrate a useful clinical role for the technique. A recent report of the combined experience at Northern General Hospital and Boston University Medical Center was directed toward addressing one of these questions: whether the use of laser thermal angioplasty can increase the initial success rate in peripheral artery total occlusion.[13] In this initial series, 50 of 56 (89%) femoropopliteal occlusions were successfully recanalized by laser thermal an-

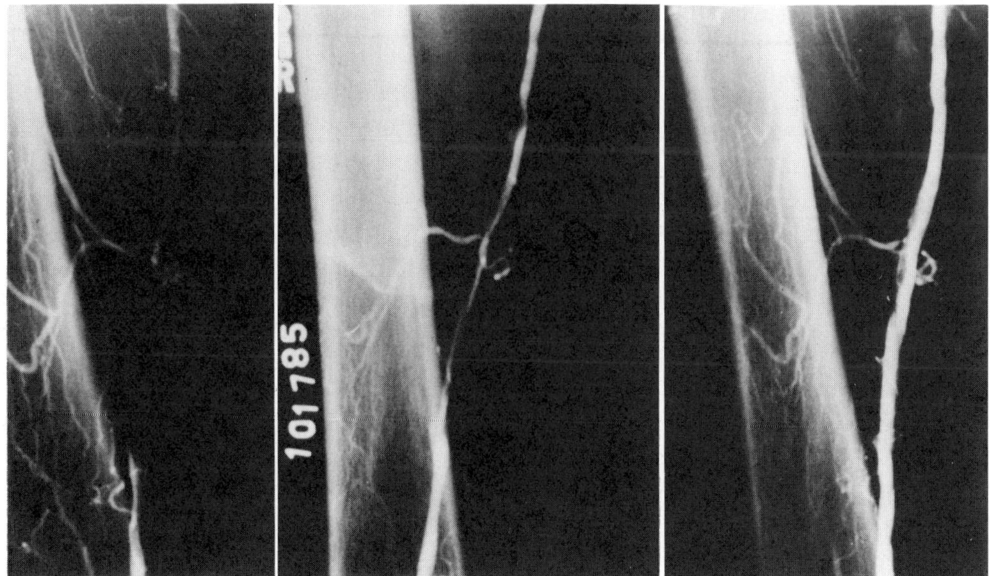

Fig. 12-5. Angiogram of a 6 cm high-grade stenosis of the superficial femoral artery *(left panel)* in which the luminal diameter was enlarged with the laserprobe *(middle panel)*. This allowed conventional balloon angioplasty to be performed more easily *(right panel)*. (Reproduced with permission of Sanborn, T.A., et al.: J. Vasc. Surg. **5**:83-90, 1987.)

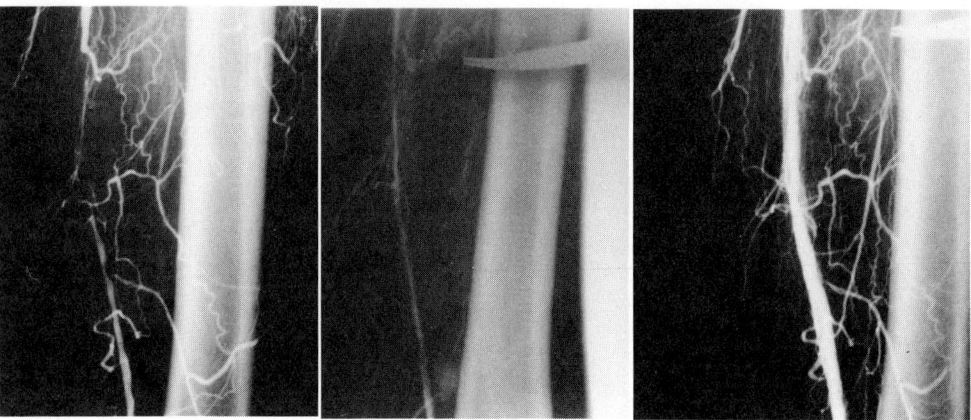

Fig. 12-6. Angiograms of a 4 cm total occlusion of the superficial femoral artery *(left panel)* that was recanalized with three pulses of 12 w of argon laser energy delivered to the laserprobe for 10 seconds duration each *(middle panel).* This was followed by balloon angioplasty to yield a good angiographic result *(right panel).* (Reproduced with permission of Sanborn, T.A., et al.: J. Vasc. Surg. **5**:83-90, 1987.)

gioplasty to provide an initial channel for subsequent balloon dilatation. Since there were two acute reocclusions, the overall initial clinical success rate in this series was 86%. These results compare quite favorably with recent large series of conventional balloon angioplasty that report initial clinical success rates of 72 to 78%.[14,15]

Interestingly, if those lesions considered easy to treat by conventional means are examined separately, the initial success rate for these 17 lesions was 100%. Thus, despite the fact that more difficult lesions were attempted in this initial series, laser-assisted balloon angioplasty resulted in minimal, nonsignificant complications, a perforation rate of only 2%, and a success rate equal to or better than previously published results for balloon angioplasty alone.

Technique Development

These results represent the early stages of development of a new technique that will obviously be modified and adapted in the future. In addition to the techniques described above, two additional modifications are worth mentioning, which related to the 0.014-inch "plus" wire attached to the laser probe.

Tip Angulation by Wire Shaping

Occasionally in tortuous lesions or at bifurcations in the artery some angulation of this straight but flexible fiberoptic and the rigid metal tip is necessary. By shaping a gentle curve in the 0.014-inch wire alongside the fiberoptic, a curve can be maintained in the laser probe and the metal tip rotated 360 degrees in a fashion similar to torque guidewires. Care must be taken, however, to be sure that this angulation is not too acute, because the curve is fixed and may make further recanalization of a straight portion of the artery more difficult. Biplane fluoroscopy or use of multiple fluoroscopic views aids in the use of these angled probes. The ability to release the angulation, as in a tip-deflecting wire, would be a useful alternative to improve the steerability of the device in the future.

Table 12-1. Comparison of 1-Year Recurrence Rate

		% Occlusions		
	% Stenoses	*<3 cm*	*4–7 cm*	*>7 cm*
Laser-assisted balloon angioplasty	5	7	24	42
Balloon angioplasty alone				
Krepel, et al.[16]	20	7	50 (>3 cm)	
Hewes, et al.[15]	19+	33+	18+	32+
Murray, et al.[17]	28+	14+ (all occlusions)		

+, 12 to 20% redilation rate not considered recurrence.

Balloon Advancement over the Probe

In extremely difficult or tortuous lesions, another technique which has proved useful is the advancement of the balloon angioplasty catheter over the fiberoptic and the "plus" wire once the lesion has been crossed. In this situation, instead of recrossing the lesion with a guidewire that can cause a dissection, the laser probe catheter actually serves as a guidewire for the balloon catheter. This technique has been quite helpful, particularly in diffusely diseased vessels. The sterile portion of the disposable fiberoptic does have to be cut about 2 m from the distal end to disconnect it from the nonsterile proximal end that is attached to the laser generator.

Follow-up Results

When examining long-term results of peripheral angioplasty, clinical patency rates and the respective recurrence rates may vary considerably depending on the type of lesion included in various series, as well as the definition of patency.[15-17] To determine the potential benefit of laser-assisted balloon angioplasty, it is necessary to compare the results with the new technique to results with conventional balloon angioplasty alone. By using subgroup analysis of our initial long-term results in 99 femoropopliteal lesions, we recently found evidence for a potential benefit of laser-assisted balloon angioplasty (Table 12-1).[18] For example, the 1-year recurrence rates for stenoses and short 1 to 3 cm occlusions were only 5 and 7% respectively. These results were considerably better than recent balloon angioplasty series in which 1-year recurrence rates of 19 to 28% were reported for stenoses and recurrence rates of 7 to 33% were reported for short occlusions.[15-17] The definition of clinical patency is important in comparing these results, since a 12 to 20% redilation rate was not considered a recurrence in two of these recent series.[15,17] For longer occlusions, treated with laser-assisted balloon angioplasty, 1-year recurrence rates of 24% for medium-length occlusions (4 to 7 cm) and 42% for occlusions greater than 7 cm are also better than a recurrence rate of 50% for occlusions greater than 3 cm reported in the series of Krepel and co-workers.[16]

Obviously, long-term patency is determined by numerous factors and a multicentered clinical trial is warranted in order to determine whether laser-assisted balloon angioplasty can improve the patency rate in

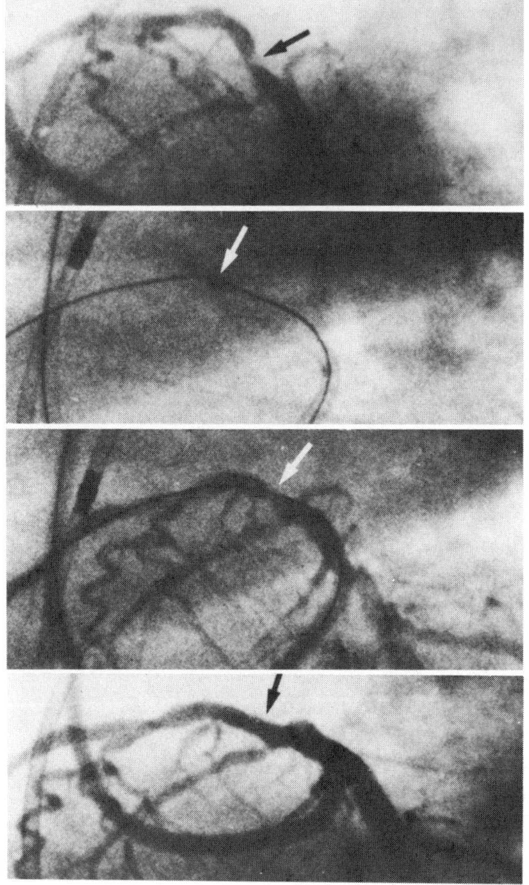

Fig. 12-7. The 60-degree anterior oblique, 10-degree caudal views of a 90% eccentric LAD coronary artery lesion *(arrows)* before treatment *(top)*, after laser thermal angioplasty with the laserprobe through the lesion and the angiographic result of laser thermal angioplasty *(middle panels)*, and after balloon angioplasty *(bottom)*. (Reproduced with permission of Sanborn, T.A., et al.: J. Am. Coll. Cardiol. **8**:1437-1440, 1986, and the American College of Cardiology.)

peripheral angioplasty. In addition, device modifications such as larger laser probes to recanalize larger channels should further improve both the initial success rate and the patency rate in peripheral angioplasty. Perhaps laser thermal angioplasty has a beneficial effect on vessel healing as suggested in the rabbit experimental model.[10]

FEASIBILITY OF PERCUTANEOUS CORONARY LASER THERMAL ANGIOPLASTY

Based on this clinical experience in peripheral vessels, clinical trials of percutaneous coronary laser thermal angioplasty were recently initiated using a specially designed 1.7 mm coronary laser-heated probe with an eccentric channel for passage over a percutaneous transluminal coronary angioplasty (PTCA) guidewire.[19,20] These preliminary studies indicated that coronary laser angioplasty could be performed percutaneously; however, a great deal of work has to be done to improve the flexibility, trackability, and profile of these early prototype devices for coronary use. Recently, lower profile 1.3 and 1.6 mm laser probe catheters with central lumens have been used clinically and they demonstrate considerable improvement in their ability to operate in more tortuous coronary arteries. Representative angiographs of our first percutaneous coronary laser thermal angioplasty procedures are shown in Fig. 12-7.

CONCLUSION

In summary, the use of flexible fiberoptics to transmit laser energy for the ablation of atherosclerotic obstructions does have significant potential in the cardiovascular areas, and initial clinical trials indicate that some of the early limitations of laser angioplasty can be solved. What remains to be determined is the exact clinical role of the emerging technology in relation to the current accepted procedures of bypass surgery and balloon angioplasty.

REFERENCES

1. Sanborn, T.A., Faxon, D.P., Haudenschild, C.C., Gottsman, S.B., and Ryan, T.J.: The mechanism of transluminal angioplasty: evidence for formation of aneurysms in experimental atherosclerosis, Circulation **68:**1136-1140, 1983.
2. Sanborn, T.A., Faxon, D.P., Haudenschild, C.C., and Ryan, T.J.: Experimental angioplasty: circumferential distribution of laser thermal energy with a laser probe, J. Am. Coll. Cardiol. **5:**934-938, 1985.
3. Abela, G.S., Normann, S.J., Cohen, D.M., Franzini, D., Feldman, R.L., Crea, F., Fenech, A., Pepine, C.H., and Conti, C.R.: Laser recanalization of occluded atherosclerotic arteries in vivo and in vitro, Circulation **71:**403-411, 1985.
4. Ginsburg, R., Wexler, L., Mitchell, R.S., and Pinfitt, D.: Percutaneous transluminal laser angioplasty for treatment of peripheral vascular disease: clinical experience with 16 patients, Radiology **156:**619-624, 1985.
5. Choy, D.S.F., Stertzer, S.H., Myler, R.K., Marco, J., and Forunial, G.: Human coronary laser recanalization, Clin. Cardiol. **7:**377-381, 1984.
6. Cumberland, D.C., Taylor, D.I., and Procter, A.E.: Laser-assisted percutaneous angioplasty: initial clinical experience in peripheral arteries, Clin. Radiol. **37:**423-428, 1986.
7. Hussein, H.: A novel fiberoptic laser probe for treatment of occlusive vessel disease, Optical Laser Technol. Med. **605:**59-66, 1986.
8. Abela, G.S., Fenech, A., Crea, F., and Conti, C.R.: "Hot tip": another method of laser vascular recanalization, Lasers Surg. Med. **5:**327-335, 1985.
9. Sanborn, T.A., Haudenschild, C.C., Faxon, D.P., and Ryan, T.J.: Angiographic and histologic follow-up of laser angioplasty with a laser probe (abstract), J. Am. Coll. Cardiol. **5:**408, 1985.
10. Sanborn, T.A., Haudenschild, C.C., Faxon, D.P., Garber, G.R., and Ryan, T.J.: Angiographic and histologic consequences of laser thermal angioplasty: comparison with balloon angioplasty, Circulation **75:**281-286, 1987.
11. Sanborn, T.A., Cumberland, D.C., Tayler, D.I., and Ryan, T.J.: Human percutaneous laser thermal angioplasty (abstract), Circulation **72:**III-303, 1985.
12. Sanborn, T.A., Greenfield, A.J., Guben, J.K., Menzoian, J.O., and LoGerfo, F.W.: Human percutaneous and intraoperative laser thermal angioplasty: initial clinical results as an adjunct to balloon angioplasty, J. Vasc. Surg. **5:**83-90, 1987.
13. Cumberland, D.C., Sanborn, T.A., Tayler, D.I., Moore, D.J., Welsh, C.L., Greenfield, A.J., Guben, J.K., and Ryan, T.J.: Percutaneous laser thermal angioplasty: initial clinical results with a laserprobe in total peripheral artery occlusions, Lancet **1:**1457-1459, 1986.
14. Zietler, E., Richter, E.I., and Seyferth, W.: Femoropopliteal arteries. In Cotter, C.T., Gruentzig, A., Schoop, W., Zeitler, E., editors: Percutaneous transluminal angioplasty, Berlin, 1983, Springer-Verlag.
15. Hewes, R.C., White, R.I., Murray, R.R., Kaufman, S.L., Chang, R., Kadir, S., Kinninson, M.L., Mitchell, S.E., and Auster, M.: Long-term results of superficial femoral artery angioplasty, Am. J. Radiol. **146:**1025-1029, 1986.
16. Krepel, V.M., van Andel, G.J., van Erp, W.F.M., and Breslau, P.J.: Percutaneous trans-

luminal angioplasty of the femoropopliteal artery: Initial and long term results, Radiology **156:**325-328, 1985.

17. Murray, R.R., Hewes, R.L., White, R.I., Mitchell, S.E., Auster, M., Chang, R., Kadir, S., Kinnison, M.L., and Kaufman, S.L.: Long segment femoropopliteal stenoses: Is angioplasty a boom or a bust? Radiology **162:**473-476, 1987.
18. Sanborn, T.A., Cumberland, D.C., Welsh, C.L., Greenfield, A.J., and Guben, J.K.: Laser thermal angioplasty as an adjunct to peripheral balloon angioplasty: one year follow-up results (abstract), Circulation **76:**IV-30, 1987.
19. Sanborn, T.A., Faxon, D.P., Kellett, M.A., and Ryan, T.J.: Percutaneous coronary laser thermal angioplasty, J. Am. Coll. Cardiol. **8:**1437-1440, 1986.
20. Cumberland, D.C., Starkey, I.R., Oakley, G.D.G., Fleming, J.S., Smith, G.H., Goiti, J.J., Tayler, D.I., and Davis, J.: Percutaneous laser-assisted coronary angioplasty, Lancet **2:**214, 1986.

Chapter 13

Spark Erosion and Its Combination with Sensing Devices for Ablation of Vascular Lesions

Cornelis J. Slager, MSc
Nicolaas Bom, PhD
Patrick W. Serruys, MD
Johan C.H. Schuurbiers
Waldina V.A. Vandenbroucke, MD
Charles T. Lancée, PhD

For the recanalization of occluded arteries by means of plaque ablation, an electrical technique called spark-erosion has been developed. In-vitro tests have shown that well-defined holes can be produced easily in fibrous, collagenous, and lipid plaques, with minimal thermal side effects. Since the method is not selective by its nature, in-vivo application requires an additional guidance technique to avoid arterial perforation.

For this purpose, the potential use of sensing techniques such as tissue impedance measurement and intraarterial ultrasonic imaging are being tested. The main advantages of spark erosion are that it is a well-controllable, low-cost, and highly effective tissue ablation technique. Currently many research efforts are directed toward the development of new interventional techniques to be performed in the cardiac catheterization laboratory for the removal of obstructions in the coronary arteries. Such techniques should allow treatment of total or partial obstructions not accessible by the current balloon dilatation techniques. Hopefully the removal of the occluding material will also improve the long-term patency rate when compared with balloon dilatation alone.

The newer methods range from purely mechanical, such as atherectomy,[1] abrasive drilling,[2] and dynamic angioplasty,[3] to melting and/or vaporization of the plaques through local application of thermal energy. As a source of energy for vaporization several types of lasers have been used.[4,5] Energy is delivered to the obstructed area through light-conducting glass fibers.

As we demonstrated before, vaporization of

arteriosclerotic plaques can be achieved with a much simpler electrical technique called "spark erosion."[6] In industry spark erosion is used under the name of "electrical discharge machining" for the fabrication of intricate holes in metals. Basically this method involves the generation of small electrical sparks between a stamp electrode and the material to be processed. Each spark melts a small amount of material. By a series of sparks a controlled quantity can be removed. The resulting hole in the material corresponds exactly with the shape of the stamp electrode. Accuracies less than 0.1 mm are easily obtained.

Radiofrequency cutting, widely applied in operating theaters, is based on the same fundamental electrical erosion principles. However, it also incorporates purposely introduced side effects, such as dehydration and coagulation of adjacent zones in the tissue to achieve hemostasis. To apply the spark erosion technique successfully for the vaporization of atheromatous material, that is, with minimal thermal side effects, the radiofrequency cutting technique cannot be used as such.

One of the main problems of such tissue removal techniques is to prevent arterial perforation. Arterial curvature and the eccentricity of the obstructions in relation to the arterial wall require proper steering of the catheter tip.

Optimally the new methods should be made selective, so that normal wall tissue should not be affected by the removal technique. Because this has not been achieved with the currently proposed laser vaporization techniques, modification of the bare fiber tip was introduced[7,8] to reduce the risk of vessel wall perforation. A technically much more complicated laser approach using a multifiber catheter collects spectroscopic data to ablate the arterial obstruction in a selective way[9] in order to guide the vaporization technique through the arterial lumen. For the application of spark erosion its possible combinations with sensing techniques like tissue impedance measurement and intraarterial ultrasonic imaging are discussed in this chapter.

ELECTRICAL GENERATOR AND ELECTRODES

To avoid potential disturbance of the natural heart rhythm, spark erosion is applied in a pulsed mode. In this way, local energy delivery can be triggered by the electrocardiogram in order to apply the vaporization pulses selectively in the refractory period of the cardiac cycle. A single pulse can last 0.6 to 10 ms. During this period a square-wave alternating voltage is generated with a peak-to-peak value of 1400 V at a frequency of 500 kHz. For safety reasons the generator is battery-operated but can still deliver a maximal peak power of several kilowatts into a load of 60 ohm. To prevent the generator from delivering direct current, the output stage is coupled to the load by capacitors. One output terminal is connected to the active electrode, an example of which is shown in Fig. 13-1. Dimensions of this electrode determine the diameter of the new lumen to be produced. The upper limit of the diameter is approximately 2.5 to 3 mm. In all cases, a return electrode is necessary. This can be a relatively small metal skin electrode; it is also possible to let the return electrode be part of the spark erosion catheter.

RESULTS

Tissue Ablation

When using the spark erosion technique on human atherosclerotic tissue, small holes with diameters equal to that of the electrode can easily be obtained. It can be calculated[6] that during a single 10 ms period the total amount of energy delivered to the tissue approximates

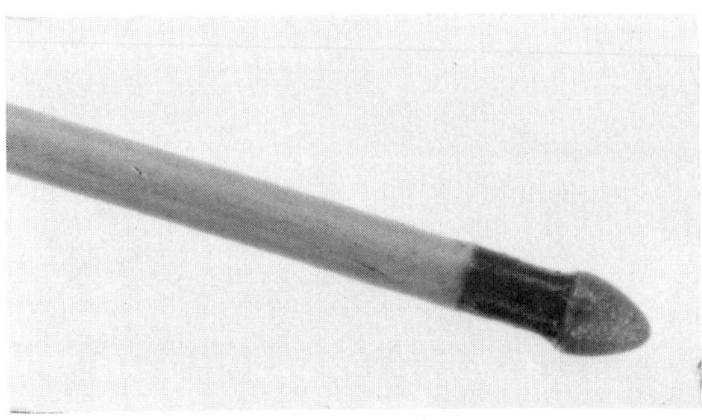

Fig. 13-1. Example of a spark erosion electrode, 1.5 mm in diameter, mounted at the tip of a catheter.

1.7 J. With this amount of energy a 1.5 mm circular electrode can produce an average ablation depth of 0.2 mm. Different types of tissue (fibromuscular, collagenous, and fibrofatty) show similar results. On mainly calcified lesions no effect can be observed.

Histologic examination showed relatively smooth edges and only a very small rim of coagulated tissue with a general thickness below 40 μm and no necrotic debris inside the holes (Fig. 13-2). In plaques containing mainly lipids the coagulative zone could reach to a distance of 200 μm.

Probably the minimal thermal side effects are the result of the powerful eroding capacities of the individual sparks and can be explained as follows. During a sparking period of some milliseconds, thousands of sparks can be generated between the electrode and the tissue. Each individual spark produces at its microscopically small target point a power density high enough to raise the local temperature over 100° C within a fraction of a microsecond. Subsequently the tissue water content starts boiling so fast that a kind of microexplosion follows that leads to ablation and fragmentation of the targeted area. After ablation some gas bubbles can be seen to escape locally. Preliminary data of a gas chromatography study show that the gas consists of hydrogen, oxygen, carbon dioxide, and a range of small hydrocarbons.

ANIMAL STUDIES

The possible effects of the spark erosion technique on the electrocardiogram and the electrical activity of the heart were studied in seven anesthetized closed-chest pigs, in which a spark erosion catheter was positioned 2 to 5 cm from the ostium in one of the main branches of the coronary arteries. The electrocardiogram and aortic pressure from a catheter-tip manometer were recorded continuously. Sparks in the coronary artery were generated over periods of 10 ms, triggered by the R wave of the electrocardiogram.

Ten tests were carried out on each of the seven animals. Ten pulses were generated immediately after the peak of the R wave on the electrocardiogram. In all cases no effects on cardiac rhythm or aortic blood pressure could be observed. In the next sequence of tests, 10 pulses were given at a different time delay after the R wave. Pulses generated at a delay of 300 ms or more after the R wave generally introduced an ectopic beat. Ventricular fibrillation did not occur.

STEERING OF SPARK EROSION

Separate spark erosion tests on normal wall tissue showed vaporization results similar to those obtained on atherosclerotic tissue. Most lesions are built up in an asymmetric way and as a consequence the position of the remaining lumen is eccentric with respect to the outer arterial wall. Mainly for this reason intraluminal spark erosion application generally requires an additional steering technique to prevent perforation of the normal part of the

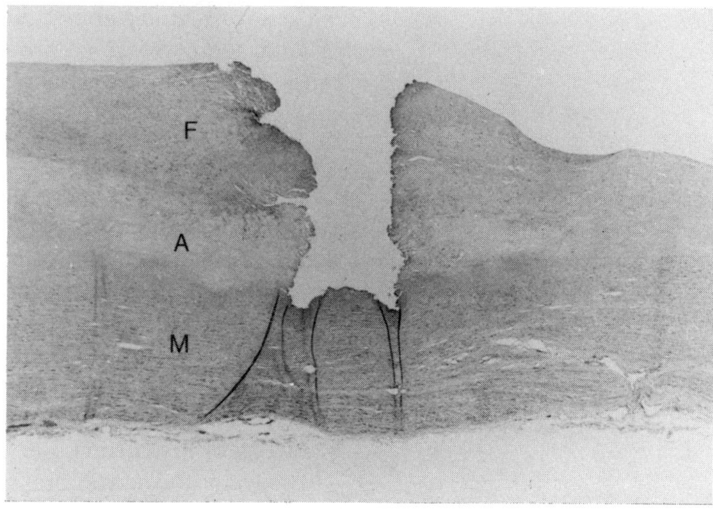

Fig. 13-2. Histologic preparation of a section through the aortic wall showing an atheromatous plaque covered by a fibrous cap and a 1.5 mm wide crater produced within it by spark erosioning. The small darker-stained zone at the crater edge shows that thermal side effects are minimal. (Hematoxylin eosin stain; × 12.) (A, atheromatous material; F, fibrous cap; M, media.)

wall. Because tissue vaporization only occurs very close to the sparking electrode, several potential constructions can be devised for local application of the sparking process in a selected region.

For example, a catheter tip as shown in Fig. 13-3, having two isolated electrodes, can be used for selecting the spark erosion process to occur in two opposite directions. Each electrode is connected by a different electrical conductor to the generator. Such a catheter tip has been tested under visual control on segments of human femoral arteries freshly obtained at autopsy, which showed an almost total eccentric occlusion. In Fig. 13-4, A and B the widened lumen in the atherosclerotic plaque was achieved by sparking with only one of the two electrodes of such a catheter tip. The endothelial wall nearest to the media shows no sign of any thermal damage. The opposite plaque side shows microscopic irregularities and discoloration as a sign of side effects of the spark erosion process.

Extension of the multielectrode tip configuration to three or more electrodes is feasible, while still maintaining sufficient flexibility of the catheter. Another solution can be achieved with a single eccentric electrode on a steerable, rotating catheter tip. A tip electrode with a small central hole that can be advanced over an isolated guidewire is also feasible.

SENSING METHODS

To guide a spark erosion catheter having a single rotating tip or a number of selectable tip electrodes safely through a complexly narrowed artery, additional means are required to sense the position of the catheter tip in relation to the atherosclerotic plaque and the outer vessel wall.

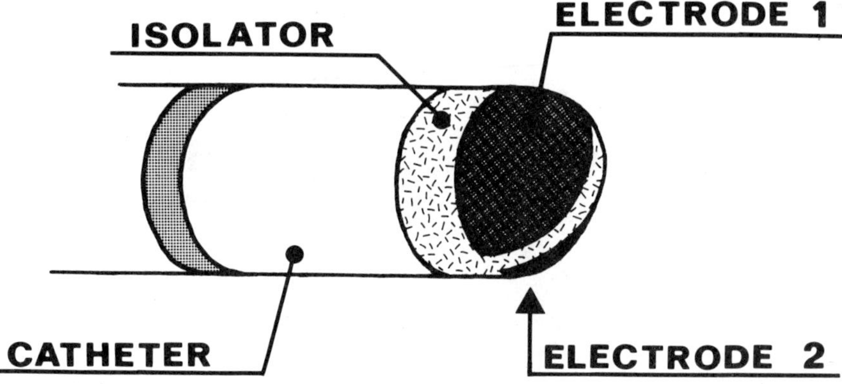

Fig. 13-3. Catheter tip with two separately selectable electrodes.

Tissue Impedance Measurement

As an attractive parameter for sensing the position of a spark erosion catheter-tip electrode in relation to an atherosclerotic plaque, we have extensively studied the electrical impedance of tissue. If the electrical impedance of an atherosclerotic plaque differs sufficiently from that of the normal wall, such a principle would have great potential for application of the catheter tip. On a series of 13 human aortic segments, freshly obtained at autopsy, the electrical impedance was measured at 56 different atherosclerotic locations and at 11 spots on the normal wall. In the measured frequency range of 5 to 500 kHz, the impedance of all tissue types was almost purely resistive. A calibrated salt bridge electrode having an aperture of 0.35 mm was used for the measurements. Histologic examination was used to classify the different types of tissue at all measuring-spots. The frequency distribution of the electrical resistivity at 100 kHz of different types of tissue is shown in Fig. 13-5. As can readily be observed, the majority of lesions consist of fibrous tissue that shows a specific resistance value being close to the normal range of 150 to 250 ohm cm. Only lesions with a superficial layer consisting of fatty or calcified deposits showed up with significant higher resistivity values than normal wall tissue. Especially calcified areas have the highest resistivity at 1400 ohm cm. This value may even be underestimated as a result of technical difficulties with the measuring method. Even a very thin wet layer on the surface of tissue with a high resistivity may cause an important amount of superficial current leakage. From this study we concluded that tissue impedance will only be of limited value as a local sensing parameter for the guidance of spark erosion.

Intraarterial Ultrasonic Imaging

The insight gained from the tissue impedance measurements, as well as from experiments with transluminal angioscopy, lead to the conviction that sensing techniques that only provide data of the superficial endothelial tissue layer will not be optimal for intraluminal guidance of the spark erosion ablation technique. For this reason study of the feasibility of high-frequency intraarterial ultrasonic imaging is a logical next step. A photograph of a first ultrasonic imaging prototype transducer, designed for in-vitro intraluminal studies is shown in Fig. 13-6. A 1 mm diameter, 20 MHz piezoelectric element is mounted at the axis position of a 2.5 mm diameter rigid steel rod. To allow for a sufficiently long dead zone

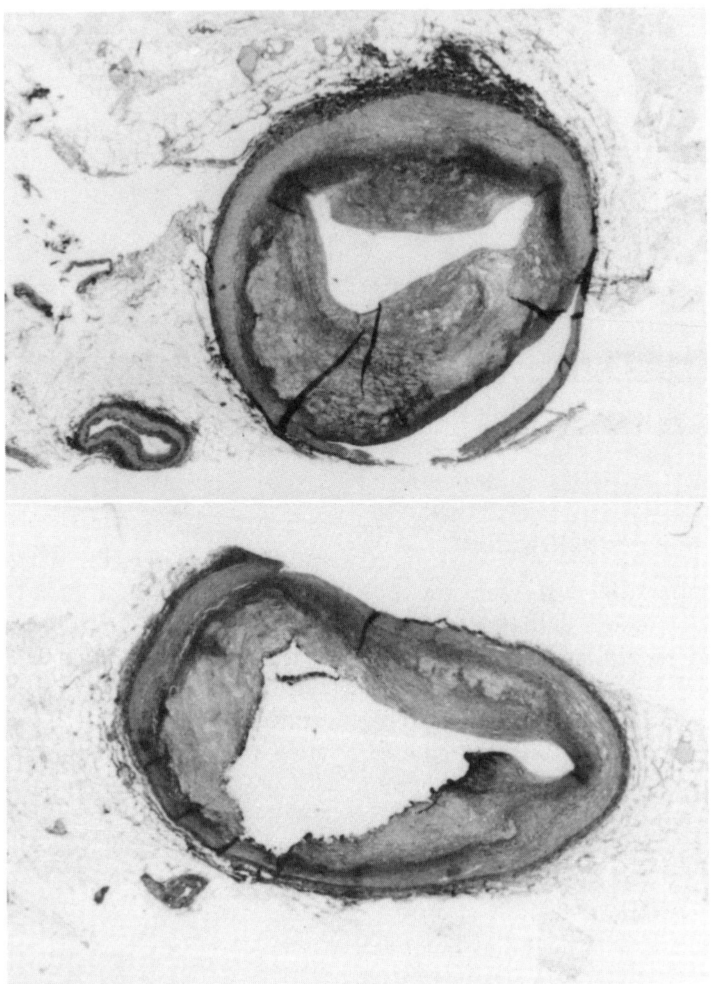

Fig. 13-4. A, Transverse section through a narrowed part of a coronary artery. **B,** Using a spark erosion electrode as drawn in Fig. 13-3, part of the lumen closely localized to the plane shown in Fig. 13-4A was widened by sparking only toward one side. (Elastic–van Giesen stain; × 22.)

between the tissue and the element, the ultrasonic beam is reflected by a mirror. The complete rod was mounted in an assembly and rotated stepwise by a stepping motor. An ultrasound intraarterial image obtained from a specimen of the carotid artery is shown in Fig. 13-7.

Constructions combining spark erosion and ultrasonic imaging[11] are currently being developed. A 2 mm diameter prototype of such a possible combination is shown in Fig. 13-8. Three tip electrodes are intended to be used for the selection of the sparking direction. A single piezo element is mounted axially in the frontal tip and the mirror is the rotating element to sweep the ultrasonic beam over 360

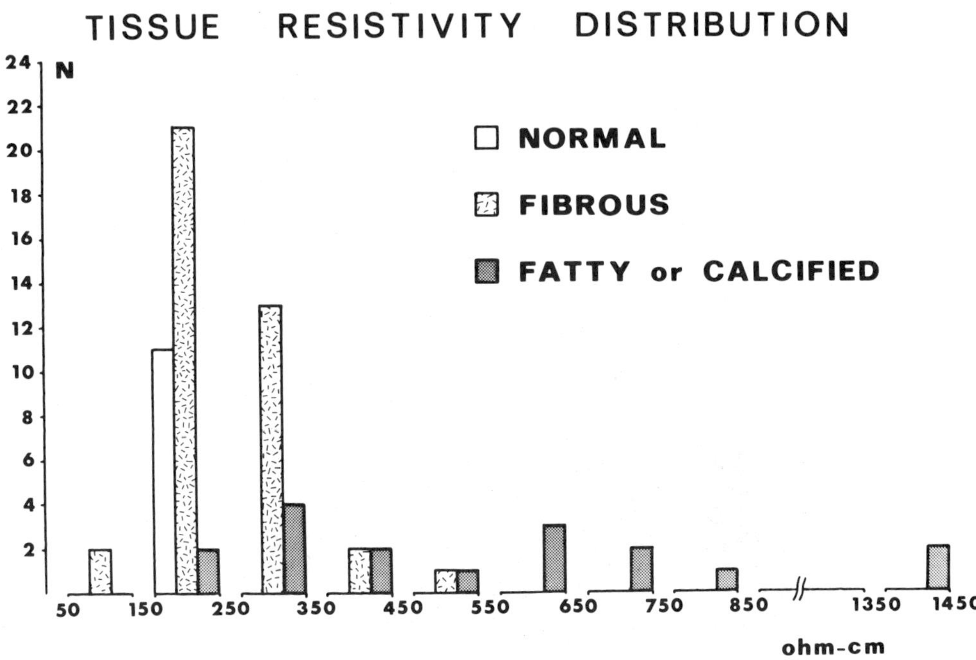

Fig. 13-5. For a total of 69 measuring spots the distribution over different specific resistance ranges is depicted in this histogram. Normal tissue is in the range of 150 to 250 Ohm cm. Of the fibrous tissue group, 16 measurements show a higher resistivity than the normal wall, 21 are in the normal range, and 2 are below normal. On fatty or calcified plaques, 15 out of a total of 17 measurements show a much higher specific resistivity than the normal group.

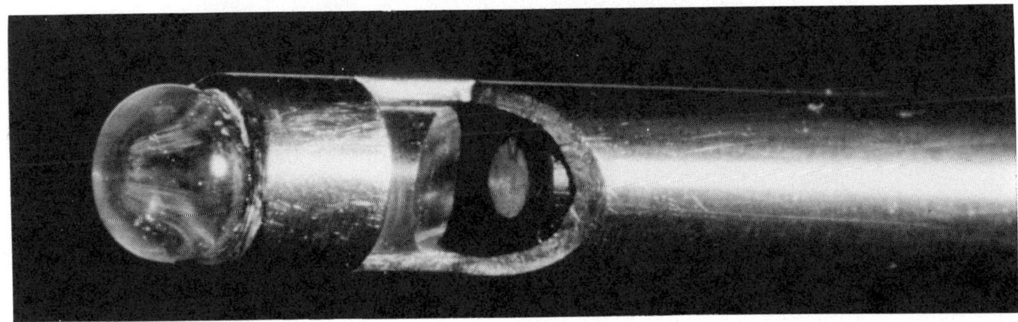

Fig. 13-6. Rigid transducer assembly driven by a stepping motor as used for rotational cross-sectional ultrasonic imaging.

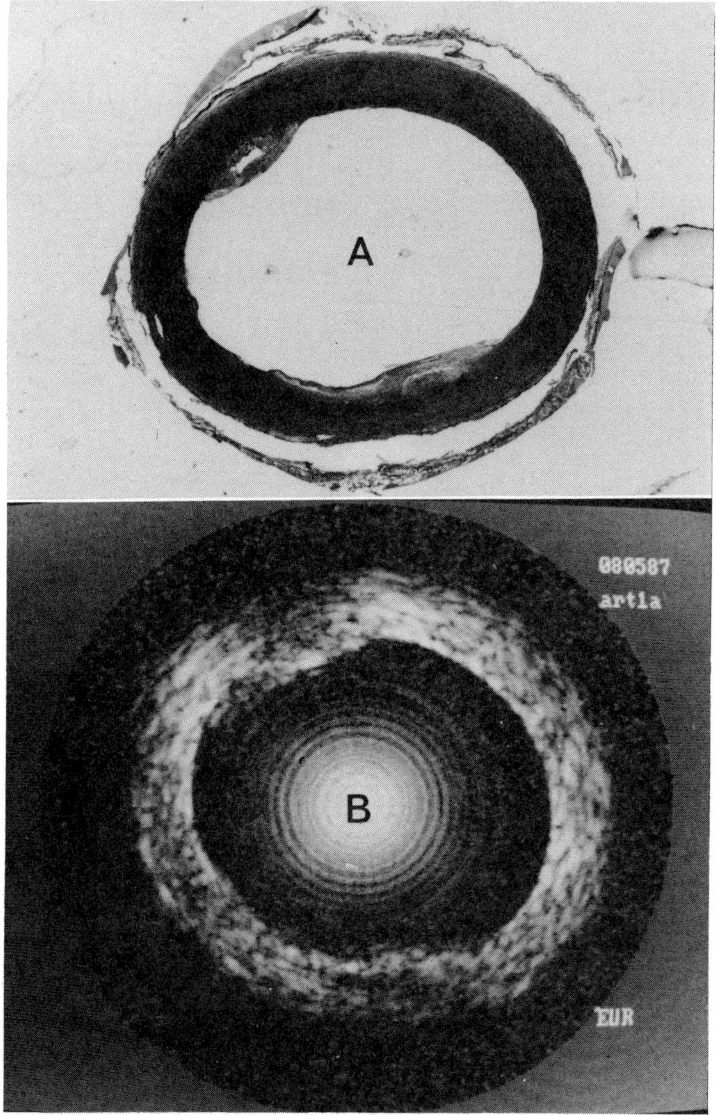

Fig. 13-7. First imaging results of an arterial specimen **(A)** and the corresponding intraarterial echo image **(B)**.

degrees. Although in this construction the imaging plane has to be positioned behind the erosion plane, probably adequate guidance can still be derived from the visualization of the media-adventitia border and its relative position to the catheters' axis. The prototype shown needs some further adaptations on a few technical details before actual testing of the combined action of spark erosion and ultrasonic imaging can take place.

DISCUSSION

For the transluminal removal of atherosclerotic plaques the application of laser energy

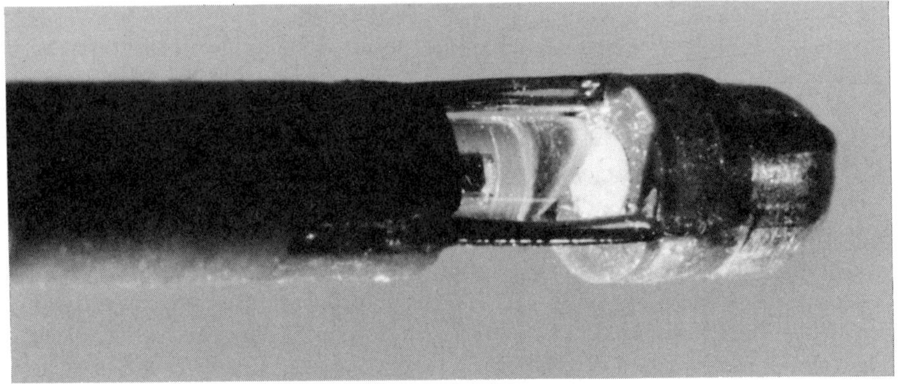

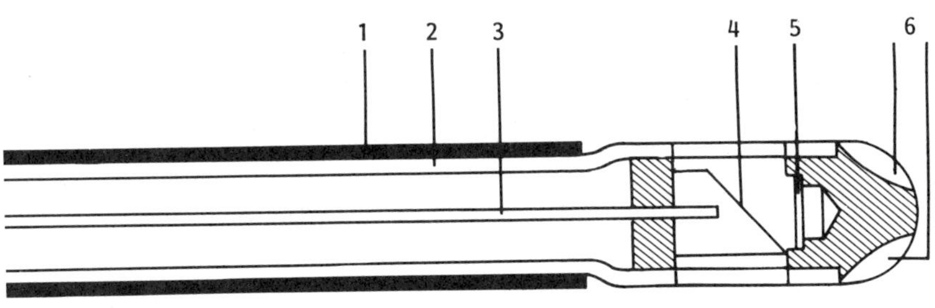

Fig. 13-8. Schematic drawing and photograph of a potential spark erosion/ ultrasonic imaging combination. Outer diameter is 2 mm.

guided through a fiberoptic delivery system is studied on a wide scale. One of the most attractive features of the laser would have been selective application by local enhanced absorption in atherosclerotic plaque compared with a negligible absorption in the normal wall. However, this operating principle has not been proved yet to be useful for recanalization of an occluded artery by a laser catheter without the risk of arterial perforation. Until now the most successful recanalization technique with a low perforation rate has been based on application of thermal energy from a heated metal catheter tip.[7] Although the laser has been used almost exclusively for heating such a tip, new, lower cost, nonlaser approaches[12,13] will probably come up for this purpose in the near future. No literature is available on the basic mechanism and the secondary heat-induced effects of the hot-tip recanalization procedure. Probably processes such as tissue desiccation and melting of lipids play a dominant role, while real tissue ablation is minimal. This could explain the low perforation risk of this procedure. However, the accompanying heat-induced tissue damage may be high. Whether these side effects will be detrimental to reach a low restenosis rate must become clear from ongoing studies in this area.[14] From our experiments with spark erosion[6] we learned how to reduce secondary heat damage to the tissue and how to accentuate tissue vaporization. Whether the production of such a clean-cut hole through an arterial obstruction will be of decisive importance to get a long-lasting recanalization result must be the subject of further study.

Electrical side effects on the heart's natural activity did not appear to be an obstacle for an ultimate cardiologic application of spark erosion. It must be studied whether this safety is preserved during myocardial ischemia. In the pig study mentioned earlier ectopic beats could be induced by applying spark erosion pulses at a delay of 300 ms or more after the R wave. Apparently, alternating current is able to stimulate nerve and/or muscle tissue despite the applied high frequency of 500 kHz. Recently started experiments to study the healing response of the iliac artery in rabbits after spark erosion application also revealed that electrical stimulation of nerves and/or muscles may accompany the spark erosion pulses. In particular the application of the spark erosion technique in peripheral arteries requires further study of this phenomenon.

The local production of gas bubbles and other tissue debris needs further investigation. As has been observed also with laser application, cutting in atherosclerotic plaques can be accompanied by the production of a nonnegligible amount of debris.[15] The most recent, more powerful version of our spark erosion generator has a number of selectable settings to study the effects of various electrical and timing parameters on the production of gas and debris.

The main problem, however, facing the construction of any intraarterial tissue removal technique based on the vaporization principle is probably the need to find an adequate guidance system. Concentric lesions can be approached easily, for example, a conical tip electrode passing over an isolated guidewire. For the removal of eccentric lesions a system will be required that combines a steering technique for the spark erosion process together with some sensing method. Since the spark erosion effect only occurs in a very limited region near the sparking electrode, steering of the process can be achieved by adequate positioning of the electrode against the atherosclerotic plaque.

As a potentially very attractive sensing parameter we have studied electrical tissue impedance. The electric resistivity measurements showed that the resistivity of fatty and calcified atherosclerotic plaques differs significantly from the normal wall values. Despite the fact that many of the fibrous lesions consist of only a relatively thin fibrous cap covering high-ohmic fatty deposits, the resistivity values obtained for these lesions show a significant overlap with those of the normal wall. The reason for this is that impedance measurements mainly yield data of the superficial tissue layer. By applying guarding techniques the impedance method may be improved to produce data of the deeper tissue layers. However, such methods are prone to other artifacts, for example, the normal arterial wall may show up with an apparently raised resistivity because of the high impedance of the embedding arterial fat.

Intraarterial ultrasonic imaging has the interesting potential of visualizing the catheter position in relation to the outer arterial wall. Our first experience with the integration of spark erosion and an intraarterial ultrasonic imaging device has shown that this is technologically feasible. In-vitro tests of the ultrasonic imaging technique delivered detailed images that closely correspond with the real anatomy.

To conclude, as for other vaporizing methods, spark erosion needs to be combined with a sensing method in order to identify the area to be vaporized. For this purpose intraarterial ultrasonic imaging seems to be an optimal technique. By its nature spark erosion can easily be applied at well-defined user selectable areas. With the exception of calcified lesions, the most frequently occurring atherosclerotic plaques can be ablated in a controllable way. Whether electrical stimulation and the production of gas and/or debris requires modification of the technique needs further study. Also tissue healing response after spark erosion is not yet known, but as has been demonstrated, the damage to adjacent tissue can be kept very minimal.

ACKNOWLEDGMENTS

This work has been supported in part by the Dutch Heart Foundation under grant No. 84.073 and by the Interuniversity Cardiology Institute of the Netherlands.

REFERENCES

1. Simpson, J.B., Johnson, D.E., Braden, L.J., Gifford, H.S., Thapliyal, H.V., and Selmon, M.R.: Transluminal coronary atherectomy (TCA): results in 21 human cadaver vascular segments (abstract), Circulation **74:**II-202, 1986.
2. Ritchie, J.L., Hansen, D.D., Vracko, R., and Auth, D.: In vivo rotational thrombectomy: evaluation by angioscopy, Circulation **74:**II-457, 1986.
3. Kensey, K., Nash, J., Abrahams, C., Lake, K., and Zarins, C.K.: Recanalization of obstructed arteries using a flexible rotating tip catheter (abstract), Circulation **74:**II-457, 1986.
4. Abela, G.S., Normann, S., Cohen, D., Feldman, R.L., Geiser, E.A., and Conti, C.R.: Effects of carbon dioxide, Nd-YAG, and argon laser radiation on coronary atheromatous plaques, Am. J. Cardiol. **50:**1199-1205, 1982.
5. Isner, J.M., Donaldson, R.F., Deckelbaum, L.J., Clarke, R.H., Laliberte, S.M., Ucci, A.A., Salem, D.N., and Konstam, M.A.: The excimer laser: gross, light microscopic and ultrastructural analysis of potential advantages for use in laser therapy of cardiovascular disease, J. Am. Coll. Cardiol. **6:**1102-1109, 1985.
6. Slager, C.J., Essed, C.E., Schuurbiers, J.C.H., Bom, N., Serruys, P.W., and Meester, G.T.: Vaporization of atherosclerotic plaques by spark erosion, J. Am. Coll. Cardiol. **5:**1382-1386, 1985.
7. Sanborn, T.A., Faxon, D.P., Haudenschild, Ch.C., and Ryan, T.J.: Experimental angioplasty: circumferential distribution of laser thermal energy with a laser probe, J. Am. Coll. Cardiol. **5:**934-938, 1985.
8. Fourrier, J.L., Marache, P., Brunetaud, J.M., Mordon, S., Lablanche, J.M., and Bertrand, M.E.: Laser recanalization of peripheral arteries by contact sapphire in man (abstract), Circulation **74:**II-204, 1986.
9. Cothren, R.M., Hayes, G.B., Kramer, J.R., Sacks, B., Kittrell, C., and Feld, M.S.: A multifiber catheter with an optical shield for laser angiosurgery, Laser Life Sciences **1:**1-12, 1986.
10. Closed-chest pig study
11. Slager, C.J.: Echo-vonkerosie recanalisatie inrichting, Dutch Patent Application No. 8700632, March 17, 1987.
12. Lu, D.Y., Leon, M.B., Bowman, R.L., Bethesda NHLBI: A prototype catalytic thermal tip catheter: design parameters and in vitro tissue studies (abstract), J. Am. Coll. Cardiol. **9:**187A, 1987.
13. Lu, D.Y., Leon, M.B., Bowman, R.L., Bethesda NHLBI: A prototype electric thermal tip: design parameters and in vitro studies (abstract), Circulation **74:**II-496, 1977.

14. Cumberland, D.C., Sanborn, T.A., Taylor, D.I., Moore, D.J., Welsh, C.L., et al.: Percutaneous laser thermal angioplasty: initial clinical results with a laser probe in total peripheral artery occlusions, Lancet **1**:1457-1459, 1986.

15. Grewe, D.D., Castaneda-Zuniga, W.R., Nordstrom, L.A., Gray, R.J., Friedberg, H.D., et al.: Debris analysis after laser photorecanalization of atherosclerotic plaque, Semin. Intervent. Radiol. **3**:53-60, 1986.

Chapter 14

The Excimer Laser: From Basic Science to Clinical Application

Frank Litvack, MD
James S. Forrester, MD, FACC
Warren S. Grundfest, MD
Frederick W. Mohr, MD
Thanassis Papaioannou, MSc

EXCIMER LASER ANGIOPLASTY IN HUMANS

We have recently begun excimer laser angioplasty in humans. In contrast to other lasers[1-4] the excimer delivers very brief, high-energy pulses that create microscopically precise cuts. There is virtually no evidence of thermal injury. Although the potential impact of the excimer laser on the practice of angioplasty is substantial, there are some important problems yet to be resolved. In this chapter, we reduce the complexities of the excimer laser and fiberoptic technology to the essentials required for the practice of interventional cardiology, and describe our first clinical experiences using this device in occlusive atherosclerotic disease of humans.

PHYSICAL CHARACTERISTICS OF THE EXCIMER LASER

"Excimer" is a contraction of "excited dimer," which means two identical atoms in an excited state. The four most important excimer gases are ArF, KrF, XeF, and XeCl, all of which produce short-wavelength ultraviolet laser light. We use the 308 nm XeCl laser because it is most practical for intravascular use. The device itself consists of a metal cylinder containing XeCl gas mixed with nitrogen, an electrical power source, a heat exchanger, and a coupler to transmit the energy from the cylinder to a fiberoptic and a catheter-based fiberoptic delivery system. The length of the metal cylinder is a multiple of 308 nm wavelength. At each end of the cylinder are parallel mirrors that serve as a resonator for the laser light. One mirror allows a portion of the 308 nm light to enter the coupler, which focuses it onto the fiberoptic delivery system.

CONVERSION OF ELECTRICAL ENERGY TO EXCIMER LASER LIGHT

Lasers are typically very inefficient: only 1 to 4% of the electrical input is converted into light; the remainder becomes heat. When electrical energy enters the gas chamber the electron energy of the XeCl molecules is transiently increased above the normal ground state. The excited, higher energy level is unstable.

When the excited electrons return to ground energy level, they emit precisely the same quantum energy just absorbed, but now the energy is in the form of radiation. The wavelength of the emitted radiation is determined by the quantum of energy previously absorbed. For XeCl gas, the wavelength emitted is 308 nm, which is light in the ultraviolet spectrum. As these energetic photons of 308 nm of light travel through the cylinder, they strike other XeCl molecules, and the same process of excitation and energy release is repeated. The reflection of light back and forth between the mirrors serves to cause an enormous escalation in the light energy within the cylinder.

Because the relationship between wavelength and energy is reciprocal, the short ultraviolet wavelength pulse has much higher energy per pulse than conventional longer wavelength medical lasers such as argon, Nd:YAG, or carbon dioxide (CO_2). The key features of the excimer laser for medical application, therefore, are its short-duration pulse (10 to 200 nanoseconds) and its high energy per pulse (e.g., 50 to 100 mJ/mm^2).

THE LASER-TISSUE INTERACTION: CONTINUOUS VERSUS PULSED ENERGY

Continuous wave and pulsed lasers have quite different effects on tissue. We have used high-speed image analysis and continuous temperature measurements to characterize laser-tissue interaction. Continuous wave lasers cause tissue ablation in a continuum of overlapping phases: blanching, melting, vaporization with visible particle ejection, carbonization, and lateral tissue expansion.[5] Histologic studies show that the vascular tissue immediately develops a cone-shaped crater with a carbonized surface. Beneath the surface are concentric zones of protein denaturation and tissue vacuolization. Thermographic camera studies clarify the mechanism of histologic injury. In vascular tissue we found that the peak temperature at the point of impact reached 160° C during 2 seconds of continuous-wave argon-ion irradiation. The temperature of adjacent tissue at a distance from the point of impact also increased. For instance tissue 2.5 mm from the impact point reached 80° C within 2 seconds.[6] This charred, ragged endothelial surface is not desirable in vascular application because it leads to thrombosis, and thermal diffusion is not desirable because it leads to perforation. Thus in the past several years it has become increasingly clear that unmodified continuous wave lasers are not well suited for vascular use, despite their ability to rapidly vaporize atheroma. As a result of this understanding, laser research has concentrated on ablating tissue while limiting thermal injury.

An appealing solution to laser-induced thermal injury is the delivery of energy in very short pulses. Pulsed XeCl excimer laser tissue ablation appears to occur as a discrete event with each short-duration, high-energy pulse when viewed by high-speed filming at 5000 frames per second. There is no melting or boiling, and no visible ejection of particulate debris. The margins of the incision are precisely regular and conform exactly to the laser beam configuration at the site of impact (Fig. 14-1). These differences suggest that greater operator control of the ablation process, greater precision of cutting, and reduced risk of spasm and thrombosis might be expected in vascular application.

The mechanism responsible for the histologic differences between the thermal and excimer laser families has been elucidated by studies of the temporal and spatial distribution of temperature. Using a thermographic camera, Mohr and co-workers found that temperature at the impact point of continuous wave lasers exceeded 225° C, whereas the maximal temperature using the excimer laser was 63.5° C. The spatial distribution of temperature was equally quite different. At 1 mm from the point of impact of thermal laser energy, temperatures were 100 to 115° C, whereas with the excimer laser the temperature was 40° C. For this reason, the cuts made by the excimer laser are microscopically precise.

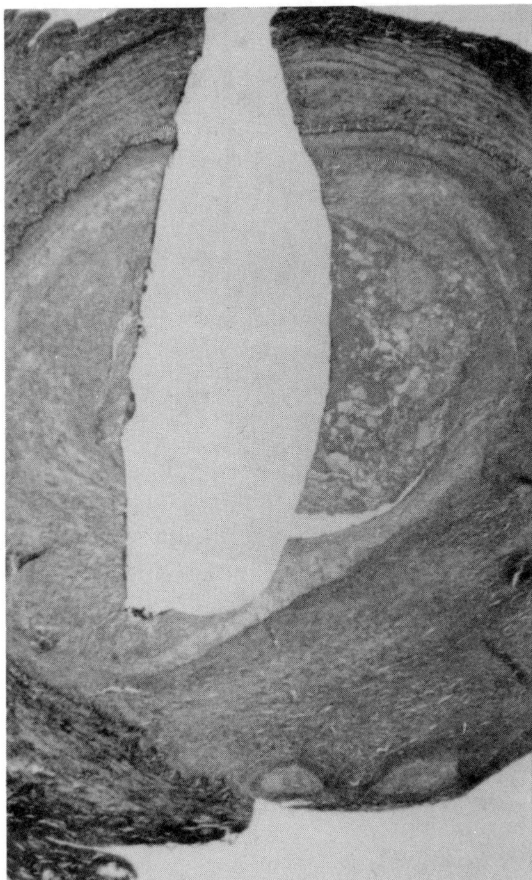

Fig. 14-1. Cross-section of a recanalized atherosclerotic artery after excimer irradiation at 193 cm, 15 nsec pulse width, 100 mJ pulses (200 mJ/mm^2), and 20 Hz. Very precise incision margins without any evidence of thermal injury are seen.

THE MECHANISM OF EXCIMER LASER ACTION

There are two theories about the absence of thermal injury with short-duration laser pulsing, and they are not mutually exclusive. The first theory invokes thermal diffusion. Excimer laser pulses penetrate only a few micra of tissue. They are also very brief. Both factors limit tissue diffusion of heat. Advocates of the thermal diffusion theory point out that the high energy of the excimer laser pulse vaporizes tissue instantly, leaving no time for heat buildup in adjacent tissue. Finally limitation of thermal injury by short-duration pulses is not limited to the 308 nm wavelength. Both Isner[7] and Grundfest and associates[8] markedly induced histologic thermal injury using a Q-switched Nd:YAG laser at a low repetition rate.

The second possible mechanism responsible for absence of thermal injury is "photodecomposition."[9,10] Photodecomposition occurs when sufficient energy is absorbed to displace an ulceration, that is, to cause an ion to form. This ionization ruptures molecular bonds, and thus material is ablated by a nonthermal process. Physicists point out that the lack of thermal injury is not unique to the XeCl laser, but rather it is typical of all high-pulse energy ultraviolet wavelengths, which are those that have sufficient energy to ionize materials. Regardless of mechanism, it is clear that the precision of the XeCl incision in vascular tissue is due to several factors: high-pulse energy, short-pulse duration, limited tissue penetrance, and possibly photodecomposition.

These physical principles can be summarized in terms of an interventional cardiologist:

1. The short-wavelength energy of the excimer laser is intensely absorbed at the atheroma surface and does not diffuse into adjacent, nontarget tissue. The effect is precise cutting, at the rate of a few micra per pulse. The precise incision makes it more suited for small vessels, in which a minimally traumatic approach may be essential to eliminate both thrombus formation and restenosis.[11]
2. The high energy of the excimer laser can instantly vaporize atheroma. As a result of its short duration and limited penetrance of the atheroma, the XeCl laser leaves very little thermal injury beneath the cut surface.
3. Because there is no lateral diffusion of energy, increasing the number of pulses does not increase the width of the incision but only its depth (Fig. 14-2).
4. The high energy of the XeCl pulse allows it to destroy atheroma constituents that are resistant to lower energy lasers. The excimer laser can effectively ablate calcified plaque unlike conventional thermal lasers.

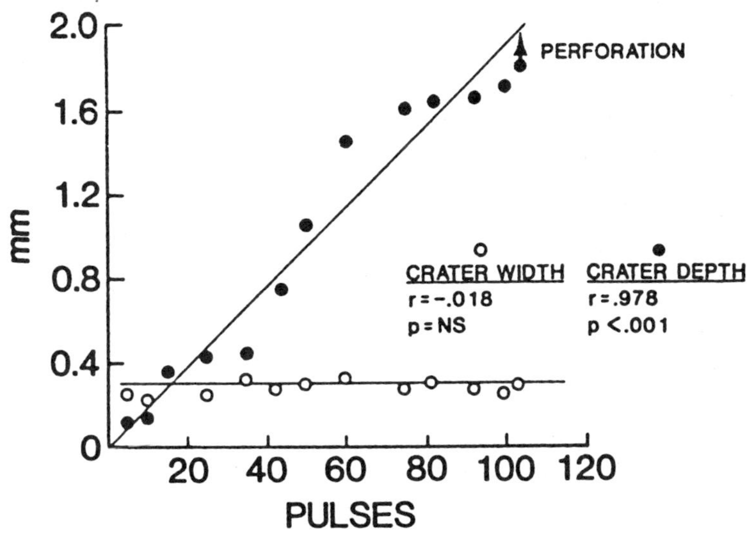

Fig. 14-2. Correlation of depth and width of incision versus number of pulses after excimer irradiation of atherosclerotic tissue at 308 nm. The depth of incision increases linearly with increasing number of pulses, whereas width remains constant.

OPERATOR CONTROL OF LASER ACTION: ENERGY DENSITY AND REPETITION RATE

Control of the amount and speed of tissue ablation is maintained by the operator through regulation of energy density and repetition rate. Energy density is the laser beam's energy per unit area at the impact site, typically expressed in mJ/mm^2. Our group and others have defined the relationship between energy density and tissue ablation by studying the dose-response curves for normal and atherosclerotic arterial tissue. This relationship is called ablation curve for each laser. It is a useful concept for the interventional cardiologist. There is a minimum energy density required to produce tissue ablation. Below this threshold level, vascular tissue is only blanched or charred. An ablation threshold of 14 to 18 mJ/mm^2 for the 308 nm XeCl laser has been reported for vacular tissue.[12] As the energy density of the 308 nm beam is increased beyond 14 to 18 mJ/mm^2 there is a progressive increase in the rate of atheroma ablation. At a certain energy density, however, the measured rate of tissue ablation reaches a plateau. For vascular tissue, this is approximately 100 mJ/mm^2. The threshold minimum and this value establish the ablation range. Within this range, the operator can increase the rate of vascular tissue ablation either by increasing the energy density or by increasing the repetition rate (Fig. 14-3).

The ablation range should be treated as a concept rather than a fixed quantity because it varies greatly with the target tissue. With the XeCl laser, for instance, there is a threefold difference in ablation rate between normal human myocardium (0.35 mm per pulse) and scarred myocardium (0.10 mm per pulse). The

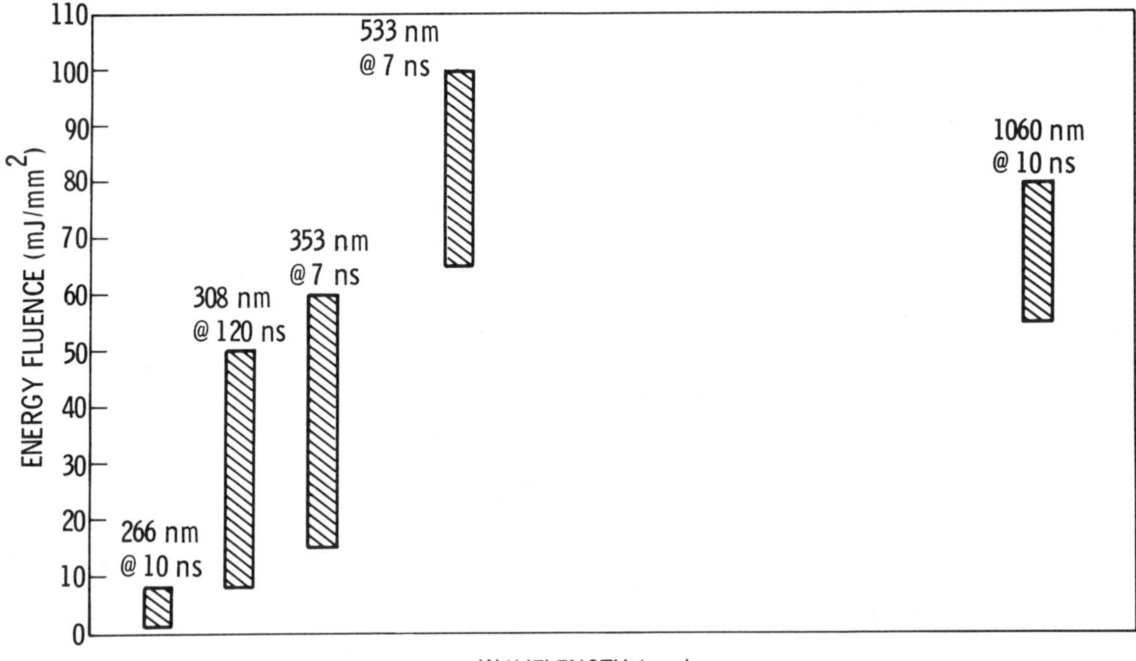

Fig. 14-3. Graph demonstrating the ablation thresholds as a function of fluence (mJ/mm^2) of different wavelengths.

practical importance of the concept, however, is that when one operates outside the ablation range thermal injury can be induced, even with the XeCl laser. There are four circumstances in which thermal injury occurs: when the energy density lies outside the ablation range, when the repetition rate exceeds 100 Hz, when irradiation is protracted over time, and when the beam is not focused.

THE FIBEROPTIC DELIVERY SYSTEM

With the possible exception of direct delivery in an operating room, laser energy for vascular application must be delivered to the target by fiberoptics. For the excimer laser in particular this requirement represented a major problem in system development. Energies within the ablation range destroyed the optical fiber by a process called dielectric (or electron avalance) breakdown. In this process the laser pulse activates the electrons of the fiberoptic material. The fiberoptic breakdown process is increased by shortening pulse duration. It therefore becomes a particular problem when nanosecond pulses are employed, as is typical for the XeCl laser.

The problem has proved to be resolvable. We discovered that we could markedly increase the pulse duration of the XeCl laser, yet remain within the nanosecond range, without changing ablation rate.[13] This finding turned out to be critically important, because when we increased the pulse duration from 10 to 100 ns, fiberoptic destruction ceased to be a problem for energies within the ablation range. We are now able to transmit high excimer laser energy density with the longer pulse duration. The useful generalization is that the pulse duration we use must be longer than that which induces fiberoptic breakdown, but shorter than that which causes thermal tissue damage. We are fortunate that the 308 nm excimer laser has a fairly wide range of effective pulse duration. Within the ablation range, a pulse of 100 to 250 ns is effective. With our current lasers, we can deliver 100 mJ/mm^2, 100 ns pulses without fiberoptic damage.

These tradeoffs involving energy density and pulse duration are particularly important for human intravascular use because small-diameter fibers are more prone to dielectric damage, but are also more flexible. Since prolongation of pulse duration reduces the damage to fiberoptics, this in turn allows the fabrication of very small diameter, flexible fibers. We can then place several very small diameter fibers in a catheter delivery system that has both flexibility and the ability to create a new orifice of sufficient diameter to restore blood flow. In our first clinical trials, discussed later, we have used two systems. For complete occlusions, we have used a single 600 μm diameter fiberoptic passed through a guiding catheter. For stenoses, we have used a multifiber, over-the-wire system (Fig. 14-4). The over-the-wire system is preferable, we believe, because it adds an important measure of operator control. The over-the-wire system causes the fiberoptic tip to be constantly oriented along the long axis of the blood vessel, and it seems to eliminate the risk of placing the tip against the side of the vessel wall.

THE PRODUCTS OF EXCIMER ABLATION

Laser irradiation of atheroma produces gaseous hydrocarbons and CO_2 regardless of wavelength.[14,15] If photodecomposition is important in the action of 308 nm excimer laser energy, we could also expect that unstable submolecular fragments such as free radicals and diatomics would be released. These have not been detectable by gas chromatography. Particulate debris can also be created when the irradiated tissue is calcified, for example, during irradiation of cardiac valves.[16] DeJesus and co-workers[17] found 30 to 1240 μm debris during 351 nm excimer laser irradiation. Both

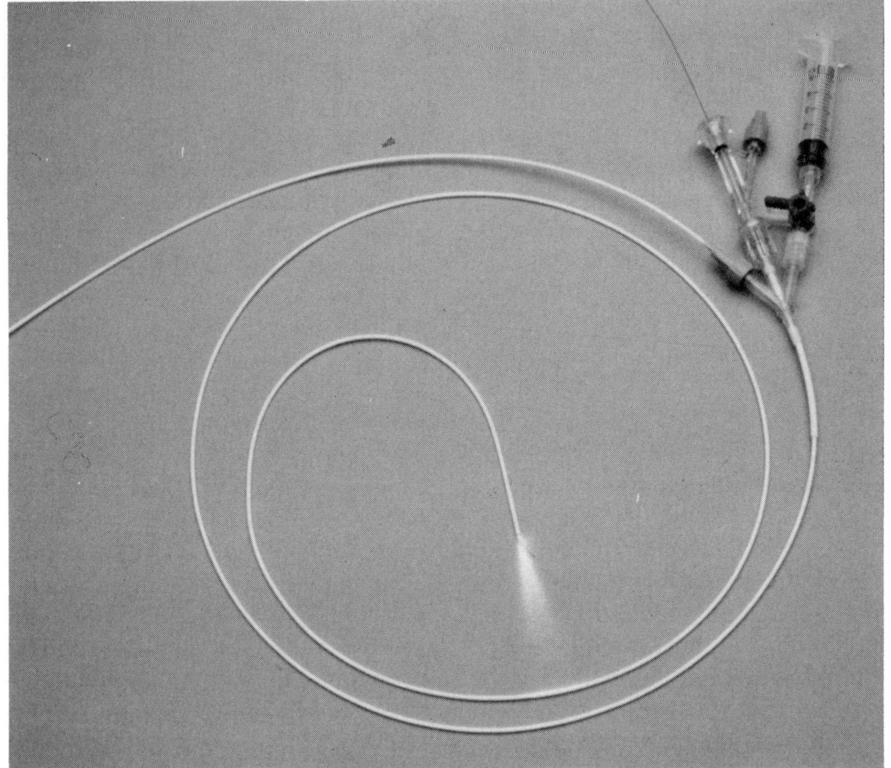

Fig. 14-4. The flexible, over-the-wire fiberoptic used for stenotic small vessels. We believe this type of device may provide sufficient safety to allow intracoronary use.

the size and amount of the particles increase when higher energy densities or high repetition rates are employed. In our limited clinical experience with ablation inside blood vessels, we have not found that distal embolization of particulate debris is a problem.

THE MUTAGENICITY OF ULTRAVIOLET LASER ENERGY

Ultraviolet light is ionizing radiation, as described earier in our discussion of the photodecomposition theory. Ionization can induce genetic change. Therefore 308 nm excimer laser light is at least potentially mutagenic at the target site. The mutagenic effect of ultraviolet light is wavelength-dependent. The mutagenic potential of ultraviolet radiation peaks near 254 nm, caused by avid absorption of this wavelength by deoxyribonucleic acid (DNA).[18,19] The dose of 308 nm ultraviolet laser energy required to induce mutation is in the range of 100 to 1000 times greater than that for 254 nm.[20] Our in-vivo histologic studies of healing (discussed below) after 308 nm laser irradiation give no evidence suggestive of mutagenic effects, and we believe that the mutagenic changes after 308 nm XeCl laser energy during vascular ablation will not be observed.

THE ACUTE AND CHRONIC HISTOLOGIC RESPONSE TO EXCIMER LASER INJURY

There is nothing unique in the response of the blood vessel surface to injury induced by lasers. As with mechanical trauma, healing appears to be related to the magnitude of initial injury. Gerrity and associates[21] studied healing after CO_2 laser ablation of vascular endothelium in atherosclerotic swine. Two days after the procedure, there was a small crater filled with platelet-fibrin thrombi, and the tissue adjacent to the crater was infiltrated with white blood cells. Two weeks following the procedure, the vessel surface was reendothelized by small, closely packed cells. At the pit of the crater, there was smooth-muscle cell proliferation and collagen production. Eight weeks after the procedure, the lesion was slightly depressed, and new endothelium covered a fibrous cap. Thus it is possible to ablate an atheroma without inducing thrombotic occlusion and to have the vascular surface return to a near-normal state.

Nevertheless, there are definite differences in healing both acute and late injury among lasers.[22,23] These differences relate to the depth of tissue penetration. We compared healing after extensive argon and excimer laser irradiation of the normal vascular surface in 25 dogs. We used a template to produce comparable ablation areas. Excimer laser energy was delivered by fiberoptics at 30 to 40 mJ/mm^2 per pulse, and continuous-wave argon ion energy was delivered by fiberoptics at 5 W. In acute injury the argon laser produced thermal injury, but excimer irradiation did not. Argon-treated aortas had extensive medial necrosis at 24 to 72 hours, and at 4 weeks there was medial scarring, intimal proliferation, and extensive transmural necrosis. In contrast, at 24 to 72 hours excimer-irradiated aortas had only localized fibrin deposition on the incised surface and an intimal inflammatory infiltrate. By 4 weeks the arteries had healed so normally that the incision site could not be identified by gross examination. Thus we believe that for any given surface area of tissue ablation, the healed area after 308 nm excimer laser injury is likely to return more closely to normal because both the initial surface is less damaged and adjacent tissue damage is less severe.

IN-VIVO EXCIMER LASER ANGIOPLASTY

Excimer laser angioplasty has been used to open completely occluded canine femoral arteries. We used the 600 μm fiberoptic delivery system. Although it was not difficult to open completely occluded vessels, we found that below the knee, mechanical perforation could be induced by the stiff fiberoptic itself. Our experience is similar to that reported by Leon and associates,[24] who also had a problem of mechanical perforation during excimer laser irradiation, secondary to inflexibility of the fiberoptic delivery system. Thus prior to human application we believe that excimer laser angioplasty without thermal injury is feasible in small arteries, but that the tradeoff between flexibility and larger diameter in our fiberoptic delivery systems remain a problem. We have developed a more flexible system and have begun testing it in humans.

EXCIMER LASER ANGIOPLASTY IN HUMANS

We have now performed our first five cases of excimer laser–assisted balloon angioplasty in humans (Fig. 14-5) using our more flexible fiberoptic waveguides. These studies, all in the femoral-popliteal system, indicate that the procedure is feasible and that complete vascular obstructions can be rapidly opened using the excimer laser–fiberoptic delivery system (Fig. 14-6). All patients had severe symptomatic peripheral vascular disease in the legs, with one- or two-block claudication. All be-

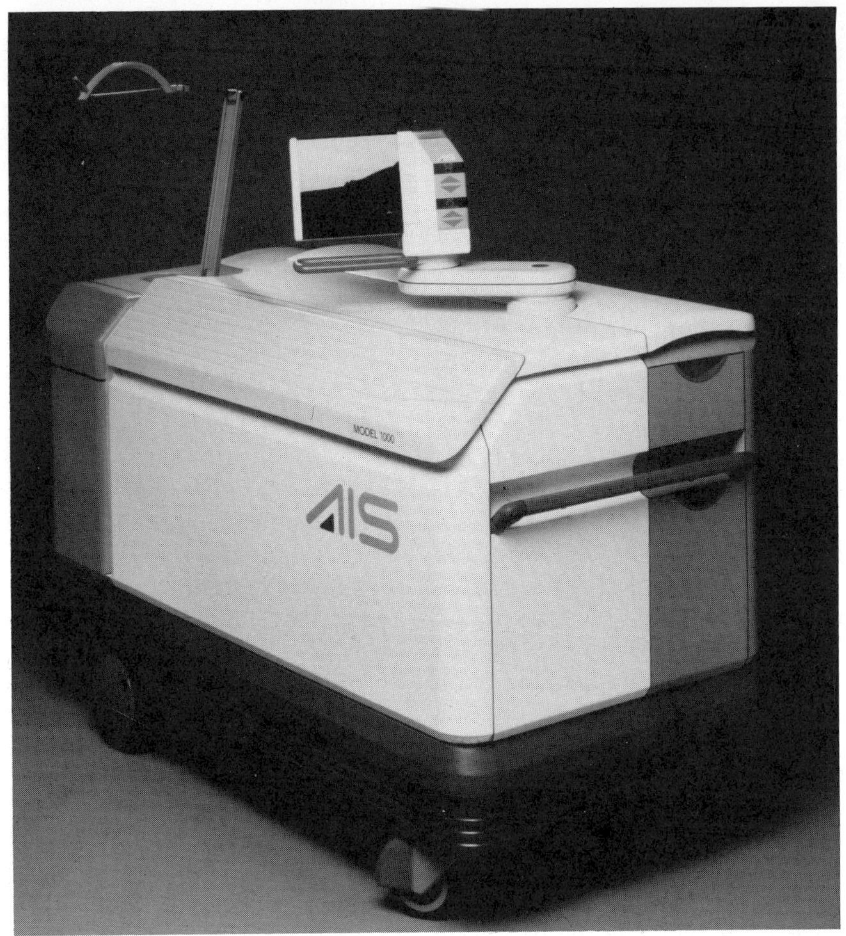

Fig. 14-5. Picture of the first clinical prototype of the long-pulsed XeCl excimer laser (Jet Propulsion Laboratories) used at Cedars-Sinai Medical Center.

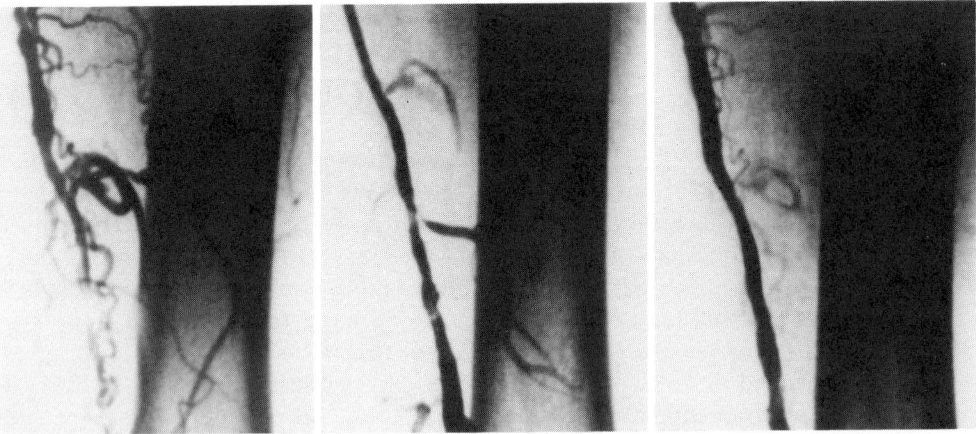

Fig. 14-6. The superficial femoral artery of a patient before (total obstruction, *left panel*), during, and after excimer laser angioplasty. After opening the complete obstruction *(middle panel)* the procedure was completed by balloon angioplasty *(right panel)*.

came asymptomatic after the procedure, which was angiographically successful in each case. The ankle-brachial index also increased in each case. Our longest follow-up is 5 months; all our patients remain asymptomatic.

We are aiming to begin intraoperative coronary application. The major impediment to percutaneous coronary use is the need to develop an even more flexible, multifiber, over-the-wire system. We are aiming for flexibility comparable to an angioplasty guidewire. We believe this is technically feasible. Thus the role of the excimer laser in treatment of atherosclerotic vascular disease is yet to be determined. Nevertheless, we believe that at the very least it will be useful in the treatment of occlusive peripheral vascular disease, and may have a role in the future of coronary angioplasty.

ACKNOWLEDGMENTS

Supported in part by the Grand Sweepstakes, Imperial Grand Sweepstakes, Medallions and the National Institutes of Health, Bethesda, Maryland.

REFERENCES

1. Choy, D.S.J., Stertzer, S.H., Myler, R.K., et al.: Human coronary laser recanalization, Clin. Cardiol. **7**:377-381, 1984.
2. Cumberland, D.: Peripheral and coronary percutaneous laser assisted balloon angioplasty: clinical results. In 3rd European Laser Assisted, Amsterdam, 1986, Lasers in Medicine.
3. Ginsburg, R., Kim, D.S., Guthamer, D., et al.: Salvage of an ischemic limb by laser angioplasty: description of a new technique, Clin. Cardiol. **7**:54-58, 1984.
4. Sanborn, T.A., Cumberland, D.C., Greenfield, A.J., et al.: Six months follow-up of laserprobe assisted balloon angioplasty, Circulation **74**(suppl. 11):1819A, 1986.
5. Grundfest, W., Litvack, F., Forrester, J.S., et al.: Comparison of tissue effects of pulsed ultraviolet lasers to continuous wave YAG and argon lasers.
6. Grundfest, W., Litvack, F., Doyle, L., et al.: Comparison of in vitro and in vivo thermal effects of argon and excimer lasers for laser angioplasty, Circulation **74**(suppl. 11):813A, 1986.
7. Isner, J.: The paradox of thermal ablation without thermal injury. In Proceedings 3rd European Laser Assisted, Amsterdam, 1986.
8. Grundfest, W.S., Litvack, F., Forrester, J.S., et al.: Laser ablation of human atherosclerotic plaque without adjacent tissue injury, J. Am. Coll. Cardiol. **5**:929-933, 1985.
9. Srinivasan, R.: Ablation of polymers and biological tissue by ultraviolet lasers, Science **234**:559-565, 1986.
10. Garrison, B.J., and Srinivasan, R.: Laser ablation of organic polymers: microscopic models for photochemical and thermal processes, J. Appl. Phys. **57**:2909-2914, 1985.
11. Forrester, J.S., Litvack, F., and Grundfest, W.: Laser angioplasty in cardiovascular disease, Am. J. Cardiol. **57**:990-992, 1986.
12. Singleton, J.S., Paraskevopoulos, G., Jolly, G.S., et al.: Excimer lasers in cardiovascular surgery: ablation products and photoacoustic spectrum of arterial wall, Appl. Phys. Lett. **48**:878-880, 1986.
13. Litvack, F., Grundfest, W., Goldenberg, T., et al.: Pulsed laser angioplasty: wavelength power and energy dependencies relevant to clinical application. (In Press.)
14. Grewe, D.D., Castaneda, W.R., Nordstrom, L.A., et al.: Debris analysis after laser photorecanalization of atherosclerotic plaque, Semin. Intervent. Radiol. **3**:53-60, 1986.
15. Isner, J.M., Clarke, R.H., Donaldson, R.F., et al.: Identification of photoproducts liberated by in vitro argon laser irradiation of atherosclerotic plaque, Am. J. Cardiol. **55**:1192-1198, 1985.
16. Mohr, F.W., Lenz, W., Kusserow, S.V., et al.: Excimer lasers for angioplasty and cardiac

valve repair, Lasers Surg. Med. **3:**93-97, 1987.

17. DeJesus, S.T., Isner, J.M., Rogione, A.J., et al.: Reductions in peak pulse energy diminish particulate debris resulting from excimer plaque ablation, Clin. Res. **34:**855A, 1986.
18. Jacobson, E.D., Krell, K., and Dempsey, M.J.: The wavelength dependence of ultraviolet light induced cell killing and mutagenesis in L5178Y mouse lymphoma cells, Photochem. Photobiol. **33:**257-260, 1981.
19. Wells, R.L., and Han, A.: Action spectra for killing and mutation of Chinese hamster cells exposed to mid- and near-ultraviolet monochromatic light, Mutat. Res. **129:**251-258, 1984.
20. Colella, C.M., Bogani, P., Agati, G., et al.: Genetic effects of UV-B: mutagenicity of 308 nm light in Chinese hamster V79 cells, Photochem. Photobiol. **43:**437-442, 1986.
21. Gerrity, R.G., Loop, F.D., Golding, L.A., et al.: Arterial response of laser operation for removal of atherosclerotic plaques, J. Thorac. Cardiovasc. Surg. **85:**409-421, 1985.
22. Litvack, F., Doyle, F., Grundfest, W., et al.: In vivo excimer laser ablation: acute and chronic effects on canine aorta, Circulation **74**(suppl. 11):1438A, 1986.
23. Higginson, L.A.J., Farrel, E.M., Valley, V.M., et al.: In vivo excimer laser ablation: acute and chronic effects on canine aorta, Circulation **74**(suppl. 11):1438A, 1986.
24. Leon, M.B., Smith, P.D., and Bonner, R.F.: In-vivo excimer laser angioplasty: design criteria and preliminary animal results, Circulation **74**(suppl. 11):32A, 1986.

Chapter 15

Laser Balloon Angioplasty

J. Richard Spears, MD, FACC

The occasional occurrence of abrupt reclosure and the high incidence of restenosis greatly limit the safety, as well as efficacy, of percutaneous transluminal coronary angioplasty (PTCA).[1-3] As a result many patients, including most patients with ischemic heart disease who are not refractory to medical therapy, are not candidates for PTCA, and the clinical decision-making process regarding potential benefits versus risks of PTCA is often complex and difficult in individual cases.

In this chapter a new technique termed "laser balloon angioplasty" (LBA) is described, which may improve both the safety and efficacy of angioplasty. An important hypothesis to be tested with LBA is that a relatively large, smooth lumen following angioplasty will be associated with predictably satisfactory result, both in the short and long term.[4,5]

CONCEPT OF LASER BALLOON ANGIOPLASTY

During balloon inflation, 1.06 μm of continuous wave Nd:YAG laser irradiation is delivered over approximately 20 seconds directly to the arterial wall in contact with and surrounding the balloon (Fig. 15-1). Absorption of the radiation by tissues results in a temperature rise in the arterial wall to an 80 to 130° C range. Balloon inflation is maintained for 20 to 30 seconds after cessation of laser irradiation to allow tissue temperature to return to baseline before deflation. Several thermal effects are sought as a result of this procedure, and they are described below.

Fusion of Disrupted Arterial Tissues

Fracture of a rigid neointimal shell, although allowing subsequent full expansion of an angioplasty balloon, can result in the production of an intimal flap and/or an arterial dissection. Rupture of vasa vasorum within the arterial wall could also cause tissue separation from an expanding intramural hematoma even in the absence of plaque fracture. Acute luminal compromise may thereby result in some cases, and in many other cases the irregular luminal geometry may be associated with local rheologic patterns of flow separation that may be at least partially responsible for chronic deposition of microthrombi on multiple exposed luminal surfaces.[5]

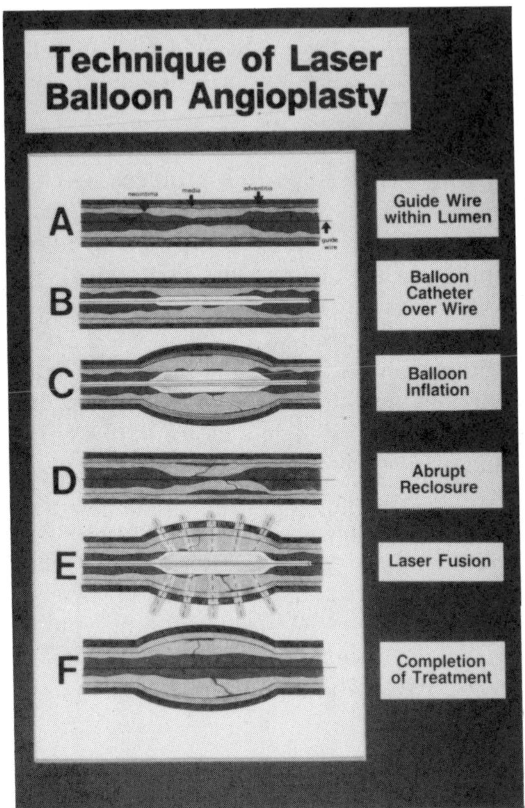

Fig. 15-1. Technique of laser balloon angioplasty (LBA) following conventional angioplasty. During balloon inflation, laser energy is directed in a cylindrical pattern directly to tissues to a depth of about 3 mm surrounding the balloon (E). Allowing the arterial wall temperature after laser exposure to normalize before balloon deflation facilitates thermal fusion of separated tissue layers and results in reduction of viscoelastic recoil. Additional potentially useful effects include elimination of vasoconstriction, dehydration of plaque, and destruction of smooth muscle cells.

Thermal fusion of soft tissues for therapeutic purposes has been used in medicine for many years. High-frequency electrocoagulation, introduced clinically at the end of the last century for achieving hemostasis by thermal closure of small vessels, was shown experimentally by Sigel and associates[6,7] in the 1960s to be a potentially effective means for repair of linear incisions in arteries and veins, for coaptive closure of large vessels (greater than 1 mm in diameter), and for creation of end-to-side portacaval anastomoses. An adequate bond, capable of withstanding 600 to 900 mm Hg intraluminal pressures, was found when the coagulum formed resulted in fusion and preservation of collagen and elastic tissues. A poor thermal bond was formed when the degree of amorphous coagulum was intense and was associated with overt loss of the structural integrity of connective tissue. Because tissue is heated solely by thermal diffusion with this technique as a result of contact with an electrocautery device, large thermal gradients must be created to coagulate tissue effectively throughout the full thickness of the wall, and excessive coagulation of surface tissues therefore occurs easily.

In contrast to this indirect method of heating tissues, absorption of laser radiation by tissue is a direct method, one in which the depth of heating can be controlled by the choice of wavelength, and excessive surface heating can more easily be avoided. A variety of medical applications of photocoagulation have been developed, and in each case the biologic long-term response has generally been benign.[8-12] In fact, fibrosis from collagen deposition appears to be less prominent at sites of vascular and other soft tissue anastomoses created by laser-thermal fusion compared with that associated with conventional suture techniques.

For performance of LBA, an Nd:YAG laser emitting 1.06 μm of continuous wave radiation was chosen for several reasons to thermally fuse together arterial tissue layers disrupted by conventional PTCA. The depth of penetration of radiation at this wavelength is approximately 3 mm in a variety of soft tissues, including atheromatous plaques, so that the full thickness of both the normal and diseased wall of the major coronary artery segments can be heated sufficiently. The scattering coefficient of arterial tissue at 1.06 μm is large compared with the absorption coefficient, as it is for other soft tissues, so that the Nd:YAG laser is an effective tool for producing diffuse, volume heating of tissue. Finally, the relatively large volume of tissue to be heated with the use of a 3 mm diameter, 2 cm long LBA balloon and a 1.5 mm long cylindric diffusing tip requires a laser capable of delivering 10 to 40 W of power, which is easily attainable with commercially available Nd:YAG lasers.

Reduction of Viscoelastic Recoil

Following conventional PTCA, the residual lumen diameter is rarely as large as that of the inflated balloon, in part because of the inherent viscoelasticity of arterial tissue.[13] Even a mild residual stenosis may be important. For example, a 30% residual diameter stenosis, which is ordinarily regarded as a satisfactory PTCA result, is a 50% stenosis by area. The latter would be doubled if no residual stenosis could be achieved, and the stenosis rate might thereby be reduced. One could simply use a larger balloon size to overstretch the tissue and thus reduce elastic recoil, but two problems are likely consequences of this approach. First, Steele and colleagues[14] have found experimentally that, when the normal arterial wall is stretched with balloon inflation to a diameter approximately 20% greater than resting values, tears in the media are created that can result in thrombosis. Second, since the normal layers of the arterial wall are usually more compliant than the neointima, a shear stress may occur at the plaque-wall junction in both the circumferential and longitudinal directions following fracture of the neointimal shell and continued balloon inflation. The use of a larger balloon may exaggerate this stress, and the risk of abrupt reclosure from partial plaque dehiscence or of propagation of a dissection may increase. The experience that balloon inflation in highly curved arterial segments is more likely to be associated with an extensive dissection is probably an example of the problem posed by balloon stretching of adjacent tissues having differential compliance.

A long balloon inflation (longer than 5 minutes) may not solve this problem, even if a weak bond between separated tissue layers can be achieved with this approach, because similar shear stresses may also occur on balloon deflation that could disrupt a weak bond.

Ordinarily, soft tissues shrink when heated; however, when arterial tissue is heated under isometric tension (e.g., tissue surrounding a balloon filled with incompressible fluid) and allowed to cool, shrinkage is minimal; in fact an actual increase in tissue length can be achieved over resting length by this maneuver. By reducing elastic recoil with LBA, any shear stresses at the plane of tissue separation that might have occurred on balloon deflation during PTCA should be reduced.

Elimination of Active Vascular Tone

Following PTCA, vasomotor tone in the dilated segment is likely to increase for several reasons. Loss of the endothelium halts production of endothelial relaxing factor, thought to be nitric oxide.[15,16] Moreover, the potent vasoconstrictor thromboxane A_2 may be locally released from platelets that adhere to the denuded luminal surface.[17,18] Patients are usually advised, therefore, to take coronary vasodilators for at least several months after PTCA, until sufficient time has elapsed for regeneration of the endothelial lining to occur.

Thermal destruction of smooth muscle cells from LBA renders the arterial wall incapable of responding to vasoactive substances, so that administration of a coronary vasodilator after LBA specifically for prevention of vasospasm of the dilated segment may not be necessary. Although the LBA-treated segment is thus an inert conduit acutely, changes in lumen dimensions will still occur with variations in distending intraluminal pressure. The arterial wall is rendered somewhat less compliant by photocoagulation,[19] but it is not a rigid tube. An interesting observation is that, in contrast to arteries anastomosed with sutures, arteries at the site of laser-thermal anastomoses in growing swine enlarge over time proportionally with the increased physiologic demand.[20]

Tissue Dehydration

Kaltenbach and co-workers[21] have shown that some fluid can be expressed from human postmortem atherosclerotic arteries by prolonged application of a high-tissue pressure. However, one would expect that tissue rehydration would quickly occur in the clinical setting. During LBA, preliminary studies done by me and my colleagues (see in-vitro studies section) suggest that a 15 to 20% weight reduction in postmortem atheromatous tissue will occur with a 20-second Nd:YAG laser exposure similar to what will be used clinically. Additional reduction in plaque volume can be expected with additional laser doses. The weight loss is due solely to the rapid evaporation of water, thus leaving intact all of the structurally supporting tissues, such as collagen and elastin layers. An important feature of this effect appears that the photocoagulated wall, at least in vitro over a 1-week period, remains relatively impermeable to water, so that significant rehydration does not occur.

LASER BALLOON ANGIOPLASTY STUDIES

Experimental studies that have been performed in our laboratory are summarized below.

In-Vitro Studies[22-26]

The majority of the in-vitro studies done by me and my colleagues to date have been designed to study the effect of a wide variety of parameters, both laser and biologic, on the strength of thermal bonds between separated layers of human postmortem atherosclerotic aortic sections. Eleven millimeter diameter disks of aorta were excised and, after manual separation of the neointima from the media, the two layers were reapposed under a known tissue pressure applied with a glass slide. Nd:YAG continuous wave laser radiation at 1.06 μm was delivered perpendicularly to the luminal surface over a 3 mm diameter nominal spot from a 400 μm core silica fiberoptic. Tissue temperature at the adventitial surface was monitored continuously with a thermistor. We have found that the presence of the thermistor does not change the temperature rise in the tissue and that the adventitial temperature is only approximately 10 to 15° C lower than that at the neointima-media junction.

Initially, a constant laser power of 10 to 25 W was used to heat the tissue to a temperature within an 80 to 130° C range. Since approximately 10 seconds were required to achieve a target tissue temperature, and since the temperature continued to rise throughout a 20- to 30-second exposure duration, it seemed desirable to find an alternative laser power format that would allow the tissue to be heated more rapidly, and thereafter to achieve a stable plateau temperature. A decremental power format was therefore investigated wherein an initially high power was employed for 5 seconds to achieve the desired temperature, and stepwise decremental downward ramping was used for the subsequent 15 seconds to maintain a constant temperature (Fig. 15-2). To our surprise, we found that the mean weld strength achieved with the decremental power format was considerably higher than the constant power format despite the achievement of similar peak temperatures between the two groups (Fig. 15-3). In addition, the energy required to achieve similar peak temperatures was markedly lower when the decremental power format was used. A possible

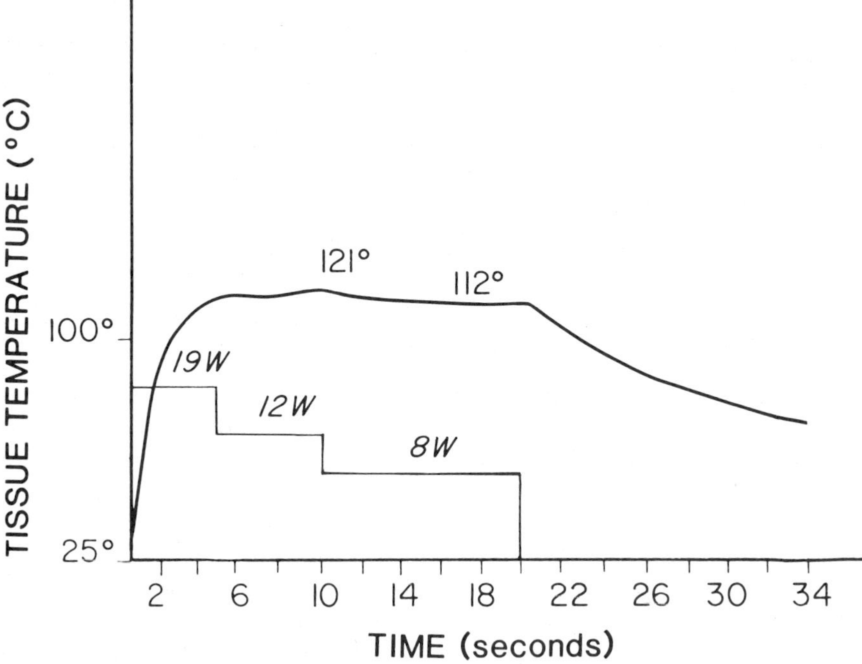

Fig. 15-2. Decremental power format used to achieve a rapid rise in tissue temperature and a stable plateau temperature thereafter. (Reprinted with permission from Anand, R.K. et al.: *Lasers in Surg. Med.* **8**:40, 1988.)

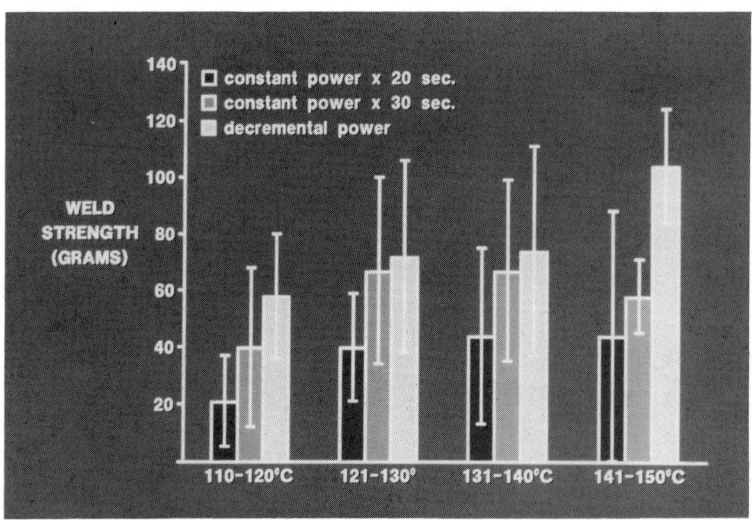

Fig. 15-3. Comparison of mean weld strength achieved with the decremental versus constant power format. The former produced stronger welds at a lesser energy cost. (Reprinted with permission from Anand, R.K. et al.: *Effect of Lasers Surg. Med.* **8**:40, 1988.)

explanation for the latter observation may be that the rapid temperature rise was accompanied by less energy wasted in thermal diffusion to adjacent tissue. The reason for the improved weld strength with this power format is unknown, but the rate of heating of collagen may affect the efficiency of thermal denaturation. Schober and associates[27] have shown by electron microscopy that the mechanism of laser-thermal fusion of vascular tissue may be interdigitation of collagen fibrillar substructures as a result of thermal breakage of noncovalent bonds (a denaturation process) and subsequent reformation of similar bonds between adjacent collagen fibers.

In view of the multiple advantages of the decremental power format, this regimen has been utilized in most of our other experimental studies and we will utilize it in the clinical setting.

Modifications of biologic variables have had remarkably very little impact on the efficacy of laser-thermal fusion of atherosclerotic aortic tissue layers.[24] Heavily calcified plaques can be welded to medial layers as easily as fibrous plaques, and weld strength is unaffected by the presence or absence of blood between tissue layers. At least mild tissue pressure, approximately 7 psi, is required for successful thermal fusion of tissues, but adequate thermal welds can be achieved at all levels of tissue pressure likely to be encountered clinically. Tissue thickness over a 0.5 to 2.5 mm range has little effect on the ability to create laser-thermal welds, so that the majority of plaques encountered in human coronary arteries should be amenable to treatment. It should be noted that it will probably be unnecessary during the clinical performance of LBA to thermally weld tissue to a depth greater than 2.5 mm, even if plaque thickness exceeds its value. Thermal sealing of all tissue tears at the luminal surface with reinforcement by coagulation and fusion of underlying tissues to a depth of 2.5 mm should be successful in abolishing ports of entry of blood into the arterial wall, and therefore in preventing the propagation of an intimal flap or dissection.

Other than the necessity for at least mild tissue pressure, the only parameters that we could identify as having an important impact on the efficacy of laser-thermal fusion of arterial tissue were tissue temperature and exposure duration. Considering the fact that laser-induced fusion of tissue is a thermal process, it is not surprising that the temperature history of the tissue is critical to the success of the technique.

In general we have found that a linear relationship exists between weld strength and a plateau adventitial tissue temperature achieved over an 80 to 150° C range for arterial wall 0.7 to 1.0 mm in thickness (Fig. 15-4). Below 80° C, no measurable welds could be achieved, and a temperature of 95° C, was necessary to have predictably successful welds. Above 150° C, rapid desiccation of tissue followed by vaporization and carbonization of luminal surface layers occurred. A useful temperature range therefore appears to be 95 to 130° C, and laser doses will be used clinically that produce comparable temperatures at a depth of approximately 1 mm from the luminal surface.

Even with the decremental power format, the first 5 seconds of a laser exposure is required just to achieve the desired tissue temperature, so that the strength of welds achieved with this short-exposure duration is quite poor. For exposure durations longer than 5 seconds, a curvilinear relationship exists between exposure duration and weld strength irrespective of the plateau tissue temperature achieved.[26] A 20-second exposure is considerably more efficacious than a 10-second exposure, while a 30-second exposure produces only slight further improvement in weld strength. During the anticipated clinical performance of LBA, a 20-second exposure duration will be used, since the slight improvement afforded by a 30-second expo-

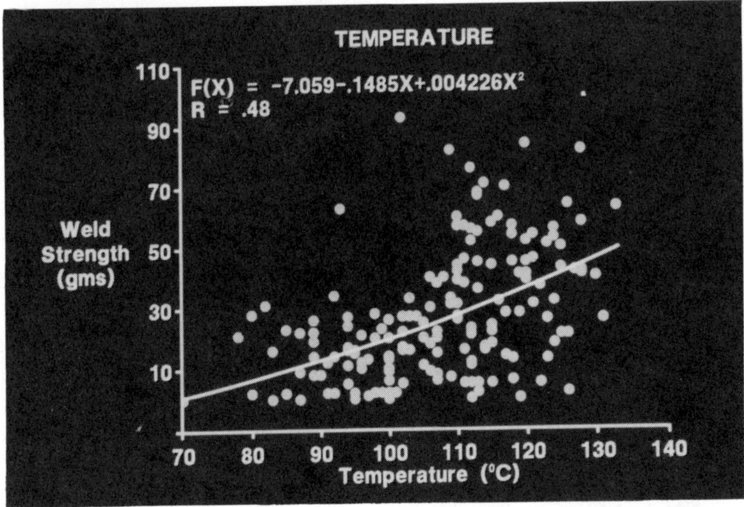

Fig. 15-4. Relationship between plateau adventitial temperature and weld strength of separated human postmortem atherosclerotic aortic intima-media pairs. (Reprinted with permission from Jenkins, R.D. et al.: *Lasers Surg. Med.* **8;** 1988.)

sure is probably unnecessary and would be accompanied by a longer period of coronary occlusion with the inflated balloon.

An important finding in the in-vitro studies was the wide variability in weld strength despite attempts to rigorously control all variables. Other investigators have likewise found a similar variation in thermal bond strength of laser-induced anastomoses of a variety of soft tissues. Soft tissues are thermally bonded by virtue of microscopic multifocal zones of adherence along the plane of tissue separation (Fig. 15-5), and it is likely that the sum-total strength of these zones will be affected by minor variations in the topographic and compositional match of the juxtaposed surfaces at both the gross and microscopic levels. Consistent with this concept has been the finding that, when a single plaque-media pair is subjected to the same laser dose and repetitive tissue layer separation during weld strength testing, the intrasample variability in weld strength achieved is similar to intersample variability, presumably as a result of random minor variations in the points of contact between the tissues. Fortunately it is likely that even the relatively weak welds, when a 95 to 130° C plateau temperature is achieved with a 20-second laser exposure, will be adequate clinically. In the event that an intimal flap or dissection persists because of a weak thermal bond, repetitive laser exposures can be performed many times at the same laser dose with the expectation that at least one of the additional exposures will produce a stronger thermal bond.

In-Vivo Studies

Before successfully demonstrating the potential efficacy of using laser energy to weld separated arterial tissue layers, we studied the acute and chronic biologic effects of heating the circumferentially intact, normal arterial wall in vivo. At the time laser balloon angioplasty was conceived, other investigators had emphasized that thermal injury adjacent to tissues targeted for laser vaporization was

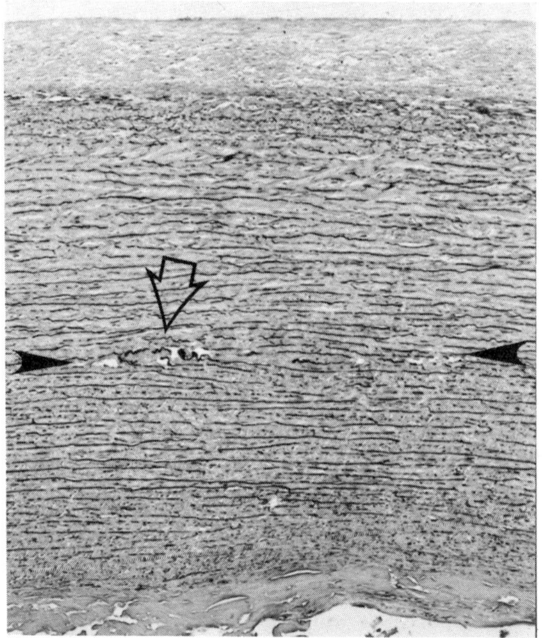

Fig. 15-5. Human postmortem plaque-media pair subjected to cw Nd:YAG (1.06 μm) thermal fusion shows multifocal zones of adherence *(arrow)* with preservation of structural detail throughout arterial wall. (Elastin stain; × 60.) (Reprinted with permission from Jenkins, R.D. et al.: *Lasers Surg. Med.* **8:** 1988.)

undesirable and might result in perforation, aneurysm formation, and thrombosis. In fact when plaque varporization with laser energy is a goal, great precision is desirable in order to ablate only targeted tissue, and techniques that produce more precise craters will be associated with less thermal injury to adjacent tissue. In addition, intense thermal injury is more likely to create a charred, irregular luminal surface, and even milder degrees of thermal injury will be associated with undesirable tissue shrinkage when isometric tension is not applied during heating. It was important, therefore, to assess whether the thermal "injury" associated with temperatures below the threshold for vaporization (i.e., temperatures that would be necessary for tissue fusion) would be tolerated by the normal arterial wall.

In six anesthetized dogs, LBA was performed with a Silastic balloon in an ipsilateral carotid artery, and conventional balloon angioplasty was performed in the contralateral carotid artery with the same balloon as a control.[28] The balloon was inflated to approximately 5 mm at 2 atm, resulting in an approximate 20% increase in resting luminal diameter. Thermal energy was delivered to the arterial wall during balloon inflation primarily by heating a chromophore solution in a balloon to 90° C with fiberoptically delivered argon ion irradiation. Adventitial temperature plateaued at 70° C during a 1- to 2-minute laser exposure. Although this manner of heating the arterial wall differs from the current LBA system, wherein Nd:YAG laser radiation is minimally absorbed by the balloon and its contents and is used to heat arterial tissue directly, the histologic appearance of coagulation necrosis with loss of structural detail was identical to that noted with the current LBA technique. Angiography was performed before, immediately after, and at 1 day, 1 week, 2 weeks, 1 month, 6 months, and 1 year after the procedure, with one dog being sacrificed for histologic examination at each interval (except 2 weeks). The only complication was an instance of thrombosis in an LBA-treated artery that occurred between 1 day and 1 week after the procedure; however, given the fact that only a 5 mm length of artery was thermally treated, corresponding to the midportion of the 2.5 cm long balloon, most of the dilated ipsilateral segment was actually treated only with conventional balloon angioplasty. Steele and co-workers[14] have shown a 15% incidence of thrombosis in pig carotid arteries inflated to 20% above resting diameter with the conventional balloon angioplasty technique, and it is therefore unknown to what extent thermal injury predisposed to the thrombosis. Noteworthy is that anticoagulation consisted solely of 2000 units of heparin given during the angioplasty procedure. In the remaining five dogs, LBA produced a greater increase in lumen diameter than conventional angioplasty at all time periods. Neointimal formation was mild bilaterally at 6 months and 1 year, and fibroblast infiltration in the media with collagen deposition appeared to have increased only slightly beyond 1 month after LBA.

A more recent study of LBA with direct Nd:YAG laser irradiation of the arterial wall in 42 rabbit iliac arteries[29] was encouraging in terms of the lack of thrombogenicity at doses even higher than what will be used clinically. No instance of thrombosis occurred in any of these studies, mild neointimal proliferation occurred to an equal extent between LBA and control (conventional balloon angioplasty) iliac segments, and when a moderate laser dose was used the increase in angiographic luminal dimensions associated with LBA, which was greater than that associated with conventional angioplasty, persisted at the 1 month follow-up period.

Studies in 17 dogs, wherein a clinical LBA catheter and Nd:YAG laser delivery system was tested in vivo on normal coronary arteries, have recently yielded encouraging results similar to those of the previous studies.[30] Even after multiple laser exposures in adjacent coronary segments were performed, no significant adverse effects on the arterial lumen occurred. Viscoelastic recoil was reduced acutely, and no significant change in angiographic lumen diameter over a 1 month period of time was noted. A mild vasoconstrictor response to ergonovine could be induced 1 day and 1 week after coronary instrumentation, but LBA-treated segments showed no such response, so that the angiogram had the appearance of a "cast" of the inflated, cylindrically shaped LBA balloon in the coronary artery.

Clinical LBA Catheter System

A 3 mm balloon angioplasty catheter has been developed by Bard, Inc. (USCI Division of C.R. Bard, Inc.) for performance of laser balloon angioplasty. The catheter looks quite similar to a standard PTCA catheter, but a third channel in the catheter shaft allows passage of a 100 μm core silica fiberoptic that terminates in a helical diffusing tip within the balloon. A 1.5 cm long cylindric pattern of irradiation is produced by the diffusing tip, so that all arterial tissue in contact with the fully inflated balloon is heated; the proximal distal ends of the balloon receive minimal or no direct laser exposure. The position of the diffusing tip is fixed permanently within the balloon, outside the central channel, so that the operator does not have to be concerned with manipulation of a fiberoptic. A standard 0.014-inch conventional guidewire is used with the LBA catheter, including during laser exposure.

The materials of the balloon components were selected to minimize 1.06 μm radiation absorption. As a result virtually all of the emitted radiation is delivered to the arterial wall, and the contrast medium–filled balloon is heated primarily only by contact with the heated tissues. The balloon material is PET (a type of polyethylene terephthalate), similar to that used in USCI high-pressure PTCA catheters.

The relatively low profile (0.036 inch), flexibility, and trackability of the LBA catheter system would allow its use as a primary dilatation catheter. However, in the initial clinical studies, the LBA catheter will be used only after completion of the conventional portion of a PTCA procedure.

Performance of an LBA procedure is quite similar to a PTCA procedure, with the following exceptions. During balloon inflation, the guiding catheter is flushed with normal saline or D_5W to reduce the hematocrit of blood trapped inside branches by the inflated balloon to 12% or less. No significant coagulation of blood can occur from laser exposure when blood is hemodiluted to at least this level (unpublished observations), and side-branch occlusion can thereby be avoided. The balloon inflation pressure that results in full inflation of the balloon and is at least 4 atm will be used, since at least mild tissue pressure is required to thermally weld together separated layers of tissue. The central channel is flushed with normal saline at approximately 0.25 ml/second during balloon inflation and throughout the 20-second laser exposure, in order to prevent excessive heating of the guidewire and to ensure that no blood, which would strongly absorb the laser radiation, remains in the central channel. The balloon is deflated 20 to 30 seconds after termination of laser exposure to allow normalization of the arterial wall temperature; otherwise balloon deflation, before tissue cooling, would result in some thermal contraction of the tissue. Thus the entire procedure requires 50 to 60 seconds to perform properly.

A 20-second decremental stepwire laser power format will be preprogrammed by the operator with a Quantronix continuous wave Nd:YAG laser delivery system, to which the fiberoptic channel of the LBA catheter is easily attached. Multiple safety features have been built into the laser delivery system, so that the proper laser dose is delivered in a highly "user friendly" manner.

Proposed Clinical Trial

A Food and Drug Administration (FDA)–approved clinical trial of percutaneous, coronary LBA will first be conducted with a small number of patients to study the safety of the procedure, as determined by angiographic follow-up 1 day and 1 month after the procedure. Assuming safety is demonstrated, a multicenter trial will then be initiated wherein patients will be randomized into either conventional PTCA alone or PTCA plus LBA. Computerized image processing of digitized angiographic images will be used to quantitate luminal dimensions objectively and accurately from angiograms[31-32] obtained initially and 6 months after the procedure, in order to determine whether LBA provides a better luminal result, both acutely and chronically, than PTCA alone.

ACKNOWLEDGMENT

This work was supported in part by NHLBI grant No. HL387349.

REFERENCES

1. Cowley, M.J., Dorros, G., Kelsey, S.F., van Raden, M., and Detre, K.M.: Acute coronary events associated with percutaneous transluminal coronary angioplasty, Am. J. Cardiol. **53:**12C, 1984.
2. Kent, K.M., Bentivoglio, L.G., Block, P.C., Bourassa, M.G., Cowley, M.J., Dorros, G., Detre, K.M., Gosselin, A.J., Gruentzig, A.R., Kelsey, S.F., Mock, M.B., Mullin, S.M., Passamani, E.R., Myler, R.K., Simpson, J., Stertzer, S.H., van Raden, M.J., and Williams, D.O.: Long-term efficacy of percutaneous transluminal coronary angioplasty (PTCA): report from the National Heart, Lung, and Blood Institute PTCA Registry, Am. J. Cardiol. **53:**27C, 1984.
3. Meier, B., King, S.B., III, Gruentzig, A.R., Douglas, J.S., Hollman, J., Ischinger, T., Galan, K., and Tankersley, R.: Repeat coronary angioplasty, J. Am. Coll. Cardiol. **4:**463, 1984.
4. Hiehle, J.F., Jr., Bourgelais, D., Shapshay, S., Schoen, F.J., and Spears, J.R.: Nd:YAG laser fusion of human atheromatous plaque-arterial wall separations in vitro, Am. J. Cardiol. **56:**953, 1985.
5. Spears, J.R.: PTCA restenosis: potential prevention with laser balloon angioplasty (LBA), Am. J. Cardiol. **60:**61B, 1987.
6. Sigel, B., and Dunn, M.R.: The mechanism of blood vessel closure by high frequency electrocoagulation, Surg. Gynecol. and Obstet. **121:**823, 1965.
7. Sigel, B., and Acevedo, F.J.: Electrocoaptive union of blood vessels: a preliminary experimental study, J. Surg. Res. **3:**90, 1963.
8. Little, H.L., Zweng, H.C., Jack, R.L., and Vassiliadis, A.: Techniques of argon laser photocoagulation of diabetic disk new vessels, Am. J. Ophthalmol. **82:**676, 1976.
9. Protell, R.L., Siverstein, F.E., and Auth, D.C.: Laser photocoagulation for gastrointestine bleeding, Clin. Gasteroenterol. **7:**766, 1970.
10. Noe, J.M., Barsky, S.H., Geer, D.E., and Rosen, S.: Port wine stains and the response to argon laser therapy: successful treatment and the predictive role of colour, age, biopsy, Plast. Recontr. Surg. **65:**130, 1980.
11. Gomes, O.M., Macruz, R., Armelin, E., Ribeiro, M.P., Brum, J.M.G., Bittencourt, D., Verginelli, G., and Zerbini, E.J.: Vascular anastomosis by argon laser beam, Tex. Heart Inst. J. **10:**145, 1981.
12. White, R.A., Abergel, R.P., Lyons, R., Klein, S.R., Kopchok, G., Dwyer, R.M., and Uitto, J.: Biological effects of laser welding on vascular healing, Lasers Surg. Med. **6:**137, 1986.
13. Roach, M.R., and Burton, A.C.: The reason for the shape of the distensibility curve of arteries, Can. J. Biochem. Physiol. **35:**681, 1957.

14. Steele, P.M., Chesebro, J.H., Stanson, A.W., Holmes, D.R., Jr, Dewanjee, M.K., Badimon, L., and Fuste, V.: Balloon angioplasty: natural history of the pathological response to injury in a pig model, Circ. Res. **57**:105, 1985.
15. Palmer, R.M., Ferrige, A.G., and Moncada, S.: Nitric oxide release accounts for the biological activity of endothelium-derived relaxing factor, Nature **327**:524, 1987.
16. Ignamo, L.J., Byrns, R.E., Buga, G.M., Wood, K., and Chaudhuri, G.: Pharmacologic evidence of endothelium-derived relaxing factor in nitric oxide: use of pyrogallol and superoxide dismutase to study endotholium-dependent and nitric oxide elicited smooth muscle relaxation, Exp. Ther. **244**:181, 1988.
17. Halushka, P.V., Dollery, C.T., and MacDermot, J.: Thromboxane and prostacyline in disease: a review, Q. J. Med. **52**:461, 1983.
18. Chierchia, S., and Patrono, C.: Role of platelet and vascular eicosanoids in the pathophysiology of ischemic heart disease, Fed. Proc. **46**:81, 1987.
19. Fasano, V.A., Ponzio, R.M., Benech, F. and Sicurco, M.: Effects of laser source (argon, Nd:YAG, CO_2) on the elastic resistance of the vessel wall: histological and physical study, Lasers Surg. Med. **3**:45, 1983.
20. Frazier, O.H., Painvin, A., Morris, J.R., Thomsen, S., and Neblett, C.R.: Laser-assisted microvascular anastomoses: Angiographic and anatomopathologic studies on growing microvascular anastomoses: preliminary report, Surgery **97**:585, 1985.
21. Kaltenbach, M., Beyer, J., Walter, S., Klepzig, H., and Schmidts, L.: Prolonged application of pressure in transluminal coronary angioplasty, Cathet. Cardiovasc. Diagn. **10**:213, 1984.
22. Jenkins, R.D., Sinclair, I.N., Anand, R.K., and Spears, J.R.: Laser balloon angioplasty: thermal profile for in vitro welding of neointimal arterial separations (abstract), J. Am. Coll. Cardiol. **9**:105A, 1987.
23. Anand, R.K., Sinclair, I.N., Jenkins, R.D., Hiehle, J.F., Jr., James, L.M., and Spears, J.R.: Laser balloon angioplasty: effect of constant temperature vs constant power on tissue weld strength. Lasers Surg. Med. **8**:40, 1988.
24. Sinclair, I.N., Anand, R.K., Kalil, A.G., Jr., Schoen, J.F., Bourgelais, D., and Spears, J.R.: Laser balloon angioplasty: factors affecting plaque-arterial wall thermal "weld" strength, Circulation **74** (suppl. 2):II-203, 1986.
25. Spears, J.R., Leonard, B.M., Sinclair, I.N., Jenkins, R.D., and James, L.M., Sinofsky, E.L.: Reversible plaque optical property changes during repetitive CW Nd:YAG laser exposure. (In press.)
26. Jenkins, R.D., Sinclair, I.N., Anand, R.K., James, L.M., and Spears, J.R.: Laser balloon angioplasty: effect of exposure duration on shear strength of welded layers of postmortem human aorta, Circulation **76**:IV-46, 1987.
27. Schober, R., Ulrich, F., Sander, T., Durselen, H., and Hessel, S.: Laser-induced alteration of collagen substructure allows microsurgical tissue welding, Science **232**:1421, 1986.
28. Serur, J.R., Sinclair, I.N., Spokojny, A.M., Paulin, S., and Spears, J.R.: Laser balloon angioplasty (LBA): effect on the carotid lumen in the dog, Circulation **72** (suppl. 3):III-144, 1985.
29. Jenkins, R.D., Sinclair, I.N., Leonard, B.M., Sandor, T., Schoen, F.J., and Spears, J.R.: Laser balloon angioplasty vs balloon angioplasty in normal rabbit iliac arteries. (In press.)
30. Sinclair, I.N., Jenkins, R.D., James, L.M., Sinofsky, E.L., Wagner, M.S., Sandor, T., Schoen, R.J., and Spears, J.R.: Laser balloon angioplasty of dog coronary arteries in vivo. (In press.)
31. Spears, J.R., Sandor, T., Als, A.V., Malagold, M., Markis, J.E., Grossman, W., Serur, J.R., and Paulin, S.: Computerized image analysis for quantitative measurement of vessel diameter from cineangiograms, Circulation **68**:443, 1983.
32. Sandor, T., D'Adamo, A., Hanlon, W.B., and Spears, J.R.: High precision quantitative angiography, IEEE Trans. Med. Imag., MI-6:258-265, 1987.

Chapter **16**

Percutaneous Mitral Valvotomy:
The Double Balloon Technique

Muayed Al Zaibag, MBChB, FRCP, FACC

Rheumatic heart disease, with its sequela of mitral valve stenosis, is still prevalent in many countries, including Saudi Arabia. Therefore, following the introduction by Kan and associates[1] of balloon valvotomy for pulmonary valve stenosis, and the early Japanese work by Inoue and co-workers[2] in dilating the mitral valve with a "handmade" balloon catheter, it was natural for our attention to turn to the potential use of this technique in the management of our patients with rheumatic mitral valve stenosis, many of whom are relatively young.

PRELIMINARY INVESTIGATIONS

In collaboration with our surgical colleagues, we dilated the stenotic rheumatic mitral valve in two patients by inflating two balloon catheters placed inside the valve under direct vision during surgery. This trial showed clearly that the inflated balloons did indeed dilate the valve—it split one or both fused commissures; in one case a secondary chorda tendinea was ruptured.[3] On the basis of this evidence we progressed to the dilatation of stenotic rheumatic mitral valves by the use of balloon catheters introduced percutaneously.

From the morphology of the mitral valve (having two commissures) we anticipated that the inflation of two balloons within the valve orifice would split the fused commissures by exerting a more lateral force than the radial pressure that would be exerted by a single inflated balloon. We also thought that the incomplete obstruction of the valve orifice by two balloons during balloon inflation would allow venting of blood through the valve, thus maintaining a reasonable blood pressure.

We always intended to use the long transseptal sheath to deliver the balloon antegradely across the mitral valve. Our rationale was that the presence of a transseptal sheath, kept in situ until the completion of the entire procedure, would minimize the trauma to the atrial septum, compared to the septal defects that would be produced by using the balloon catheters alone, particularly when withdrawing the deflated and wrinkled balloons. They would also reduce the possibility of accidentally dilating the septal puncture by retrograde slippage of these large inflated balloons. We believed that if such iatrogenic septal defects persisted they would not only generate new disease, but also interfere with the accurate calculation of the mitral valve area achieved immediately following dilatation, giving a false illusion of success and leading to a potentially higher incidence of early restenosis. Therefore, from the first case and afterward we used two transseptal sheaths through which we advanced the two balloons across the septum; the sheaths would be withdrawn only after completion of the hemodynamic studies following dilatation. Further advantages of the sheaths and the two balloon catheters soon became obvious as we developed the technique. Aware of the obvious difficulty in selecting the appropriate balloon-size combination to dilate the mitral valve, in contrast to that for the aortic or pulmonary valves, we deliberately chose a combination of small balloons, both 12 mm in diameter and 3 cm in length (Meditech, Mansfield/Boston Scientific), for the first two of our patients who underwent percutaneous balloon mitral valvotomy. All the balloon catheters used in these and subsequent procedures were manufactured by Meditech.

Although we successfully introduced the balloons along the guidewires across the mitral valve through 12F transseptal sheaths, and achieved an apparent degree of valve dilatation following balloon inflation, the residual left atrial/left ventricular (LA/LV) gradients were still significant. However, despite the lack of complications, we were reluctant at this stage to use larger balloons. The two patients were therefore referred for open heart surgery, which was performed within a week. Direct examination of the valves during surgery confirmed limited splitting of the fused commissures, and also revealed that the septal punctures were 4 to 5 mm longitudinal slits, each requiring a single stitch for closure.

Following this confirmation of the ineffective dilatation of the valve by the two 12 mm balloon combination, although minimal septal trauma and no evidence of damage to the annulus was noted, we moved confidently to the use of two larger balloons of 15 mm diameter, which we could also introduce through the 12F transseptal sheaths.

By using this combination of a larger balloon size, a 100% increase in mitral valve area (MVA) was achieved in the subsequent seven patients, from a mean of 0.7 $\pm$ 0.2 cm^2 to 1.4 $\pm$ 0.3 cm^2, assessed by using two independent measures, namely the Gorlin formula and 2-D echocardiograms. The increase persisted at the short-term (6 weeks) follow-up study (Table 16-1).[3] This improvement in the mitral valve area was also confirmed by the increase in the A_2-opening snap interval, demonstrated by phonocardiograms (Table 16-1). The principal conclusions from this early work were that this procedure was feasible, with no complications, and may offer an alternative to surgery in the management of rheumatic mitral valve stenosis. The protocol used for these seven patients has been subsequently modified slightly with our increased experience, and will be referred to later.

Although there had been marked symptomatic improvement associated with the

Table 16-1 Mean MVA (cm^2) by Gorlin Formula and 2-D Echocardiogram, with A_2-OS Interval (msec), Before *(B)*, After *(A)*, and 6 Weeks After *(F)* Balloon Valvotomy.*

	MVA (Gorlin)	*MVA (Echo)*	*A_2-OS (Phono)*
B	0.7 $\pm$ 0.2	0.7 $\pm$ 0.2	71 $\pm$ 9
A	2.0 $\pm$ 0.8	1.5 $\pm$ 0.2	98 $\pm$ 18
F	1.4 $\pm$ 0.3	1.4 $\pm$ 0.2	96 $\pm$ 15
	p <0.005	p <0.005	p <0.005

**No. = 7 patients.*

A_2-OS, Interval between A_2 and opening snap.

100% increase in the MVA, we were convinced that further increases in valve area were needed to raise the procedure to the status of proven therapy. Encouraged by the above findings, we began a small prospective study to compare the results of various combinations of balloon sizes.[4] A total of 35 patients were involved, divided into 4 groups, as illustrated in Table 16-2. All 4 groups were improved symptomatically after successful valve dilatation. Size 14F long transseptal sheaths were used to accommodate the larger balloons of 18 to 20 mm diameter. Throughout the clinical trial we collaborated with Cook (Europe) to manufacture the large sheaths to our requirements.

The important conclusion from this second study was that use of larger balloons produced larger valve areas. The lack of statistical significance between the MVA results achieved in groups I and III may be due to the small number of patients, but there was a significant difference between groups I and IV. The incidence of mitral regurgitation, assessed by angiogram, is shown in Table 16-2. Incidentally, of the 35 patients, 12 had a trace of incompetence before dilatation.

CURRENT PATIENT SELECTION

After the first 20 cases had been successfully performed, we removed certain restrictions in patient selection, namely, the lower age limit of 15 years, a history of previous surgical valvotomy, some degree of mitral calcification, and the presence of mild mitral regurgitation or atrial fibrillation.

Our current criteria are severe symptomatic rheumatic mitral stenosis, with no other valve lesion of significance requiring surgery; no history of thromboembolic events; and no detectable left atrial clot by 2-D echocardiogram or angiography.

Table 16-2 Achieved MVA Using Various-sized Combinations of Balloon Catheter

	Patient Groups			
	Gr I	*Gr II*	*Gr III*	*Gr IV*
Patients per group	7	10	10	8
Balloon combination (mm)	15 +15	15 +18	15 +20	20 +20
Mean age (yr)	23	25	28	39
Mean BSA (m^2)	1.4	1.5	1.6	1.6
Predilatation MVA	0.7 ± 0.2	0.7 ± 0.2	0.8 ± 0.2	0.9 ± 0.2
Postdilatation MVA (6 weeks)	1.4 ± 0.3*†	1.5 ± 0.3	1.8 ± 0.4†	2.0 ± 0.5*
MR (angiogram) (grades 1 to 4)				
Before	0	0	0	3
6 weeks after	2	3	4	4‡

*p <0.03.
†p=*Not significant.*
‡*(+ 1 grade 2/4).*
MVA, Mitral valve area in cm² by Gorlin formula; BSA, body surface area; MR, mitral regurgitation.

CURRENT PROTOCOL

Cross-sectional echocardiography (2-D echocardiography) is done with a Hewlett Packard phased array system, with 3.5 to 5 MHz transducers. Standard views are obtained and images recorded for subsequent analysis. The mitral valve area is calculated by the short-axis parasternal view. Continuous wave Doppler studies using a composite transducer are performed using a Toshiba machine and the MVAs are calculated using a method described by Hatle and Angelson.[5] The results are recorded before valvotomy, on the next day, at 6 weeks, at 6 months, and at 12 months after the balloon valvotomy, and thereafter annually. They are reviewed independently by cardiologists working regularly in the noninvasive laboratory.

The protocol includes recording of pulmonary arterial pressure, and pulmonary capillary wedge pressure, corroborated by direct left atrial pressure, using fluid-filled catheters. Using simultaneous LA/LV pressure measurements, the mean diastolic and end diastolic gradients are obtained. The calculation of the mitral valve area is by the Gorlin formula, using a mean of 5 consecutive cardiac cycles for patients in sinus rhythm, and 10 cycles for those in atrial fibrillation. These measurements, together with left ventricular and left atrial angiography plus an oximetry series, are performed before and immediately following the procedure, and again after a 6- to 8-week interval. The angiography and oximetry required for the detection of any iatrogenic left-to-right atrial shunting are performed at the 6- to 8-week follow-up study. In the event of a shunt being detected, these procedures would be repeated at the 1-year follow-up study.

A consent form is signed after full discussion of the procedure with the patient and a close relative, including a discussion of possible complications and the prospects of success. All patients are anticoagulated with warfarin for the 6 to 8 weeks preceding the procedure, regardless of rhythm. Warfarin is stopped 2 days before admission, when intravenous heparin infusion is started. This is withheld 6 hours before the start of the balloon dilatation. Oral medication of digoxin and diuretics is given as required. Beta blockers are also given to reduce the resting heart rate to around 60 beats per minute, lowering the transmitral gradient; they are also noted to reduce the induction of ventricular arrhythmias during manipulation of the guidewires in the ventricle.

To prevent disturbance by voiding during the procedure, all patients have an indwelling urethral catheter inserted, which is withdrawn 6 hours after the completion of balloon dilatation. Prophylactic intravenous (IV) antibiotics are started before the procedure and continued for a 48-hour period. In addition to the routine premedication (diazepam 10 mg orally), 2.5 to 5 mg of morphine is given intravenously just before insertion of the transseptal sheaths, and a mixture of up to 40 to 50% nitrous oxide with oxygen inhalation is also administered if required. This combination of sedation enables the procedure to be performed smoothly and with minimal discomfort for the patient.

TECHNIQUE

The technique of percutaneous mitral double balloon valvotomy is here described in detail. Using local anesthesia (1% lidocaine), two 8F short venous sheaths (USCI) are inserted into the right femoral vein through punctures at least 2 cm apart, and a third one is inserted into the left femoral vein. A 7F thermodilution catheter is inserted through the left femoral venous sheath into the pulmonary artery. A 7F pigtail catheter is then inserted through the left femoral artery. Using this catheter, a left ventriculogram is performed in RAO 30, to assess possible mitral regurgitation. Radiopaque markers are placed on the anterior and lateral chest wall for orientation. Through either of the right venous sheaths, a 7F Berman angiocatheter is inserted into the pulmonary artery to perform the pulmonary angiogram and its levophase in biplane anteroposterior (AP) and lateral views, to outline the left atrium and rule out the presence of left atrial clots. The outline of the left atrium, the radiopaque markers, and the shaft of the pigtail catheter in the aorta are now marked directly on the AP and lateral television (TV) monitors to assist in the transseptal puncture (Fig. 16-1).

After establishing the baseline hemodynamics and performing angiography, a 14F transeptal sheath and dilator (Cook Europe) is positioned in the superior vena cava over a 0.038-inch Teflon-coated guidewire, through the upper right femoral vein puncture. The left atrium is entered using a Brockenbrough needle under biplane fluoroscopy and continuous atrial pressure recording, assisted by the marking on the TV monitors. A hand injection of contrast media is made through the needle to outline the upper limit of the left atrium more clearly, after which the dilator and sheath are advanced over the needle. By carefully adhering to this prescribed sequence of maneuvers, our staff safely perform many transseptal punctures for diagnostic and therapeutic procedures with no complications. Our dilator is specially manufactured to allow a 2.5 cm distal protrusion of the Brockenbrough needle (Fig. 16-2,A and B), giving more control in crossing a septum that may be thickened and distorted by the enlarged left atrium in an adult compared with that of children with congenital heart disease.

Once the sheath is appropriately positioned in the left atrium, the needle is completely withdrawn. A 20 ml syringe is connected to the hub of the dilator; as the dilator is withdrawn from the sheath, 10 to 20 ml of blood is aspirated to ensure that the sheath is filled with fresh blood from the left atrium and to aspirate any possible clot from inside the dilator. Following the withdrawal of the needle

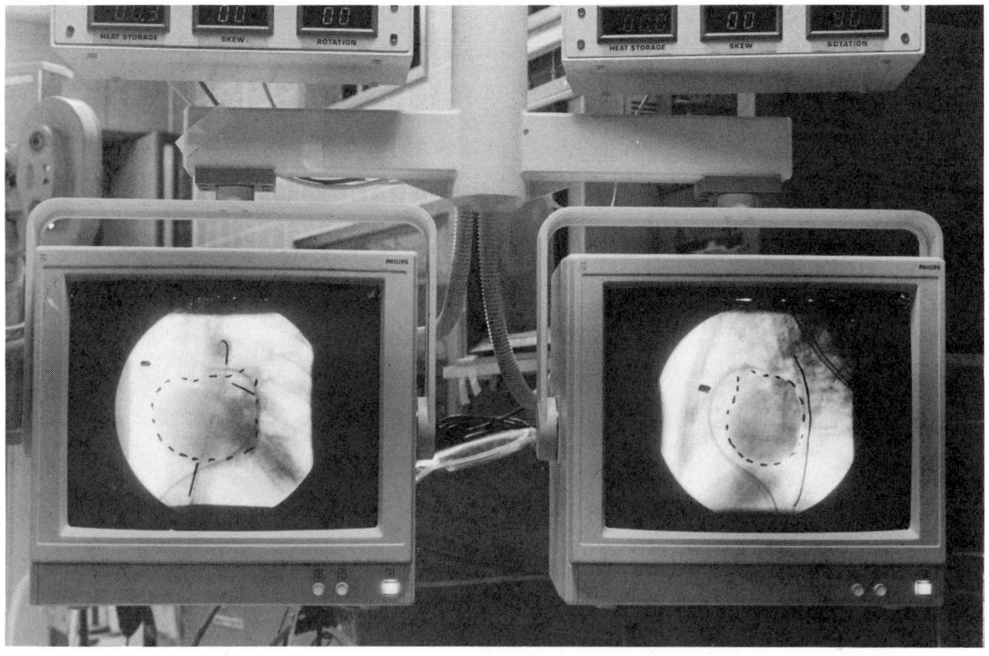

Fig. 16-1. AP and lateral video monitors illustrating the method of marking the left atrium.

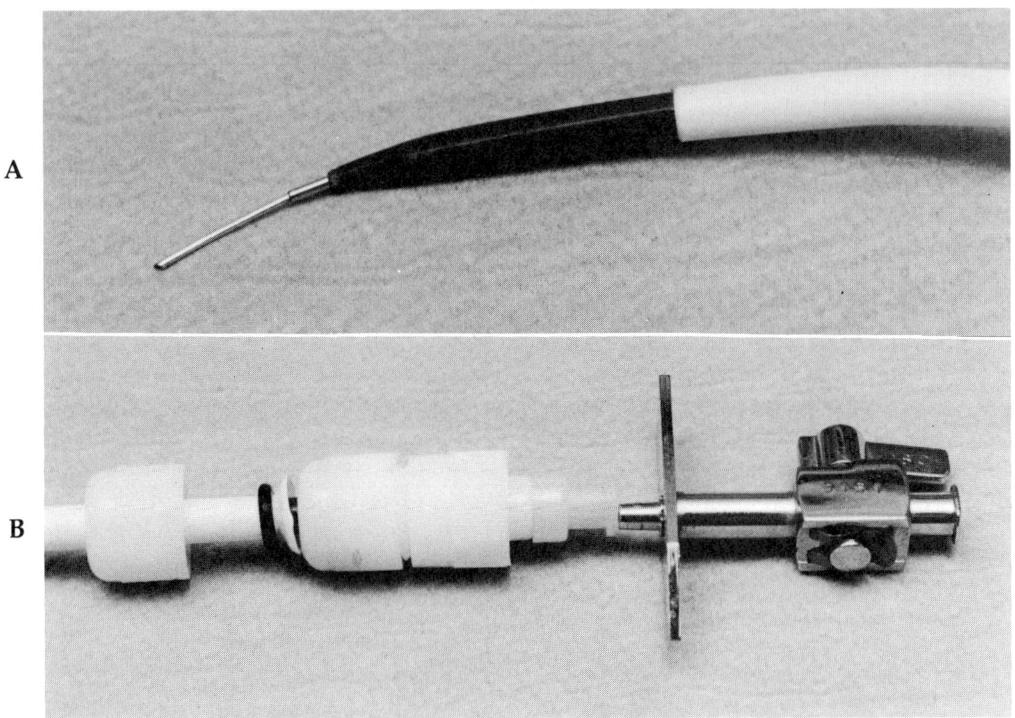

Fig. 16-2. **A,** Distal and **B,** proximal end of transseptal needle, dilator, and sheath.

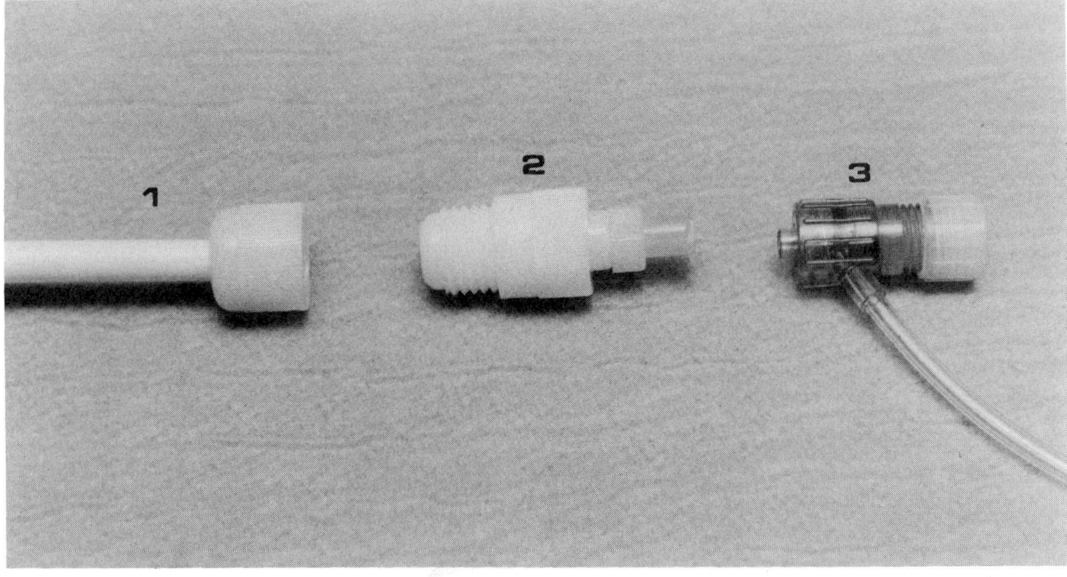

Fig. 16-3. 1, 14F sheath with collar; **2,** hub; **3,** small (Kimal) hemostatic valve with side arm.

and dilator from the sheath, and allowing a few milliliters of blood to issue from the proximal end of the sheath (to flush any possible clot), a Tuohy-Bourst hemostatic valve (Kimal Scientific) is connected to the hub of the sheath (Fig. 16-3). A hand injection of contrast medium is again made directly through the side arm of the hemostatic valve into the left atrial cavity to further rule out a left atrial clot and confirm the relative position of this first puncture in the septum, thus providing guidance for the second transseptal puncture. Heparin, 1000 units in 10 ml of normal saline, is injected through the side arm of the sheath and the three-way tap is then locked to hold this concentrated heparin solution in the sheath while the second transseptal puncture is performed.

A second 14F transseptal sheath is positioned in the left atrium through the lower right femoral puncture using the same steps. At this point heparin (200 units/kg body weight, including the first 1000-unit solution) is given in a divided dose through both sheaths. Although not essential, the ACT is monitored (Haemocrom 400), in the catheter laboratory; a level of 250 to 350 seconds is maintained.

A 7F right coronary Judkins catheter is inserted through the first sheath, over a 0.038-inch Teflon-coated straight guidewire, and advanced across the mitral valve to the left ventricular cavity (Fig. 16-4). The guidewire is then replaced by a curved, preshaped 0.038-inch Teflon-coated exchange guidewire (260 cm) that is positioned near the left ventricular

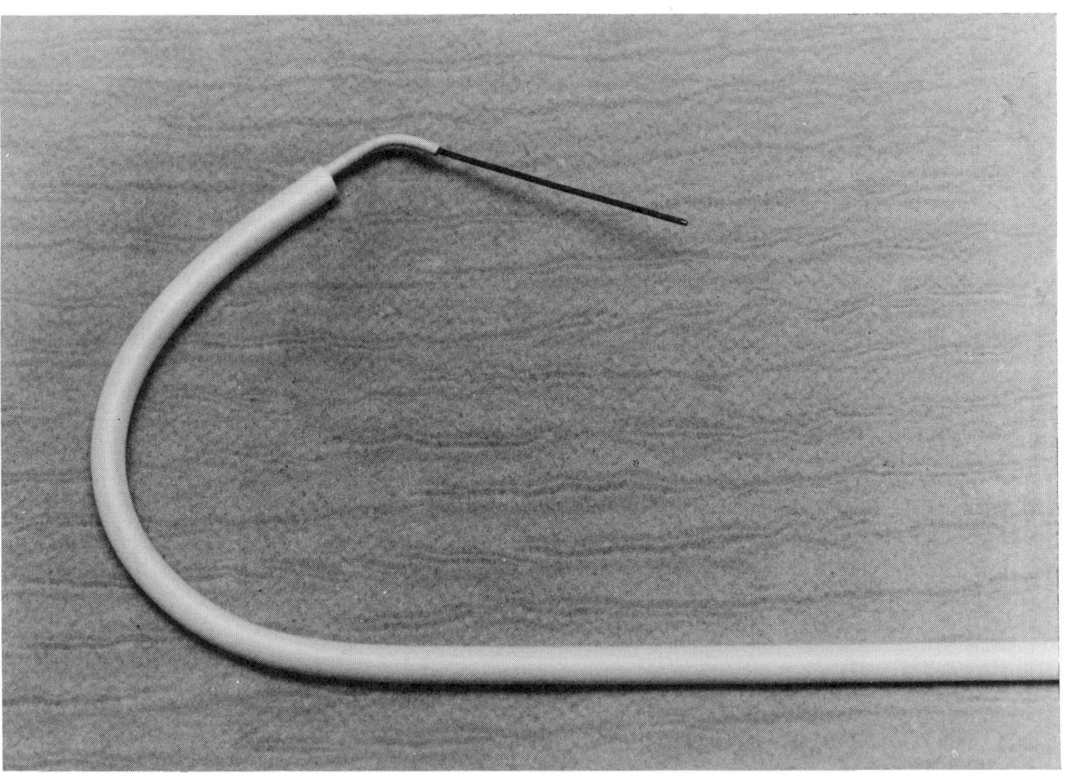

Fig. 16-4. Illustration of a 0.038-inch straight guidewire, right coronary Judkins catheter, and 14F sheath.

apex. Note that it is not necessary to position the guidewire in the aorta. The Judkin catheter is then removed. The second exchange guidewire is then placed in a similar position in the left ventricle through the second sheath using the same steps.

Each sheath is then clamped by a rubber-shod clamp (Fig. 16-5) to prevent blood loss while disconnecting the Tuohy-Bourst hemostatic valve and hub, leaving the exchange guidewires in the left ventricle. The socket of the valve is left connected to the end of the sheath. A deflated, 3-cm-long Meditech balloon catheter, 18 to 20 mm in diameter, is advanced along each guidewire (Fig. 16-6) (the rubber-shod clamp being removed as the balloon catheter is advanced) and positioned within the sheath, just above the mitral valve orifice. On the 9F shaft of each balloon catheter, a specially designed hemostatic valve (Cook Europe) is already positioned before insertion over the exchange guidewire, to be engaged with the valve socket on the end of the sheath without delay (Fig. 16-6). The latest transseptal sheaths are manufactured from material that retains the preshaped curve (Fig. 16-5) to direct the Judkin catheters and the balloons easily into the mitral valve orifice, thereby also minimizing the manipulation of wires and catheters in the left atrium.

The balloon catheters are then advanced consecutively through the mitral valve under biplane fluoroscopy (RAO and lateral views). The position of the balloons across the mitral valve is confirmed by detection of the balloon indentation during the first inflation. Both balloons are simultaneously inflated up to 5 atm, with continuous aortic pressure monitoring, for around 6 to 10 seconds. During balloon inflations the sheaths play a significant role in an important maneuver, the purpose of which is to prevent possible perforation of the left ventricular apex by the tip of the balloon catheter. A gentle and steady backward tension is maintained on both balloon catheters while holding both sheaths firmly in position at the groin puncture. By this means, the proximal end of the inflated balloon will im-

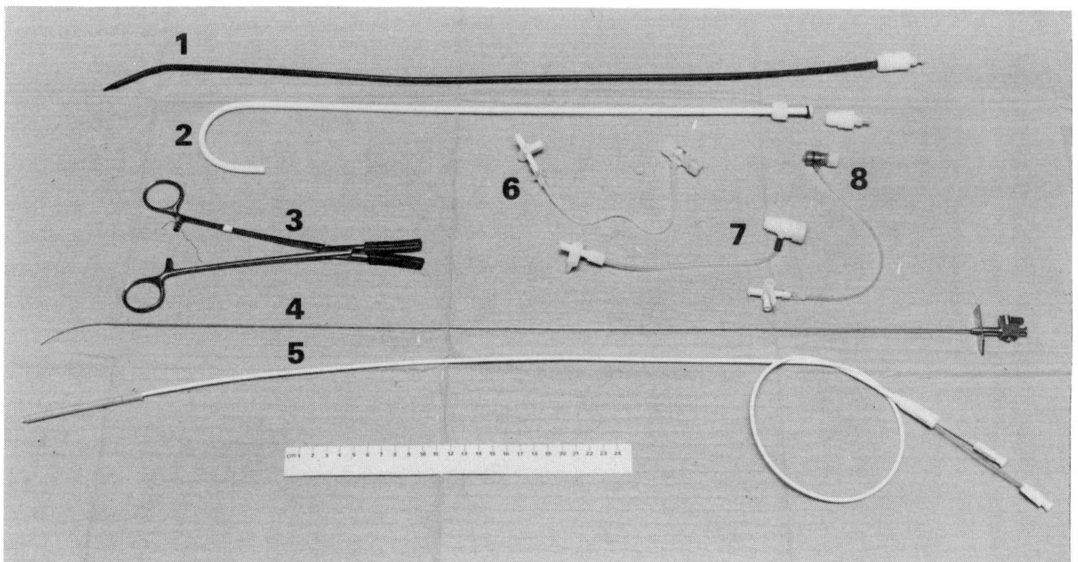

Fig. 16-5. 1, Transseptal dilator; **2,** transseptal sheath; **3,** rubber-shod clamp; **4,** transseptal needle; **5,** balloon catheter; **6,** prototype large hemostatic valve; **7,** large (Cook) hemostatic valve; and **8,** small (Kimal) hemostatic valve.

pinge on the distal end of the sheath, thus locking the balloons in position across the stenotic mitral valve and preventing the tough, sharp distal end of the balloon catheter from stabbing the left ventricular apex if the balloons slip distally during inflation (Fig. 16-7). The positioning of the preshaped exchange guidewire into the aorta, as advocated by other workers, has never seemed to be logical to us, for it is not firm enough to prevent the distal end of the balloon catheter from damaging or even perforating the left ventricle if the balloon forcibly slips forward during inflation, with its potentially fatal complications. We rely on the anchor of the sheaths rather than the hawser of the guidewires! Fig. 16-8 shows the overall view at this stage of the procedure.

A successful result is judged at the time by loss of balloon indentation (Fig. 16-9) in almost all patients. In a small number of patients this is not visualized, although they produce a successful result. Success is confirmed later by the hemodynamic changes, which are determined from the reduction of the gradient across the mitral valve, using the capillary wedge and left ventricular end diastole (LVED) pressures, through the thermodilution and pigtail catheters. To enable these provisional measurements to be made, the balloon catheters are temporarily withdrawn ("parked") into the sheath above the mitral valve orifice, leaving only the preshaped guidewires in the left ventricular cavity. This will also improve the blood flow through the valve by removing any obstruction. If a significant gradient persists, the balloons can be readvanced from the sheaths along the guidewires for further inflations. The inflations are repeated until a satisfactory result is achieved, or the procedure is abandoned. Up to 16 inflations have been performed with no complications, but the average is around 5 inflations for each procedure.

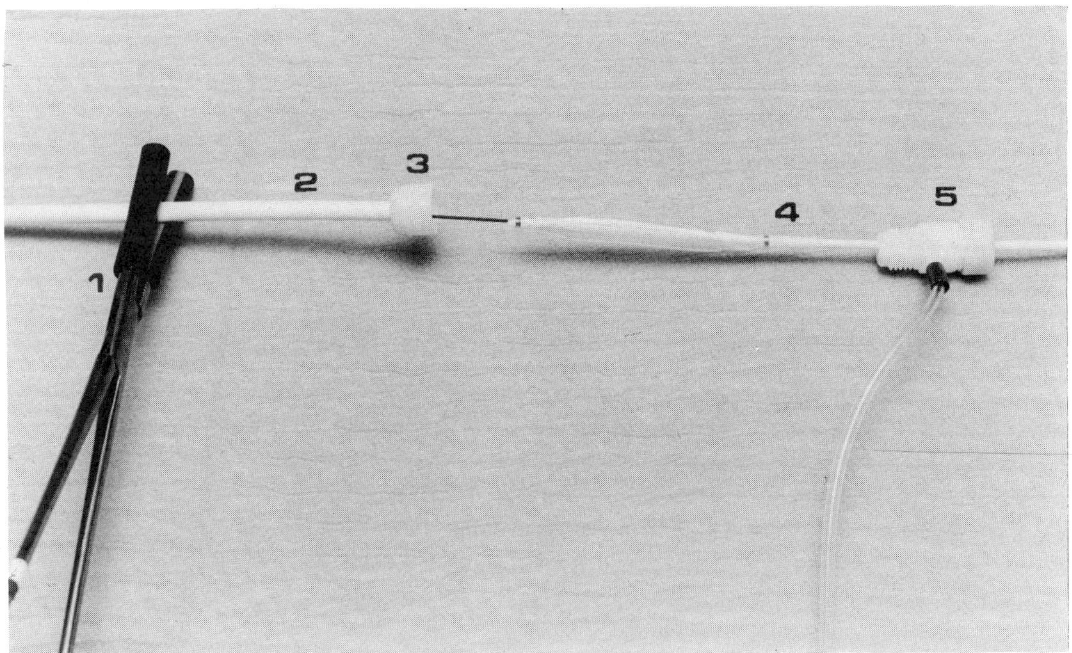

Fig. 16-6. 1, Rubber-shod clamp; **2,** 14F sheath with socket; **3,** Socket; **4,** 9F balloon catheter over the guidewire; **5,** Large (Cook) hemostatic valve on the shaft of the 9F balloon catheter.

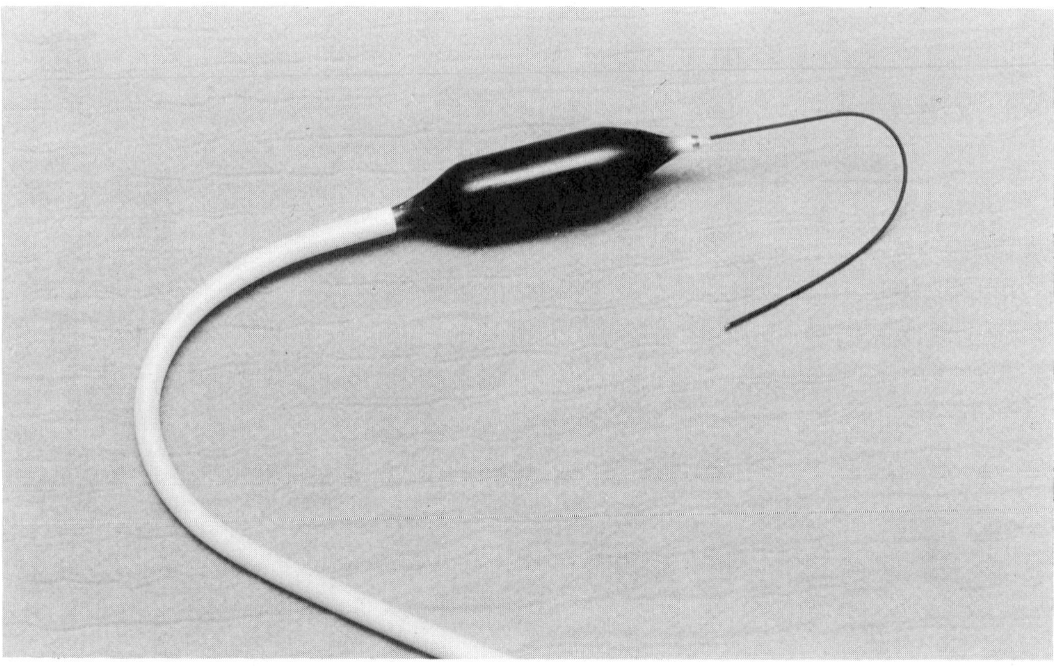

Fig. 16-7. Illustration demonstrating the locking of the inflated balloon against the distal end of the 14F transseptal sheath, controlling balloon movement. Note the curved preshaped exchange guidewire.

During the few seconds of balloon inflation, the aortic systolic pressure is always maintained around 40 to 50 mm Hg. Apart from occasional nausea, none of the patients experienced symptoms requiring attention during balloon inflation. It would seem appropriate here to mention a further advantage of the sheaths. If for any reason a balloon catheter must be replaced, for example following balloon rupture or the need to substitute larger balloons, the availability of the sheath in position makes this a simple matter.

Following the achievement of a satisfactory dilatation, the balloons are withdrawn from the sheaths, followed by the guidewires, keeping the three-way tap attached to the side arm of the hemostatic valve in the "open" position, thus allowing the deflated balloon to clear the contents of the sheath as it is withdrawn. The rubber-shod clamps are reapplied across the sheaths while disconnecting the special hemostatic valve, removing the balloons and reconnecting the Tuohy-Bourst hemostatic valves. The side arm of the latter is then connected to the pressure recording lines. We then measure the mitral valve gradient by simultaneous direct LA and LV pressures, followed by cardiac output calculation using the thermodilution catheter already in position. A final LV angiogram is performed and the sheaths are withdrawn into the right atrium. Heparinization is then reversed by an appropriate dose of IV protamine. To facilitate the complete withdrawal of the firmly preshaped transseptal sheaths and to prevent damage to the wall of the IVC by the passage of the sheath, the previously used dilator is inserted over a guidewire through the sheath into the right atrium. The sheaths, dilators, and guidewires are then

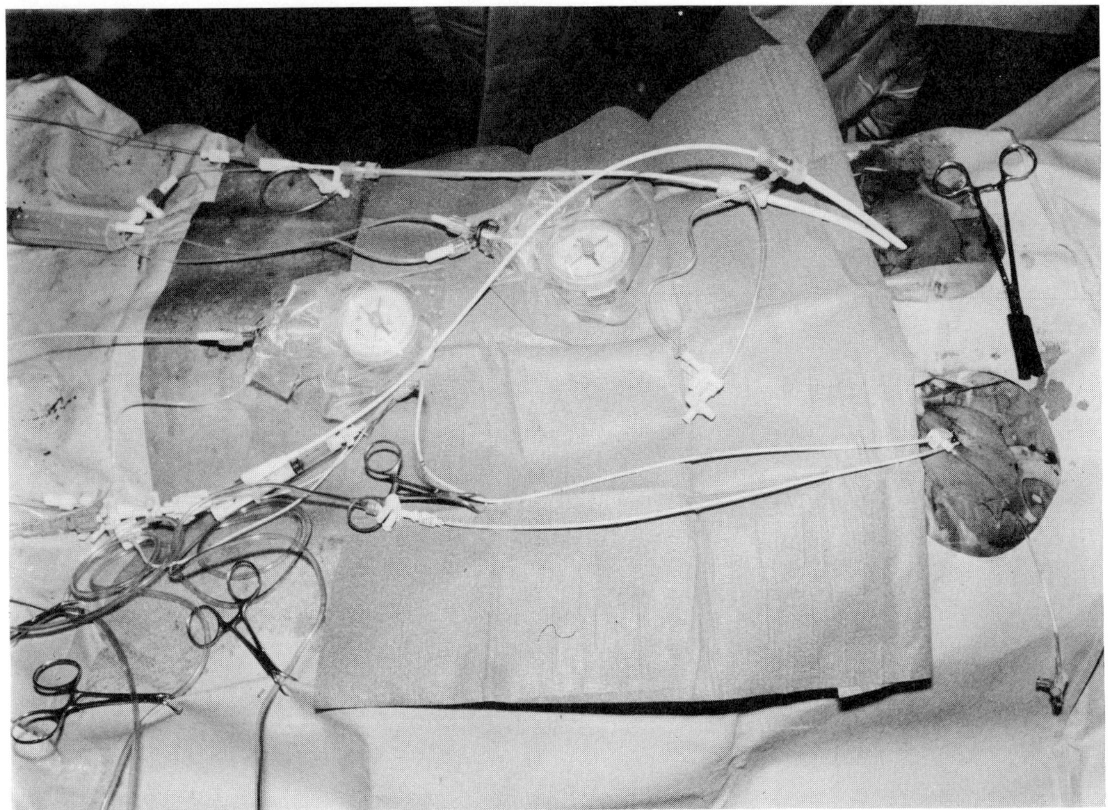

Fig. 16-8. General view of the procedure showing the two 14F transseptal sheaths inserted 2 cm apart into the right femoral vein, ready for balloon dilatation.

completely withdrawn together. The thermodilution catheter with its short venous sheath, and the pigtail catheter, are withdrawn. Pressure is applied to both groins until the bleeding stops. The patient is returned to the general cardiac ward and is usually discharged from the hospital within 24 to 48 hours.

CUMULATIVE RESULTS

Table 16-3 contains the cumulative total results of 60 successful procedures in which the 6- to 8-week follow-up study is complete. The increase in valve area of more than 100% persists at 6-week follow-up. In 14 other procedures we failed either to advance the sheath through the septum or to cross the stenotic mitral valve. These problems were mainly due to the initial difficulties we encountered in obtaining a reliable transseptal sheath that would pass easily through the septum and also retain its preshaped curve inside the left atrium, to facilitate easier crossing of the mitral valve. Now we are using much improved sheaths and the more recent results demonstrate their obvious advantages. Of those 14 patients in whom effective dilatation was not achieved, 12 had subsequent elective open heart surgery and two underwent a second, successful balloon dilatation, using the latest sheaths.

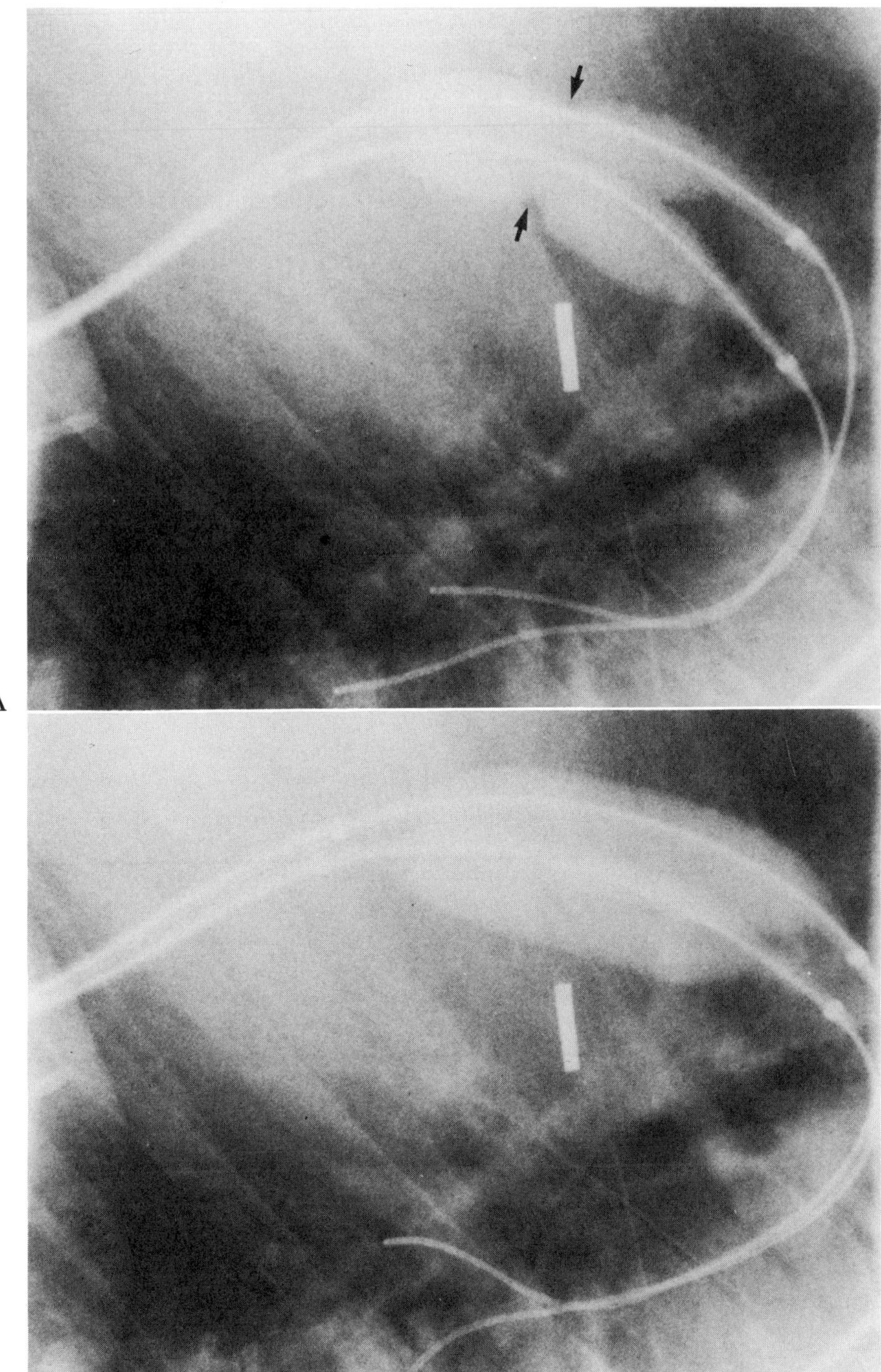

Fig. 16-9. Two transatrial balloons positioned across the mitral valve. **A,** Indentations seen in both balloons *(arrows)* during early inflation. **B,** Loss of balloon indentation following successful mitral balloon valvotomy.

Table 16-3 MVA Measurement in Balloon Mitral Valvotomy of 60 Patients

	2-D Echocardio-gram	*Doppler*	*Gorlin*
Predilatation	0.8 ± 0.2*	0.8 ± 0.1	0.8 ± 0.2
Postdilatation	1.7 ± 0.3*	1.7 ± 0.3	1.7 ± 0.4
(6 wk)	$p < 0.005$	$p < 0.005$	$p < 0.005$

**Mitral valve area (MVA) in cm^2.*

LONG-TERM FOLLOW-UP RESULTS

To determine the long-term efficacy of balloon mitral valvotomy, we are following our patients objectively, using a protocol that involves blind calculation of the MVA by two independent methods, namely 2-D echocardiography and Doppler echocardiography, at 6 and 12 months' postdilatation periods, and annually thereafter. Cardiac catheterization has been performed at the 12 months' study only in those four patients who showed persistent minor left-to-right atrial shunting by angiography, although not by oximetry, at the 6 weeks' examination. In all four cases this shunt had disappeared at the 12 months' study (Fig. 16-10).

All of the first 30 consecutive patients who underwent successful double balloon mitral valvotomy, with a mean age of 29 years, had improved to New York Heart Association (NYHA) Class I at the 1-year follow-up study. The one patient who remained in Class III at the 6 weeks' study, and who had coexisting bronchial asthma, had become asymptomatic at the 1-year stage. At her second year follow-up she was pregnant. Table 16-4 highlights the fact that on objective assessment of the results of balloon dilatation by calculated MVA, there is no evidence of restenosis at the 1-year follow-up study.

Like other workers, we have found that percutaneous balloon valvotomy is also feasible in cases of restenosis after surgical valvotomy. Of the five successful cases in this category to date, four have been studied at 6 to 12 months' follow-up and the increase in MVA has been maintained. The fifth patient is still awaiting the 1-year follow-up study. Three of this group of 5 patients had mitral valve calcifications. One patient not only had heavy calcification, but also had undergone two previous surgical valvotomies, 17 years and 6 years before successful mitral balloon valvotomy.

COMPLICATIONS

The benefits of this procedure have been chronicled, but mention must be made of the three cases from our total series in which we have encountered complications. After an apparently straightforward dilatation, with commissural splitting seen on fluoroscopy, one patient developed a giant v wave in the left atrial pressure tracing, which was subsequently confirmed by LV angiogram to be due to severe mitral regurgitation (MR) grade 4/4. The patient was asymptomatic, and the mean LA pressure remained around 30 mm Hg—the same level as before balloon dilatation. The lack of symptoms, even with the patient supine, was probably due to the chronically high LA pressure from the mitral stenosis and the relatively large left atrium. The patient felt so well that he originally rejected surgery, but he was persuaded to accept it since we were reluctant to discharge him with such severe mitral regurgitation. When surgery was eventually performed a tear in the anterior leaflet of the mitral valve was revealed, although with no splitting of the fused commissures. The surgeon was astonished at how severely the valve was fibrosed, so much so that there was not even an attempt at repair and the valve was replaced. Following this experience

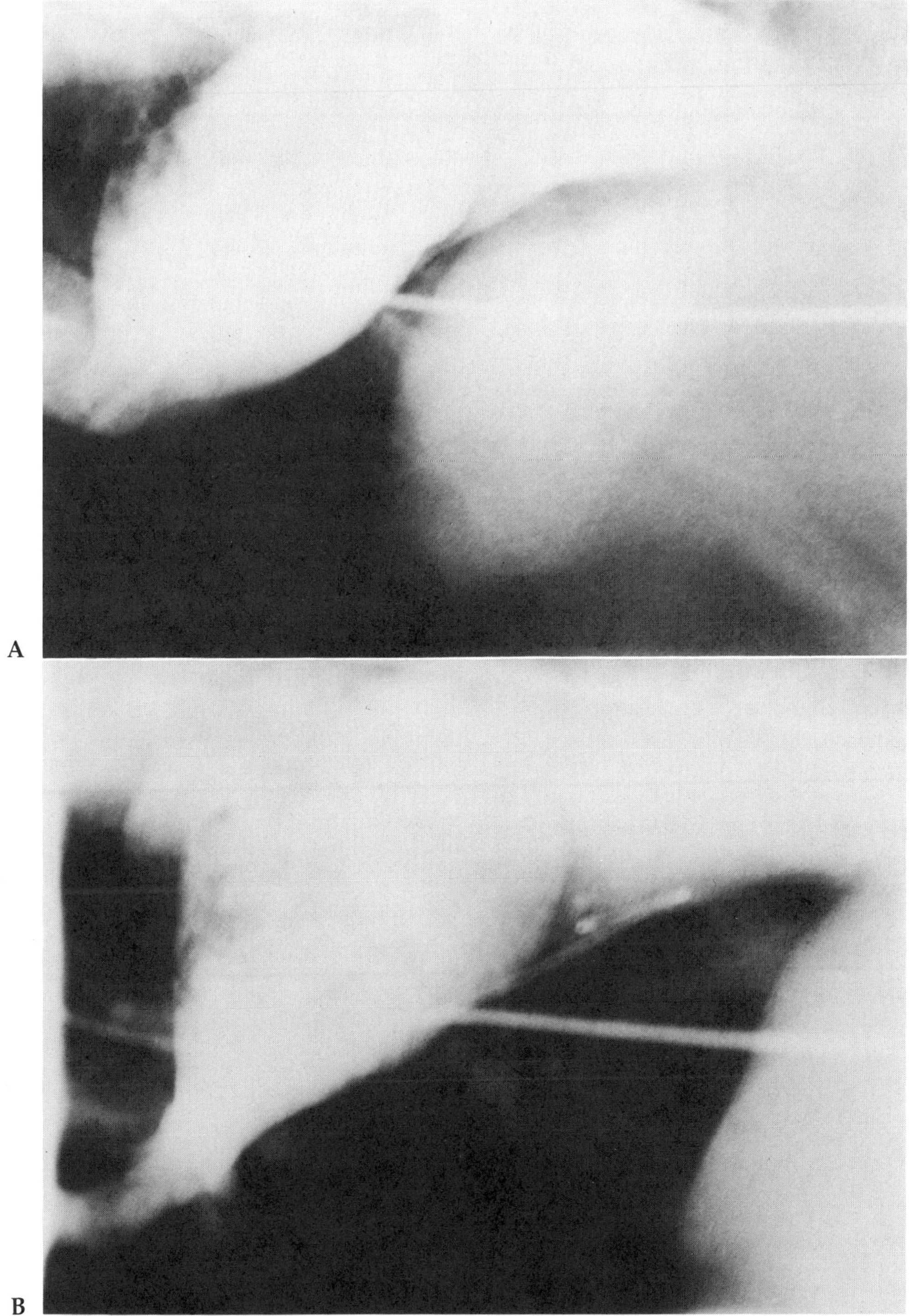

Fig. 16-10. Left atrial angiography in the LAO cranial angulation, showing **A,** left-to-right shunting at 6 to 8 weeks, and in contrast, **B,** no shunting.

Table 16-4 One-Year Follow-Up Study of 30 Patients Who Underwent Double Balloon Mitral Valvotomy

	Before	*After*	*1 Year*
NYHA Classes I and II	7*	29	30
NYHA Classes III and IV	23	1	0
MVA 2-D echocardiography	0.7 ± 0.2†	1.5 ± 0.2	1.6 ± 0.3
MVA Doppler echocardiography	0.7 ± 0.1	1.5 ± 0.2	1.6 ± 0.3
MVA Gorlin formula	0.8 ± 0.2	1.5 ± 0.3	Not done
$p < 0.001$			
MR (angiogram) (grades 1 to 4)	1	9	Not done

**Number = no. of patients.*
†Mitral valve area (MVA) measured in cm^2.
MR, Mitral regurgitation.

we are confident that even such an apparently dramatic complication can be managed successfully without resorting to immediate surgery.

The other two incidents arose from the passage of the transseptal sheaths, leading to cardiac tamponade. This was easily controlled by passage of a right coronary catheter through the sheath and through the atrial puncture into the pericardial cavity, to drain the hemopericardium calmly until the patient was taken to cardiac surgery.

We regard percutaneous balloon mitral valvotomy as an acceptable therapeutic alternative to surgery, with minimum morbidity, provided that it is performed by skilled operators. At present we believe that the use of the long transseptal sheath and the double balloon technique is justified to achieve reasonably large and persistent increases in MVA with minimal complications. Presently this procedure is offered as a first choice of therapy to those selected patients with severe rheumatic mitral stenosis.

REFERENCES

1. Kan, J.S., White, R.I., Mitchell, S.E., and Gardner, T.J.: Percutaneous balloon valvoplasty: a new method for treating congenital pulmonary valve stenosis, N. Engl. J. Med. **307**:540-542, 1982.
2. Inoue, K., Owani, T., Kitamura, F., and Miyamoto, N.: Clinical applications of transvenous mitral commissurotomy by a new balloon catheter, J. Thorac. Cardiovasc. Surg. **87**:394-402, 1984.
3. Al Zaibag, M., Ribeiro, P.A., Al Kasab, S., and Al Fagih, M.R.: Percutaneous double-balloon mitral valvotomy for rheumatic mitral-valve stenosis, Lancet 757-761, 1986.
4. Al Zaibag, M., Ribeiro, P.A., Al Kasab, S., and Habbab, M.: Percutaneous double balloon valvotomy: comparison of different size balloons (abstract), J. Am. Coll. Cardiol. **9**:82A, 1987.
5. Hatle, L., and Angelson, B.: Doppler ultrasound in cardiology: physical principles and clinical applications, Philadelphia, Lea & Febiger, 1982.

Chapter 17

Percutaneous Balloon Mitral Valvotomy

Peter Block, MD, FACC

Percutaneous mitral valvotomy (PMV) using dilating balloon catheters has become a therapeutic alternative to surgical mitral commissurotomy for some patients with mitral stenosis. The procedure has appeal since it can be done in a cardiac catheterization laboratory percutaneously, without general anesthesia and with a relatively low risk. Patients usually leave the hospital 24 to 36 hours after the procedure.

TECHNIQUE OF PERCUTANEOUS MITRAL VALVOTOMY

A transseptal puncture is first performed using standard techniques from the right femoral vein. The safety of transseptal puncture has been increased by the use of a modified Brockenbrough needle. The tip of the needle used to puncture the atrial septum is No. 22. The needle tip is advanced carefully through the foramen ovale, care being taken not to advance the larger dilator and sheath until the operator is certain of an intra–left atrial position. This is documented by pressure measurements, as well as by oxygen saturation measured from the tip of the needle after puncture. If a satisfactory left atrial position is not documented, the needle should be retracted and the sequence begun again. Heparin, obviously, should not be given until the transseptal puncture has been completed and the Mullin's sheath (8F, USCI, Billerica, Mass.) is positioned in the left atrium.

Biplane fluoroscopy can be helpful in evaluating the position of the needle tip before and after transseptal puncture. Some operators place a retrograde or pigtail catheter in the ascending aorta to help delineate aortic position and avoid inadvertent aortic puncture. If the foramen ovale is difficult to engage with the Brockenbrough needle tip, an echocardiogram in the catheterization laboratory can be helpful to document needle tip position. A Mullin's sheath is then advanced over a dilator into the left atrium. Heparinization is performed with 100 units per kg body weight given intravenously. A 7F floating balloon tipped catheter (Arrow International, Reading, Pa.) is passed through the sheath antegradely across the mitral valve. Simultaneous pressures in the left ventricle and left atrium are then measured. At the same time cardiac output is measured (either the thermodilution or the Fick technique) to allow calculation of the mitral valve area. The floating balloon catheter is then advanced, usually with the help of a guidewire, out the aortic valve and into the ascending aorta. A 0.038-inch transfer guidewire is advanced through the floating balloon catheter and advanced into the descending aorta. The floating balloon catheter and Mullin's sheath are removed, leaving the single transfer wire behind (Fig. 17-1A).

An 8 mm balloon dilating catheter (Mansfield, Mansfield, Mass.) is advanced over the guidewire to straddle the atrial septum. One or two inflations are performed to allow passage of a second transfer guidewire and larger balloon dilating catheters (Fig. 17-1B). The 8 mm balloon is removed and replaced by a double lumen catheter (8F, Mansfield, Mansfield, Mass.). This is advanced over the guidewire until its tip is in the ascending or

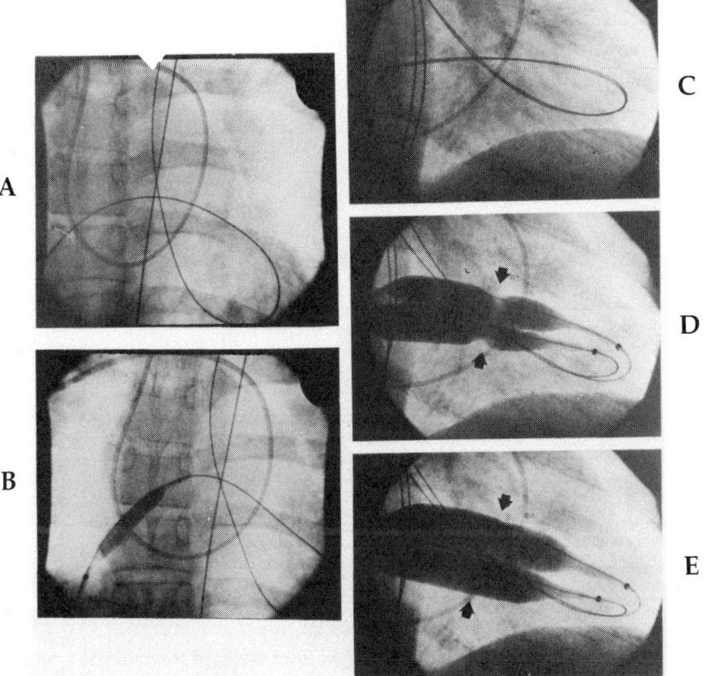

Fig. 17-1. Technique of percutaneous mitral valvotomy. **A,** Single transfer guidewire (0.038 inch) in place from the right femoral vein, across the atrial septum and mitral valve, out the aortic valve. Its tip is in the descending aorta. **B,** An 8 mm dilating balloon catheter inflated in the atrial septum. **C,** Second transfer guidewire (0.038 inch) in place parallel to the first guidewire. **D,** Two 20 mm dilating balloon catheters partially inflated across the stenotic mitral valve (note the "waist" *[arrows]*). **E,** Full inflation of the two 20 mm dilating balloon catheters. The "waist" *(arrows)* has disappeared.

transverse aorta. A second 0.038-inch transfer guidewire is then advanced through the second, empty lumen. Its tip is advanced into the descending aorta parallel to the first guidewire. The double lumen catheter is removed leaving the two guidewires behind (Fig. 17-1C). Twenty-millimeter dilating balloon catheters are then advanced over each guidewire and placed in position to straddle the stenotic mitral valve. Two to three simultaneous balloon inflations are performed with a handheld 60 ml Luer-lock syringe containing one-third contrast and two-thirds saline. Frequently a "waist" can be seen in the balloons as they are first inflated (Fig. 17-1,D and E). If the balloons are correctly positioned across the mitral valve, inflation obstructs left ventricular inflow and leads to severe hypotension. Rapid inflation-deflation cycles lasting no more than 20 seconds are imperative to avoid prolonged hypotension and syncope (Fig. 17-2). The balloon-dilating catheters are removed, but the transfer wires are left behind. The floating balloon catheter and transseptal sheath are replaced over one of the wires into the left ventricle and atrium respectively. Repeat pressure measurements are made in the left ventricle and left atrium with simultaneous cardiac output measurements to allow calculation of the mitral valve area after PMV. The floating balloon catheter is withdrawn and a Berman 7F or pigtail 7F catheter is then advanced through the Mullin's sheath into the left ventricle. As the last step, left ventricular cineangiography is performed to evaluate mitral regurgitation. After the left

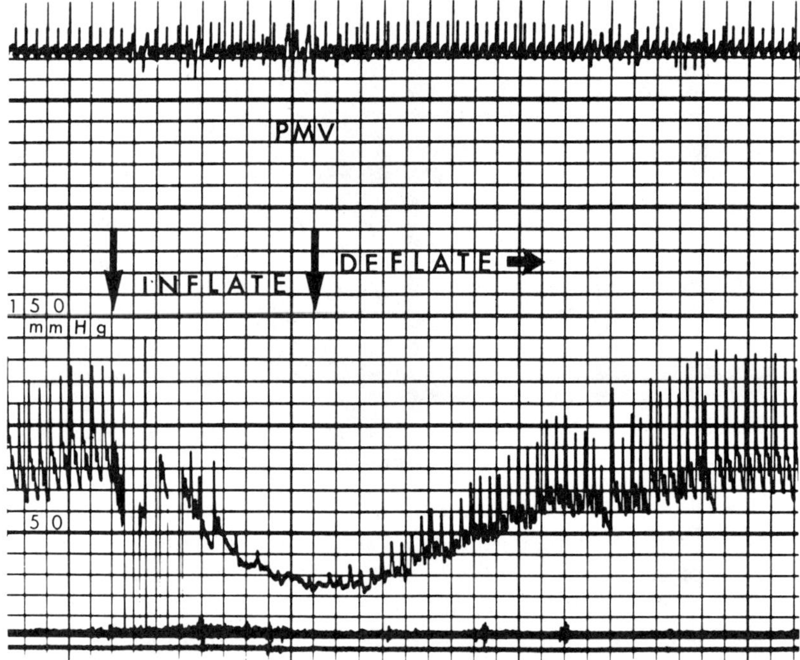

Fig. 17-2. Radial artery pressure recording before, during, *(inflate)* and immediately after *(deflate)* percutaneous mitral valvotomy with two 20 mm balloons. During inflation blood pressure drops from 120/70 mm Hg to 30/25 mm Hg. Recovery of blood pressure occurs rapidly as the balloons deflate.

atrial sheath and angiographic catheters are withdrawn, an oxygen run is performed using the Swan-Ganz catheter. If there is evidence of left-to-right shunting through the atrial septum, cardiac output should be repeated using the Fick technique. The elevated right-sided output produced by the left-to-right shunt spuriously increases the calculated mitral valve area.

Twenty-millimeter balloon-dilating catheters are usually used as a first choice. A 25 mm and 15 mm balloon-dilating catheter combination can also be used to enlarge the mitral orifice further. Left atrial pressure should be lowered to less than 14 mm Hg (giving a mitral gradient of 6 mm Hg or less). Percutaneous mitral valvotomy should not be considered satisfactory unless left atrial pressure is reduced to this level.

RESULTS

The initial experience with PMV included patients with many different kinds of mitral valve morphology and severity of mitral valve stenosis. The results are shown in Table 17-1 and Fig. 17-3. The mean mitral valve area increased from 0.8 ± 0.1 to 1.7 ± 0.2 cm (p <0.0001). The mitral valve gradient in the entire group fell from 19 ± 1 mm Hg to 7 ± 1 mm Hg (p <0.0001). Cardiac output rose approximately 1 L per minute and pulmonary artery pressure dropped significantly, as did pulmonary vascular resistance. With experience and careful patient selection (see below), mitral valve area should be increased to 2 cm^2 or more in all patients.

Complications of Percutaneous Mitral Valvotomy

There are many potential complications of PMV. They include the production of mitral regurgitation, thromboembolic events, problems related to transseptal catheterization (tamponade, creation of a left-to-right shunt through the atrial septum) and rhythm disturbances. In our first 75 patients, 1 patient (1.3%) died at emergency surgery of right-sided heart failure caused by severe pulmonary hypertension. One additional patient had an acute inferior myocardial infarction as a result of atherosclerotic coronary artery disease 24 hours after a successful PMV. Embolic events occurred in two patients (2.7%). Two patients had heart block at the time of balloon inflation and one of them required a permanent pacemaker. One patient developed severe mitral regurgitation. However, this pa-

Table 17-1 Results of Percutaneous Mitral Valvotomy (75 Patients)

	Before PMV	*After PMV*
Valve area	0.8 ± 0.1 cm^2	1.7 ± 0.2*
Mitral gradient	19 ± 1.0 mm Hg	7 ± 1*
Cardiac output	3.8 ± 2.4 L/min	4.6 ± 0.2
Mean PA pressure	41 ± 2 mm Hg	27 ± 2*
Pulmonary resistance	338 ± 45 dynes/sec/cm$-^5$	260 ± 33*

*= p <0.0001.
PA, Pulmonary artery.

tient has not required surgery in a 2-year follow-up. Approximately half of the patients who underwent PMV had no change in the degree of their mitral regurgitation. The other half had an increase in mitral regurgitation of approximately one grade. None of the patients required urgent or emergency surgery because of the production of severe mitral regurgitation and heart failure. Left-to-right shunting could be measured by oximetry immediately after PMV in six patients. However, oximetry studies 24 hours later demonstrated no left-to-right shunting in any of these patients.

Selection of Patients

Reports of the results of cardiac surgery for mitral stenosis have shown that the best results of surgical mitral commissurotomy are in patients with minimally calcified valves and maintenance of valvular mobility.[1-4] Clinically, the presence of an opening snap was frequently the predictor of a good mitral split. Therefore, one would anticipate that the best results of PMV are in patients with minimally calcified or noncalcified valves, without severe subvalvular fibrosis, and with good mobility and minimal thickening of the valve leaflets.[5,6] Patients with a history of previous mitral commissurotomy done surgically, some valvular calcification, severe pulmonary hypertension, mild (grade 2+/4+) mitral regurgitation, or left ventricular dysfunction should *not be excluded* from consideration for PMV. The presence of insignificant other valvular disease that does not need repair and the presence of nonsurgical coronary artery disease or other associated disease states are not contraindications. Patients who have severe

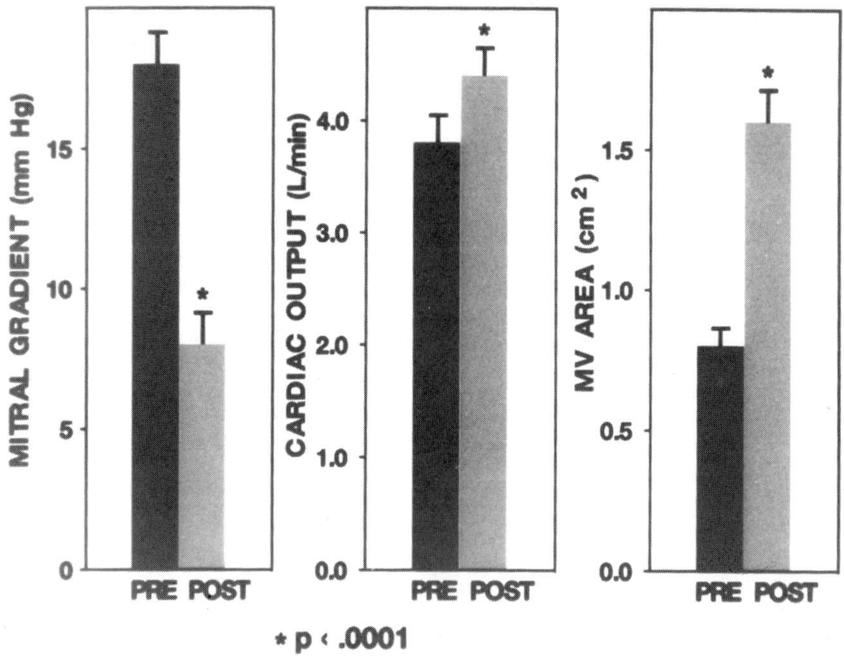

Fig. 17-3. Hemodynamic changes after percutaneous mitral valvotomy.

pulmonary hypertension secondary to mitral stenosis need careful monitoring during PMV to avoid hypovolemia, hypotension, and right-sided heart failure.

Multiple stepwise regression analysis of factors that predict the best results after PMV identified the following:

1. Minimal valve calcification
2. Mobile mitral valve
3. Minimal subvalvular fibrosis
4. Minimal valvular thickening

These four factors can be evaluated noninvasively using echocardiographic techniques. All patients who are potential candidates for PMV should first have a careful echocardiographic examination.[7] An "echo score" can be generated by grading the four factors 1 to 4+ (Table 17-2). For example, a patient with no mitral valve calcification, a mobile mitral valve, no subvalvular fibrosis, and minimal valve thickening would have a score of 1 for each factor—a total score of 4. Conversely, a patient with severe mitral valve calcification, a rigid mitral valve, a thickened mitral valve, and severe subvalvular fibrosis would have a score of 4 for each factor and a total score of 16 (Fig 17-4). Multiple regression analysis has shown that patients who have an echo score of 8 or less have a high likelihood of a good result from PMV. In our series, valve area increased from 0.9 ± 0.1 cm^2 to 2.0 ± 0.1 cm^2 in this subgroup of patients (Fig. 17-5). The echo

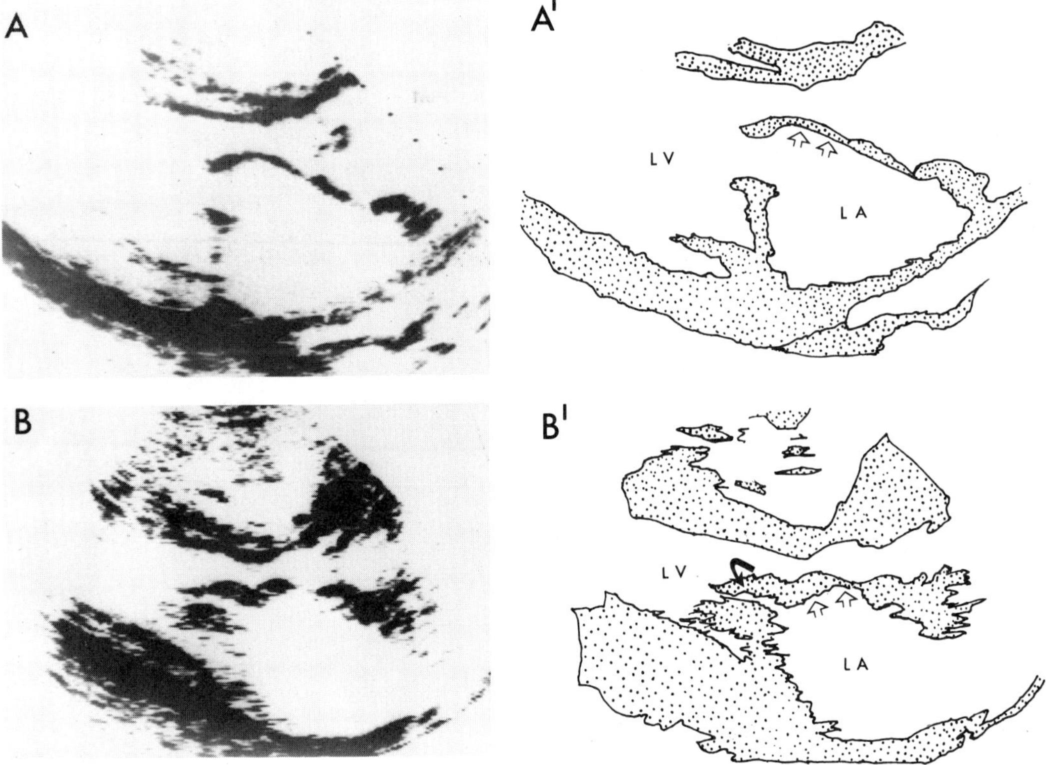

Fig. 17-4. Echocardiograms and outline diagrams of a mitral valve favorable for PMV *(A; A')* and not favorable for PMV *(B; B')*. The favorable valve has thin, mobile leaflets *(arrows, A')*, the unfavorable valve has thick, rigid leaflets *(B')*, severe subvalvular thickening *(curved solid arrow, B')*, and calcification. (LA, left atrium, LV, left ventricle.)

Table 17-2 Determination of Echo Score

	Minimal	*Severe*
Valve rigidity	1	4
Valve thickening	1	4
Calcification	1	4
Subvalvular thickening	1	4
ECHO SCORE TOTAL	4	16

Score of 1 for each factor in minimal disease, and a score of 4 for each factor in severe disease.

score also appears to be predictive of long-term results. If the echo score is 8 or less, the initial result should be good and follow-up at 1 year has demonstrated little if any restenosis. If, however, the echo score is greater than 8, even if the initial result is good, there is a higher incidence of restenosis (20% compared with 7%) at 1 year. Contraindications to the procedure are the following: high echo score, presence of left atrial thrombus, recent untreated thromboembolic event, severe associated coronary disease in a patient who is a candidate for combined mitral valve surgery and coronary bypass surgery, severe associated regurgitant disease of the aortic or mitral valve, and the presence of left ventricular thrombus (Table 17-3).

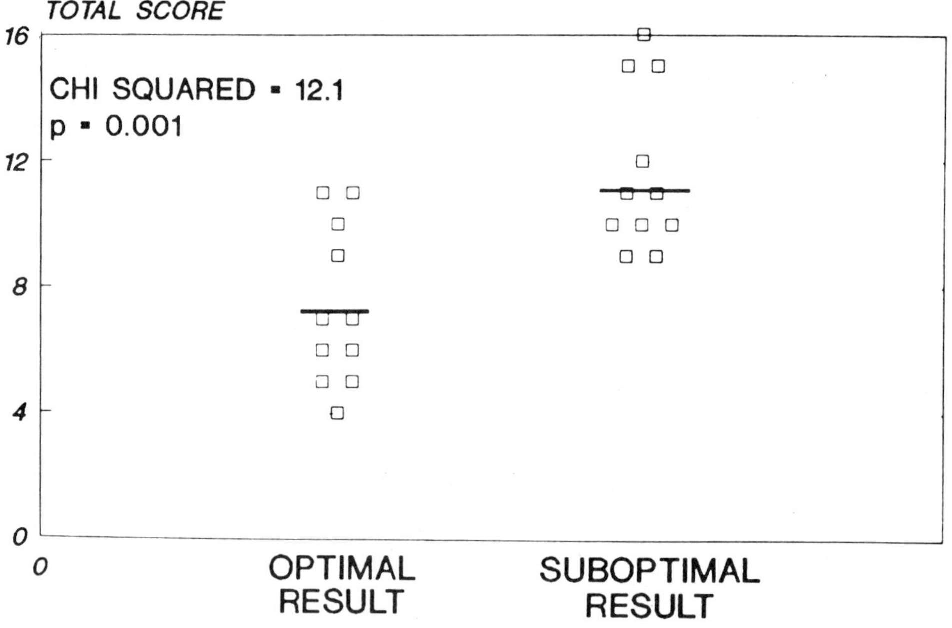

Fig. 17-5. Echo score (abscissa) of patients plotted against the valve area increase after PMV. "Optimal" results = increase in valve area of more than 25% and more than 1 cm^2; "suboptimal" results = increase in valve area of less than 25% or to less than 1 cm^2.

Table 17-3 Indications and Contraindications for PMV

Factors Favorable for PMV

1. Echo score of 8 or less
2. Young age
3. Presence of opening snap
4. Normal sinus rhythm
5. No calcification of valve

Factors Unfavorable for PMV

1. Echo score of 10 or more
2. Age greater than 70
3. No opening snap
4. Atrial fibrillation (long-standing)
5. Calcification of valve
6. Severe subvalvular fibrosis
7. Thickened atrial septum (>3 mm)

Contraindications to PMV

1. Left atrial thrombus
2. Recent (3 mo) thromboembolic event
3. 2+ grade or higher grade of mitral regurgitation
4. Left ventricular thrombus
5. Associated surgical coronary or other valve disease

Appendix A Setup for Mitral Valvuloplasty

20	Gauze sponges
2	16 oz flush basins
1	16 oz basin (for 50 ml contrast solution to 100 ml dextrose and water)
1	6-cup plastic basin
1	O.R. basin
10+	Towel clips
2	Large curved hemostatic forceps
1	Small straight hemostatic forceps
1	No. 11 blade and handle
4	12 ml plastic syringes
1	30 ml plastic syringe
2	60 ml plastic syringes
3	Pressure tubing
4	Stopcocks
2	Telfa dressing pads
1/2	No. 1040 Steri-drape
2	No. 038-260-3J exchange guidewires
1	No. 032-145-3J guidewire (use with Arrow International floating balloon catheter)
1	Double lumen catheter (Mansfield)
1	Arrow International floating balloon catheter (7F)
1	Berman angiographic catheter (7F)
1	No. 8591 transseptal introducer set
1	No. 3994 Brockenbrough transseptal needle

CONCLUSION

Percutaneous mitral balloon valvotomy is a safe and effective procedure and offers an alternative to surgical mitral commissurotomy in selected patients with mitral stenosis.[5] Careful echocardiographic evaluation to develop an echo score should be done on each patient before commitment to PMV. Patients with an echo score of 8 or less (mobile valve, little calcium, little valve thickening, little subvalvular fibrosis) should have a good result and should have little or no restenosis in long-term follow-up. Patients with echo scores of more than 8 may have a good result, but the restenosis rate is higher. Nevertheless, the option of an attempt at PMV should be given to most patients who have symptomatic mitral stenosis that requires mechanical repair.

REFERENCES

1. Block, P.C., Palacios, I.F., Jacobs, M.L., and Fallon, J.T.: Mechanism of percutaneous mitral valvotomy, Am. J. Cardiol. **59**:178-179, 1987.
2. Commerford, P.J., Hastie, T., and Beck, W.: Closed mitral valvotomy: actuarial analysis of results in 654 patients over 12 years and analysis of preoperative predictors of long-term survival, Ann. Thorac. Surg. **33**:473-479, 1982.
3. Gross, R.I., Cunningham, J.N., Jr., Snivley, S.L., Cantinella, F.P., Nathan, I.M., Adams, P.X., and Spencer, F.C.: Long-term results of open radical mitral commissurotomy: ten year follow-up study of 202 patients, Am. J. Cardiol. **47**:821-825, 1981.
4. Kirklin, J.W., and Barrett-Boyes, B.G.: Mitral valve disease with or without tricuspid valve disease. In Cardiac surgery, New York, 1986, John Wiley & Sons, Inc.
5. Palacios, I.F., Block, P.C., Brandi, S., Blanco, P., Casal, H., Pulido, J.I., Munoz, S., D'Empaire, G., Ortega, M.A., Jacobs, M., and Vlahakes, G.: Percutaneous balloon valvotomy for patients with severe mitral stenosis, Circulation **75**:778-784, 1987.
6. McKay, R.G., Lock, J.E., Safian, R.D., et al.: Balloon dilation of mitral stenosis in adult patients: post-mortem and percutaneous mitral valvuloplasty studies, J. Am. Coll. Cardiol. **9**:723-733, 1987.
7. Hermann, H.C., Williams, G.C., Vbascal, V., Weyman, A.E., Block P.C., Palacios I.F.: Percutaneous mitral balloon valvotomy for patients with mitral stenosis: analysis of factors influencing early results, Accepted for publication.

Chapter 18

Percutaneous Double Balloon Valvotomy for Patients with Severe Mitral Stenosis

Carlos E. Ruiz, MD
John W. Allen, MD
Pamela J. Kaiser, MPH
Francis Y.K. Lau, MD

In this chapter we describe a methodology for treating severe mitral stenosis with percutaneous double balloon valvotomy (PDBV) developed at Loma Linda University and White Memorial Medical Center in Los Angeles. Our experience, based on a series of over 90 procedures performed between 1985 and 1987, has led us to view PDBV as an effective, less costly, nonsurgical alternative for patients who have clinical indications for surgical mitral valvotomy.

HISTORY

Although the incidence of rheumatic heart disease has markedly decreased in the United States,[1,2] it continues to be the primary underlying cause of mitral stenosis. A high prevalence of mitral stenosis in developing nations is common,[3,4] and some recent reports indicate that the incidence of rheumatic fever in the United States is beginning to increase.

Open mitral valve commissurotomy remains the popular treatment of choice for stenotic disease in many places around the world. An alternative procedure, nonsurgical balloon valvotomy, was first reported by Inoue and associates.[5] Other investigators have also reported single balloon methods[6,7] and, in a small number of patients, double balloon techniques.[8] A drawback of the double balloon procedure is perhaps the higher cost and the potential for creating larger atrial septal defects. We have modified and simplified the technique in an attempt to minimize both the procedure time and the concomitant risks. We also feel that there are theoretic reasons for making the double balloon technique safer and more effective than the single balloon approach to valvotomy.

PATIENT SELECTION

Appropriate patients for the PDBV are symptomatic, New York Heart Association (NYHA) Class II or above, without any absolute contraindications for a transseptal catheterization. Such contraindications would include interrupted inferior vena cava, documented or suspected intracardiac clots, and recent history of thromboembolism (within 6 months). Patients with pliable leaflets, without mitral valve calcification, and without subvalvular involvement are the best candidates for PDBV. Optimal results in our series were obtained among patients with no calcification, or among those with 1+ to 2+ calcification (4-point scale). However, valve area was increased significantly even among those patients with heavily calcified mitral valves (Table 18-1).

All patients with an enlarged left atrial cavity and chronic atrial fibrillation should be fully anticoagulated for at least 2 months before the procedure, as previously recommended by Palacios and co-workers.[9]

At this time there is no accurate diagnostic tool available to exclude patients with small atrial clots. Careful echocardiographic analysis by an experienced echocardiographer must be carried out in all patients before PDBV to identify and rule out patients at high risk for emboli.

Two-dimensional (2-D) Doppler echocardiography should be utilized to determine what portions of the mitral apparatus are involved: commissures, leaflets, and/or subvalvular structures. The patient's response to balloon dilatation will be influenced by which of these aspects are involved. The ideal patient would be one with minimal leaflet thickening, generous doming, and reduced transverse diameter without mitral regurgitation or extraleaflet stenosis. A marginal candidate would be a patient with severe leaflet stenosis, minimal or no doming, markedly thickened or calcified leaflets, minimal reduction in transverse orifice diameter, heavy subvalvular involvement with marked fibrosis or calcification, and moderate mitral regurgitation.

PERCUTANEOUS DOUBLE BALLOON VALVOTOMY PROTOCOL

In patients with chronic atrial fibrillation, and for those who are on oral anticoagulant therapy, warfarin is discontinued 72 hours before the procedure and a heparin drip is begun. Heparin is discontinued 4 hours before the transeptal puncture and reinitiated (150 units per Kg body weight) when the catheters are in place in the left atrium.

With the cardiac surgical theater on standby, patients are taken to the catheterization laboratory where both groins are surgically prepared and properly draped. The left femoral vein is approached using the Seldinger technique with an 18-gauge needle. An 8F Hemaquet sheath (USCI, Billerica, Mass.) is advanced into the femoral vein. A thermodilution Swan-Ganz catheter is then advanced and pressures are obtained from the right atrium, right ventricle, and pulmonary artery. A 7F Hemaquet sheath is placed in the left femoral artery by the same Seldinger technique and a 7F pigtail catheter is advanced to the ascending aorta, where pressures are again recorded. Using the same percutaneous approach, the right femoral vein is then cannulated with the intention of accessing the left atrium by the transseptal technique.

Transseptal catheterization is accomplished from the right femoral vein using standard technique, a modified Brockenbrough needle, and an 8F Mullins' transseptal sheath-dilator (USCI, Billerica, Mass.). A biplane cinefluoroscopy x-ray unit, rather than a single-plane unit, is highly recommended to facilitate the correct placement of the needle before the transseptal puncture and thereby to minimize the risks of cardiac perforations (Fig. 18-1).

Table 18-1 **P.D.B.V. FOR SEVERE M.S IMMEDIATE OUTCOME**

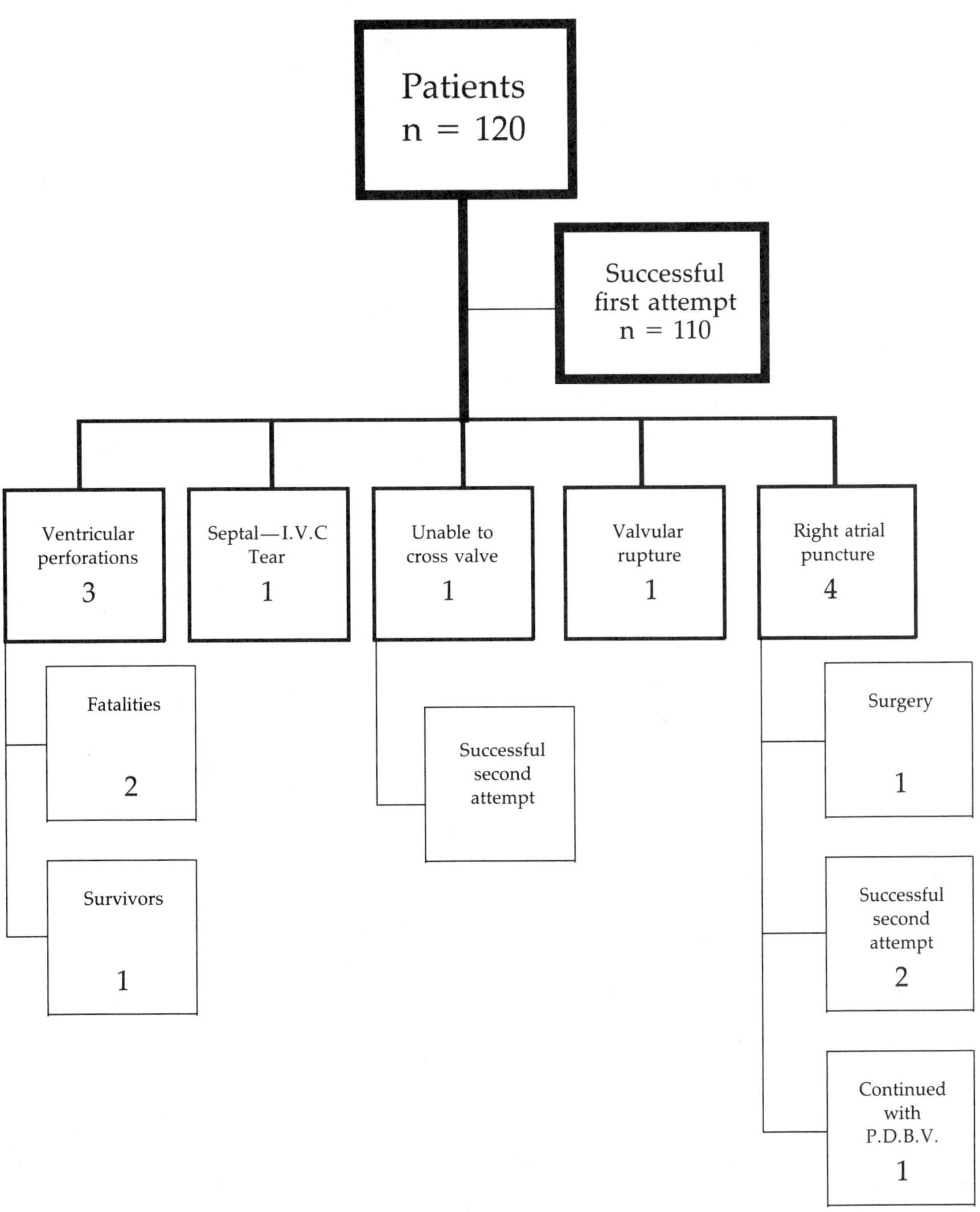

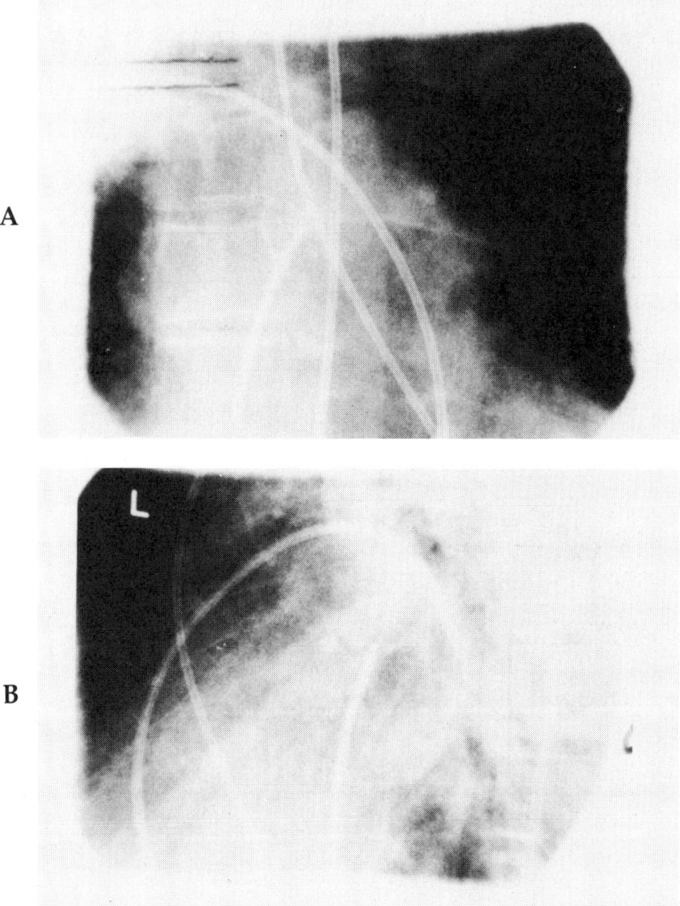

Fig. 18-1. Transseptal needle properly oriented against the interatrial septum before the puncture. **A,** Straight anteroposterior view; **B,** Lateral view.

Once the transeptal needle has successfully crossed the interatrial septum, continuous pressure monitoring is done through the needle to obtain left atrial pressure readings. Before advancing the Mullins' sheath, we obtain a blood sample to confirm the left atrial oximetries. Contrast medium is injected through the needle to determine the distance to the left atrial wall and to judge the room available to advance the sheath.

Baseline hemodynamic measurements include a diagnostic oxygen saturation series, and systemic arterial, left ventricular, pulmonary artery, pulmonary capillary wedge and left atrial pressures. The mean gradient across the mitral valve is measured using the Mullins' sheath and the retrograde pigtail catheter, which has been advanced across the aortic valve into the left ventricular cavity. Simultaneous cardiac output measurements are obtained by thermodilution. When significant tricuspid insufficiency is present, a green-dye technique can be used with injection into the main pulmonary artery and sampling from the ascending aorta. The mitral valve area is then calculated by the Gorlin formula; pulmonary vascular resistance is derived from the simultaneous measurement of mean pulmonary artery pressure, mean left atrial pressure, and cardiac output.

After collection of baseline hemodynamic data, the Mullins' transseptal sheath is advanced into the left ventricle by a slight pullback and counterclockwise manipulation. Care must be taken not to pull back too far. Should the sheath accidentally be drawn into the right atrium, the patient's anticoagulation would preclude making a new puncture through the septum in most cases.

Unlike other techniques, for this procedure the guidewires are not advanced to the descending aorta because the size of the balloon catheters provides sufficient stability along the longitudinal axis of the left ventricle to secure both balloons across the mitral apparatus. The duration of the procedure and the patient's exposure to radiation are therefore considerably shortened.

A 260 cm, specially shaped (2 1/2 turns) exchange wire (Med-Rad Co., Pittsburgh, Pa.) is advanced and placed at the apex of the left ventricle (Fig. 18-1A) by way of the Mullins' transseptal sheath. A 7F catheter (8 mm diameter by 3 cm length) dilating balloon (Meditech Inc., Watertown, Mass.) is advanced over the guidewire through the Mullins' transseptal sheath, all the way to the left atrium. The sheath is then pulled back over the shaft of the septostomy balloon catheter to allow expansion of the balloon. The inflated balloon is pulled back through the septum (Fig. 18-2), maintaining the guidewire in the same position in the left ventricle. After septostomy, the Mullins' sheath is readvanced into the left ventricle and a second identically shaped exchange wire is advanced and positioned next to the first one (Fig. 18-3). The transseptal sheath is then withdrawn. The first valvotomy balloon catheter (Mansfield Scientific Inc., Mansfield, Mass.) is ad-

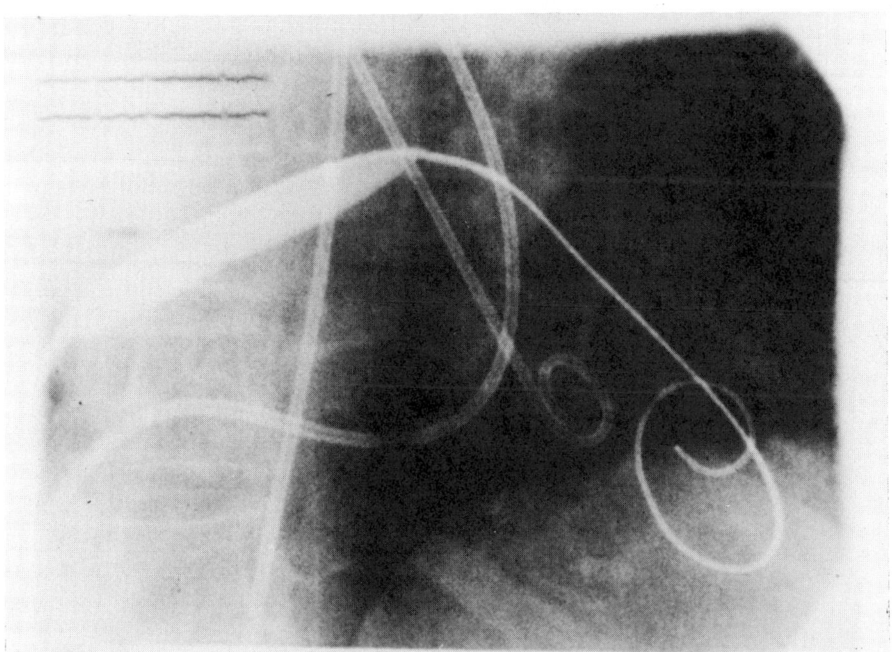

Fig. 18-2. Septostomy balloon catheter across interatrial septum. Notice the indentation of the septum in the contour of the balloon *(arrow)*.

vanced over one of the wires and positioned across the mitral valve, leaving a large double loop of the preshaped wire extending out of the tip of the balloon catheter and positioned in the apex of the left ventricle. A second balloon dilatation catheter is advanced over the second wire and positioned parallel to the first one across the mitral valve. The two balloon catheters are then inflated by hand simultaneously (Fig. 18-4, A and B) until the "waist" of the stenotic valve over the balloons' silhouette disappears (Fig. 18-4, C and D). Inflation times range from 20 to 120 seconds. Two to four inflations are usually done.

A

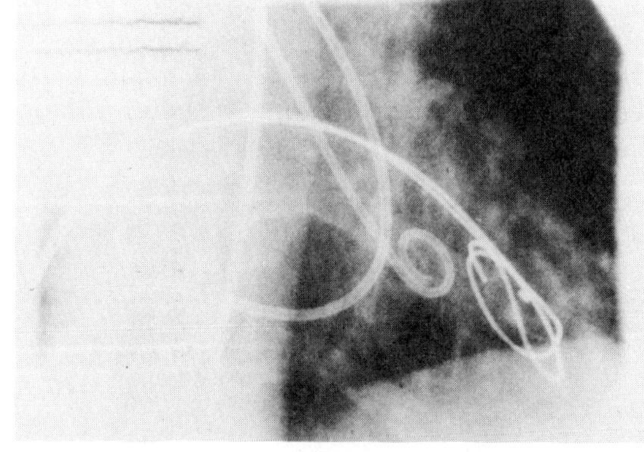

B

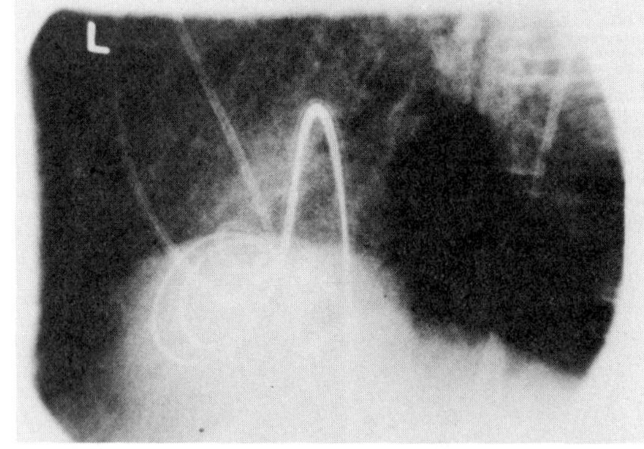

Fig. 18-3. Two specially shaped exchange guidewires already across and positioned at the apex of the left ventricle. **A,** Anteroposterior view; **B,** Lateral view.

A balloon length of 5.5 cm and a diameter of 20 mm is typically used in normal-size adults to achieve an oversizing of the annulus of between 10 to 27% (average oversize is 20%). In no instance should the mitral annulus be oversized more than 30% as measured by 2D-echocardiography.

The use of two simultaneously inflated balloons permits a safe oversizing of the annulus by 25%. Because the area occupied by the two balloons does not exceed the valvular orifice area, the longitudinal diameter of the valvular apparatus can be safely overstretched and a more effective splitting of the fused commissures can be obtained (Fig. 18-5). The free space between balloons allows the continued flow of blood across the valve during maximum inflation, resulting in improved hemodynamic stability during inflation. In our recently reported (16) series of 60 patients, postdilatation valve areas were 50% larger, or more, in all patients. These results are better than those reported by other authors[6,9,10] utilizing a single balloon technique.

Immediately after the procedure, the balloon catheters are removed and a pigtail catheter is advanced transseptally over the guidewire to the left ventricle. Pullback pressures are recorded from the left ventricle to the left atrium. Simultaneous recordings of pressures are obtained from both cavities, using the retrograde left-ventricular pigtail catheter and the transseptal left-atrial pigtail catheter. Simultaneous cardiac output measurements, pulmonary artery pressures, and systemic hemodynamic measurements are also recorded. Left atrial cineangiography in the cranial (LAO) projection is performed to evaluate the angiographic presence of any left-to-right shunt. Left ventriculography is done to evaluate the severity of mitral regurgitation. Oximetric data are used to assess the presence of a left-to-right shunt through the atrial septostomy.

The procedure is routinely completed in less than 2 hours and most patients are discharged home within 24 hours.

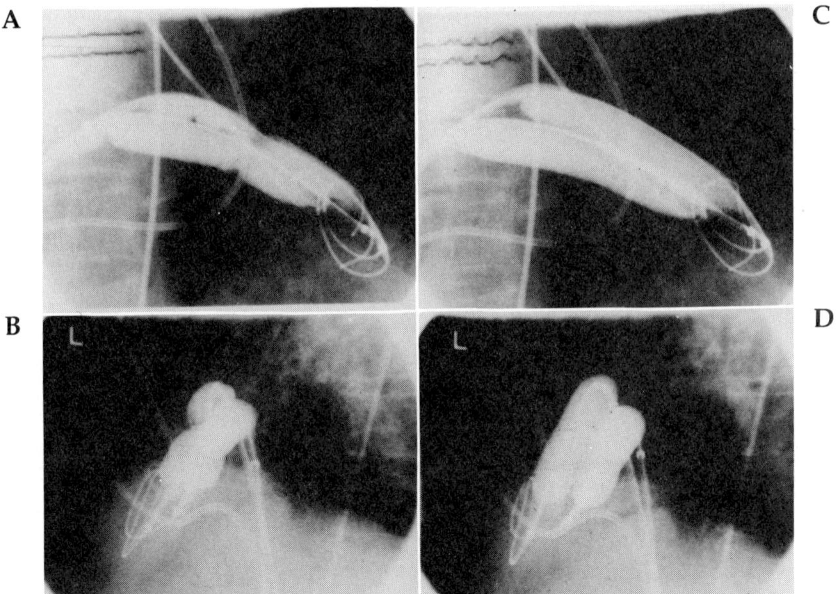

Fig. 18-4. View of two balloons during inflation. Balloons are parallel to each other and across the mitral valve. The exchange guide-wires with a specially preshaped double-loop extend out of the tip of the balloon catheters and lodge at the apex of the left ventricle. During inflation the "waist" produced by the stenotic valve on the balloons' silhouette is seen. **A,** Anteroposterior view and **B,** lateral view. After full inflation of both balloons the fused commissures are cracked and the waist on the balloon silhouette has disappeared (**C,** anteroposterior view and **D,** lateral view).

HEMODYNAMIC CONSEQUENCES OF PDBV

Hemodynamically successful PDBV was achieved in all but one patient in the reported series of our first 60 cases (Table 18-1).[16] The mean mitral valve gradient decreased, cardiac output increased, effective valve area increased, mean pulmonary artery pressure decreased, and mean left atrial pressure decreased significantly (Fig. 18-6). In noncalcified or minimally calcified valves that are still very pliable with no severe involvement of the subvalvular structures, the hemodynamic response, as well as the echocardiographic results, after PDBV can be rather spectacular (Fig. 18-7). As we previously reported,[16] although the procedure seems effective even in heavily calcified valves with subvalvular involvement the results obtained, nevertheless, are suboptimal (Table 18-1), and therefore those patients should probably be considered better surgical candidates unless a major contraindication to surgery exists.

The double balloon technique geometrically approaches the shape of the mitral annulus configuration. The predilection of the two balloons to fit into the commissure may be a rea-

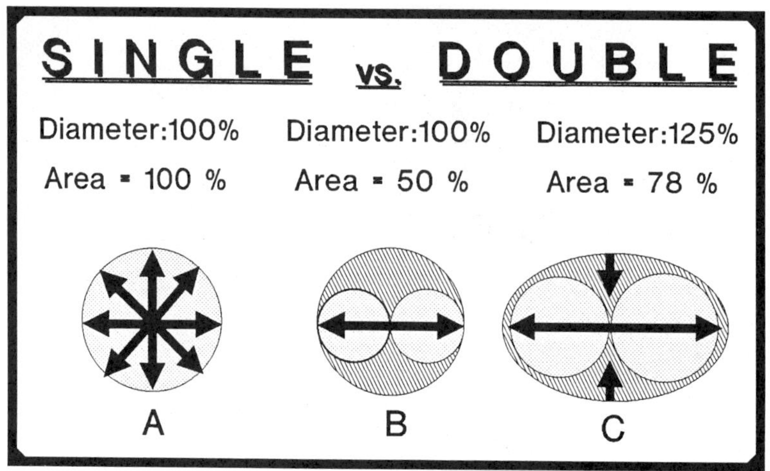

Fig. 18-5. For a given cross-sectional diameter a single circle generated from this diameter will have a 50% larger surface area **(A).** However, if from the same diameter one generates two circles using each radius as the diameter for each of the new circles, the total cross-sectional diameter remains unchanged while the total area generated by the sum of the two new circles is 50% smaller than the original circle **(B).** This allows one to oversize the longitudinal diameter of this stretchable ring as much as 125% and it still would not occupy the total inner area of the original ring **(C).**

son for the greater efficiency of this technique in opening the stenotic valve.

PROCEDURE TOLERANCE AND COMPLICATIONS

The procedure is usually very well tolerated by the patient under local anesthesia. Using the double balloon technique allows hemodynamic support during balloon inflations in a sufficient manner to make the patient feel only some light-headedness, since the systemic arterial blood pressure is commonly above 80 mm Hg and blood flow has been shown to occur around the inflated balloons by color flow Doppler analysis during balloon inflation (Fig. 18-8), unless the mitral valve area is less than 0.5 cm^2, in which case the systemic blood pressure may drop more during balloon catheter passage or inflation across the valve.

Several major complications can be associated with PDBV, including the creation of acute severe mitral insufficiency by tearing the mitral valve leaflet or any of its delicate structures. However, in our experience of over 90 cases only one young postpartum patient suffered a large tear of the anterior leaflet at the point of the fused anterior commissure. The severe acute mitral regurgitation required emergency surgery to repair it (Fig. 18-9). In addition a lesser degree of mitral regurgitation appeared or worsened in 20% of our patients, less than a grade III/IV, that required no surgical intervention.

About 10% of patients had preexisting mitral insufficiency that improved or disappeared with PDBV.

We experienced two procedure-related

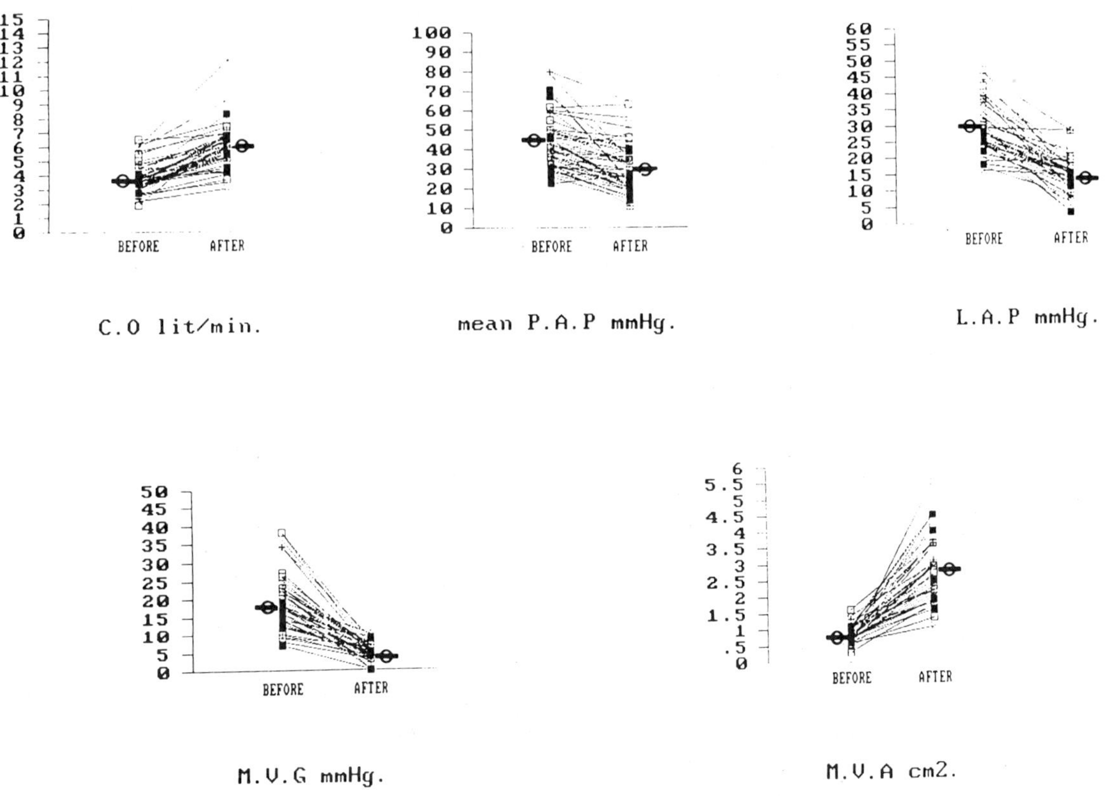

Fig. 18-6. Hemodynamic changes before and after PDBV.

deaths, both secondary to large left ventricular perforations induced by the dilatation balloon catheters. Both patients were over 60 years of age and one had a heavily infiltrated myocardium with myeloma tumor.

A major potential risk of PDBV for patients who are in atrial fibrillation, who have large left atrial cavities, and who have calcific mitral valves is the mobilization of a clot during the procedure, resulting in a catastrophic cerebrovascular embolic accident. In our experience we have had no major cerebrovascular accidents, although three of our patients suffered mild transient ischemic attacks. In one case this appeared 18 hours after the valvulotomy and the other occurred during the procedure. All resolved in less than 12 hours leaving no neurologic deficits. Surprisingly all three patients were in normal sinus rhythm and fully anticoagulated during the procedure. No embolic phenomena were detected in any of the patients who were in atrial fibrillation during the procedure.

A small left-to-right shunt developed at the atrial septostomy level in 12% of patients, and in only one patient the oximetric study revealed a shunt of 1}:1.6, which 6 weeks later was nondetectable by Doppler studies. No patients developed conduction abnormalities.

Four patients developed a traumatic pericardial effusion during the attempt to perform the transseptal approach and the procedure was aborted, but two patients came back a week later and underwent uneventful PDBV of their mitral valve.

Atrial and ventricular arrhythmias induced by catheters, wires, and balloon-dilating catheters were common in all patients, but usually were well tolerated.

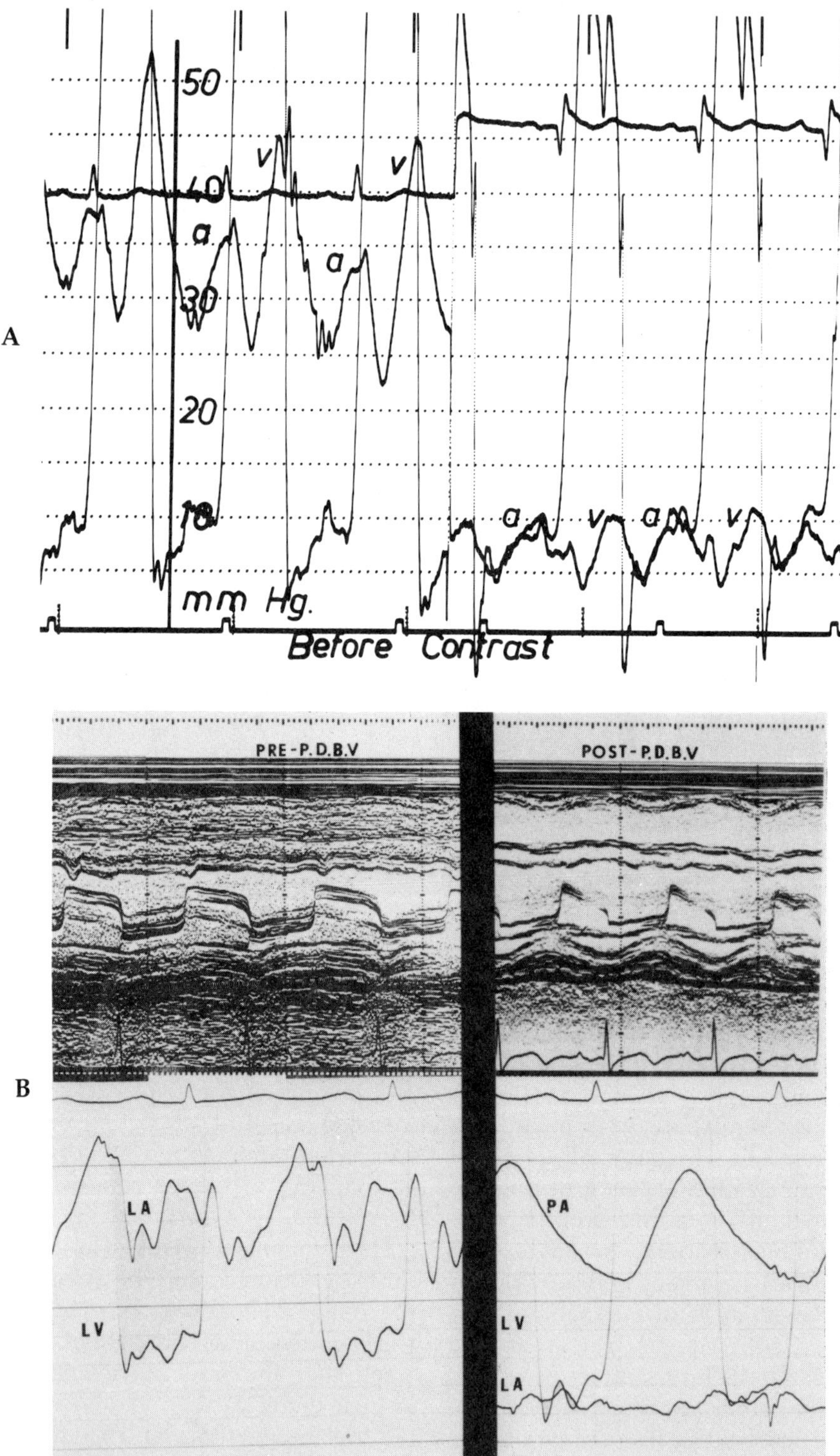

Fig. 18-7. Typical examples of the mitral valve gradient before **(A)** and after **(B)** PDBV M-mode echocardiographic changes after valvotomy and correlation with the hemodynamic changes.

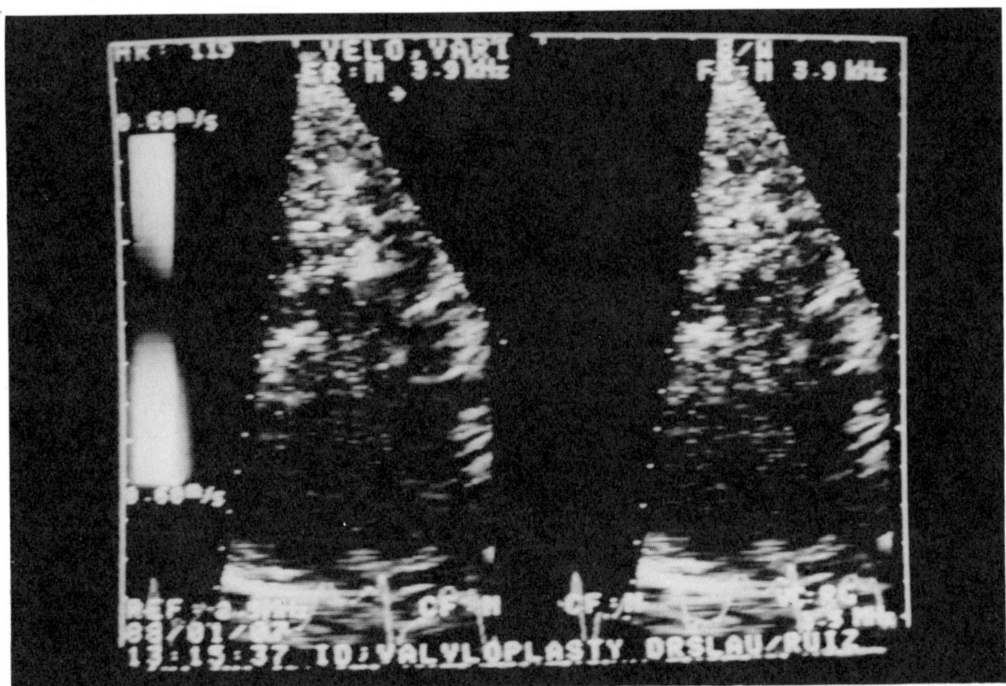

Fig. 18-8. Color flow Doppler mapping of the mitral valve during full inflation of both dilatation balloons across the stenotic valve showing blood flow around the inflated balloons.

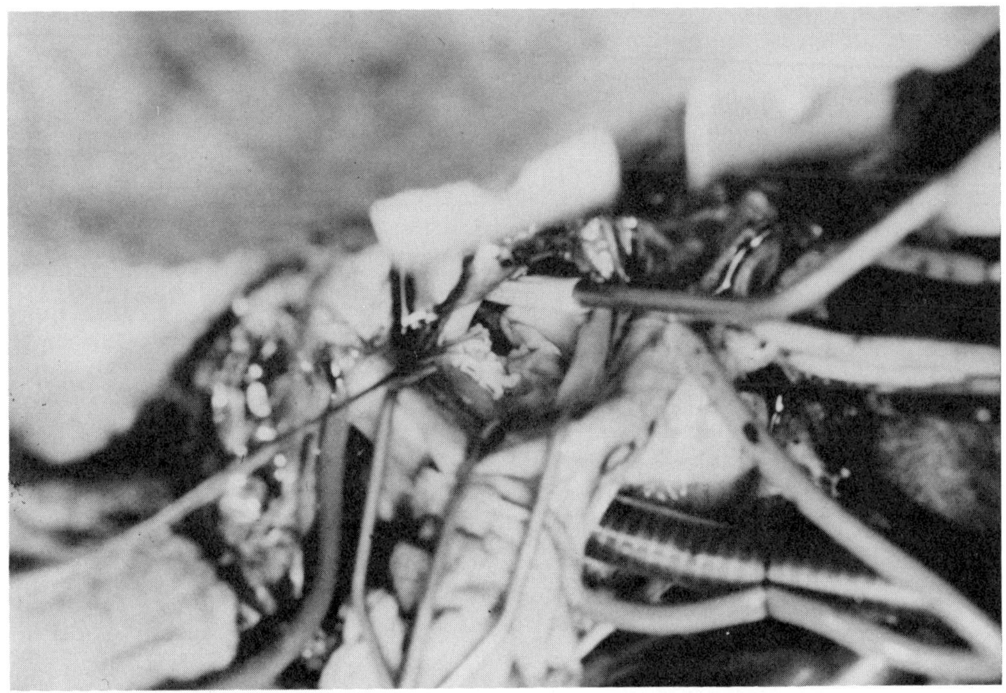

Fig. 18-9. Repaired anterior mitral valve leaflet after it was torn by one of the balloon valvotomy catheters.

CLINICAL IMPLICATIONS

A major advantage of PDBV over surgical commissurotomy is that restenosis can possibly be redilated at a later time, as long as mitral insufficiency is not a major hemodynamic complication. The restenosis rate associated with PDBV cannot yet be assessed because the procedure is so new. While significant rates of restenosis may occur after PDBV, we suspect they will probably be lower than rates seen with the single balloon technique, or will most likely develop at a later stage.

Economically important is the fact that the hospital cost associated with PDBV is much lower than with surgical alternatives; however, the cost-effectiveness on a long-term basis still needs to be determined. The patient's hospital stay is shorter, and certainly the convalescent period before being able to return to work should also be much shorter. The economic advantages of PDBV may be especially significant in countries where this kind of disease is common.

We believe that PDBV is an effective, palliative procedure for severe mitral stenosis, that the long-term results should not differ much from those found in patients who undergo closed surgical commissurotomies, and that the technique can be safely performed by professionals familiar with transseptal cardiac catheterization. This procedure requires the coordinated efforts of the catheterization laboratory, noninvasive cardiology, and cardiovascular surgery teams. It is a special technique that under no circumstance should be considered to be an extension of PTCA.

Appendix A Equipment List

The following is a list of the equipment that we currently use to perform PDBV, as well as the manufacturers of such equipment.

7F and 8F Hemaquet sheaths (USCI division, C.R. Bard Inc., Billerica, Mass.)

8F thermodilution Swan-Ganz catheter (American-Edwards, Santa Ana, Calif.)

7F Pigtail catheter (Cordis, Miami, Fla.)

Modified Brockenbrough transseptal needle (Cook Co., Bloomington, Ind.)

8F Mullins' transseptal sheath (USCI division, C.R. Bard Inc. Billerica, Mass.)

160 cm × 0.032-inch Teflon-coated wire (Cook Co., Bloomington, Ind.)

260 cm × 0.038-inch tapered cord exchange wire (Med-Rad Co., Pittsburgh, Pa.)

8F Berman wedge catheter (Arrow International Inc., Reading, Pa.)

7F balloon dilatation catheter for the septostomy with a 3 cm × 8 mm balloon (Meditech Inc., Watertown, Mass.)

9F balloon dilatation catheters with 5.5 cm × 15, 18 or 20 mm balloon (Mansfield Scientific Inc., Mansfield, Mass.)

REFERENCES

1. Roberts, W.C.: Morphologic features of the normal and abnormal mitral valve, Am. J. Cardiol. **51**:100s, 1983.
2. Gordis, L.: The virtual disappearance of rheumatic fever in the United States: lessons in the rise and fall of disease. T. Duckett Jones Memorial Lecture, Circulation **72**:1155, 1985.
3. Markowitz, M.: Observations on the epidemiology and preventability of rheumatic fever in developing countries, Clin. Ther. **4**:240, 1981.
4. Community control of rheumatic heart disease in developing countries. 1. A major health problem, W.H.O. Chron. **34**:336, 1980.
5. Inoue, K., Owani, T., Nakamura, T., Kitamura, T., and Miyamoto, N.: Clinical application of transvenous mitral commissurotomy by a new balloon catheter, J. Thorac. Cardiovasc. Surg. **87**:394, 1984.
6. Lock, J.E., Khalilullah, M., Shrivasta, S., Bahl, V., and Keane, J.F.: Percutaneous catheter commissurotomy in rheumatic mitral stenosis, N. Engl. J. Med. **313**:1515, 1985.
7. Babic, U.U., Pejcic, P., Djurisic, Z., Vucinic, M., and Grujicic, S.M.: Percutaneous transarterial balloon valvuloplasty for mitral stenosis, Am. J. Cardiol. **57**:1101, 1986.
8. Zaibag, M.A., Kasab, S.A., Ribeiro, P.A., and Fagih, M.R.: Percutaneous double balloon mitral valvotomy for rheumatic mitral valve stenosis, Lancet **1**:757, 1986.
9. Palacios, I., Block, P.C., Brandi, S., Blanco, P., Casal, H., Pulido, J.I., Munoz, S., D'Empaire, G., Ortega, M.A., Jacobs, M., and Vlahakes, G.: Percutaneous balloon valvotomy for patients with severe mitral stenosis, Circulation **75**:778, 1986.
10. McKay, R.G., Lock, J.E., Safian, R.D., Come, P.C., Diver, D.J., Baim, D.S., Warren, S.E., Mandell, V.E., Royal, H.D., and Grossman, W.: Balloon dilatation of mitral stenosis in adult patients: postmortem and percutaneous mitral valvuloplasty studies, J. Am. Coll. Cardiol. **9**:723, 1987.
11. Mullins, C.E.: Perforation of the left ventricle induced by the guidewire and the balloon dilatation catheter with the wires positioned in the descending aorta. Personal communication.
12. John, S., Bashi, V.V., Jairaj, P.S., Muralidharan, S., Ravikumar, E., Rajarajeswari, T., Krishnaswami, S., Sukumar, I.P., and Rao, P.S.S.: Close mitral valvotomy: early results and long-term follow-up of 3724 consecutive patients, Circulation **68**:891, 1983.
13. Nathaniels, E.K., Mencure, A.C., and Scanell, J.G.: A fifteen year follow up study of closed mitral valvuloplasty, Ann. Thorac. Surg. **10**:27, 1970.
14. Ellis, L.B., Singh, J.B., Morales, D.D., and Harken, D.E.: Fifteen-to-twenty year study of one thousand patients undergoing closed mitral valvuloplasty, Circulation **48**:357, 1973.
15. Block, P.C., Palacios, I.F., Jacobs, M., and Fallon, J.: The mechanism of successful mitral valvotomy in humans, Am. J. Cardiol. **59**:178, 1987.
16. Ruiz, C.E., Lau, F.Y.K.: Percutaneous double balloon valvotomy in sixty consecutive patients with severe mitral stenosis, Submitted for publication.

Chapter 19

Percutaneous Balloon Mitral Valvuloplasty in 156 Patients
A French Cooperative Study

Alec Vahanian, MD
Jérome Petit, MD
Jean Pierre Bassand, MD
Jacques Boschat, MD
Antoine Gommeaux, MD
Frédéric Collet, MD
Yves Chabrillat, MD
Jacques Berland, MD
Gerard Drobinski, MD
Michel E. Bertrand, MD

Over the last 5 years, balloon dilatation treatment has appeared as a rapidly evolving technology. After the growing success of coronary angioplasty, it was natural that an attempt should be made to dilate stenotic cardiac valves. Thus catheter balloon valvuloplasty was applied to congenital pulmonary stenoses, coarctation of the aorta, and aortic and mitral valve stenoses. The technique of percutaneous mitral valvuloplasty through a transseptal approach was described by Inoue and associates in 1984.[1] Lock and colleagues[2] and Kveselis and associates[3] applied the technique to adolescents with critical mitral stenosis, while Zaibag,[4] McKay,[5,6] Palacios,[7,8] and Vahanian,[9] and their co-workers extended the initial indications to older patients. In 1986 a working group of the French Cardiac Society decided to open a National Registry to collect data concerning this technique, which was performed in the 10 medical centers of France listed in Appendix A. This study reports the results of percutaneous mitral valvuloplasty in 156 patients with mitral stenosis.

MATERIAL AND METHODS

The patient population included 156 patients who had symptomatic mitral stenosis. However, mitral valvuloplasty was performed in only 133 patients, since 23 attempts using other procedures were unsuccessful or complicated before valvuloplasty was initiated. The failures resulted mainly from the impossibility of crossing the septum (3 patients) or the mitral valve (12 patients). Six patients developed a hemopericardium and two patients had cerebral gas embolism without clinical consequences.

Thus the valvuloplasty was performed in 133 patients (102 women and 31 men) with a mean age 40 ± 15 years (range 9 to 79 years). Thirty-four patients were in New York Heart Association (NYHA) Class II, 90 patients in Class III, and 9 patients in Class IV. Ninety-one patients were in normal sinus rhythm and 42 patients had atrial fibrillation. Eleven patients had a history of peripheral arterial embolism. All patients underwent right-sided and left-sided heart catheterization, measurement of cardiac output, and left cineventriculography for detection of mitral regurgitation, which was graded qualitatively from grades 1+ to 4+. In 20 patients, the decision to perform valvuloplasty was related to surgical contraindications (age or poor general physical condition in eight patients, extracardiac disease in seven patients, and refusal of surgery in five patients).

PROCEDURE

Transseptal left-sided heart catheterization was performed from the right common femoral veins with an 8F Mullins transseptal sheath and Brockenbrough needle. Anticoagulation with heparin was achieved in each case. Single balloon valvuloplasty was done in 25 patients. Sixteen of these patients were treated using a Trefoil balloon catheter. In two patients, the balloon diameter was less than 20 mm in diameter. Most often (108 patients), valvuloplasty was done with two balloons; the Trefoil balloon catheter plus a conventional balloon catheter was used in 57 patients. After valvuloplasty the balloons were removed and hemodynamic measurements and left ventricular cineangiography were repeated. Right-sided heart oximetry was performed to detect significant left-to-right shunt in most of the patients. The duration of the procedure averaged 133 ± 45 minutes (a range of 70 to 315 minutes).

RESULTS

Before valvuloplasty was performed the mitral valve gradient was 16 ± 8 mm Hg and the cardiac index was 2.7 ± 0.6 L/min/m^2. The pulmonary capillary wedge pressure was 21 ± 12 mm Hg. The mitral valve area was calculated from hemodynamic measurements using the Gorlin's formula[11] and was 1.0 ± 0.2 cm^2. Twenty-nine patients had grade 1+ mitral regurgitation and three patients had grade 2+.

MODIFICATIONS INDUCED BY VALVULOPLASTY

Table 19-1 and Fig. 19-1 list the changes in hemodynamic variables produced by percutaneous mitral valvuloplasty. The average mitral valve gradient decreased from 16 ± 8 mm Hg to 6 ± 2 mm Hg (p <0.01). Pulmonary capillary wedge pressure decreased from 21 ± 12 mm Hg to 10 ± 6 mm Hg (p <0.01). Cardiac index was slightly but significantly increased from 2.7 to 2.9 L/min/m^2.

A significant increase of mitral valve area was observed (from 1 ± 0.2 to 2.0 ± 0.4 cm^2)

Table 19-1 Hemodynamic Variables Before and After Valvuloplasty

	Before Valvuloplasty	*After Valvuloplasty*
PCWP (mm Hg)	21 ± 12	10 ± 6*
Cardiac index (L/min/m^2)	2.7 ± 0.6	2.9 ± 0.6†
Mitral valve gradient (mm Hg)	16 ± 8	6 ± 2*
Mitral valve area (cm^2) (Hemod)	1.0 ± 0.2	2.0 ± 0.4*
Mitral valve area (cm^2) (Echo)	1.04 ± 0.23	1.9 ± 0.4*

*p <0.01.
†p <0.05.
PCWP, Pulmonary capillary wedge pressure; Hemod, evaluation of the valve area with Gorlin's formula; Echo, evaluation with echo Doppler.

(p <0.01). Echo Doppler (110 patients) by Henry and co-workers[12] demonstrated an increase of the same magnitude (from 1.04 ± 0.23 cm^2 to 1.9 ± 0.4 cm^2). Of the 29 patients with grade 1+ mitral regurgitation before valvuloplasty, there was no change in 24 patients, but the severity of mitral regurgitation increased from grade 1+ to grade 2+ in 2 patients and up to grade 3+ in 3 patients. Sixteen of 74 patients without mitral regurgitation had grade 1+ mitral regurgitation after the procedure (Fig. 19-2). Twenty-one patients (16%) had faintings or syncope during the procedure. After the procedure, 13 patients (10%) had a left-to-right shunt and in 5 patients the ratio of pulmonary output to systemic output was greater than 1.5.

COMPLICATIONS DURING THE PROCEDURE

There was no patient mortality before discharge from the hospital. Transient and reversible stroke occurred in four patients (3%), two patients had hemopericardium, and 1 patient (0.7%) had local hematoma at the groin needing surgical repair.

COMMENTS

These series are taken from the largest in the literature: Zaibag and associates,[4] 9 patients; Palacios and co-workers,[7,8] 35 patients and McKay and associates,[5,6] 18 patients. The French percutaneous transluminal coronary angioplasty (PTCA) registry demonstrates that percutaneous mitral valvuloplasty produces significant hemodynamic improvement. However, it should be noted that the mitral valve area after valvuloplasty was only 2 cm^2, a value which is usually considered the limit of severe mitral stenosis. Furthermore, after the procedure 18 patients had a valve area less than 1.5 cm^2; these hemodynamic changes are in agreement with previous reports. However, the modesty of the mitral valve area enlargement suggests that this procedure should be considered a palliative technique. Although the long-term follow-up results are unknown, it would be logical to admit that it could be compared with the results obtained using surgical closed-chest mitral commissurotomy.[13-15] The postmortem studies of McKay,[6] Kaplan,[16] and Reifart,[17] and their associates suggest that the increased valve area obtained by balloon dilation resulted from a separation of fused commis-

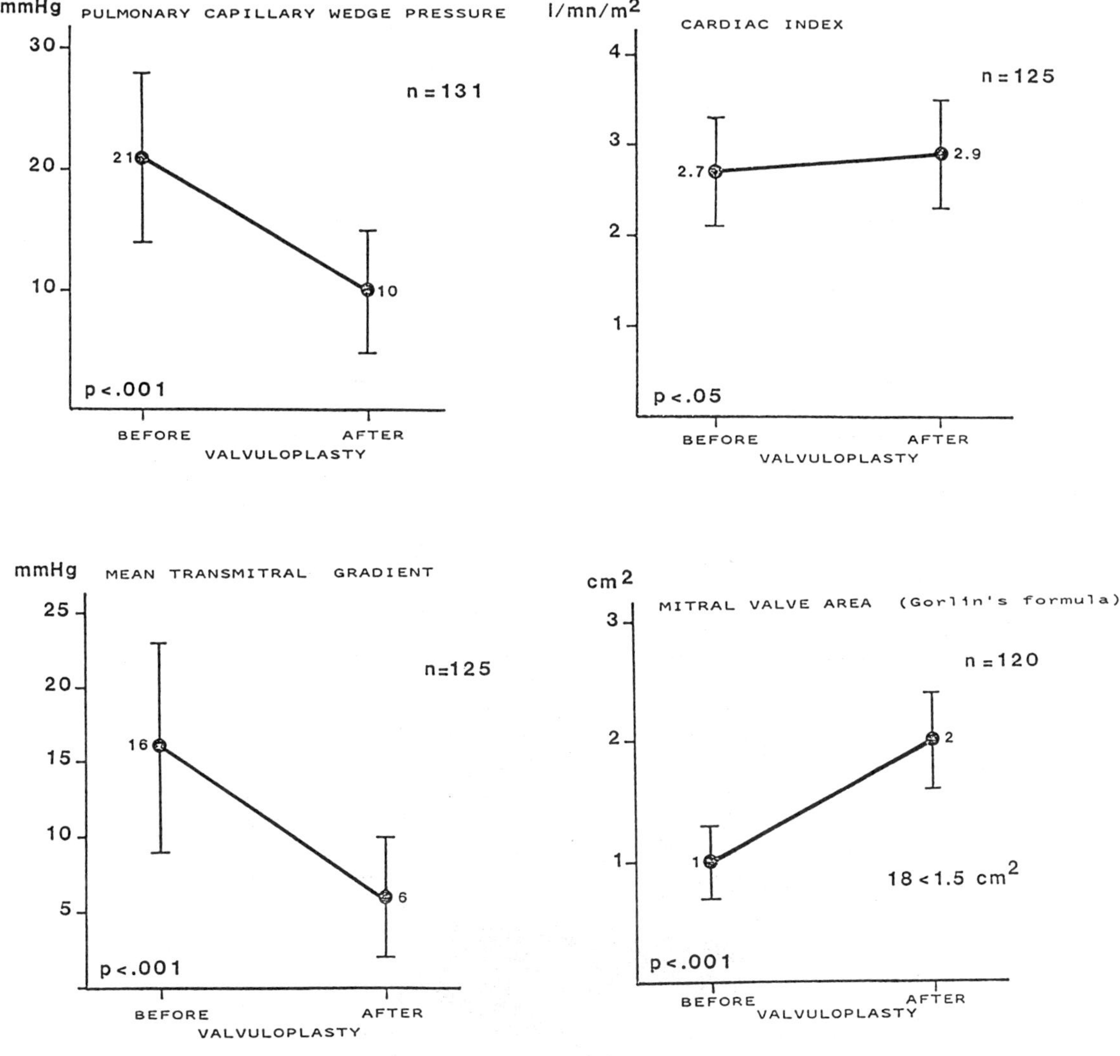

Fig. 19-1. Changes in hemodynamic variables produced by percutaneous mitral valvuloplasty.

sures and fracture of nodular calcium within the valve leaflets. Today the double balloon technique is the most commonly used and allows a larger dilation of the orifice. Moreover, the combination of Trefoil and conventional balloons affords a better stability in the orifice. An increasing or a severe new mitral regurgitation is rarely observed, but it is recommended that patients with previous mild mitral regurgitation should not be considered for the double balloon procedure. In our series, most of the complications are related to the left-sided heart transseptal catheterization. Therefore, only well-skilled teams should perform this technique and it should be noted that only four teams in our series had, before their attempt at valvuloplasty, expert experience with transseptal catheterization technique.

Our series was obtained with a certain number of patients coming from various countries. In France the incidence of rheumatic disease is so low that only a small number of patients could be treated by percutane-

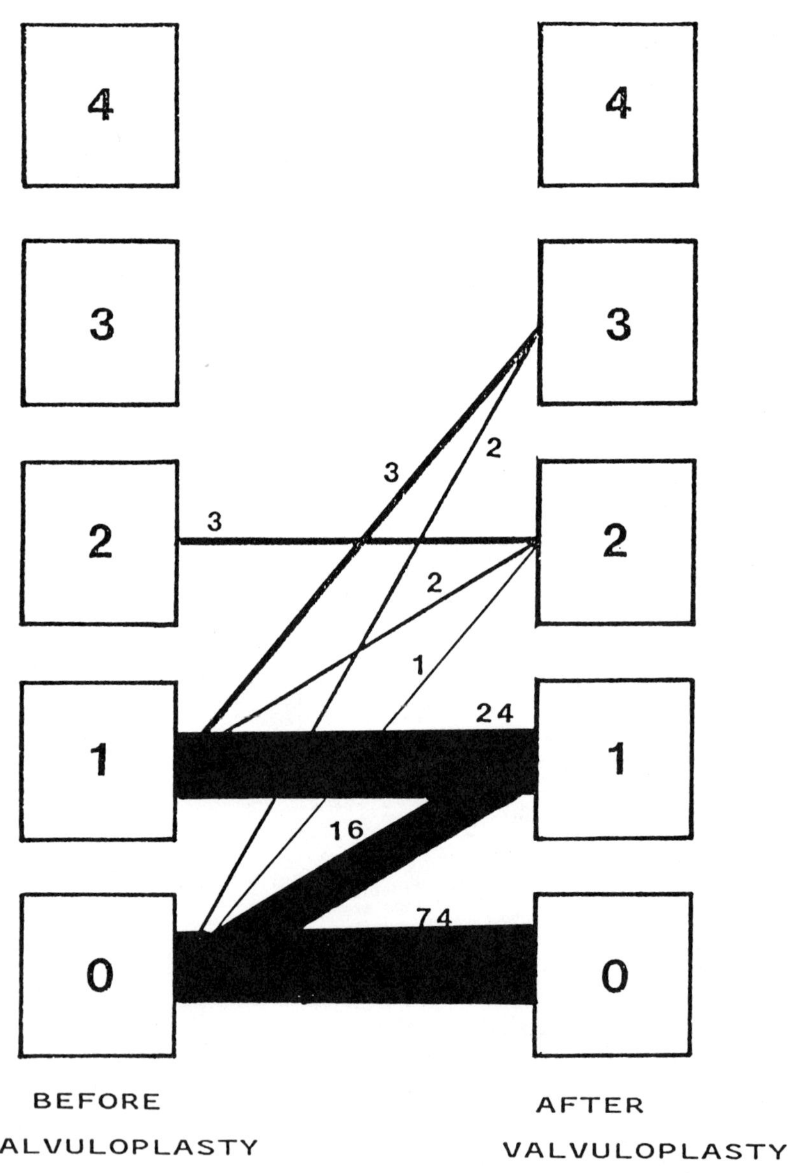

Fig. 19-2. Mitral regurgitation before and after valvuloplasty.

ous balloon mitral valvuloplasty. However, in several countries, especially Africa and India, rheumatic valvular diseases are prevalent and in these countries the percutaneous balloon mitral valvuloplasty technique will certainly be useful. The encouraging short-term results of this study suggest that this technique may become one of the treatments of choice in these countries.

Appendix A. Ten French Medical Centers Where Patients Were Enrolled

Besançon: Dr. Bassand

Brest: Dr. Boschat

Caen: Dr. Gommeau

Lille: Dr. Bertrand

Marseille (2 centers): Dr. Collet and Dr. Chabrillat

Rouen: Dr. Berland

Paris (3 centers): Drs. Vahanian, Petit, Drobinski

REFERENCES

1. Inoue, K., Owaki, T., Nakamura, T., Kitamura, F., and Miyamoto, N.: Clinical application of transvenous mitral commissurotomy by a new balloon catheter, J. Thorac. Cardiovasc. Surg. **87**:394-402, 1984.
2. Lock, J.E., Khalilollah, M., Shrivastava, S., Bahl, V., and Keane, J.F.: Percutaneous catheter commissurotomy in rheumatic mitral stenosis, N. Engl. J. Med. **313**:1515-1518, 1985.
3. Kveselis, D.A., Rocchini, A.P., Beekman, R., Snider, A.R., Crowley, D., MacDonald, D., et al.: Balloon angioplasty for congenital and rheumatic mitral stenosis, Am. J. Cardiol. **57**:348-350, 1986.
4. Zaibag, M.A., Alkasab, S., Ribeiro, P.A., and Al Fagih, M.R.: Pércutaneous double balloon mitral valvulotomy for rheumatic mitral valve stenosis, Lancet **2**:757-761, 1986.
5. McKay, R.G., Lock, J.E., Safian, R.D., Mandell, V.S., Baim, P.S., Diver, D.J., Royal, H.R., Come, P.C., and Grossman, W.: Percutaneous balloon valvuloplasty in adult patients with critical mitral stenosis (abstract), Circulation **74** (Suppl. 2):II-209, 1986.
6. MacKay, R.G., Lock, J.E., Keane, J.F., Safian, R.D., Ardesty, J.M., and Grossman, W.: Percutaneous mitral valvuloplasty in an adult patient with calcific rheumatic mitral lesions, J. Am. Coll. Cardiol. **7**:1410-1415, 1986.
7. Palacios, I.F., Lock, J.E., Keane, J.F., and Block, P.C.: Percutaneous transvenous balloon valvotomy in a patient with severe calcific mitral stenosis, J. Am. Coll. Cardiol. **7**:1416-1419, 1986.
8. Palacios, I., Block, P., Brandi, S., Blanco, P., Casal, H., Pulido, J.I., Munoz, S., D'Empaire, G., Ortega, M.A., Jacobs, M., and Vlahakes, G.: Percutaneous balloon valvotomy for patients with severe mitral stenosis, Circulation **75**:778-784, 1987.
9. Vahanian, A., Slama, M., Cormier, B., Michel, P.L., Savier, C.H., and Acar, J.: Valvuloplastie mitrale percutanée chez l'adulte, Arch. Mal. Coeur **79**:1896-1902, 1986.
10. Babic, U., Pejcic, P., Durisc, Z., Vucinic, I., and Grujucici, S.: Percutaneous transarterial balloon valvuloplasty for mitral valve stenosis, Am. J. Cardiol. **57**:1101-1104, 1986.
11. Gorlin, R., and Gorlin, G.: Hydraulic formula for calculation of area of stenotic mitral valve, other cardiac valves and central circulatory shunts, Am. Heart J. **41**:1-29, 1951.
12. Henry, W.L., Griffith, J.M., Michablis, L.L., and Epstein, S.: Measurement of mitral orifice area in patients with mitral valve disease by real time, two dimensional echocardiography, Circulation **51**: 827-831, 1975
13. John, S., Bashi, V.V., Jairaj, P.S., Muralidharan, S., Ravikumuar, E., Rajarjeswari, T., Sukumar, I.P., and Sundar Mao, P.S.S.: Closed mitral valvotomy: early results and long term follow up of 3274 consecutive patients, Circulation **68**:891-896, 1983.
14. Breyer, H.R., Mills, A.S., Hudspeth, S.A., Johnston, R.F., Watts, E.L., Nomeir, M.A., and Cordell, R.A.: Open mitral commissurotomy: long term results with echocardiographic correlation, J. Cardiovasc. Surg. **26**:46-52, 1985.
15. Housman, L.B., Bonchek, L., Lambert, L., Grunkemeier, G., and Starr, A.: Prognosis of patients after open mitral commissurotomy: actuarial analysis of late results in 100 patients, J. Thorac. Cardiovasc. Surg. **73**:742-745, 1977.
16. Kaplan, J., Isner, J., Karas, R., Halaburka, K.R., Konstan, M.A., Hougen, T.J., Cleveland,

R.J., and Salem, D.N.: In vitro analysis of mechanisms of balloon valvuloplasty of stenotic mitral valves, Am. J. Cardiol. **59**:318-324, 1987.

17. Reifart, N., Nowak, B., Baykut, D., Bussman, W.D., and Kaltenbach, M.: Experimental mitral valvuloplasty of fibrotic and calcified valves with balloon catheter (abstract), J. Am. Coll. Cardiol. **5**:448, 1985.

Chapter 20

Aortic Valvuloplasty: Techniques, Results, and Perspectives

The Rouen Experience

Alain Cribier, MD
B. Letac, MD

We attempted for the first time percutaneous transluminal aortic valvuloplasty (PTAV) for severe aortic stenosis in adult patients in September 1985, after successful balloon dilatation had been reported in pulmonic and aortic valve stenosis[1-3] and in rheumatic mitral stenosis.[4] At the beginning, PTAV was done as an ultimate lifesaving procedure in patients with severe life-threatening aortic stenosis for whom valve replacement was definitely rejected because of an unacceptably high surgical risk owing to both old age and major myocardial deterioration.[5] Improvement in valve opening was demonstrated by the decrease in the left ventricular–aortic pressure gradient and by the increase in calculated aortic valve area. The good hemodynamic results were later confirmed by a dramatically rapid and lasting clinical improvement in these critically ill patients. Subsequently, we reported the results of PTAV in our first large series of 92 elderly patients,[6] mean age of 75 years, who were very ill (73% in New York Heart Association [NYHA] Classes III and IV) including 15 patients who were considered to be moribund at the time of the procedure. These patients either had a clearly high surgical risk or had a definite contraindication for valve replacement. Whereas a mortality of 44 to 60% per year has been reported in natural history studies of similar patients,[7-9] the procedure performed in the hospital had a mortality of only 3% in our series of patients who had PTAV. Only eight additional patients died in the 18 weeks' follow-up, during which time most patients continued to show sustained dramatic improvement.

Other centers have reported their experience with PTAV, confirming our initial results.[10-14] We were thus encouraged to routinely offer valvuloplasty to nonsurgical or high surgical risk adult patients with severe aortic stenosis. The procedure has likewise gained wide acceptance and despite the recent development of this investigational technique, there are now over 700 cases in the French Registry (with 250 from our center, Centre Hospitalier Régional & Universitaire de Rouen), and it can be estimated that 2000 cases have probably been performed worldwide.

Because of the good results in very ill, elderly, high surgical risk patients, we recently have begun to evaluate the possibility of extending the indications of PTAV to younger patients with increased surgical risk, as well as to patients who were good surgical candidates but who refused surgery or who wanted to defer surgery in favor of PTAV. The increase in aortic valve area obtained was higher and the complication rate was lower in this group of younger patients. It is still too early, however, to determine the long-term effects and restenosis rate in these patients. Clearly the indications for this new and rapidly evolving technique have not yet been firmly established.

IMMEDIATE RESULTS AND EVOLUTION OF THE TECHNIQUE

Our objective in performing percutaneous transluminal aortic valvuloplasty is to obtain the largest possible aortic valve area. In our series of 218 patients we were able to achieve an increase in aortic valve area from 0.52 cm^2 to 0.93 cm^2. This was associated with a decrease in the peak-to-peak gradient from 72 to 29 mm Hg (Fig. 20-1).

It is important to point out that through our experience in performing aortic valvuloplasty, and by learning more about the mechanism of dilatation, there has been a change in our goals and a continued evolution in technique. When we first started performing PTAVs we successively inflated several balloons of increasing size (15 mm, 18 mm, and then 20 mm diameter) across the aortic valve until a good result was achieved. At that time we

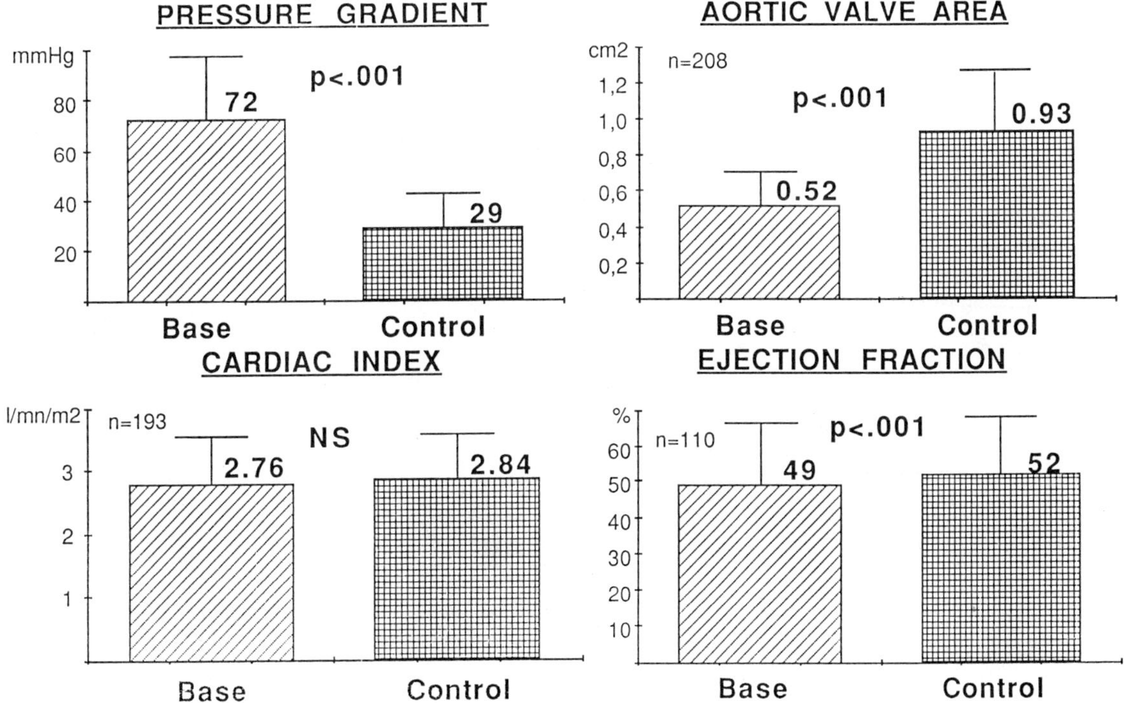

Fig. 20-1. Baseline and immediate post-PTAV hemodynamic results in 218 patients.

thought that a reduction of the peak transvalvular gradient to less than 40 mm Hg was a good result. However, we soon realized that the reduction in gradient alone could not be considered the determinant of a good result. Since the gradient across the valve is dependent on ventricular loading and contractility, as well as on systemic arterial resistance, we subsequently defined the quality of the result on the basis of the increase in calculated aortic valve area. This was important to us when evaluating our early experience with PTAV, because by simply determining the systolic gradient we were led to overestimate the quality of the result, when indeed, despite a marked decrease in the gradient, the patient still had a pronounced degree of aortic stenosis.

We have become more persistent in our attempts to increase the valve area as we have learned more about the mechanism of action of the dilating balloon.[10,15] The mechanisms of balloon valvuloplasty include the separation of fused commissures, the fracture of calcific nodular deposits in the valve leaflets, and to a limited degree stretching of the valve cusps (Fig. 20-2). Postmortem studies that we have done have shown that the 20 mm diameter balloon (with an effective dilating area of 3.14 cm^2) does not always fully open the valve leaflets of the aortic valve, although in some cases full valve opening is obtained. In the presence of a large aortic annulus the use of two balloons side by side or the use of a larger balloon size (23 mm or even 25 mm) may be required. In approximately 25% of our last 58 patients, the increase in the aortic valve area after dilatation with the 20 mm diameter balloon was insufficient. We therefore continued the procedure by using either the double balloon technique (15 mm + 18 mm or 15 mm + 20 mm, for a total cross-section of 4.3 cm^2 or 4.9 cm^2, respectively) or more frequently a single 23 mm diameter balloon (cross-section of 4.2 cm^2) (Figs. 20-3 and 20-4). By using larger diameters we were able to obtain a final valve area at or above 0.9 cm^2 in 62% of these last 58 patients, and above 1 cm^2 in 31%. By comparison, the final valve area was equal to or greater than 0.9 cm^2 in only 39% of our previous cases. In fifty-six of our last 58 cases there was an increase in valve area of 75% or more. In comparison, this percentage was reached in only 42% of our previous cases. Poor results (less than 50% increase in valve area) were observed in 21% of our last 58 patients and in 38% of our previous cases (Fig. 20-5). Although we have found the larger diameters useful, we still recommend a

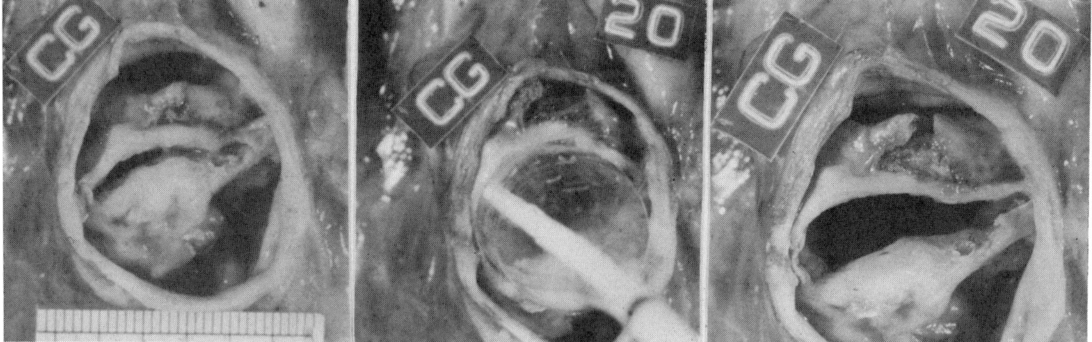

Fig. 20-2. Postmortem balloon dilatation (20 mm size) of a severely stenosed bicuspid aortic valve. *Left panel,* Before balloon inflation, note the massively calcified leaflets and fusion of the commissures. *Middle panel,* Inflation of the 20 mm balloon. *Right panel,* After inflation there is a full opening of the commissures and fracture of the calcified plaque resulting in marked enlargement of the aortic valve orifice.

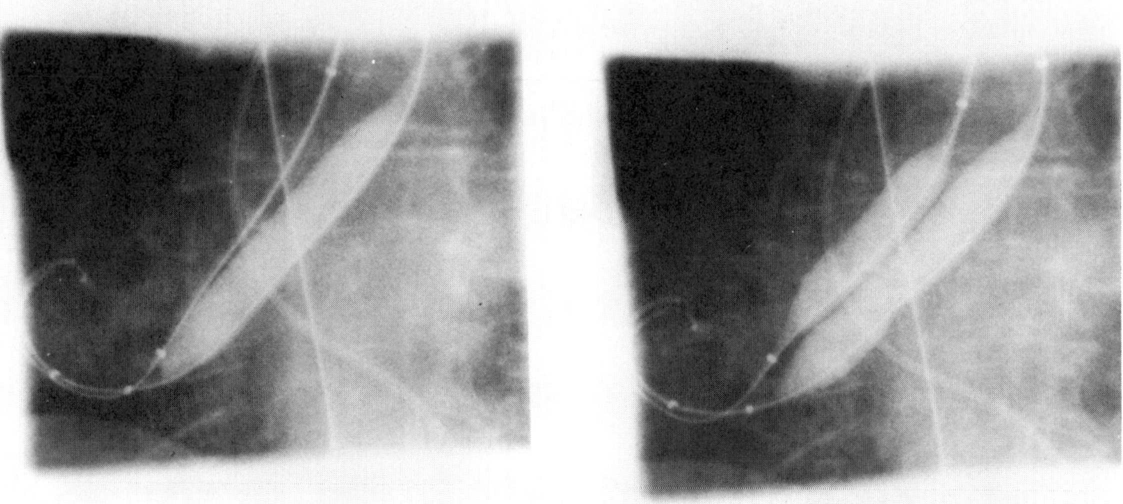

Fig. 20-3. After insufficient results with 20 mm balloon inflations, two balloon catheters (15 mm and 20 mm) were simultaneously inflated side by side.

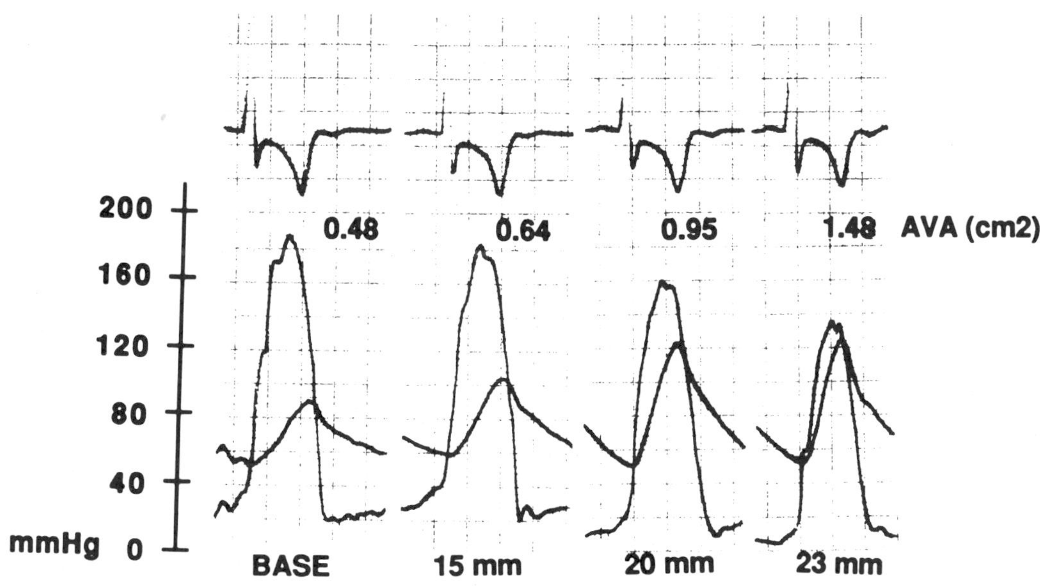

Fig. 20-4. Improvement in peak-to-peak transvalvular gradient and aortic valve area following valvuloplasty using balloons of 15 mm, 20 mm, and finally 23 mm diameter. Note that the gradient decreased from 120 to 40 mm Hg after using the 20 mm balloon. A further decrease to 10 mm Hg was obtained after inflating the 23 mm balloon. Note also the further gain of 50% in the valve area after inflation of the 23 mm balloon (0.95 to 1.48 cm^2).

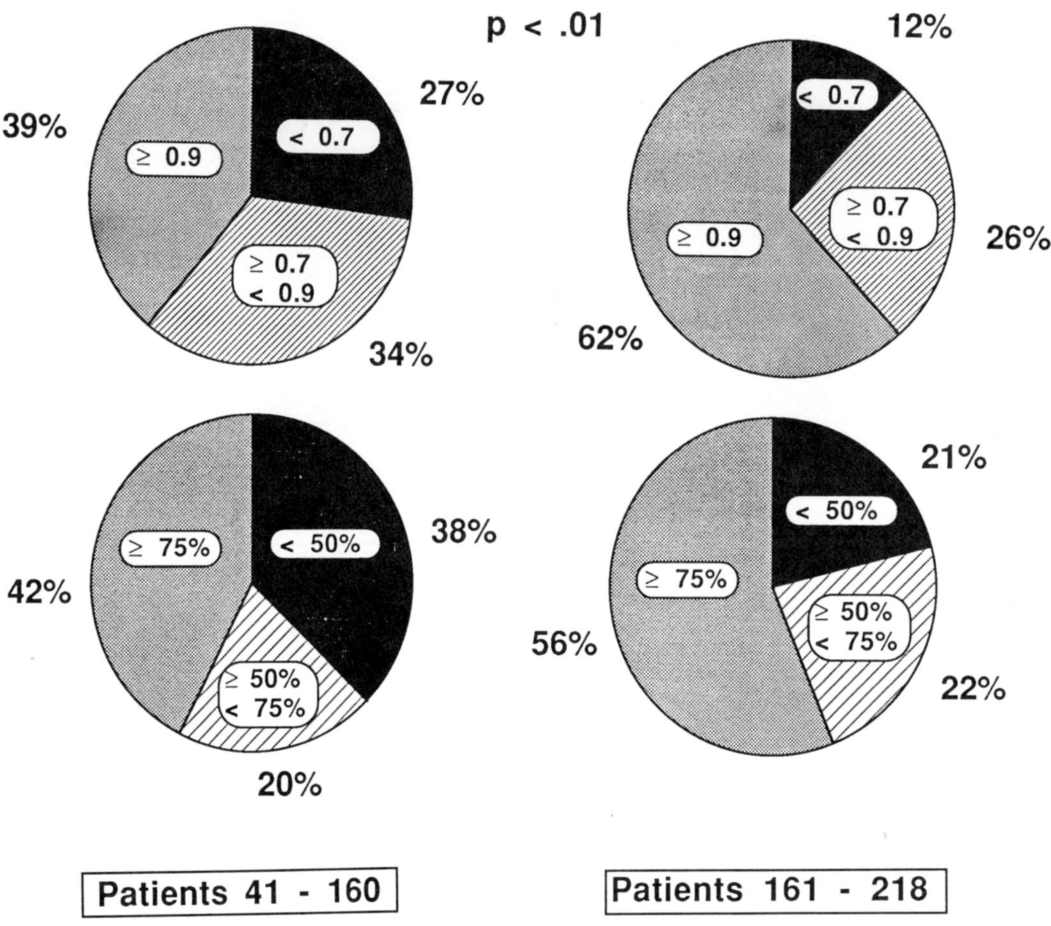

Fig. 20-5. Distribution of postvalvuloplasty valve area (cm^2) in the upper panels, and percentage increase in valve area in the lower panels, comparing the results in patients relatively early in our experience after the initial learning curve (patients 41 to 160) with the latest results (patients 161 to 218).

step-by-step increase in the balloon sizes in order to reduce the risk of serious complications such as massive aortic regurgitation or rupture of the aortic annulus.

As our goals and strategy have evolved, so has the technique. We began our experience using balloon catheters with a 9F shaft that had been designed for dilatation of the peripheral arteries and for congenital pulmonic valve stenosis. Specifically the protocol included the administration of 0.5 mg of atropine intravenously, and then baseline hemodynamic assessment using a thermodilution Swan-Ganz catheter positioned in the pulmonary artery through a femoral vein. A 7F pigtail catheter was inserted into the femoral artery through an 8F sheath and was then positioned in the ascending aorta for continuous monitoring of the aortic pressure. The same catheter was used to obtain a supravalvular aortogram immediately before and after the procedure. Through an 8F sheath, a 7F Sones catheter was inserted into the contralateral femoral artery over a 0.035-inch straight guidewire and this was used to cross the aortic valve. However, if there was a large aortic

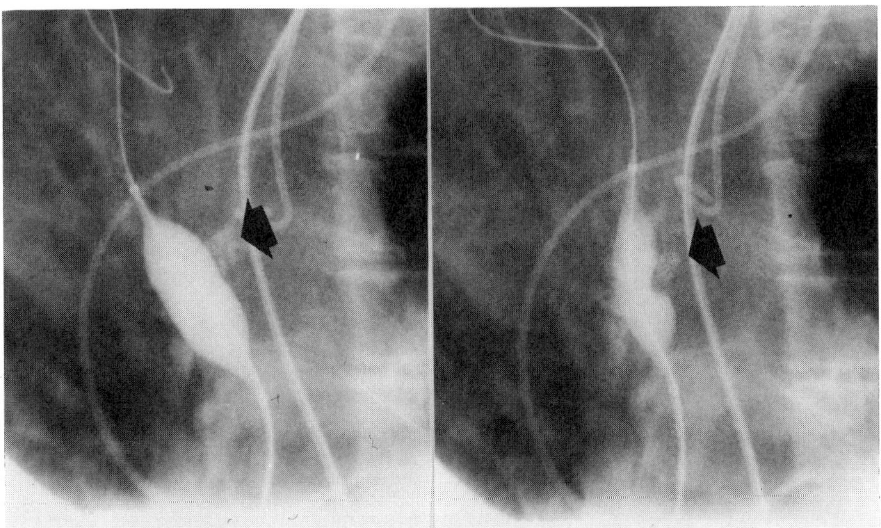

Fig. 20-6. Single-size, 18 mm balloon showing a "waist" caused by calcification in the stenotic valve when the balloon is first inflated across the aortic valve. The balloon becomes cylindric when maximally inflated, and the waist disappears.

root and vertical orientation of the aortic valve orifice, a 7F Amplatz left coronary artery catheter was preferentially used. The peak-to-peak and mean transvalvular systolic pressure gradients were measured while the cardiac output was being determined using the thermodilution method. The aortic valve area was estimated during the procedure using the simplified method of Hakki,[16] but was always calculated for the final result according to Gorlin's formula[17] after the procedure was done. A left ventricular angiogram was obtained in the 30-degree right anterior oblique (RAO) projection for the assessment of left ventricular function.

Following the ventriculogram, the pigtail catheter was removed over a 0.038-inch-diameter, 270-cm-long guidewire and exchanged for the first balloon dilatation catheter, which had been carefully purged of air. Because these patients can be very sensitive to excessive discomfort at the femoral entry site resulting in excessive vagal reactions, additional local anesthesia was administered and a strong negative pressure was applied with a 20 ml syringe to maximally deflate the balloon in order to reduce its profile and to minimize manipulations during the transcutaneous insertion. We were able to use the femoral approach in 90% of our cases. We used a brachial artery cutdown approach only when there was occlusion or severe tortuosity of the femoral or iliac arteries.

In only the very first patients were small balloon diameters of 8 mm, 10 mm, or 12 mm used. Subsequently balloons 3 cm or 4 cm long with inflated diameters of 15 mm, 18 mm, or 20 mm were used. The 15 mm diameter balloon always passed easily through severely stenosed valves and was used for the first dilatation. The balloon was usually inflated for 60 seconds if the systolic aortic pressure remained above 60 mm Hg, and the duration shortened if there was a further decrease in pressure. The balloon was inflated two or three times before exchanging it for an 18 mm balloon, also used for two or three inflations, and then the 18 mm balloon was exchanged for a 20 mm balloon if necessary.

With experience, it was possible to stabilize

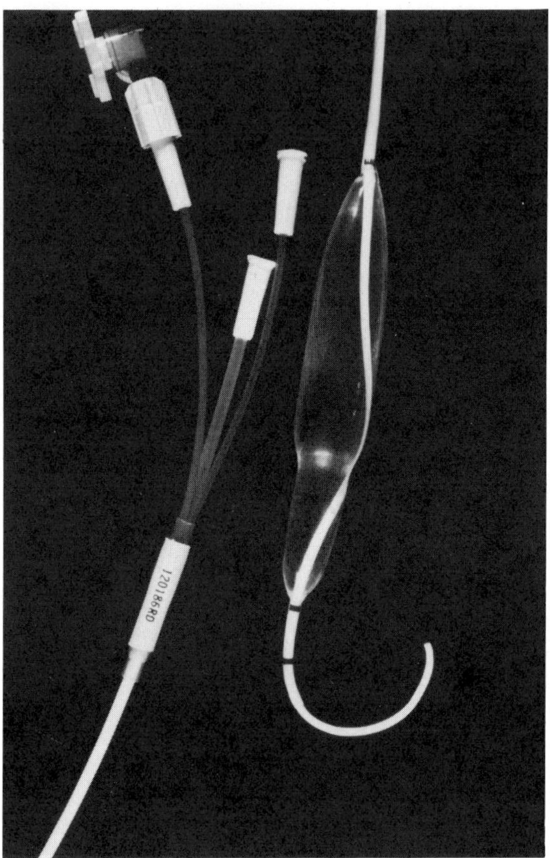

Fig. 20-7. The Mansfield triple lumen, double-size catheter has a large pigtail curve at the tip. This balloon has a proximal diameter of 20 mm, a distal diameter of 15 mm, and a total length of 5.5 cm. There are double markers distal to the balloon tip to aid in positioning the catheter for measurement of the transvalvular gradient without balloon artifact.

the inflated balloon in the aortic valve orifice (Fig. 20-6). This was accomplished by applying opposing forces to the balloon by pushing both on the balloon catheter and on the exchange wire placed through the lumen of the catheter, with the distal extremity of the wire preshaped into an exaggerated pigtail curve that comes in contact with the left ventricular endocardium. This shaping of the wire extremity is crucial in preventing perforation of the myocardium.

The inflation pressure of the balloon was measured only in the first few cases. The maximal inflation pressure before rupture varied between 4 to 6 atm. The variability may in part be due to damage to the balloon if it contacts sharp calcific deposits in the valve. We always tried to obtain the maximal balloon size and rigidity by observing the shape of the balloon on the fluoroscope. All the balloon's "waist" at the valve orifice must disappear and the balloon should appear cylindric or, better, overdistended. To reach the absolute maximal diameter, we often try to burst the balloon at the end of the last inflation of each larger balloon size. There was no complication associated with bursting of the balloons since they are carefully purged of air, and since by design the balloons burst with a longitudinal tear.

Technique has markedly improved with the development of a specially designed aortic valvuloplasty catheter that we now use routinely (Figs. 20-7 and 20-8). This is a triple lumen 9F catheter with a 7F tip shaped into a large pigtail-type curve. There is a distal lumen for pressure measurement and angiography. The proximal lumen located 10 cm above the balloon is used for continuous monitoring of central aortic pressure. The balloon has a proximal segment 3 cm long and 20 or 23 mm in diameter when inflated. There is an abrupt taper to the distal segment, which is 2 cm long and 15 or 18 mm in diameter when inflated. Using this catheter it is possible to dilate first with the distal segment (15 or 18 mm) and then with the proximal segment (20 or 23 mm). This reduces the need to exchange catheters to carry out a dilatation with progressively increasing sizes. Also the procedure is further simplified because the central pressure is monitored, the transvalvular gradient is measured, and angiography is performed with the same catheter.

This newly designed catheter also reduces the complications associated with the procedure. The low profile reduces the trauma at entry into and at withdrawal from the femoral artery. Trauma to the artery is also re-

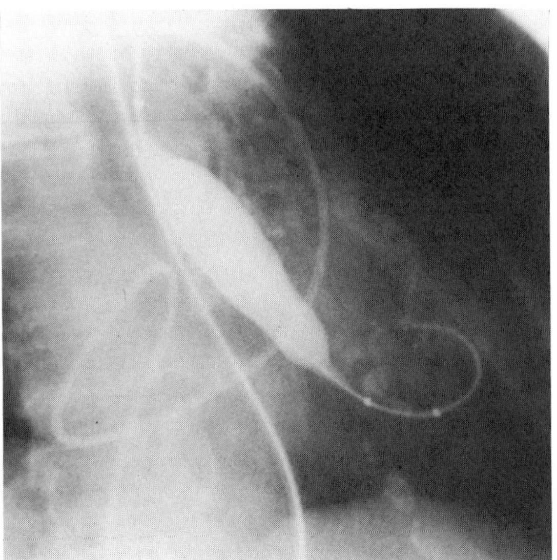

Fig. 20-8. The Mansfield double-size balloon catheter with 20 mm diameter proximal segment inflated across the valve.

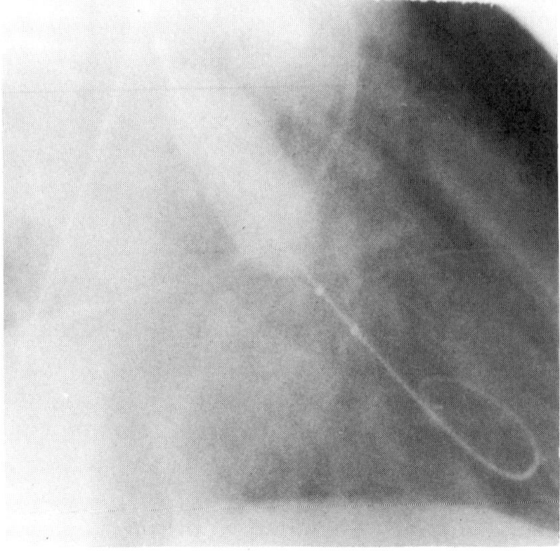

Fig. 20-9. The use of the single-size, 23 mm balloon to further increase the aortic valve area.

duced by the fewer exchanges required. This also decreases the vagal stimulus to the patient by reducing manipulation at the groin. The catheter can also be used through a 14F sheath.

The distal extremity of the catheter has a protective curve to reduce myocardial injury. However, because of the length of the balloon and tip combined, one must be cautious when dilating with the proximal segment in patients who have a small left ventricular cavity. In such patients, a similarly constructed catheter with a single balloon size (15 mm, 18 mm, 20 or 23 mm) could be preferentially used (Fig. 20-9).

We also now use a 0.038-inch extra stiff guidewire for better tracking of the balloon across the valve and to obtain a more stable position of the balloon in the aortic valve orifice. Although the distal extremity of the wire is very flexible and can be preshaped into a large curve, this wire can be dangerous. The junction of the stiff core and flexible distal segment could form into an acute angle with a risk of penetration into the myocardium and perforation of it. Therefore the wire must be kept positioned inside the catheter lumen during balloon inflations. Also during catheter exchanges over this wire, the junction between the stiff core and the flexible distal segment should always be kept away from the ventricular apex.

These refinements in equipment and technique have enabled us to perform PTAV more quickly, more safely, and more efficiently. Valvuloplasty can now often be performed in 30 to 40 minutes immediately following the diagnostic cardiac catheterization.

PROCEDURE-RELATED COMPLICATIONS

Procedure-related mortality in our series has been low despite the populations of elderly and very sick patients. Only 1 of 218 patients died in the catheterization laboratory during the procedure and she was a 92-year-old woman in critical condition. There were nine other patients who died in the hospital following the procedure, but four of these were patients who had been in extremely severe cardiac failure before the procedure and they did not recover. The remaining deaths were due to stroke (one patient), gram-negative sepsis (two patients), internal hemorrhage (one patient), and cardiac arrest under general anesthesia for surgical repair of a femoral artery complication (one patient). The patient who had a lethal stroke caused by a massive cerebral hemorrhage also had cancer of the breast with metastasis to the brain. The total procedure had an intrahospital mortality of 4.5% (10 patients). It is interesting to note, however, that during the same period of time there were 16 comparably ill patients who died while waiting for their scheduled valvuloplasty procedure.

Nonfatal complications included stroke (three patients), tamponade (three patients), hemodynamically important aortic regurgitation (one patient), and myocardial infarction (one patient). The cause of stroke in three patients was undertermined. Although a calcific embolism was feared, it could not be documented. The three cases of cardiac tamponade were due to myocardial perforation by the catheter tip or by the guidewire. The treatment for this consists of immediate pericardiocentesis. The incidence of this complication should be minimized by preshaping the distal extremity of the wires into an exaggerated curve, by careful manipulation of the wire during balloon inflation and during catheter exchanges, and by the use of pigtail-tipped balloon catheters. Aortic regurgitation has not been a significant complication. A massive regurgitation did occur after the use of a 23 mm balloon in only one patient, a 78-year-old woman who subsequently had uneventful valve replacement. The patient who had a myocardial infarction had severe diffuse coronary disease.

Complications at the femoral entry site have been frequent. There were 26 patients (13%) who had postprocedure hematomas and 9 patients with persistent bleeding or arterial thrombosis requiring surgical repair. Heparin, initially given intravenously at a dose of 10,000 units at the beginning of the procedure, has been progressively limited to a total dose of 2000 to 3000 units added to the catheter flushing solutions. This has markedly shortened the postprocedure femoral compression time to 20 minutes on the average, with no increase in the thromboembolic complication rate. There has been a definite reduction in the complication rate caused by vascular trauma since we have been using the new-design catheter because of its low profile and because it has also reduced the need for catheter exchanges.

Finally, as in all new invasive techniques, there exists a learning curve that obviously has an impact on the complication rate. As the teams performing the procedure gain experience, and as the technology of the valvuloplasty devices improves, the morbidity and mortality of the procedure should diminish further.

CLINICAL FOLLOW-UP

The long-term results following optimal aortic valvuloplasty remain an important but as yet unanswered question. We have clinical follow-up information at an average of 8 months obtained from the first 148 patients in our series, including the very first patients in whom the procedure was attempted.

During this interval of clinical follow-up 24 patients died. Nineteen (80%) of these patients were in NYHA functional Class IV at the time of valvuloplasty. Seven of the patients died during the first month. Only one of the patients had been a surgical candidate, but this patient, a 68-year-old woman, had definitely refused surgery. Two other patients under 70 years old died, one had liver cancer and the other had severe diffuse coronary artery disease with previous myocardial infarctions. The average age of the other 21 patients who died was 79 years. The majority of these patients died as a result of heart failure. The mean ejection fraction of these patients was

38% and it is possible that valvuloplasty could not reverse their myocardial deterioration. However, in these patients severe aortic stenosis persisted after the dilatation with a post-PTAV mean aortic valve area of 0.65 cm^2. Those patients who had PTAV early in our experience undoubtedly had insufficient dilatation by our current criteria.

In the majority of the survivors, however, there was marked, sustained clinical improvement. Before the procedure, 87 of the patients had symptoms categorized as NYHA functional Class III or Class IV. At 8 months follow-up there were only 14 Class III or Class IV patients. Of the 67 patients who had angina, the symptoms disappeared or improved in 50. The remaining 17 patients with unchanged angina had severe diffuse coronary artery atherosclerosis not suitable for surgery or angioplasty. There were no recurrences of syncope.

HEMODYNAMIC FOLLOW-UP

Repeat hemodynamic assessment has been done in 52 patients. In 41 patients repeat catheterization was scheduled at the time of the initial dilatation and was carried out as a routine examination despite their persistent clinical improvement at an average of 4.5 ± 2.8 months after the valvuloplasty procedure. However, since the objective of the late repeat-catheterization was to assess the restenosis rate, the 8 patients of this group who clearly had an insufficient post-PTAV increase in valve area (less than 25% increase) were eliminated and the late hemodynamic results were considered only in the 33 patients who had a more adequate initial dilatation. In 11 patients, the catheterization was done because of a recurrence of symptoms and the procedure was carried out 6 ± 3 months after the initial dilatation.

We defined restenosis as 50% or more loss of the postvalvuloplasty gain in the aortic valve area. Using this definition, there were 8 patients (24%) with restenosis in the group of 33 patients who had routine follow-up repeat-catheterization. In the second group of patients who had recurrence of symptoms, all 11 had restenosis. It thus appears that recurrence of symptoms is associated with a very high probability of restenosis. Restenosis, however, can also be found in patients who remain asymptomatic.

CURRENT PERSPECTIVES ON VALVULOPLASTY

Based on our experience and the reports of the experience of others, it is our opinion that PTAV is a feasible technique that leads to marked clinical improvement in most symptomatic adult patients with severe aortic stenosis. PTAV is certainly a valuable treatment for all patients not being considered for valve replacement because of contraindication or unacceptably high surgical risk. Improvement in the devices used has made the procedure relatively simple for an experienced interventional cardiologist. The risk of complications is low, particularly in view of the elderly and seriously ill patients to whom the procedure is applied. The restenosis rate and long-term results, however, are still not known.

Percutaneous transluminal aortic valvuloplasty is definitely indicated in elderly patients, for example, those 80 years old or older. The procedure requires only local anesthesia and cardiac catheterization, which is obviously less traumatic than surgical valve replacement. These patients are more often able to resume normal activities for their age after only 5 or 6 days' hospitalization. Surgical publications on aortic valve replacement for aortic stenosis in elderly patients do not include reports on patients over the age of 80 in sufficiently large series.[18-20] In our series, 54 patients (25%) were 80 years old or older. Thus, comparing PTAV results and surgical outcome in so-called elderly patients is not valid until a similar series of elderly patients treated surgically is available. In fact before the PTAV era most of these very old patients who have been entered in our series would probably have never been referred for cardiac catheterization because of their age alone.

The mortality of patients with severe left ventricular dysfunction remained high in the year following valvuloplasty despite transient clinical improvement. However, most of these patients continued to have severe aortic stenosis following the procedure, despite an apparently marked decrease in peak-to-peak gradient. This probably explains the lack of prolonged clinical improvement. In these patients with a low cardiac output, the pressure gradient has to be almost totally eliminated to obtain a satisfying increase in valve area. For example, in a patient with a low cardiac output of 3.5 L/min, the gradient should be reduced to below 15 mm Hg in order to increase the valve area to 1 cm^2. With a final gradient of 30 mm Hg, considered satisfactory at first sight, the valve area would remain below 0.7 cm^2, still a severe degree of aortic stenosis. In patients with marked left ventricular dysfunction, that is, a decreased ejection fraction to or below 40%, an immediate improvement in myocardial function can be observed after PTAV. In 72 such patients of our series with an ejection fraction of 29 ± 5% on the average, it increased to 34 ± 7% ($p < 0.001$) immediately after the procedure. In 11 patients of this group who had a repeat catheterization, the ejection fraction, which had increased from 29 ± 8% to 39 ± 10% after PTAV, had further increased to 52 ± 11% ($p < 0.01$) at 5 months. This dramatic improvement in ejection fraction indirectly confirms the lasting efficacy of PTAV with persistent enlargement of the aortic orifice. Furthermore, at this point some of these patients could now be considered better candidates for valve replacement with decreased surgical risk.

Earlier in our experience, we were reluctant to perform PTAV in younger patients, particularly patients under 70 years old, unless there was a definite surgical contraindication or surgery was definitely refused by the patient. However, the good results and the low complication rate in this subgroup led us to later consider PTAV in these patients even when they were good surgical candidates, sometimes as a temporary treatment aimed at postponing surgery. In 65 patients under the age of 70, the postvalvuloplasty aortic valve area was 1.1 cm^2 on the average (above 1 cm^2 in 50% of the cases, with a mean of 1.29 cm^2). Only one patient in NYHA functional Class IV who was not suitable for surgery died in the hospital after the procedure. All other complications were markedly lowered in this subgroup of patients. Thus in experienced laboratories it could be reasonable to attempt valvuloplasty in young patients as a continuation of the cardiac catheterization procedure. Surgical valve replacement could still be considered in case of insufficient results, or in case of restenosis.

Since percutaneous transluminal aortic valvuloplasty is a new, evolving technique, definitive indications for its use cannot be given at the present time. The best indication is for patients in whom surgery cannot be considered or in whom it carries a very high risk, and also for patients who definitely refuse to be operated on. Further long-term studies are needed and randomized studies comparing PTAV with surgery can also be justified, particularly in young patients, to determine the exact place of this relatively simple, low-risk, low-cost method for treatment of acquired aortic stenosis.

REFERENCES

1. Kan, J., White, R.I., Mitchell, S.E., and Gardner, T.J.: Percutaneous balloon valvuloplasty: a new method for treating congenital pulmonary valve stenosis, N. Engl. J. Med., **307:**540, 1982.
2. Pepine, C.J., Gessner, J.H., and Feldman, R.L.: Percutaneous balloon valvuloplasty for pulmonic valve stenosis in the adult, Am. J. Cardiol. **50:**1442, 1982
3. Lababidi, Z., Wu, J.R., and Walls, J.T.: Percutaneous balloon aortic valvuloplasty: results in 23 patients, Am. J. Cardiol. **53:**194, 1984.
4. Inoue, K., Ouraki, T., Nakamura, T., Kitamura, F., and Miyamoto, N.: Clinical application of transvenous mitral commissurotomy by a new balloon catheter, J. Thorac. Cardiovasc. Surg. **87:**394, 1984.
5. Cribier, A., Savin, T., Berland, J., Saoudi, N., Rocha, P., and Letac, B.: Percutaneous transluminal valvuloplasty of acquired aortic stenosis in elderly patients: an alternative to valve replacement?, Lancet **63:**1, 1986.
6. Cribier, A., Savin, T., Berland, J., et al.: Percutaneous transluminal balloon valvuloplasty of adult aortic stenosis: report of 92 cases, J. Am. Coll. Cardiol. **9:**381, 1987.
7. Frank, S., Johnson, A., and Ross, J., Jr.: Natural history of valvular aortic stenosis, Br. Heart J., **35:**41, 1973.
8. O'Keefe, J.H., Jr., Vlietstra, R.E., Bailey, K.R., and Holmes, D.R.: Natural history of candidates for balloon aortic valvuloplasty, Mayo Clin. Proc. **62:**986-991, 1987.
9. Turina, J., Hess, O., Sepulcri, F., and Krayenbuehl, H.P.: Spontaneous course of aortic valve disease, Eur. Heart J. **8:**471-483, 1987.
10. McKay, R.G., Safian, R.D., Lock, J.E., et al.: Balloon dilatation of calcific aortic stenosis in elderly patients: postmortem, intraoperative, and percutaneous valvuloplasty studies, Circulation **74:**119, 1986.
11. McKay, R.G., Safian, R.D., Lock, J.E., Diver, D.J., Berman, A.D., Sanford, E.W., Come, P.C., Baim, D.S., Mandell, V.E., Royal, H.D., and Grossman, W.: Assessment of left ventricular and aortic valve function after aortic balloon valvuloplasty in adult patients with critical aortic stenosis, Circulation **75:**102-203, 1987.
12. Isner, J.M., Salem, D.N., Desnoyers, M.R., Hougen, T.J., Mackey, W.C., Pandian, N.G., Eichhorn, E.J., Konstam, M.A., and Levine, H.J.: Treatment of calcific aortic stenosis by balloon valvuloplasty, Am. J. Cardiol. **59:**313-317, 1987.
13. Jackson, J., Thomas, S., Monaghan, M., Forsyth, A., and Jewitt, D.: Inoperable aortic stenosis in the elderly: benefit from percutaneous transluminal valvuloplasty, Br. Med. J. **294:**83-86, 1987.
14. Drobinski, G., Lechat, P., Metzger, P., Lepailleur, C., Vacheron, A., Grosgogeat, Y.: Results of percutaneous catheter valvuloplasty for calcified aortic stenosis in the elderly, Eur. Heart J. **8:**22, 1987.
15. Roberts, W.C.: Good-bye to thoracotomy for cardiac valvulotomy, Am. J. Cardiol. **59:**198-202, 1987.
16. Hakki, A.H., Iskandrian, A.S., Bermis, C.E., Kimbiris, D., Mintz, G.S., Segal, B.L., and Brice, C.: A simplified valve formula for the calculation of stenotic cardiac valve areas, Circulation **63:**1050-1055, 1981.
17. Gorlin, R., and Gorlin, G.: Hydraulic formula for calculation of area of stenotic mitral valve, other cardiac valves and central circulatory shunts, Am. Heart J. **41:**1-29, 1951.
18. Kay, P.H., and Paneth, M.: Aortic valve re-

placement in the over seventy age group, J. Cardiovasc. Surg. **22**:312-315, 1981.

19. Murphy, E.S., Lawson, R.M., Starr, A., and Rahimtoola, S.H.: Severe aortic stenosis in patients 60 years of age and older: left ventricular function and 10-year survival after valve replacement, Circulation **64** (suppl. 2):184-188, 1981.
20. Rich, M.W., Sandza, J.G., Kleiger, R.E., and Connors, J.P.: Cardiac operations in patients over 80 years of age, J. Thorac. Cardiovasc. Surg. **90**:56-60, 1985.

Chapter 21

Techniques and Results with Trefoil or Bifoil Balloons and Long Sheaths for Percutaneous Valvuloplasty

Bernhard Meier, MD
Beat Friedli, MD

With their article on pulmonary valvuloplasty in 1982, Kan and co-workers[1] introduced percutaneous balloon valvuloplasty into human medicine. Valvuloplasty of aortic stenosis in children followed in 1984[2] and valvuloplasty of mitral stenosis in 1985.[3] Later came balloon valvuloplasty in aortic stenosis of infants first published in 1985,[4] of calcific aortic stenosis in the elderly initiated in 1985 and published in 1986,[5,6] of a bioprosthesis in tricuspid position in 1986,[7] and of a rheumatic tricuspid stenosis in 1987.[8]

The inflation of a balloon in the stenotic valve was responsible for a brief syncope in several of the initial patients with pulmonary valvuloplasty,[1,9] particularly in the absence of a patent foramen ovale.[10,11] With valvuloplasty in aortic and mitral position in adults, circulatory collapse during balloon inflation was reported to be less frequent, about 20% for aortic stenosis[12] and 30% for mitral stenosis.[13] This was explained by the irregular shape of these valves and might also be due to the fact that relatively small balloons were employed.

To allow for some transvalvular blood flow during balloon inflation, we developed together with Schneider Shiley of Zurich, Switzerland a special balloon catheter.[14,15] It consists of three angioplasty balloons mounted around the shaft at the tip of a 7F, 8F, or 9F catheter. The three balloons are inflated and deflated through a common port. Their cross-section resembles a three-leaf clover, hence the name Trefoil balloon.

Fig. 21-1 illustrates the characteristics of this type of balloon comparing it with a single balloon in an animal experiment. In-vivo animal experiments have been reported earlier.[14-16] Fig. 21-2 compares the combined cross-sectional area of Trefoil balloons and Bifoil balloons (two balloons instead of three) with that of single balloons. Since the three individual balloons of the Trefoil balloon are positioned in a triangle, their diameters do not add up completely. We select the Trefoil bal-

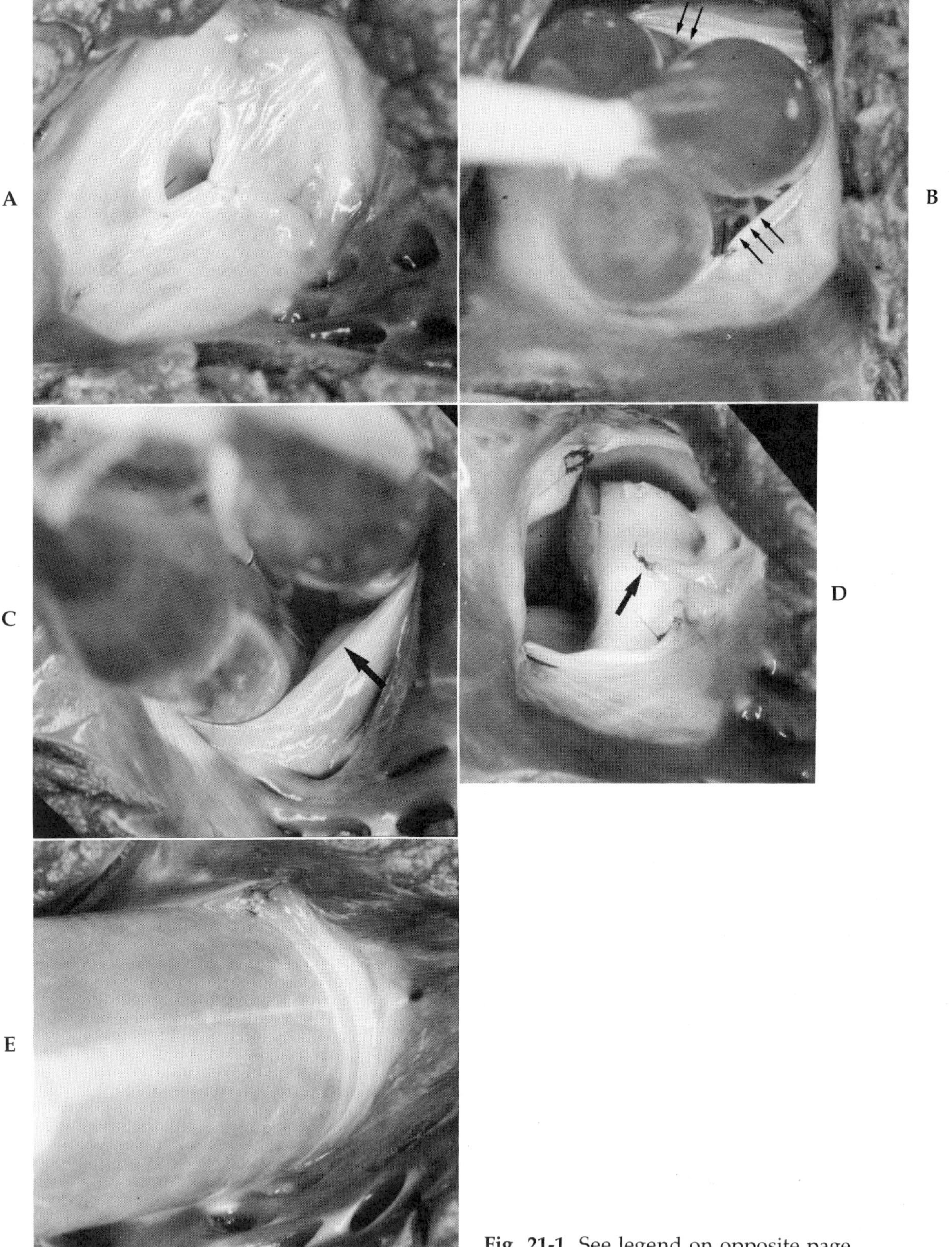

Fig. 21-1. See legend on opposite page.

loon by taking 3 × 60% of the diameter of the single balloon that would be chosen for the particular valve. For example, for a 20 mm single balloon we take a 3 × 12 mm Trefoil balloon (60% of 20 = 12).

CLINICAL APPLICATION

We have clinically evaluated Trefoil balloons since 1985.[14,15,17] In 1986 we started to introduce them through a specially developed long sheath (outer diameter up to 17F) for easier introduction and positioning of the balloon and continuous monitoring of the pressure gradient through a single puncture hole.[16]

Pulmonary Valvuloplasty

Technique

The pulmonary artery is passed with a diagnostic catheter introduced through a femoral vein. A particularly rigid 0.020- to 0.035-inch exchange wire (backup wire, solid steel manufactured by Schneider Shiley, Zurich, Switzerland) with a floppy tip is placed into a distal pulmonary artery through this catheter. Heparin (100 units per kg body weight) is given. The long sheath is advanced into the pulmonary artery or at least into the right ventricle. The balloon is introduced into the sheath, which features a self-adjusting hemostatic valve (Fig. 21-3), and advanced across the stenotic valve. The sheath is left in the right ventricle and permits continuous pressure monitoring through its side arm (Fig. 21-3). If monitoring of the pressure in the pulmonary artery is desired, it can be accomplished through the central lumen of the balloon catheter.

If no introducer sheath is used, the femoral vein has to be predilated before introducing the collapsed balloon over the exchange wire. The right ventricular pressure should be monitored with a separate catheter introduced through the opposite femoral vein.

Still frames from a biplane right ventriculogram (Fig. 21-4) and contrast medium injections into the right ventricle aid in correctly positioning the balloon.

Results

Fig. 21-5 summarizes the results (hemodynamically measured transvalvular peak-to-peak pressure gradients) in 13 consecutive patients treated using a Trefoil balloon and compares them with the results of 4 patients treated using a single balloon. The results were similar, but the procedure was better tolerated with the Trefoil balloon. This impression was confirmed by another group.[18]

There were three poor results. Two occurred with a Trefoil balloon in very dysplastic valves, which are a well-recognized reason for failed pulmonary valvuloplasty[19,20] and one with a single balloon in a patient with severe infundibular stenosis who underwent surgical infundibulectomy a few days later.

Fig. 21-1. Trefoil balloon and single balloon pulmonary valvuloplasty in a valve of a 51 kg dog (seen from the right ventricular outflow tract.) **A,** A pulmonary stenosis (0.2 cm^2 valve area) is created with No. 6-0 polypropylene suture. **B,** A 3 × 8 mm Trefoil balloon is inflated (4 bar). The arrows point to the space between the balloons for continued transvalvular blood flow. The resulting valve area was 1.8 cm^2. **C,** A 3 × 12 mm Trefoil balloon is inflated (4 bar). The arrow points to the space between the balloons. **D,** The resulting valve area is 2.8 cm^2. Some of the sutures are torn *(arrow)* and the cusps are stretched. **E,** A 19 mm single balloon is inflated (4 bar). Its cross-sectional area is smaller than that of the 3 × 12 mm Trefoil balloon in **C.** Nevertheless, the single balloon completely obstructs the valve orifice.

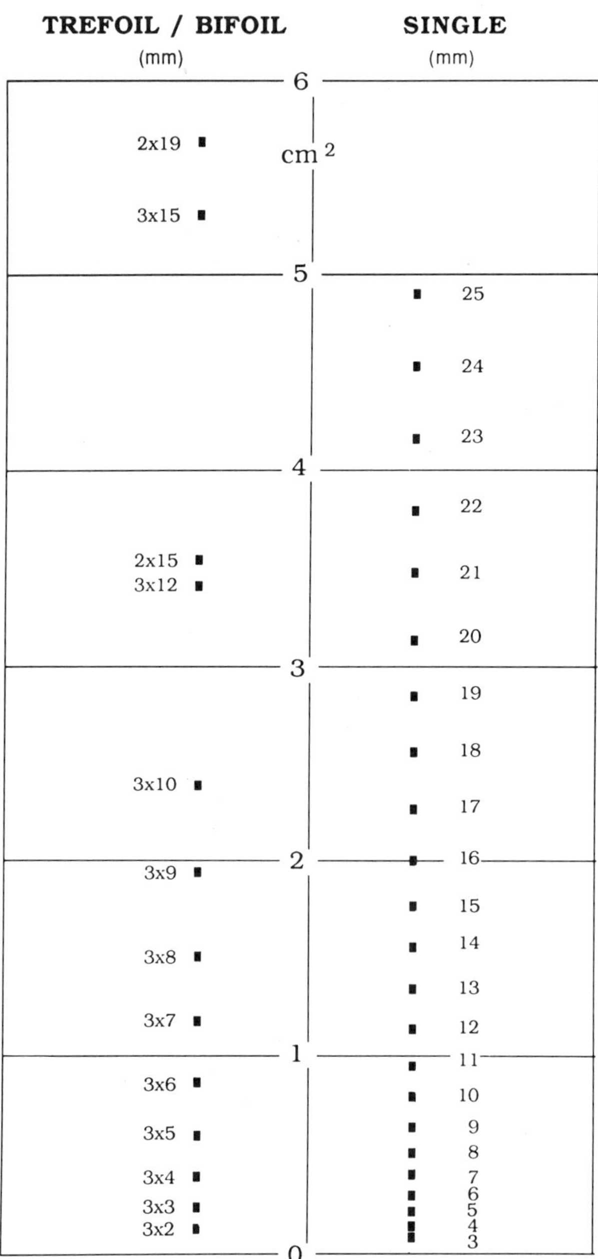

Fig. 21-2. Cross-sectional area of Trefoil, Bifoil, and single balloons. With Trefoil and Bifoil balloons, the area of the catheter and the area between the balloons are not included.

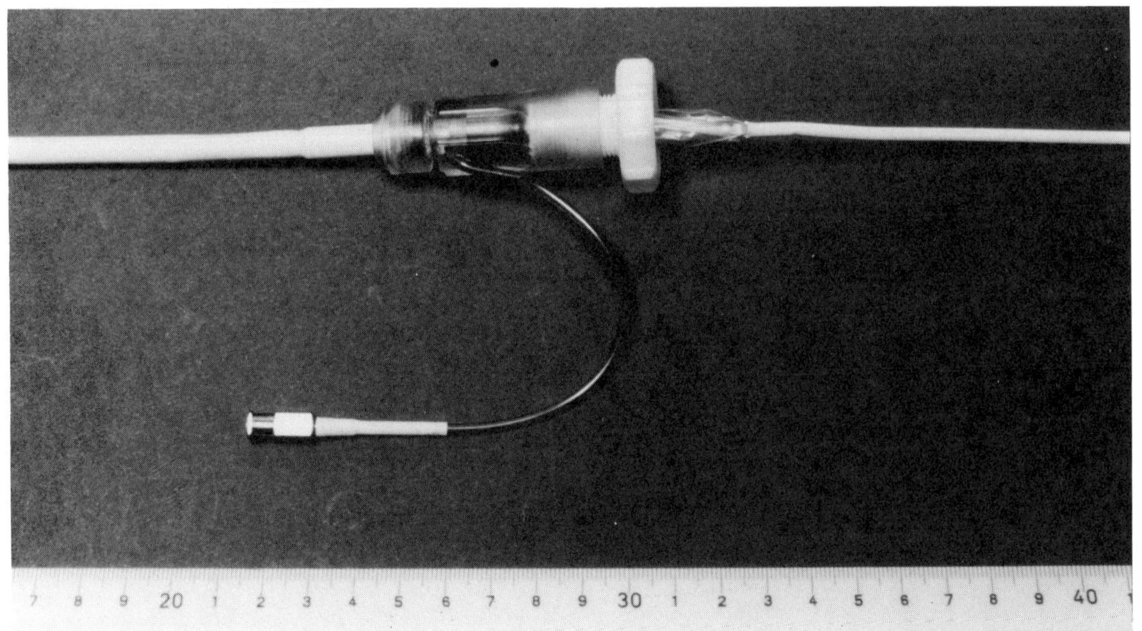

Fig. 21-3. Collapsed 3 × 12 mm Trefoil balloon entering the self-adjusting hemostatic valve of a 17F long sheath. The ruler indicates centimeters.

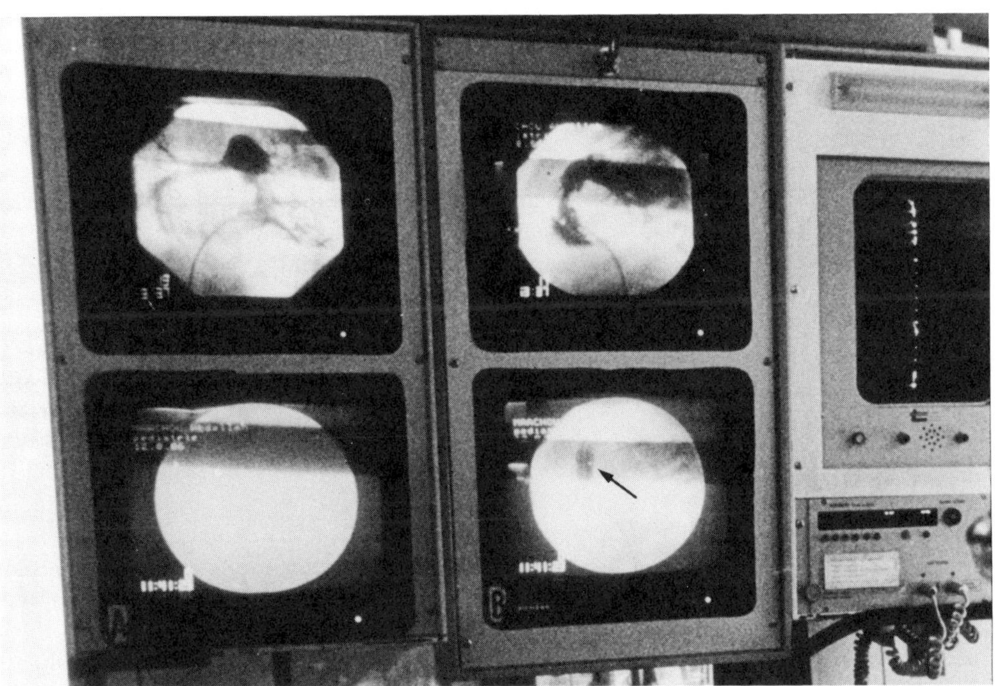

Fig. 21-4. Biplane still frames (*left*, posteroanterior; *right*, lateral view) for correct positioning of a 3 × 8 mm Trefoil balloon (arrow of live fluoroscopy monitor at the bottom right) in a 4-year-old boy with pulmonary valve stenosis. The still frames are selected by the operator (sterile remote control) with a solid state digital frame grabber (Leutron, Siemens).

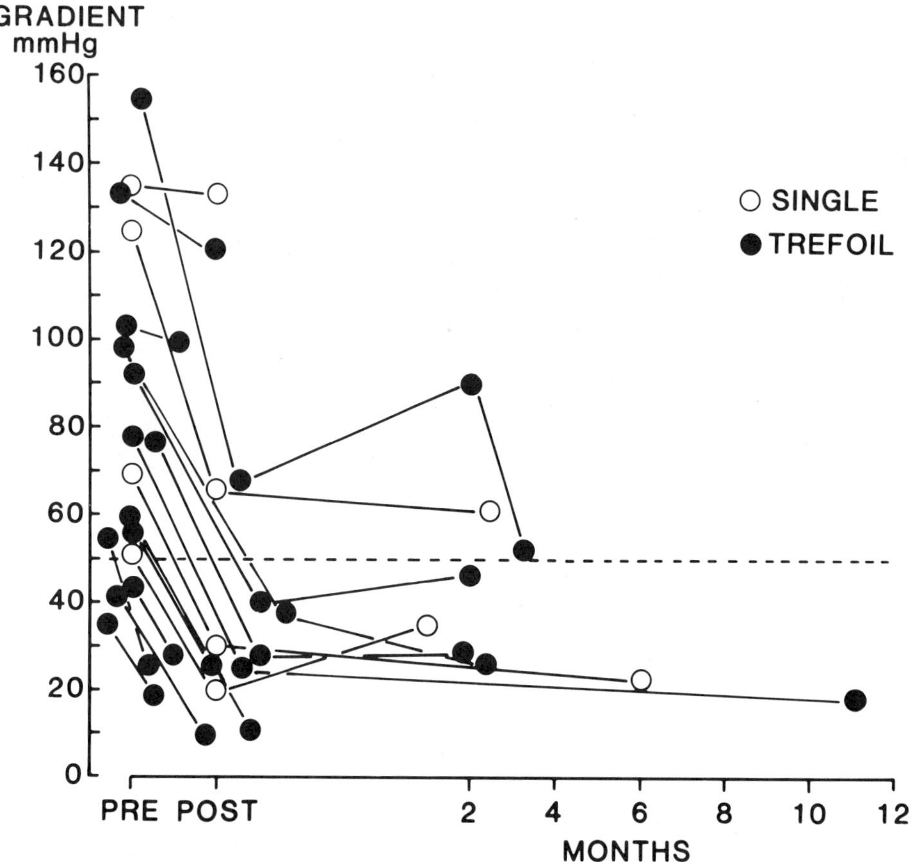

Fig. 21-5. Pulmonary transvalvular peak-to-peak pressure gradients before and after balloon valvuloplasty in 17 consecutive patients. One patient had a second valvuloplasty during follow-up for an incomplete result.

The valve was found to be widely patent at the time of operation. There was an intimal tear in the supravalvular portion of the pulmonary artery.

Aortic Valvuloplasty

Technique

The aortic valve is crossed retrogradely from a femoral artery with a diagnostic catheter and a steerable 0.035-inch straight or J-shaped wire. Then a 0.020- to 0.035-inch backup exchange wire with a U-shaped tip is placed into the left ventricle and a long sheath (100 cm, 17F) is introduced into the left ventricle or just distal to the aortic valve if the sheath's cross-section (0.3 cm^2) is obstructive. Heparin (100 units per kg body weight) is given. The obturator of the sheath (Fig. 21-6) is removed leaving the guidewire in place. Flushing is important to prevent coagulation within the sheath. A Trefoil balloon with a pigtail tip is advanced over the wire through the sheath into the ventricle. The sheath is withdrawn just proximal to the balloon, where it stabilizes the balloon and allows continuous supravalvular aortic pressure recording. The left ventricular pressure can be mon-

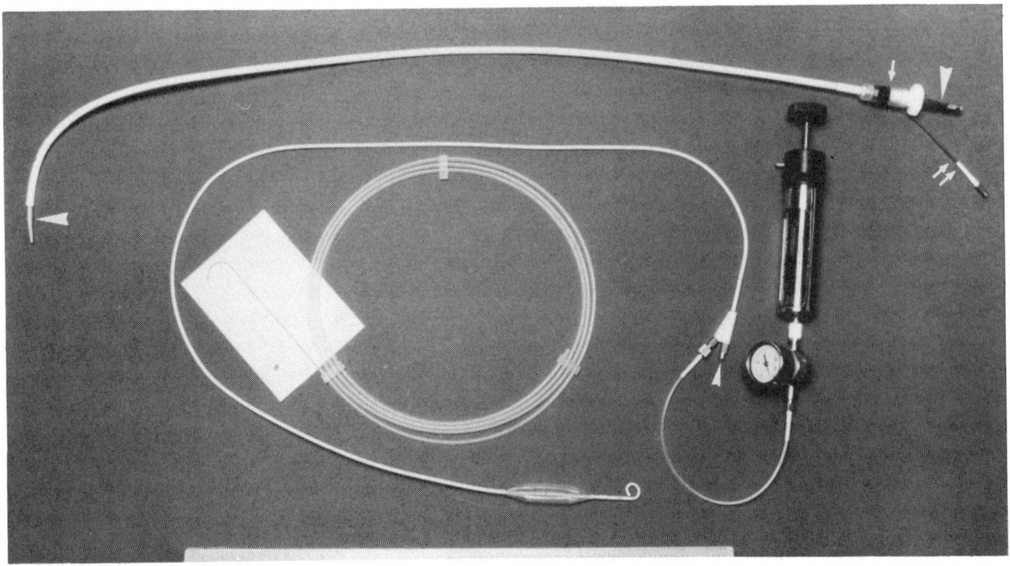

Fig. 21-6. Kit for aortic or pulmonary valvuloplasty with the long sheath technique. The obturator *(large arrowheads)* can be removed and replaced by the balloon catheter when the sheath is in place. The hemostatic valve *(arrow)* automatically adjusts from 0 to 16F. The transvalvular pressure gradient is obtained from the side arm of the hemostatic valve *(double arrow)* and the central lumen of the balloon catheter *(small arrowhead)*. The guidewire is a 300 cm, 0.035-inch solid steel backup exchange wire with a steerable floppy tip of 5 to 15 cm. The deflator is a 50 ml syringe with a screw thread on the piston rod that can be disengaged for rapid deflation. The length of the ruler is 50 cm.

itored from the pigtail tip of the balloon catheter after retracting the guidewire a few centimeters. Balloon exchanges may be performed by readvancing the sheath into the left ventricle or simply over the guidewire. Prophylactic atropine has proved salutary for preventing reactive bradycardia during balloon inflation.

Results

The immediate and some follow-up results (hemodynamically measured peak-to-peak pressure gradients) of the first 10 consecutive patients treated with this method are depicted in Fig. 21-7. Four patients were younger than 25 years, and six patients were older than 70 years and had calcific stenosis. Simultaneous coronary angioplasty was performed in two of these patients. The mean peak-to-peak pressure gradient was reduced from 70 ± 35 mm Hg to 27 ± 13 mm Hg, but in the three patients with follow-up examination (all over 70 years old with calcific stenosis) a significant recurrence of the pressure gradient was noted.

A 74-year-old patient suffered an embolic myocardial infarction (circumflex coronary artery) at the end of the procedure. A 23-year-old patient required needle pericardiocentesis for cardiac tamponade caused by left ventricular penetration of the balloon tip. The same patient underwent surgical valve replacement immediately after balloon valvuloplasty because of an aortic regurgitation of 60% of the stroke volume secondary to a flail leaflet created by valvuloplasty. The patient was found

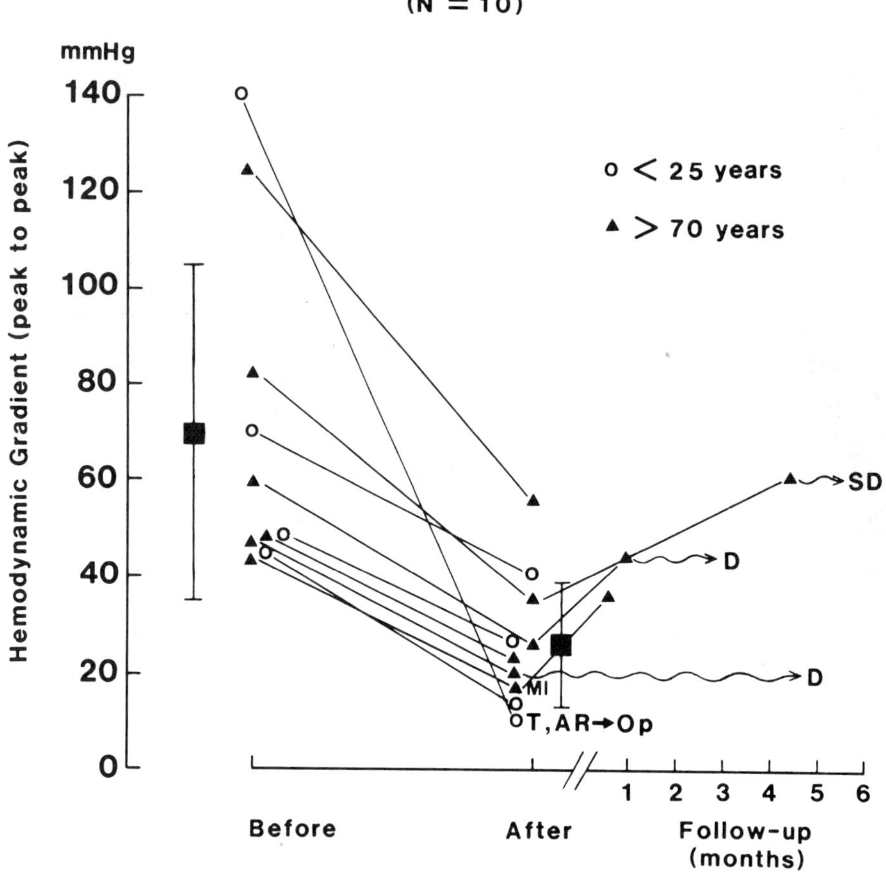

Fig. 21-7. Peak-to-peak transvalvular pressure gradient before and after aortic Trefoil balloon valvuloplasty in 10 consecutive patients. One patient had an embolic myocardial infarction (MI) and one patient needed needle pericardiocentesis for tamponade (T) and urgent operation (Op) for massive aortic regurgitation (AR) caused by a flail leaflet. Of the patients older than 70 years, 3 (50%) died (D) within a few months after the procedure. One of them (SD) died a few days after surgical valve replacement.

to have a monocuspid valve with dehiscence of about 30 degrees of the circumference starting from the cleft created by the balloon. There was no intrahospital mortality, but two patients (80 and 81 years) died a few months later and a 75-year-old patient died a few days after surgical valve replacement that became necessary 4 months after valvuloplasty because of recurrence of symptoms. The valve showed no evidence of the previous balloon dilatation.

Mitral Valvuloplasty

Technique

The access through the femoral vein and the interatrial septum was used exclusively. The transseptal puncture was performed either with a standard transseptal set or directly through the long sheath (Fig. 21-8). The 0.035-inch backup wire may sometimes guide the sheath directly into the left ventricle. If

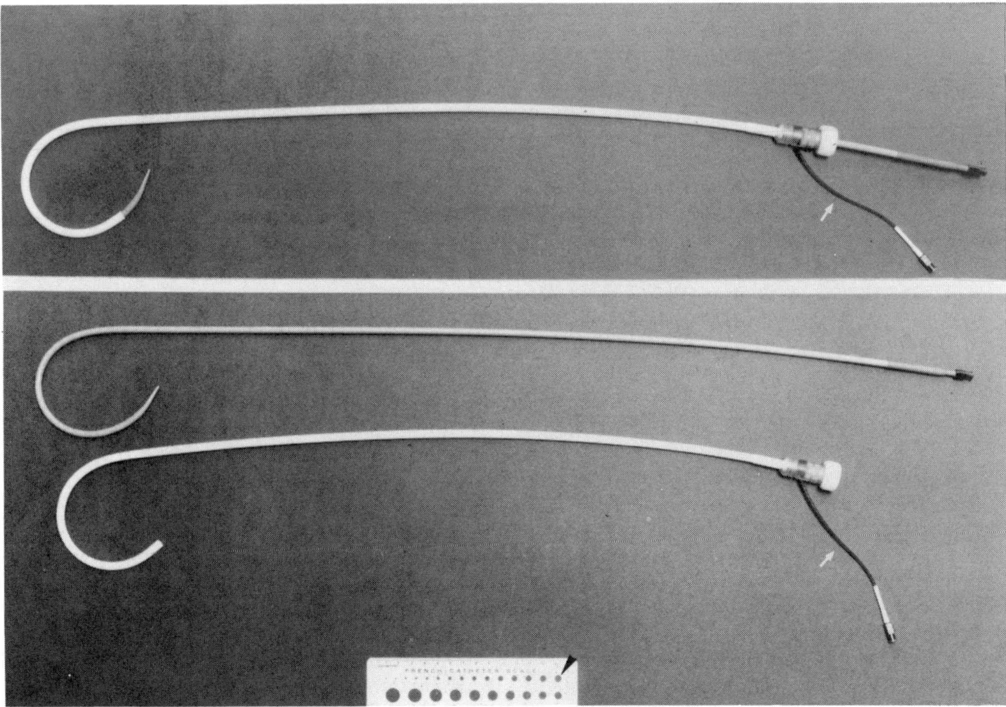

Fig. 21-8. Long sheath (17F) for mitral valvuloplasty. The obturator is removed before balloon placement *(bottom)*. The hemostatic valve with side arm *(arrow)* permits pressure monitoring in the left atrium throughout the procedure. The ruler indicates centimeters and the French (F) scale. The 17F hole is indicated by an arrowhead.

the valve is difficult to pass, a balloon-tipped catheter accepting the 0.035-inch wire or a diagnostic Judkins-shape coronary catheter may help. Heparin (100 units per kg body weight) was given after the transseptal passage. Once the sheath or at least the stiff part of the backup wire is in the left ventricle, the obturator is removed (Fig. 21-8) and replaced by the balloon catheter. During dilatation, the sheath is positioned in the let atrium just proximal to the balloon to stabilize it (Fig. 21-9). It monitors the left atrial pressure, whereas the left ventricular pressure can be monitored through the pigtail tip of the balloon catheter after retracting the guidewire a few centimeters. After withdrawal of the sheath, the oxygen saturation should be measured in the vena cava and the pulmonary artery to exclude a left-to-right shunt. Such an occurrence is unlikely with this technique, which produces a transseptal hole smaller than 0.3 cm^2. Prophylactic atropine before balloon inflation is recommended.

The 3 × 12 mm Trefoil balloon is currently the largest Trefoil balloon accepted by the 17F sheath. It may not be sufficient in some adult patients. In these cases, we used a 2 × 19 mm Bifoil balloon (Fig. 21-9).

Results

There were two technical failures among the first 10 patients (mean age 54 years, range 14 to 74 years; 3 patients with prior surgical commissurotomy) undergoing mitral valvuloplasty with this technique. One was due to defective material and the other one was due to a cerebral embolus during balloon place-

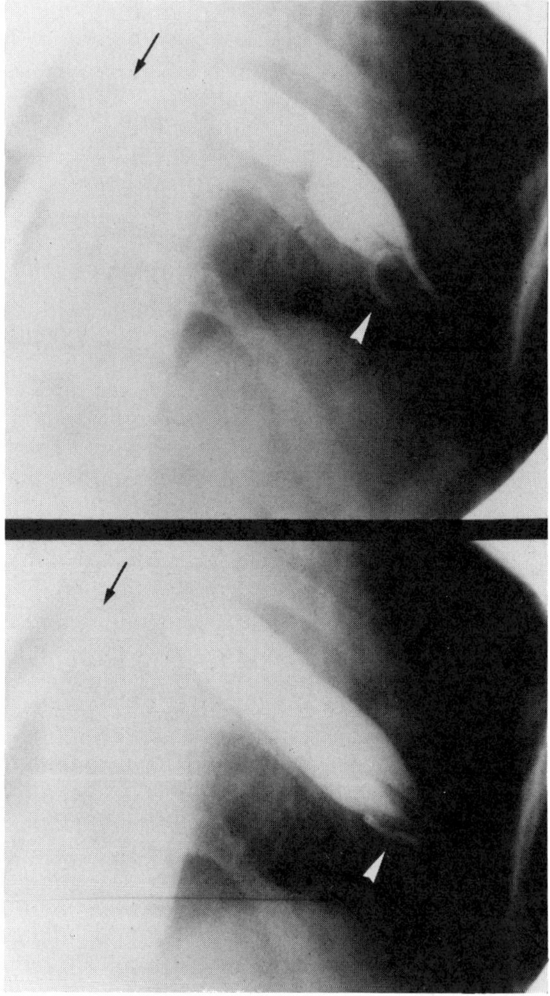

Fig. 21-9. Mitral valvuloplasty with a 2 × 19 mm Bifoil balloon and the long sheath (17F) technique in a 31-year-old woman with rheumatic mitral stenosis (right anterior oblique view). The arrow points to the tip of the sheath in the left atrium, and the arrowhead shows the pigtail tip of the balloon catheter. *Top,* Inflation at 2 bar showing an indentation by the stenotic valve. *Bottom,* Inflation at 5 bar. The two balloons are fully expanded. The mean pressure gradient was reduced from 24 to 6 mm Hg.

ment with sequelae lasting 3 weeks. In one of the eight patients in whom the balloon was actually inflated, there was no significant improvement in the pressure gradient because the balloon was too small. The mean transmitral pressure-gradient changes of the remaining seven patients are listed in Table 21-1.

In two patients with good hemodynamic results, mitral regurgitation was significantly increased and one patient needed surgical drainage for a sequestrated cardiac tamponade (the patient who had a prior commissurotomy). In this patient, control cardiac catheterization at 1 month confirmed an unchanged, minimal transmitral gradient (2 mm Hg) but persistently increased mitral regurgitation compared with her prevalvuloplasty status. She had valve replacement 6 months after balloon valvuloplasty. There was no mortality and none of the other patients underwent valve surgery during a follow-up of 8 to 18 months.

DISCUSSION

The best opening by balloon valvuloplasty of a stenosed cardiac valve should be obtainable with a single oversized balloon. Although some oversizing may be advantageous in the elastic pulmonary valve, in which subsequent insufficiency is of little importance, it has to be strongly discouraged in a heavily calcified aortic valve of an elderly patient. The thickened, calcified cusps require space in addition to the balloon within the noncompliant annulus, and aortic insufficiency should be avoided as much as possible.

The Trefoil balloon may not be as efficient in dilating a valve as a single balloon, since it does not have circumferential contact with the valve. Yet it acts almost like a single balloon while it is not yet fully inflated, that is, in a tight valve. There it exerts the same dilating power as a single balloon, but on the other hand it lacks the single balloon's advantage of maintained blood flow since the space be-

Table 21-1 Mean Transmitral Pressure Gradient in Patients with Successful Valvuloplasty

				Pressure Gradient (mm Hg)	
Sex	*Age (yr)*	*Prior Commissurotomy*	*Balloon Size (mm)*	*Before Valvuloplasty*	*After Valvuloplasty*
Male	68	−	Trefoil 3 × 12	11	7
Male	14	−	Trefoil 3 × 12	24	6
Male	53	+	Bifoil 2 × 19	16	6
Female	53	−	Bifoil 2 × 19	15	7
Female	31	−	Bifoil 2 × 19	22	2
Female	32	−	Bifoil 2 × 19	24	16
Female	50	+	Bifoil 2 × 19	22	2

tween the balloons is minimal or none. Once fully unfolded, the Trefoil balloon permits inflations of several minutes across the pulmonary or aortic valve. Flow across the mitral valve appears less sufficient, probably because of the small pressure difference in the adjacent chambers.

Apart from the hemodynamic advantage of continuous transvalvular blood flow during full inflation, the Trefoil balloon also permits higher filling pressures than a corresponding single balloon. These advantages hold true for the Bifoil balloon as well. The Bifoil balloon will probably work best in terms of valve opening and maintained blood flow if it orients itself perpendicular to the long axis of the valve to be dilated (which is commonly the mitral valve).

Other authors have reported their results with two balloons introduced individually and inflated simultaneously. This technique is more cumbersome but has the advantage of smaller entry holes. This and the fact that sufficiently large single balloons were not available prompted the use of two balloons in the pulmonary valve[21-23] and the aortic valve.[24] The easier and less traumatic passage through the interatrial septum was an additional incentive to use two balloons for mitral valvuloplasty.[25,26]

To reduce bleeding and morbidity at the puncture site in aortic valvuloplasty and to facilitate transseptal passage in mitral valvuloplasty, we have developed the long sheath technique. The diameter of the puncture hole created by the largest sheath used (17F) is about 6 mm. This is smaller than the hole created by retraction of a deflated large valvuloplasty balloon, particularly if it had been ruptured during the intervention. Moreover, the sheath has a completely smooth surface that may further diminish trauma to the puncture site. Endeavors to miniaturize the deflated balloons to allow smaller sheaths are underway.

The hemostatic valve prevents bleeding even during catheter exchanges and the side arm permits continuous pressure monitoring. The sheath facilitates negotiation of tortuous iliac vessels and passage through the interatrial septum and through the stenotic valve provided it is used with a special backup wire and provided the stiff part of this wire is across the obstacle. Because of the danger of thrombus formation within the sheath, patients have to be heparinized and the sheath has to be regularly flushed.

Our initial clinical experience with Trefoil balloons, Bifoil balloons, and the long sheath technique for percutaneous valvuloplasty demonstrates that these interventions carry significant risks, particularly in mitral valves with large left atria in chronic fibrillation. The results are very satisfactory in pulmonary valves, promising in mitral valves and aortic valves of young people, but they are disappointing in our few elderly patients with calcified aortic stenosis seen in follow-up examinations.

REFERENCES

1. Kan, J.S., White, R.I., Jr., Mitchell, S.S.E., and Gardner, T.J.: Percutaneous transluminal balloon valvuloplasty for pulmonary valve stenosis, N. Engl. J. Med. **307:**540-542, 1982.
2. Lababidi, Z., Wu, J.R., and Walls, J.T.: Percutaneous balloon aortic valvuloplasty: results in 23 patients, Am. J. Cardiol. **53:**194-197, 1984.
3. Lock, J.E., Khalilullah, M., Shrivastave, S., Bahl, V., and Keane, J.F.: Percutaneous catheter commissurotomy in rheumatic mitral stenosis, N. Engl. J. Med. **313:**1515-1518, 1985.
4. Rupprath, G., and Neuhaus, K.L.: Percutaneous balloon valvuloplasty for aortic valve stenosis in infancy, Am. J. Cardiol. **55:**1855-1856, 1985.
5. Cribier, A., Savin, T., Saoudi, N., Rocha, P., Berland, J., and Letac, B.: Percutaneous transluminal valvuloplasty of acquired aortic stenosis in elderly patients: an alternative to valve replacement?, Lancet **1:**63-67, 1986.
6. McKay, R.G., Safian, R.D., Lock, J.E., Mandell, V.S., Thurer, R.L., Schnitt, S.J., and Grossmann, W.: Balloon dilatation of calcific aortic stenosis in elderly patients: postmorten, intraoperative, and percutaneous valvuloplasty studies, Circulation **74:**119-125, 1986.
7. Feit, F., Stecy, P.J., and Nachamie, M.S.: Percutaneous balloon valvuloplasty for stenosis of a porcine bioprosthesis in the tricuspid valve position, Am. J. Cardiol. **58:**363-364, 1986.
8. Zaibag, M.A., Ribeiro, P., and Kasab, A.S.: Percutaneous balloon valvulotomy in tricuspid stenosis, Br. Heart J. **57:**51-53, 1987.
9. Lababidi, Z., Wu, J.R., and Walls, J.T.: Percutaneous balloon pulmonary valvuloplasty. Am. J. Cardiol. **52:**560-562, 1986.
10. Leisch, F., Bergmann, H., Jr., and Herbinger, W.: Patent oval foramen protects against severe hemodynamic changes during percutaneous balloon pulmonary valvuloplasty, Int. J. Cardiol. **10:**303-306, 1986.
11. Shuck, J.W., McCormick, J.D., Cohen, I.S., Oetgen, W.J., and Brinken, J.A.: Percutaneous balloon valvuloplasty of the pulmonary valve: role of right to left shunting through a patent foramen ovale, J. Am. Coll. Cardiol. **4:**132-135, 1984.
12. Cribier, A., Savin, T., Berland, J., Rocha, P., Mechmeche, R., Saoudi, N., Behar, P., and Letac, B.: Percutaneous transluminal balloon valvuloplasty of adult aortic stenosis: report of 92 cases, Am. J. Cardiol. **9:** 381-386, 1987.
13. McKay, R.G., Lock, J.E., Safian, R.D., Come, P.C., Diver, D.J., Baim, D.S., Berman, A.D., Warren, S.W., Mandell, V.E., Royal, H.D., and Grossmann, W.G.: Balloon dilatation of mitral stenosis in adult patients: postmortem and percutaneous mitral valvuloplasty studies, J. Am. Coll. Cardiol. **4:** 723-731, 1987.
14. Meier, B., Friedli, B., Oberhänsli, I., Belenger, J., Finci, L., and Rutishauser, W.: "Trefoil balloon," un nouvel instrument pour la valvuloplastie percutanée, Schweiz. Med. Wochenschr. **116:**1667-1620, 1986.
15. Meier, B., Friedli, B., Oberhänsli, I., Belenger, J., and Finci, L.: Trefoil balloon for percutaneous valvuloplasty, Cathet. Cardiovasc. Diag. **12:**277-281, 1986.
16. Meier, B., Finci, L., Niederhauser, W., Adatte, J.J., Öztürk, M., and Rutishauser, W.: Long sheath technique for balloon valvuloplasty (abstract), Circulation 1987, (in press).
17. Meier, B., Friedli, B., and Oberhänsli, I.: Trefoil balloon for aortic valvuloplasty, Br. Heart J. **56:**292-293, 1986.
18. Van den Berg, E.J.M., Niemeyer, G.M., Plok-

ker, W.T.W.M., Ernst, S.M.P.G., and de Korte, J.: New triple-lumen balloon catheter for percutaneous (pulmonary) valvuloplasty, Cathet. Cardiovasc. Diag. **12:**352-356, 1986.
19. Musewe, N.N., Robertson, M.A., Benson, L.N., Smallhorn, J.F., Burrows, P.E., Freedom, R.M., Moes, C.A.F., and Rowe, R.D.: The dysplastic pulmonary valve: echocardiographic features and result of balloon dilatation, Br. Heart J. **57:**364-370, 1987.
20. Tynan, M., Baker, E.J., Rohmer, J., Jones, D.H., Reidy, J.F., Joseph, M.C., and Ottenkamp, J.: Percutaneous balloon pulmonary valvuloplasty, Br. Heart J. **53:**520-524, 1985.
21. Ali Khan, M.A., Yousef, A.L., and Mullin, C.E.: Percutaneous transluminal balloon pulmonary valvuloplasty for the relief of pulmonary valve stenosis with special reference to double-balloon technique, Am. Heart J. **112:**158-166, 1986.
22. Rey, C., Marache, P., Matina, D., and Mouly, A.: Valvuloplastie transluminale percutanée des sténoses pulmonaires, Arch. Mal. Coeur **5:**703-710, 1985.
23. Kasab, A.S., Ribeiro, P., and Zaibag, M.A.: Use of double balloon technique for percutaneous pulmonary valvotomy in adults, Br. Heart J. **58:**136-141, 1987.
24. Dorros, G., Ruben, F.L., James, F.K., and Janke, L.M.: Percutaneous transluminal valvuloplasty in calcific aortic stenosis: the double balloon technique, Cathet. Cardiovasc. Diag. **13:**151-156, 1987.
25. Palacios, I., Block, P.C., Brandi, S., Blanco, P., Casa, H., Pulido, J.I., Munozj, S., D'Empaire, G., Ortega, M.A., Jacobs, M., and Vlahakes, G.: Percutaneous balloon valvotomy for patients with severe mitral stenosis, Circulation **75:**778-784, 1987.
26. Zaibag, M.A., Ribeiro, P., Kasab, A.S., and Al Fagih, M.R.: Percutaneous double-balloon mitral valvotomy for rheumatic mitral-valve stenosis, Lancet **5:**757-761, 1986.

Chapter 22

Balloon Valvuloplasty of Congenital Lesions

Michael R. Nihill, MD
Charles E. Mullins, MD

The era of interventional cardiology started in the mid-1960s with the work of Dotter and Judkins,[1] who dilated peripheral arterial stenoses with graded bougie catheters. At about the same time Rashkind and Miller[2] introduced a balloon catheter into the heart to enlarge the interatrial septal defect in children with transposition of the great arteries. Gruntzig and co-workers[3] combined Dotter's technique with the concept of a balloon catheter to dilate peripheral arterial, renal, and finally stenotic coronary arteries in the mid to late 1970s. The technique of balloon dilatation of peripheral and central vessel stenosis was soon applied to the pulmonary valve in the late 1970s and early 1980s. In 1979 Semb and colleagues[4] used an angiographic CO_2-inflated balloon catheter to relieve severe congenital pulmonary valve stenosis in a neonate. Shortly afterward Jean Kan and associates[5,6] and other workers[7] converted the Gruntzig balloon design to a larger scale to dilate stenotic pulmonary valves. These techniques have now been applied to dilatation of every valve within the heart,[8,9] as well as dilatation for coarctation of the aorta,[10-12] of pulmonary artery branches,[13] pulmonary veins,[14] venae cavae,[15] and even subvalvular aortic membranes.[16]

A large experience has rapidly accumulated since 1982 in the field of dilatation of congenital cardiovascular lesions. Although the length of follow-up of these first patients treated with balloon dilatation is short, the initial excellent results have been enthusiastically received by both pediatric and adult cardiologists and the technique has been applied to a variety of congenital and acquired stenotic lesions in the heart and great vessels. Short-term evaluation of up to 5 years has revealed maintenance of the initial good results; an ongoing review of the early results has led to an evolution of the technique of dilatation for various lesions.

The results of balloon valvuloplasty depend on both the pathology of the lesion as much as the technique of dilatation. For instance, congenital pulmonary stenosis can be due to fusion of the commissures of a tricuspid or bicuspid valve, a pinhole opening in a membranous-like valve, or thick myxomatous leaflets. Valve stenosis may be associated with concomitant obstructive lesions such as a small pulmonary valve annulus, supravalvular pulmonary artery stenosis, subvalvular membranous obstruction, or congenital and acquired diffuse muscular infundibular stenosis. In the majority of patients with congenital pulmonary or aortic valve stenosis, the valve is mobile, domes are in systole, and the annulus is normal size. These valves can be very effectively dilated by inflating one or two rigid balloons across the annulus. Judicious overdistention of the valve annulus can virtually abolish the gradient with no restenosis over the next 2 to 5 years.

PULMONARY VALVE STENOSIS

Technique

A right-heart catheterization was performed using the percutaneous sheath technique[17] and a careful pullback recorded from the branch pulmonary arteries across the main pulmonary artery, pulmonary valve, and annulus to the subvalvular area and then to the right ventricular inflow tract. More than one area of stenosis may be identified in this fashion.

A Cardiomarker catheter (USCI Division of C.R. Bard, Inc., Billerica, Mass.) was positioned in the right ventricular apex or outflow tract near the pulmonary annulus so that the 1 cm marks at the tip of the catheter were perpendicular to at least one plane of the biplane angiographic system (Fig. 22-1). This catheter provides an intracardiac grid to measure the pulmonary annulus at the hinge points of the valve. We also perform a right ventricular angiogram in the anteroposterior (AP) and lateral projections with the catheter at the apex so that any infundibular stenosis may be identified. From the angiogram we also identify the level of the valve annulus and place a lead-shot marker on the chest wall so that the middle of the balloon may be placed across the annulus during dilatation. The balloon diameter is selected to be 30 to 60% greater than the measured annulus diameter for pulmonary valve stenosis. Depending on the size of the child and the femoral veins, one or two balloon catheters are used.[18] When the annulus size is greater than 18 to 20 mm in diameter, the bulk of the balloon catheter on a 9F shaft is often too large to fit easily into the relatively small femoral veins of children less than 15 years of age. We do not calculate effective dilatation areas or valve orifice areas, since we have found empirically that a combined balloon diameter of 50% greater than the annulus diameter produces very effective relief of isolated pulmonary valve stenosis (Table 22-1).[18]

Table 22-1 Pulmonary Balloon Valvuloplasty Technique

1. Single balloon (53 patients)	
Annulus 8–23 mm	Mean 15.1 mm
Balloon/annulus ratio 0.63–2.0	Mean 1.17
Mean gradient reduction 70.9%	(p = NS)
2. Double balloon (33 patients)	
Annulus 5–35 mm	Mean 19.3 mm
Balloon/annulus ratio 1–1.75	Mean 1.35
Mean gradient reduction 65.2%	(p = NS)

NS, Not significant.

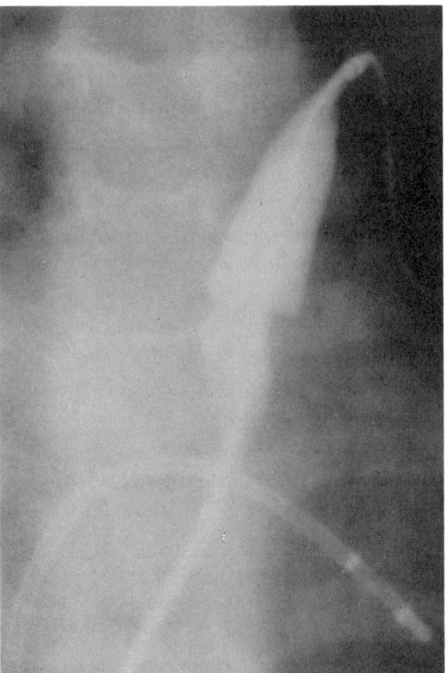
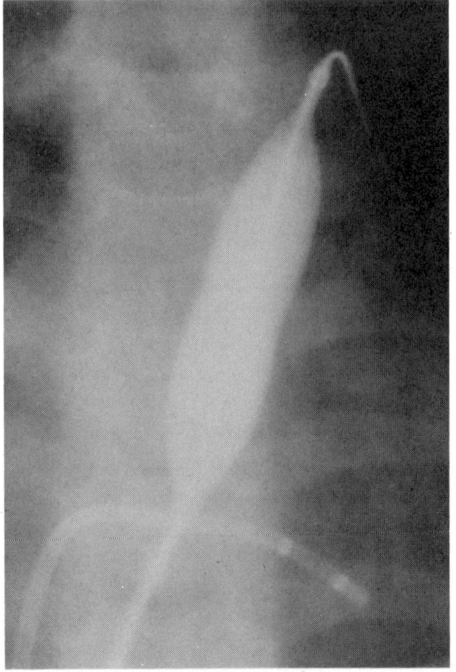

Fig. 22-1. Cardiomarker catheter in right ventricular apex. Markers are 1 cm apart. Left frame shows partially inflated balloon with indented "waist" formed by stenotic pulmonary valve. Right frame shows fully inflated balloon with disappearance of the waist as the stenosis is relieved.

An end-hole catheter was passed across the pulmonary valve, preferably into the left lower lobe pulmonary artery. A 0.038-inch Teflon-coated exchange wire (USCI Division of C.R. Bard, Inc., Billerica, Mass.; Argon Medical Corp., Athens, Tex.) with a curve formed at the floppy end was passed through the catheter and lodged in the left lower lobe pulmonary artery. The end-hole catheter and sheath were withdrawn leaving the exchange wire in place. A tightly furled balloon catheter (Mansfield Scientific Inc., Mansfield, Mass.; Medi-Tech Inc., Watertown, Mass.) was advanced percutaneously over the wire and positioned across the pulmonary annulus. If a single balloon was used, we advanced another catheter from the opposite femoral vein into the right ventricle to monitor pressure during balloon inflation and to measure a pullback gradient after the inflations. When two balloons were used from each femoral vein, a third venous access line was obtained from the brachial or axillary vein to monitor right ventricular pressure and administer drugs if necessary.[19]

The balloon catheter was inflated with a 1:5 diluted solution of contrast material. A "waist" should be seen in the midportion of the balloon, which should disappear with full inflation (Fig. 22-1). During inflation the operator must control the balloon position, for the balloon will tend to be ejected into the pulmonary artery during inflation. Likewise, when two balloons are used, one balloon may slide alongside the other into the pulmonary artery during inflation. After three to four inflations lasting 8 to 12 seconds, the balloons are withdrawn along the guidewires into the inferior vena cava and a pressure pullback is recorded from the main pulmonary artery, pausing be-

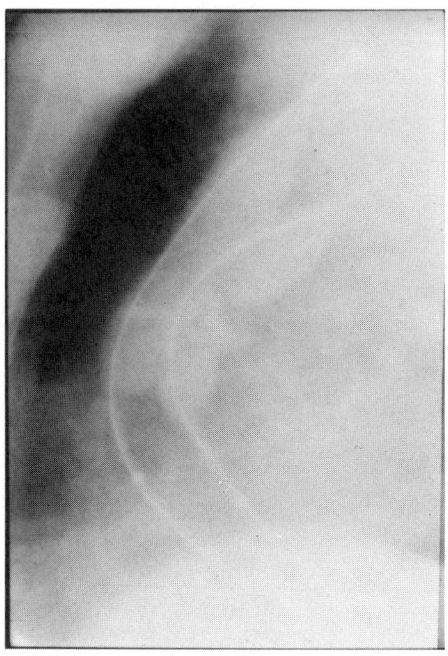

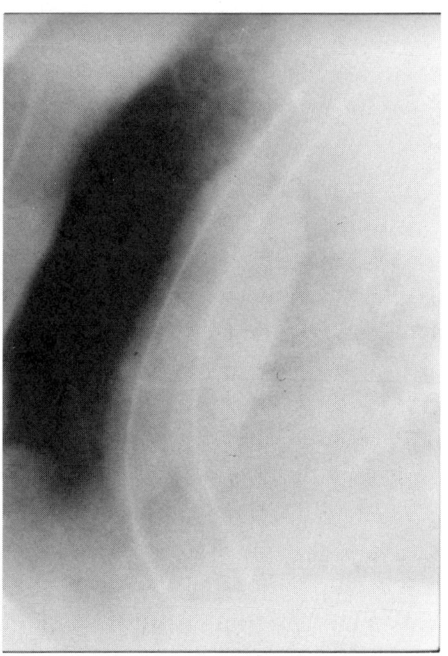

Fig. 22-2. Lateral view of two balloons across a stenotic calcified, pulmonary valve in a 71-year-old man.

low the annulus and then resuming measurement in the inflow portion. In most patients with isolated pulmonary valve stenosis, there was almost complete abolition of the valve gradient but sometimes there was a residual gradient across the infundibular portion of the right ventricle caused by septal hypertrophy or congenital infundibular stenosis.

Patients were sedated during the balloon inflation; some older patients experienced chest pain during inflation.

There was often significant tachycardia after several balloon inflations because of a rebound from the systemic hypotension produced by occlusion of the pulmonary valve. The degree of systemic hypotension is significantly less when two balloons are used or when there is an atrial septal defect or a patent foramen ovale. Two balloons side by side allow a significant amount of blood to pass around them into the pulmonary circulation. For example, a combined balloon diameter 20% greater than the annulus diameter occludes only 70% of the annulus area (Fig. 22-2). If there was significant tachycardia after balloon dilatation, we allowed some time for the heart rate to turn to predilatation levels before measuring the residual gradient. Propranolol may be administered to reduce the tachycardia induced infundibular narrowing.

Two infants had severe pulmonary valve stenosis with a dlated right ventricle and severe tricuspid regurgitation. The opening in the pulmonary valve was pinhole-sized (Fig. 22-3) and attempts to pass a full-size balloon across this could result in severe hypotension, bradycardia, and cardiac arrest. We used serial, graded dilatations starting with a small 4 to 5 mm balloon and performing progressive dilatations up to a balloon diameter 50% greater than the annulus (Fig. 22-4). We also recommend placing these children under general anesthesia with endotracheal intubation for better control of hemodynamics and respiration.

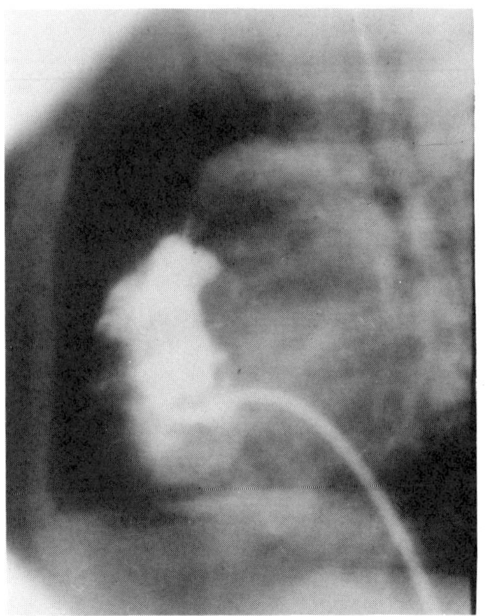
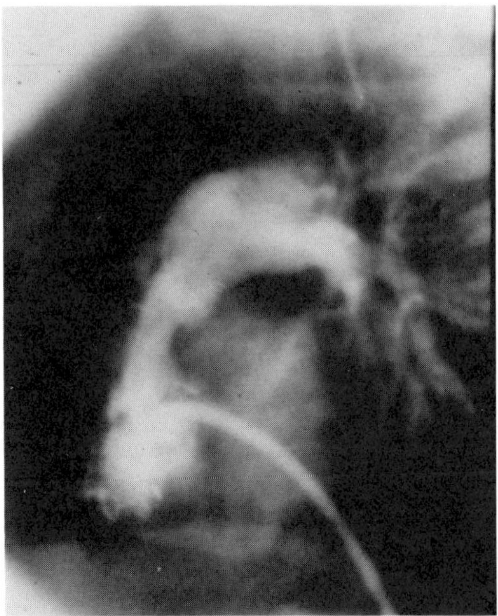

Fig. 22-3. Lateral view of right ventricular angiograms before *(left panel)* and after *(right panel)* balloon valvuloplasty in a 1-day-old infant.

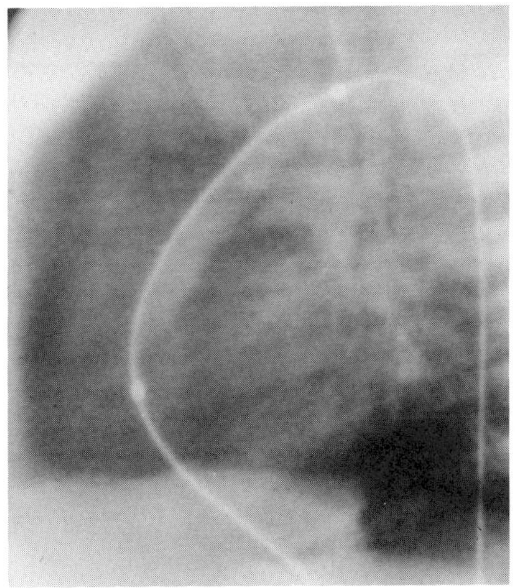
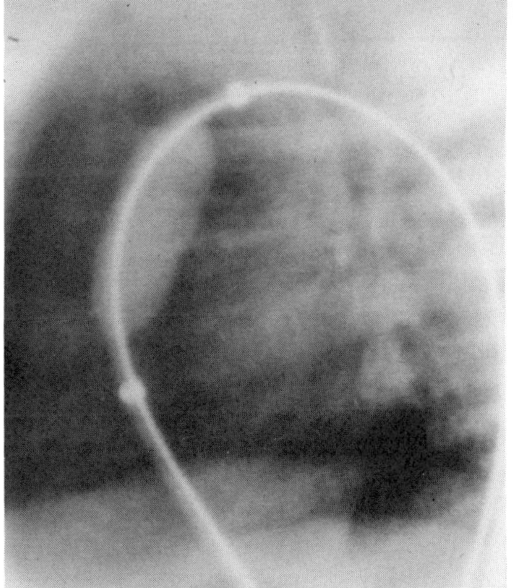

Fig. 22-4. Serial dilatation of the severely stenotic pulmonary valve of the infant in Fig. 22-3 with a 5 mm and later an 8 mm balloon catheter.

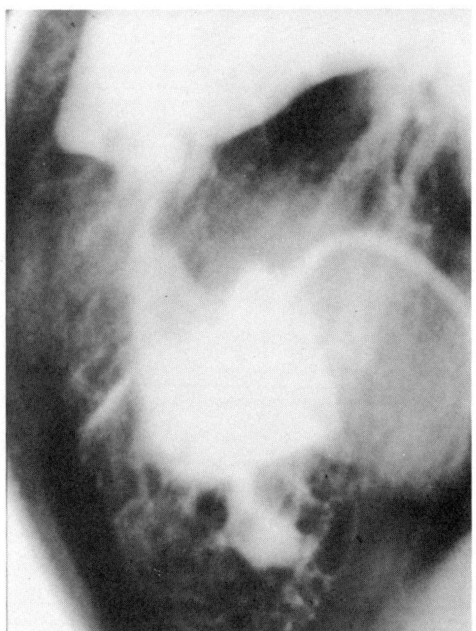

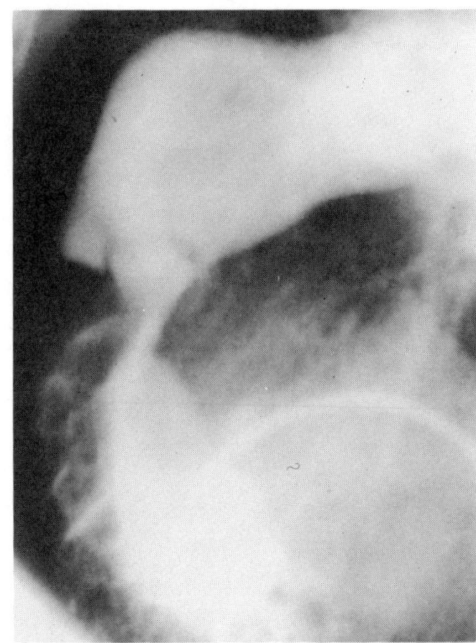

Fig. 22-5. Lateral view of a right ventricular angiogram of a patient with valve and severe infundibular pulmonary stenosis. The right-hand panel shows relief of the valve stenosis after balloon valvuloplasty while the infundibular stenosis remains.

Table 22-2 Pulmonary Balloon Valvuloplasty in 85 Patients

Patients	
Age: 1 day–76 yr	Mean: 7.6 yr
Weight: 1.11–77.5 kg	Mean: 23.12 kg
Associated defects	
Infundibular stenosis	19
Atrial septal defect	7
Pulmonary branch stenosis	6
PO valvotomy	2
Congestive heart failure, TVR	2

Patients (Table 22-2)

We have performed pulmonary valve dilatation in 85 patients ranging in age from 1 day to 76 years, with a mean age of 7.61 years. Three patients were 51, 71, and 76 years of age. Twenty patients were less than 1 year of age.

Seven patients had an atrial septal defect with associated pulmonary branch stenosis in two of these patients. Nineteen patients had markedly hypertrophied infundibular muscle or infundibular stenosis (Fig. 22-5) with an atrial septal defect present in four of these patients. Six patients had associated pulmonary branch stenosis with supravalvular pulmonary artery stenosis in three of these patients. The pulmonary annuli measured 5 to 35 mm in diameter and the balloon diameters were 5 to 25 mm. The overall ratio of the balloon diameter to the annulus diameter averaged 1.25 with a range of 0.63 to 2.0. Thirty-three patients had a double balloon dilatation with an annulus size of 5 to 35 mm (mean 19.3 mm).These patients had a balloon/annulus ratio of1.35, whereas those patients with a single balloon dilatation had a balloon/annulus ratio of 1.17.

Results (Table 22-3)

Right ventricular pressure ranged from 40 to 210 mm Hg before balloon dilatation (mean 89.43 ± 30.93 mm Hg), with a gradient of 20 to 192 mm Hg (mean 69.31 ± 31.78 mm Hg) (see Fig. 22-1). After balloon dilatation the right ventricular pressure ranged from 15 to 130 mm Hg, with a mean of 44.7 ± 20.67 mm Hg. The gradient after balloon dilatation ranged from 2 to 112 mm Hg, with a mean of 22.37 ± 19.58 mm Hg (Fig. 22-6). The percent drop in gradient ranged from 2 to 96%, with an average drop of 68.39% (see Table 22-1).

Two patients early in the series had an insignificant drop in gradient because of the use of a smaller balloon size than we currently use.

Table 22-3 Pulmonary Balloon Valvuloplasty in 85 Patients—Results

	RV Pressure (mm Hg)		*RV–PA Gradient (mm Hg)*		
	Prevalvuloplasty	*Postvalvuloplasty*	*Prevalvuloplasty*	*Postvalvuloplasty*	*% Change*
Mean	89.4	44.8	69.3	27.4	68.4
Range	40–210	15–130	20–192	2–112	2–96

RV, Right ventricular; PA, pulmonary artery.

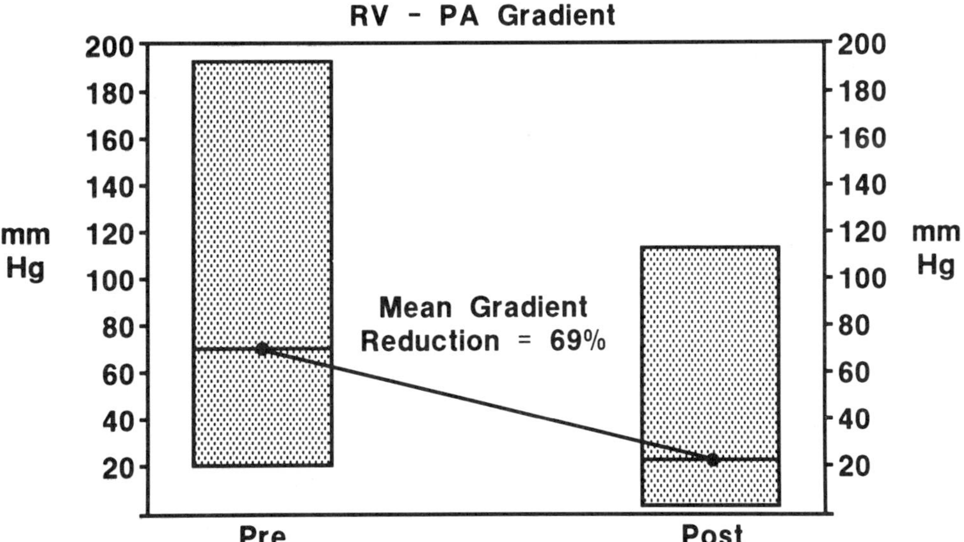

Fig. 22-6. Right ventricle to pulmonary artery peak systolic gradient before and after pulmonary valvuloplasty. The average reduction in the gradient was 69%.

Complications

There were no deaths in this series of 85 patients. Complications were minor, consisting of blood loss requiring transfusion in three infants and episodes of hypotension and bradycardia in two infants who had critical pulmonary stenosis and tricuspid regurgitation.

Conclusion

Isolated congenital stenosis of the pulmonary valve can be effectively relieved by balloon dilatation and the gradient reduced by 70 to 90% if the balloon diameter is 50% greater than the annulus diameter. Residual gradients are usually due to infundibular hypertrophy, which regresses over the ensuing 3 to 6 weeks. Follow-up studies with cardiac catheterization and Doppler echocardiography have shown no increase in the gradient.

PULMONARY VALVULOPLASTY WITH OTHER DEFECTS

Other forms of pulmonary stenosis have been treated by balloon dilatation. We have dilated the pulmonary valve in two patients who had tetralogy of Fallot, with an increase in systemic saturation from 58 to 69% and 83 to 86% (Table 22-4). Three patients with complex congenital heart disease have undergone pulmonary valvuloplasty. One patient had single-ventricle, double-outlet right ventricle and transposition; the second patient had mitral atresia, transposition, and ventricular septal defect; and the third patient had tricuspid atresia and transposition. There was a negligible increase in systemic saturation in these patients. Attempts were made to dilate the pulmonary valve in two neonates, one with Ebstein's malformation and a hypoplastic pulmonary annulus and one with absent pulmonary valve syndrome and suprasystemic pressure in the right ventricle. Both attempts were unsuccessful in relieving the pulmonary stenosis.

Obstructive prosthetic conduits from the right ventricle to the main pulmonary artery have been successfully dilated in three patients (Fig. 22-7). Gradients were reduced by 41 to 64%.

Table 22-4 Pulmonary Balloon Valvuloplasty for Miscellaneous Lesions

Rastelli conduit stenosis	3	Gradient reduction Mean 57% Range 41–64.3%
Tetralogy of Fallot	3	SaO_2 increase Mean 3.7% Range 0–11%
PVS + single ventricle	1	
PVS + mitral atresia	1	
PVS + tricuspid atresia	1	

PVS, Pulmonary valve stenosis; SaO_2, oxygen saturation.

AORTIC VALVE STENOSIS

Balloon dilatation of congenital aortic valve stenosis was carried out in 30 patients ranging in age from 12 days to 27 years (Table 22-5). Six patients previously had surgical aortic valvotomy, and one patient had a conduit from the left ventricular apex to the descending aorta because of a small aortic annulus.

Patients and Methods (Table 22-5)

The initial two patients had dilatation with a single 4 cm long balloon. This was quite successful in a 5-year-old patient with an annulus measuring 15 mm in diameter (Fig. 22-8), but it was unsuccessful in a 10-year-old patient whose annulus measured 23 mm. A 12-day-old infant with congestive heart failure and critical aortic stenosis underwent balloon dilatation using the prograde route through the foramen ovale, mitral valve, and left ven-

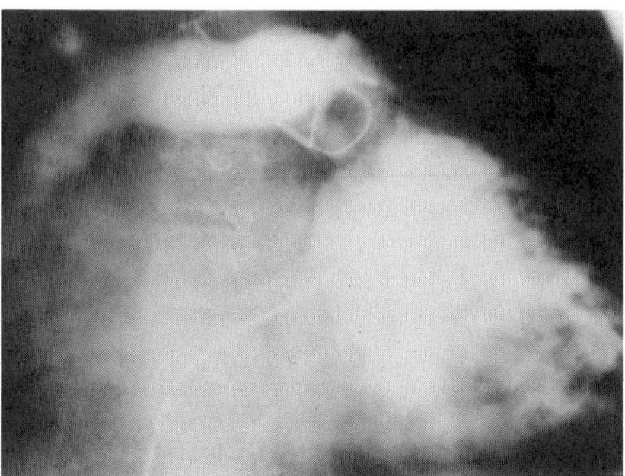

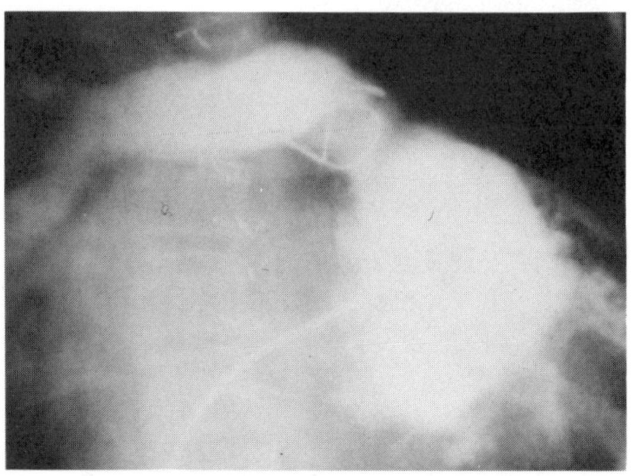

Fig. 22-7. AP right ventricular angiogram before *(top panel)* and after *(bottom panel)* balloon valvuloplasty of a stenotic bioprosthetic valve in a right ventricle to main pulmonary artery conduit.

tricular outflow tract. In the latter patient, the aortic annulus measured 7 mm. Initially a 4 mm and then a 6 mm balloon was advanced across the valve over a guidewire whose tip had been placed in the descending aorta (Figs. 22-9 and 22-10). Twenty-eight patients had dilatation with two balloons that were advanced retrogradely across the aortic valve.

After a right-sided heart catheterization, a Mullins transseptal sheath (USCI Division of C.R. Bard, Inc., Billerica, Mass.) was placed in the left atrium and a catheter advanced through the sheath into the left ventricle to monitor pressure. In three patients, a 9F

Table 22-5 Aortic Balloon Valvuloplasty in 30 Patients

Patients	
Age: 12 days–27 yr	Mean: 11.06 yr
Weight: 3.3–88.8 kg	Mean: 41.83 kg
Previous surgery: 7	
Aortic valvotomy	6
LV–Aortic conduit	1
Annulus diameter:	
7–30 mm	Mean: 21.03 mm
Balloon diameter:	
6–40 mm	
Balloon/annulus ratio:	
0.83–1.84	Mean: 1.15

LV, Left ventricular.

transseptal sheath was placed in the left ventricle to vent the ventricle to the femoral vein during balloon inflation. This has been found to be unnecessary; no untoward effects were noted when the ventricle was not vented, especially when two balloons were used. Angiograms were performed in the left ventricle in the right anterior oblique (RAO) and long axial projections to rule out subvalvular and supravalvular stenosis. A Cardiomarker (USCI Division of C.R. Bard, Inc., Billerica, Mass.) catheter was advanced retrogradely above the aortic valve for aortography, or placed in the left ventricle in infants, the diameter of the annulus was calculated in two planes, measured at the base of the doming cusps in systole. We recommend a combined balloon diameter of 10 to 20% greater than the aortic annulus measured at the base of the valves.

An end-hole catheter was advanced across the aortic valve into the left ventricle. Through this catheter, a 0.038-inch Teflon-coated exchange wire (USCI Division of C.R. Bard, Inc., Billerica, Mass.; Argon Medical Corp., Athens, Tex.) with a 180-degree curve formed at the soft end was passed into the left ventricle so that the apex of the curve was

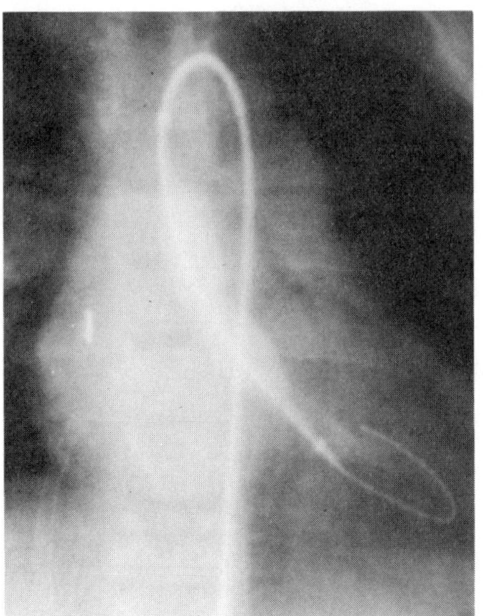
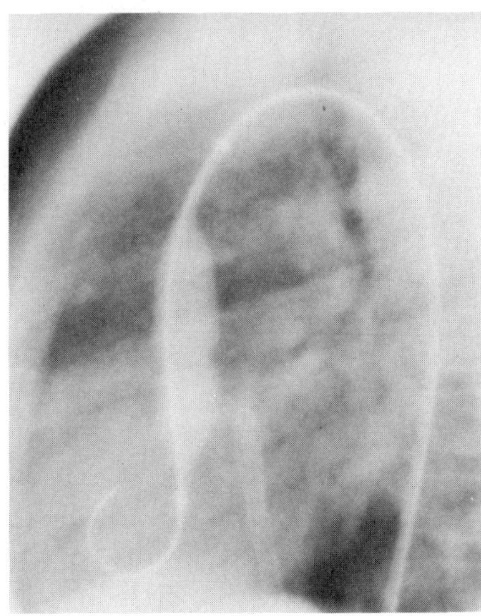

Fig. 22-8. Single balloon dilatation of aortic valve stenosis in a 5-year-old boy. A 9F transseptal sheath has been placed in the left ventricle as a vent during balloon inflation.

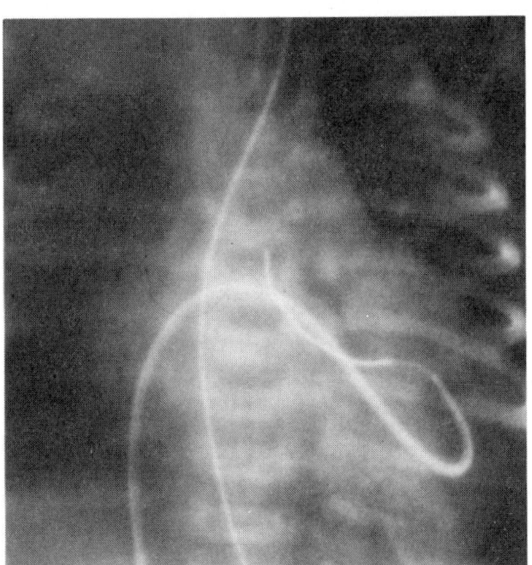
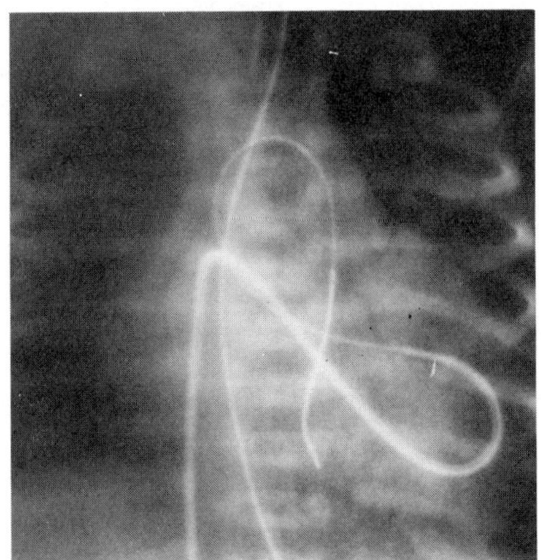

Fig. 22-9. Prograde dilatation of aortic valve stenosis in a 2-week-old infant. An end-hole catheter has been passed across the patent foramen ovale into the left ventricle and the tip deflected toward the aortic valve. A 0.018-inch guidewire was passed across the aortic valve and down the descending aorta.

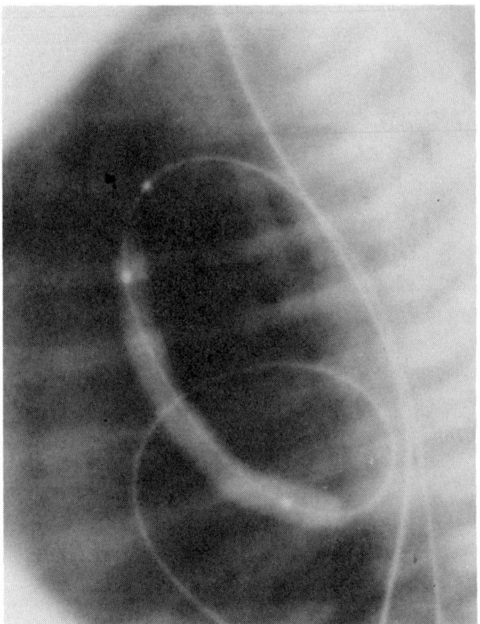
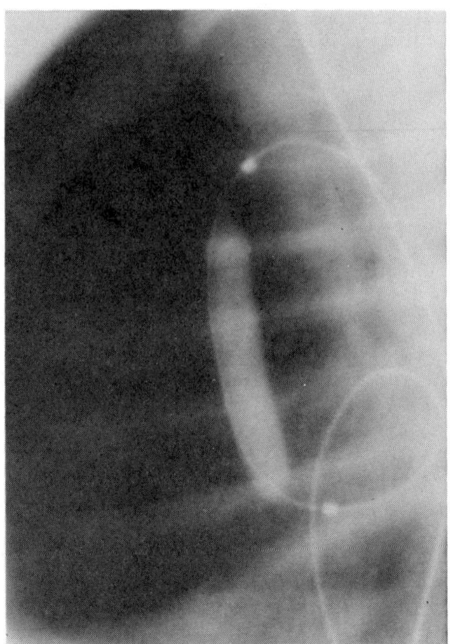

Fig. 22-10. Prograde serial dilatation of severe aortic stenosis with a 4 mm *(left panel)* and a 6 mm *(right panel)* balloon catheter in a 2-week-old infant.

at the apex of the left ventricle and the tip of the wire facing the left ventricular outflow tract (Fig. 22-11). A second end-hole catheter and wire was placed in a similar fashion in the apex of the left ventricle, and a second exchange wire advanced. With the wires in position and a stable cardiac rhythm established, the catheters were withdrawn over the exchange wires and the percutaneous sheaths and catheters were withdrawn. Tightly furled balloon catheters were inserted percutaneously over the guidewires and advanced to the aortic root. Long balloon catheters were used to dilate the aortic valve to avoid ejection of the partially inflated balloon. The length of the balloon was estimated to reach from the left ventricular apex to the midascending aorta. The balloon catheters were advanced singly across the aortic valve, and positioned to lie side by side with the midpoints at the previously marked aortic annulus. Both balloons were inflated simultaneously until the waist disappeared (Fig. 22-12). Left ventricular pressure was monitored during inflation, and in some patients a systemic pressure was monitored by a radial or brachial artery line. After an average of five inflations, both balloon catheters were withdrawn across the aortic valve and the left ventricular pressure was remeasured. In four patients, the transseptal sheath remained in the left ventricle during inflation and a balloon catheter was floated out to the ascending aorta before dilating so that simultaneous left ventricular and ascending aorta pressures could be measured. In the other patients, one of the balloon catheters was exchanged for an end-hole catheter that was advanced to the midascending aorta to record simultaneous left ventricle and ascending aorta pressure. If there was a satisfactory reduction in gradient obtained, the second balloon catheter was withdrawn and a second angiogram was obtained in the aortic root to estimate the degree of aortic regurgitation (Fig. 22-13).

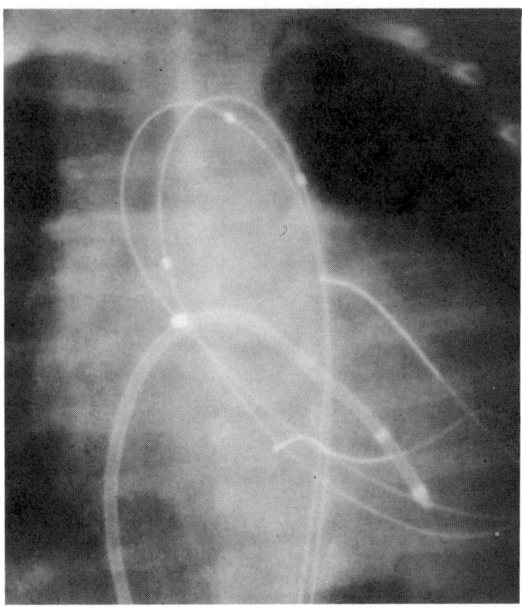

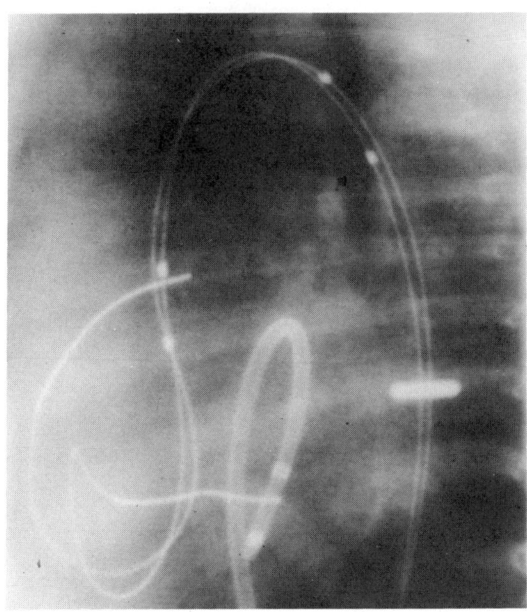

Fig. 22-11. Two exchange wires passed retrogradely into the left ventricle of a 2-month-old infant. Large curves are formed in the apex. A 6F Cardiomarker catheter is in the left ventricle to serve as an internal grid to measure the aortic annulus during angiography.

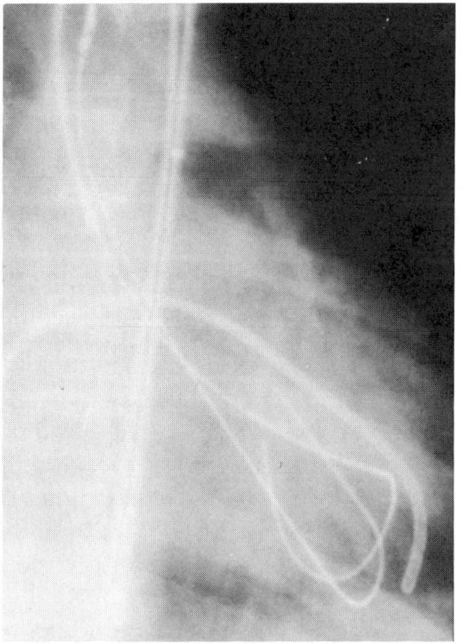

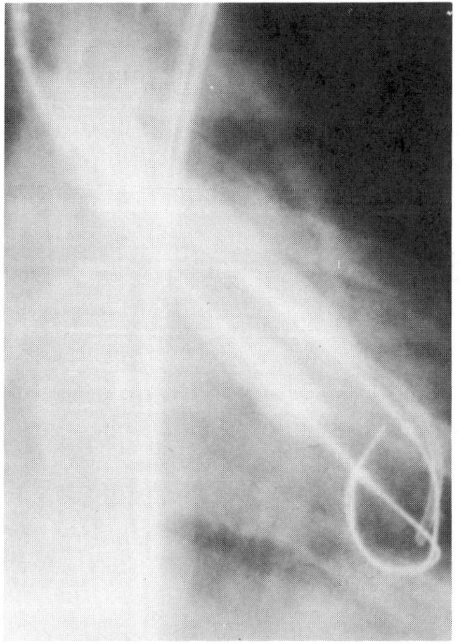

Fig. 22-12. Double balloon aortic valvuloplasty in a patient who previously had surgical valvotomy.

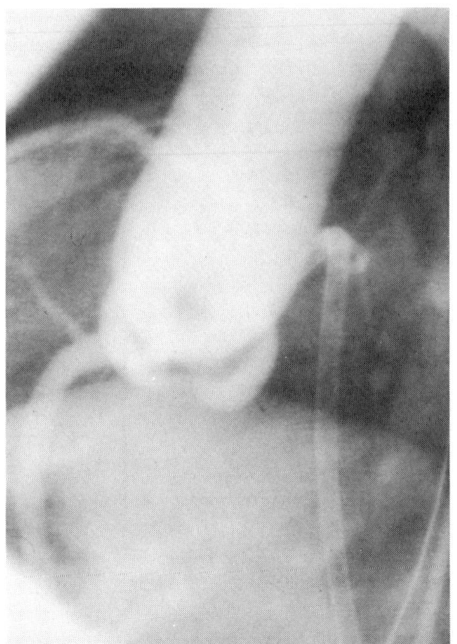
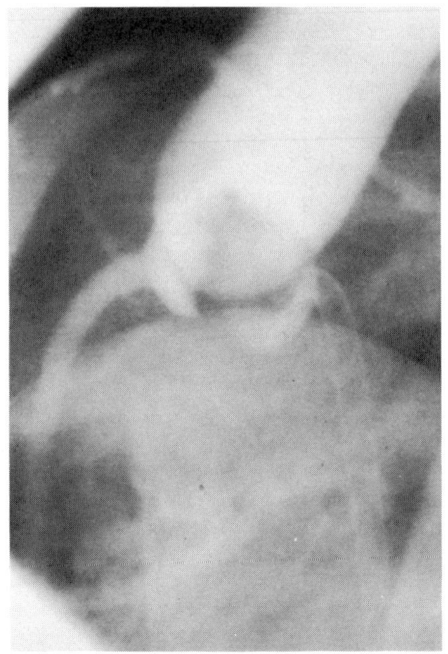

Fig. 22-13. Orifice view of aortic valve before *(left panel)* and after *(right panel)* valvuloplasty. The small circular orifice in the left panel has been converted into a large tricuspid orifice.

Table 22-6 Aortic Balloon Valvuloplasty in 30 Patients—Results

	LV Pressure (mm Hg)		*Gradient (mm Hg)*		
	Prevalvuloplasty	*Postvalvuloplasty*	*Prevalvuloplasty*	*Postvalvuloplasty*	*% Change*
Mean	177.1	136.6	73.5	27.3	62.5
Range	125–230	95–125	37–115	0–75	7–100

Results (Table 22-6)

The left ventricle/aortic gradient was reduced from a mean of 73.5 mm Hg (range 37 to 115 mm Hg) to a mean of 27.3 mm Hg (range 0 to 75 mm Hg) after balloon dilatation (Fig. 22-14). Aortic regurgitation was present in 11 patients before dilatation up to grade 1+ and was present in 17 patients after balloon dilatation. Two infants aged 12 days and 2 months were in heart failure before balloon dilatation but improved symptomatically, with a decrease in heart size and pulmonary edema and an increase in ejection fraction (Fig. 22-15). One patient with a small aortic annulus and previous left ventricle to aortic conduit had an unsuccessful dilatation and underwent surgery to enlarge the aortic annulus. Valve dilatation was unsuccessful in our first patient, who had a 23 mm annulus. She underwent surgical valvotomy.

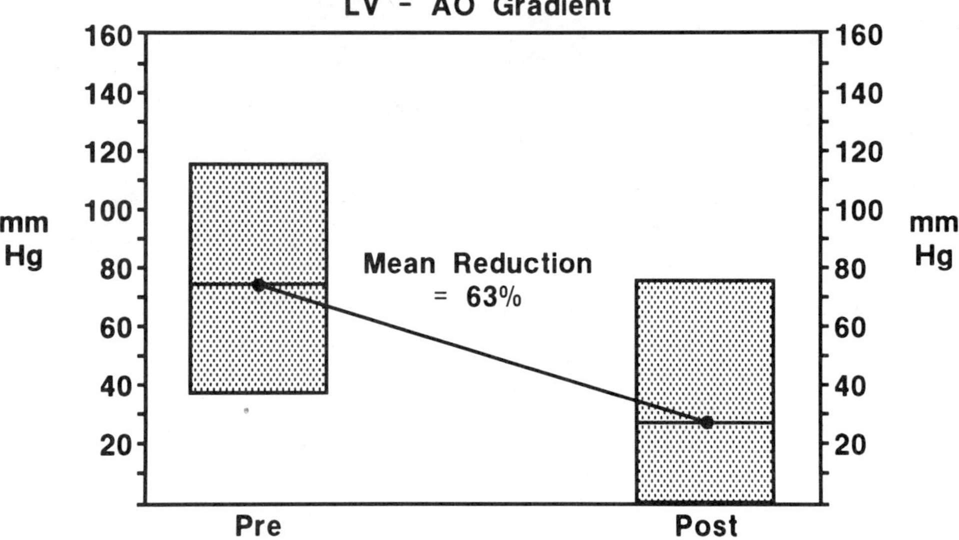

Fig. 22-14. Left ventricle to aortic peak systolic gradient before and after valvuloplasty. The average reduction in gradient was 63%.

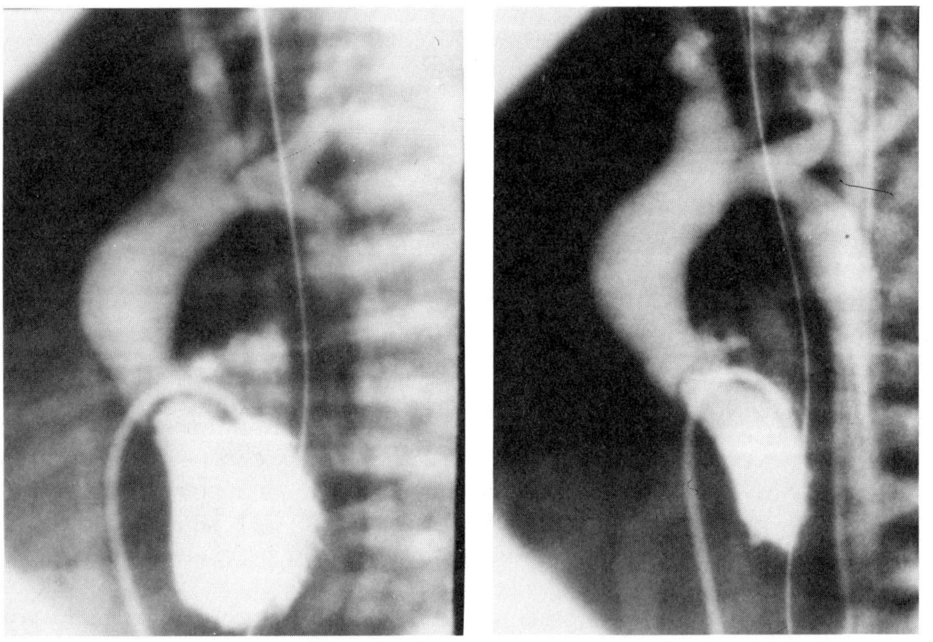

Fig. 22-15. Long avial projection of a left ventricular end-systolic frame before *(right panel)* and after *(left panel)* aortic balloon valvuloplasty in a 2-week-old infant.

Complications

Blood loss requiring transfusion occurred in one patient. Femoral pulses were decreased in 7 of 54 femoral arteries. Surgical exploration and embolectomy was required in one patient, and in the others the pulses returned with good peripheral circulation after the administration of heparin in three patients and intravenous streptokinase in three other patients. Transient left bundle branch block occurred during balloon inflation in eight patients and lasted from 30 minutes to 24 hours. In the latter part of our experience, the number of balloon inflations decreased and the incidence of left bundle branch block became infrequent and transient.

Conclusions

Balloon dilatation of congenital aortic valve stenosis can be achieved with excellent results comparable to those obtained by surgical valvotomy. There was a minimal increase in the degree of aortic regurgitation after valvuloplasty, and no patients required surgery for aortic regurgitation. Infants and children with congestive heart failure caused by critical aortic stenosis can have successful palliation and improvement in left ventricular function by balloon valvoplasty, making them more suitable candidates for surgery if necessary to achieve further reduction of the gradient.

MITRAL VALVE STENOSIS

Balloon dilatation of the mitral valve has been undertaken in 13 patients (Table 22-7). Two children had congenital mitral stenosis caused by fused commissures, and one child had a parachute mitral valve. The other valvuloplasties were undertaken with our colleagues at the Texas Heart Institute.

Patients and Methods

The technique of mitral valve dilatation is the same in children and adults. Two long balloons are used; the combined diameter is selected to equal the mitral annulus diameter measured from an apical echocardiogram or an RAO angiogram of the left atrium or left ventricle.

Table 22-7 Mitral Balloon Valvuloplasty in 13 Patients

Patients	
Age: 6–60 yr	Mean: 37.6 yr
Children 6, 8, 9 yr	
Pathology	
Parachute	1
Calcified	8
Regurgitation	10 (grade 1+)
Atrial fibrillation	5
Technique: two balloons	10 + 12 mm to 20 + 20 mm

A transseptal puncture was performed and a large 9 to 12F sheath (USCI Division of C.R. Bard, Inc., Billerica, Mass.) is advanced to the left atrium. All patients were anticoagulated. An end-hole catheter was advanced across the mitral valve to the left ventricle; thermodilution cardiac output and simultaneous pressures were measured in the left atrium and left ventricle. Angiography was performed in the left atrium in the RAO and lateral projections to measure the mitral annulus and to visualize the valve leaflets and distal orifice. Left ventricular angiography was also performed to estimate the degree of mitral regurgitation before the balloon dilatation.

Two different guidewire placements have been used in this small series. In seven patients, a large-bore balloon catheter was floated out to the aortic arch and a 0.038-inch Teflon-coated exchange wire was advanced through the balloon to the descending aorta. The balloon catheter was withdrawn and a Block double lumen catheter was advanced over the guidewire to the aortic arch or descending aorta. A second guidewire was advanced through this catheter to the descending aorta so that both wires were in one femoral vein. The double lumen catheter and sheath were withdrawn and two balloon dilatation catheters were advanced sequentially through the femoral vein and positioned across the atrial septum in the left atrium. Both guidewires were placed so that a wide loop was positioned well down into the apex of the left ventricle while the ends of the wire were in the ascending or descending aorta (Fig. 22-16). The long (6 to 8 cm) balloon catheters were advanced across the mitral valve so that the catheters pointed to the apex and not transversely across the short axis of the ventricle. Both balloons were inflated simultaneously with the midportion of the balloon across the distal orifice of the valve leaflets, making sure that none of the balloon was seated across the atrial septum. The balloons were inflated until the waist at the level of the leaflets disappeared (Fig. 22-17).

In six patients the exchange wires were not advanced into the ascending aorta and a curve at the distal floppy end of the guidewires was looped in the apex of the left ventricle with the tip of the wires pointing toward the outflow tract (Fig. 22-18). This technique can save considerable time, and the stability of the catheters was equal to those with aortic wires.

When the transseptal puncture is performed with a 10 or 12F sheath and dilator, we have not found it necessary to dilate the septum in order to pass the balloon catheters across. In children we have used a transseptal sheath from each groin, since the smaller size of the femoral vessels in children does not allow passage of two balloons through one femoral vein.

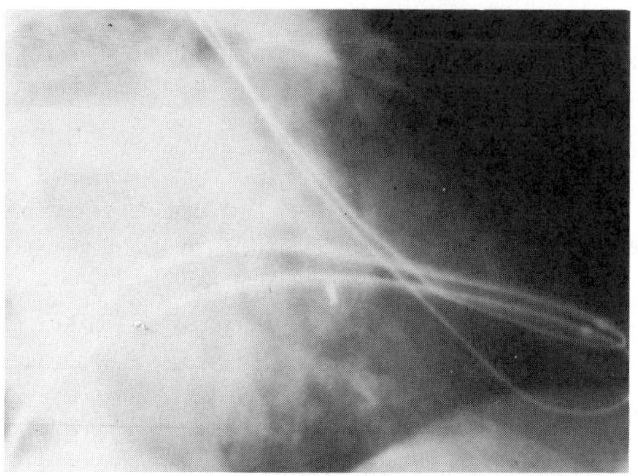

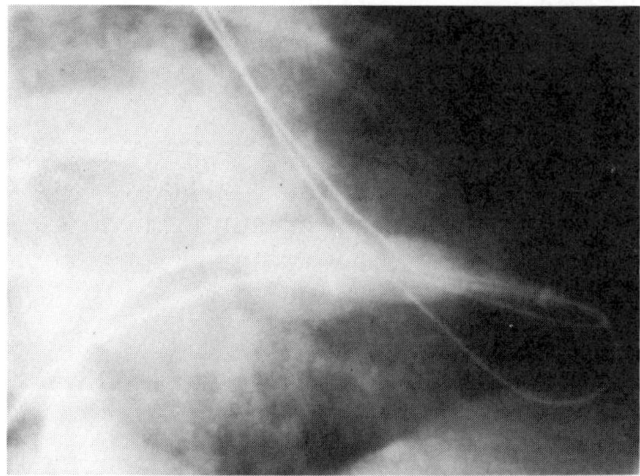

Fig. 22-16. Two balloons positioned side by side across the mitral valve. The balloons have been advanced over guidewires that have formed a loop in the apex of the left ventricle, and the ends of the wires are in the ascending aorta.

Results (Table 22-8)

The patients' ages ranged from 6 to 60 years. Balloon sizes ranged from 12 mm up to 20 mm. Six of the adult patients were in atrial fibrillation. The left atrial mean pressure to left ventricle end-diastolic pressure gradient averaged 10.33 mm Hg, with a range of 4 to 18 mm Hg before balloon dilatation, and fell to an average of 3.1 mm Hg (range 0 to 8 mm Hg) after dilatation. Those patients in sinus rhythm and an average a-wave gradient of 15.4 mm Hg (range 6 to 27 mm Hg) before ballooning had an average of 4 mm Hg (range 0 to 8 mm Hg) after dilatation.

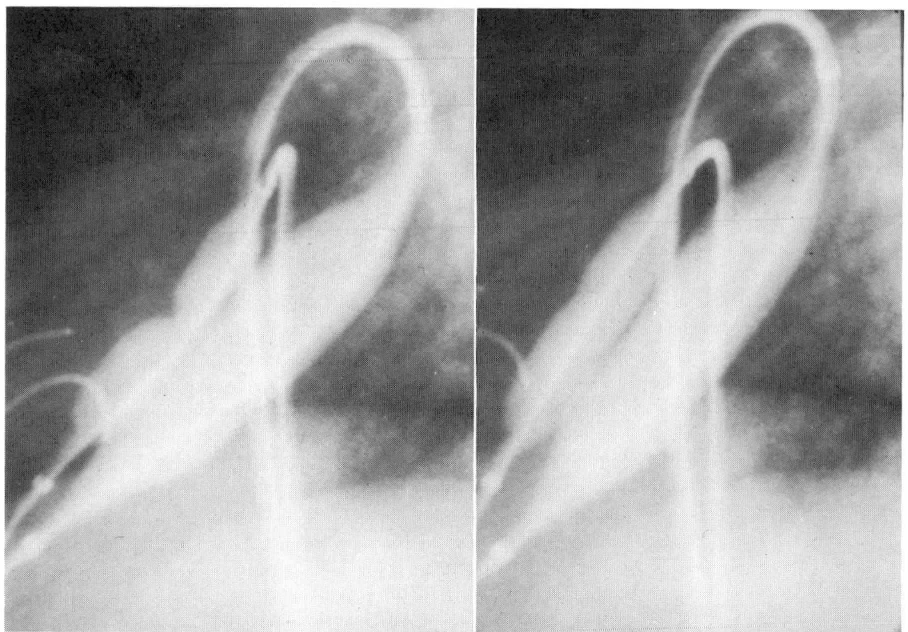

Fig. 22-17. Lateral projection of two balloons inflated across the mitral valve. The left panel shows a "waist" in the smaller balloon at the level of the stenotic orifice. The waist disappears with full inflation.

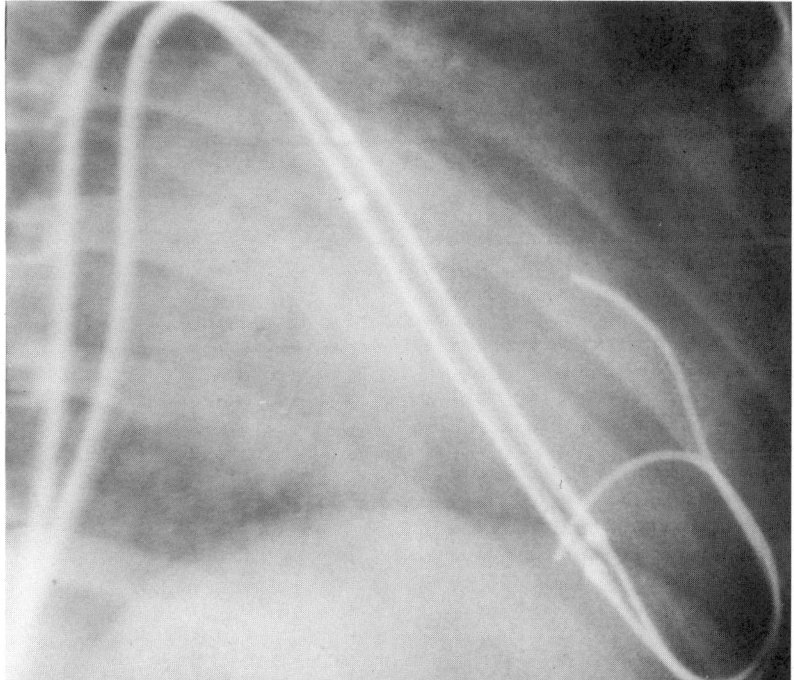

Fig. 22-18. Two balloons positioned across the mitral valve with the guidewires looped in the apex of the left ventricle and the tips pointing to the outflow tract.

Table 22-8 Mitral Balloon Valvuloplasty in 14 Patients—Results

	Mean LA Pressure–LVEDP (mm Hg) *Prevalvuloplasty*	*Mean LA Pressure–LVEDP (mm Hg)* *Postvalvuloplasty*	*% Change*
Mean	10.33	3.09	72.35%
Range	4–18	0–8	33–100

LA, Left atrial; LVEDP, left ventricle end-diastolic pressure.

Complications

One patient (not dilated) suffered a nonfatal myocardial infarction caused by a right coronary artery embolus after transseptal puncture. Pericardial hemorrhage occurred in another patient. Inflation of two balloons across the mitral valve was well tolerated with a moderate amount of systemic hypotension.

TRICUSPID STENOSIS

We have performed balloon dilatations for stenotic lesions of the right ventricular inflow tract five times. One patient had rheumatic tricuspid stenosis and previous replacement of aortic and mitral valves. His tricuspid valve was dilated on two occasions 1 year apart. Symptoms of restenosis occurred 9 months after the initial dilatation. Since the second dilatation, he has been asymptomatic for 12 months. Two patients with bioprosthetic valves in the tricuspid position underwent dilatation with relief of the gradient from the right atrium to right ventricle. One was a 54-year-old woman with a 27 mm Ionescu valve and the other a 10-year-old boy with a 33 mm porcine valve (Figs. 22-19 and 22-20). A 12-

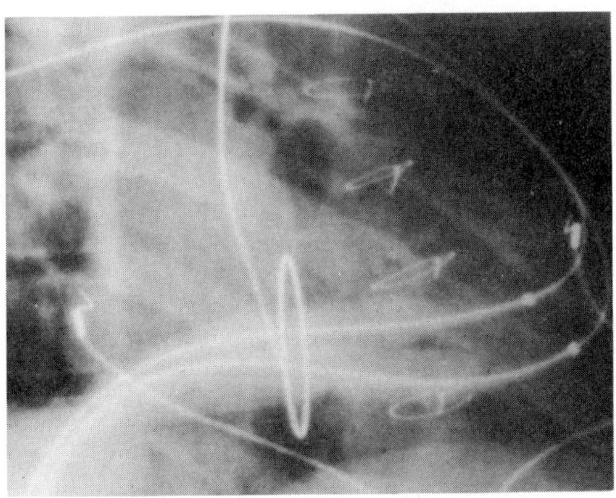

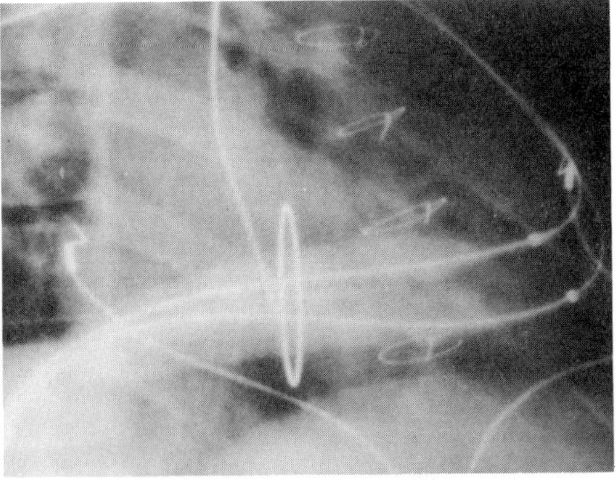

Fig. 22-19. Balloon dilatation of an obstructed prosthetic tricuspid valve.

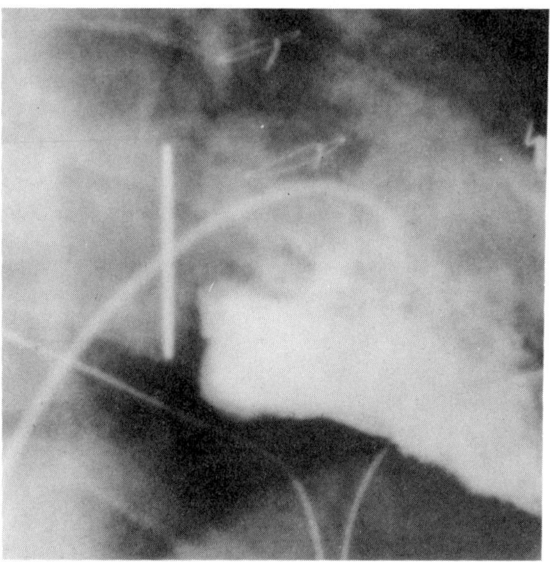

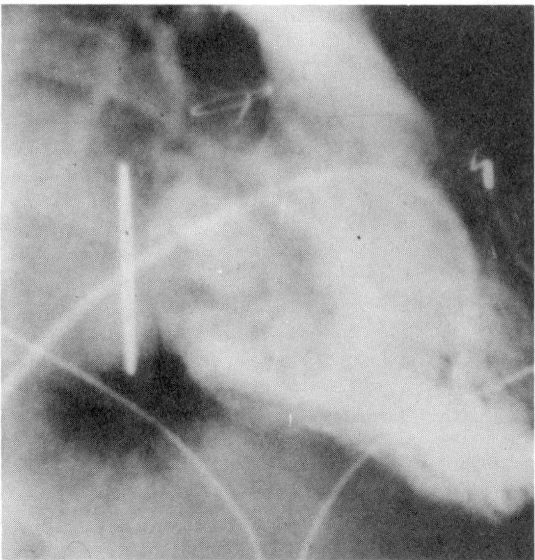

Fig. 22-20. RAO view of a right ventricular angiogram in a 12-year-old boy with an obstructed prosthetic tricuspid valve. Very restricted diastolic flow is seen in the left panel before valvuloplasty, and a much broader diastolic stream is noted after valvuloplasty *(right panel).*

year-old child had a conduit placed from the right atrium to the right ventricle as part of a Fontan operation for tricuspid atresia. She developed intimal thickening and stenosis at the proximal end of the conduit and this was successfully dilated with relief of right-sided heart failure (Fig. 22-21).

Technique

End-hole catheters are inserted in each femoral vein and passed across the tricuspid valve to the main and left pulmonary arteries. Teflon-coated exchange wires (0.038 inch) were advanced to the left pulmonary artery and the catheters and sheaths withdrawn over the guidewires. Two balloons whose combined diameter equaled the tricuspid annulus diameter were advanced over the guidewires with the distal tip of the balloons lying in the right ventricular outflow tract, and the midportion of the balloon across the annulus and tricuspid leaflets. Both balloons were inflated simultaneously. Elimination of the waist in the balloons was not possible with the prosthetic valves, but relief of the gradient occurred in both cases. When balloons are inflated across a rigid structure such as a prosthetic valve ring, balloon rupture may result in a circumferential tear of the balloon rather than the usual longitudinal tear. This may produce difficulties in withdrawing the balloon through the femoral vein because the distal part of the balloon inverts and becomes bulky or even detaches from the catheter shaft.

CONCLUSION

Balloon valvuloplasty has proved to be a very effective and safe technique in patients who have congenital stenotic lesions of the pulmonary, aortic, mitral, and tricuspid valves (Table 22-9). Balloon valvuloplasty is now the treatment of choice for isolated congenital pulmonary valve stenosis. The technique has a place as initial palliation for those children with congestive heart failure caused by severe pulmonary stenosis who have a

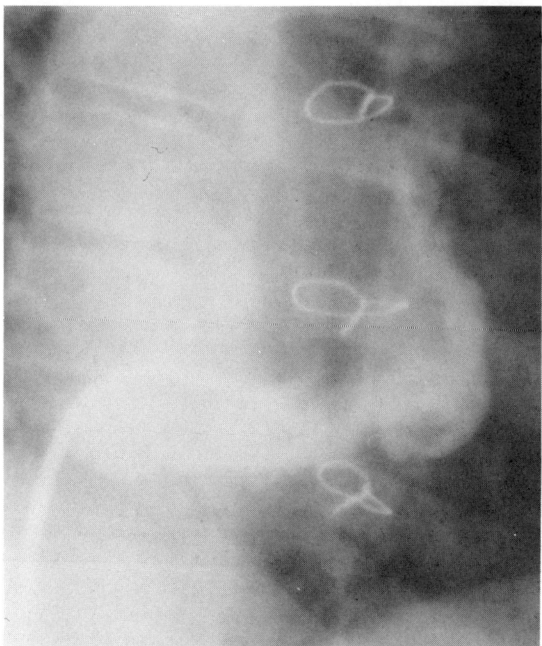

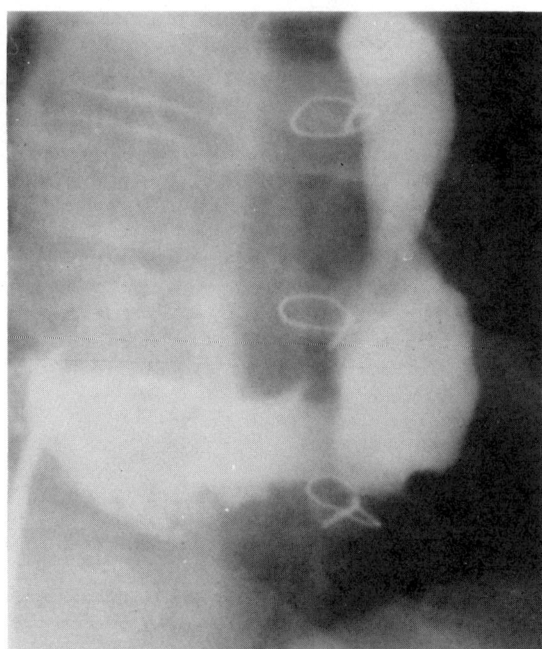

Fig. 22-21. Obstructed distal end of a conduit from the right atrium to the right ventricle in a 10-year-old girl after a Fontan operation *(left panel)*. The intimal ridges have been compressed by balloon dilatation.

Table 22-9 Selection of Balloon Size for Valvuloplasty in Children

Lesion	*Diameter Cf. Valve Annulus*	*Length*
Pulmonary valve stenosis	1.5 ×	Mid RV to bifurcation
Aortic valve stenosis	1.1–1.2 ×	LV apex to midascending aorta
Mitral valve stenosis	1.0 ×	LV apex to mid left atrium
Tricuspid valve stenosis	1.0 ×	RV outflow to low right atrium

RV, Right ventricle; LV, left ventricle.

small annulus. Likewise, balloon dilatation of stenotic valves in tetralogy of Fallot or other complex lesions may serve as an alternative temporary palliation. In these more complex lesions, the results are limited by the size of the pulmonary annulus and associated lesions, such as infundibular and supravalvular and branch pulmonary artery stenosis.

Palliation of congenital aortic valve stenosis is also amenable to balloon dilatation with results comparable to those obtained by surgical valvotomy. To ensure commissure splitting, we recommend that two balloons be used with a combined diameter of 10 to 20% greater than the aortic annulus diameter. Balloon dilatation of the aortic valve can also be performed with little increase in the degree of aortic regurgitation in those patients who have residual gradients after surgical valvotomy. Dilatation of membranous subaortic stenosis has been described by Lababidi and associates[16] but it appears that this might be limited to those subaortic membranes that are thin and close to the aortic valve.

Congenital commissural fusion of the mitral valve is rare but has been relieved by balloon dilatation using two balloons. Rheumatic mitral stenosis in children should be readily relieved as it has been in older patients, and would be the preferred method of palliation in small patients.

Bioprosthetic valves in children are notorious for undergoing degeneration and calcification resulting in stenosis and insufficiency. When these valves are used in conduits from the right ventricle to the pulmonary artery or from the right atrium to the right ventricle in a modified Fontan operation, early degeneration and obstruction of the valve may necessitate surgical removal of an otherwise adequate conduit. Balloon dilatation of conduits obstructed by "intimal peel" may enable one to postpone surgery until a time when a larger conduit can be placed.

After 5 years of trials and exploration, balloon dilatation techniques have been developed and modified to suit a variety of congenital and acquired stenotic lesions of cardiac valves, arteries, and veins. Some lesions, such as isolated pulmonary valve stenosis, will be exclusively treated by balloon dilatation, while others, such as pulmonary stenosis with a small annulus, may be initially palliated by balloon dilatation in order to improve ventricular function and cardiac output in preparation for surgical repair with cardiopulmonary bypass. Continued longitudinal follow-up and restudy of patients treated by balloon dilatation will allow guidelines to be formulated for optimal utilization of these techniques.

REFERENCES

1. Dotter, C.T., and Judkins, M.P.: Transluminal treatment of arteriosclerotic obstruction, Circulation **30:**654-679, 1964.
2. Rashkind, W.J., and Miller, W.W.: Creation of an atrial septal defect without thoracotomy: a palliative approach to complete transposition of the great vessels, J. Am. Med. Assoc. **196:**991-992, 1966.
3. Gruntzig, A., Kuhlman, U., Vetter, W., Meier, B., Lutolf, U., and Siegenthaler, W.: Treatment of renovascular hypertension with percutaneous transluminal dilatation of a renal artery stenosis, Lancet **1:**801-802, 1978.
4. Semb, B.K.H., Tjonneland, S., Stake, G., and Aabyholm, G.: Balloon valvulotomy of congenital pulmonary valve stenosis with tricuspid valve insufficiency, Cardiovasc. Radiol. **2:**239-241, 1979.
5. Kan, J.S., White, R.I., Jr., Mitchell, S.E., Anderson, J.H., and Gardner, T.J.: Percutaneous transluminal balloon valvuloplasty for pulmonary valve stenosis, Circulation **69:**554-560, 1984.
6. Mitchell, S.E., White, R.I., Kan, J., and Tolkoff, J.: Improved balloon catheters for large-vessel and valvular angioplasty, Am. J. Roentgenol. **142:**571-572, 1984.
7. Rocchini, A.P., Kveselis, D.A., Crowley, D., Dick, M., and Rosenthal, A.: Percutaneous balloon valvuloplasty for treatment of congenital pulmonary valvular stenosis in children, J. Am. Coll. Cardiol. **3:**1005-1012, 1984.
8. Lababidi, Z., Wu, J., and Walls, J.T.: Percutaneous balloon aortic valvuloplasty: results in 23 patients, Am. J. Cardiol. **53:**194-197, 1984.
9. Inoue, K., Owaki, T., Nakamura, T., and Miyamoto, N.: Clinical application of transvenous mitral commissurotomy by a new balloon catheter, J. Thorac. Cardiovasc. Surg. **87:**394-402, 1984.
10. Lock, J.E., Niemi, T., Burke, B.A., Einzig, S., and Castaneda-Zuniga, W.R.: Transcutaneous angioplasty of experimental aortic coarctation, Circulation **66:**1280-1286, 1982.
11. Lababidi, Z., Daskalopoulos, D.A., Stoeckle, H., Jr.: Transluminal balloon coarctation angioplasty: experience with 27 patients, Am. J. Cardiol. **54:**1288-1291, 1984.
12. Evans, V.L., Nihill, M.R., and Yousef, S.A.: Balloon dilatation angioplasty for coarctation of the aorta in infants, J. Am. Coll. Cardiol. **7:**46A, 1986.
13. Lock, J.E., Niemi, T., Einzig, S., Amplatz, K., Burke, B., and Bass, J.L.: Transvenous angioplasty of experimental branch pulmonary artery stenosis in newborn lambs, Circulation **64:**886-893, 1981.
14. Driscoll, D.J., Hesslein, P.S., and Mullins, C.E.: Congenital stenosis of individual pulmonary veins: clinical spectrum and unsuccessful treatment by transvenous balloon dilation, Am. J. Cardiol. **49:**1767-1772, 1982.
15. Lock, J.E., Bass, J.L., Castaneda-Zuniga, W., Fuhrman, B.P., Rashkind, W.J., and Lucas, R.V.: Dilation angioplasty of congenital or operative narrowings of venous channels, Circulation **709:**457-464, 1984.
16. Suarez DeLozo, J., Pan, M., Sancho, M., Herrera, N., Arizow, J., Franco, M., Concha, M., Valles, F., and Romanos, A.: Percutaneous transluminal balloon dilation for discrete subaortic stenosis, Am. J. Cardiol. **58:**619-621, 1986.
17. Neches, W.H., Mullins, C.E., Williams, R.L., Vargo, T.A., and McNamara, D.G.: Percutane-

ous sheath cardiac catheterization, Am. J. Cardiol. **30**:378-384, 1972.

18. Mullins, C.E., Nihill, M.R., Vick, G.W., Ludomirsky, A., O'Laughlin, M.P., Bricker, J.T., and Judd, V.E.: Double balloon technique for dilatation of valvular or vessel stenosis in congenital and acquired heart disease, J. Am. Coll. Cardiol. **10**:107-114, 1987.
19. Hesslein, P.S., Mullins, C.E., Kugler, J.D., and Gillette, P.C.: Percutaneous sheath brachial vein cardiac catheterization in children, Cathet. Cardiovasc. Diagn. **6**:197-205, 1980.

Chapter 23

Elective Coronary Angioplasty and Aortic Valvuloplasty Using Semipercutaneous Cardiopulmonary Support

Robert A. Vogel, MD, FACC
Carl L. Tommaso, MD
Steven R. Gundry, MD

Over the past 10 years coronary angioplasty has become widely utilized for the treatment of coronary artery disease.[1] More recently balloon valvuloplasty has been introduced for the management of aortic, mitral, and pulmonic valvular stenosis.[2] Both interventions have risk/benefit ratios that make them acceptable for treating selected patients. Coronary angioplasty is associated with an approximate 5% risk of acute arterial closure.[3] This complication is usually managed with emergent coronary artery bypass surgery, which in this instance is associated with a 2 to 10% mortality.[4] Patients whose target vessels supply large amounts of myocardium and those with substantially reduced left ventricular function are often not considered angioplasty candidates because of the hemodynamic collapse associated with vessel occlusion. At times intraaortic balloon pumping is used prophylactically in conjunction with angioplasty in high-risk patients.[5,6] Balloon pumping is also often utilized following angioplasty-induced vessel closure in order to hemodynamically stabilize patients as they are transported to the operating room. Intraoperative angioplasty has also been performed in cardiopulmonary bypass surgery as adjunctive therapy to surgical revascularization.[7]

Balloon valvuloplasty of the aortic valve has been performed successfully in patients who have high operative risk or operative contraindication. Balloon inflation across the aortic valve is associated with substantial reduction of cardiac output, hypotension, and ventricular arrhythmias. Since aortic valvuloplasty is generally performed in older patients and in those who have significant concomitant medical illnesses, this intervention has associated morbidity and mortality. To reduce the problems associated with high-risk coronary angioplasty and aortic valvuloplasty, we have prophylactically placed patients on semipercutaneous cardiopulmonary bypass in the cardiac catheterization laboratory before the performance of these interventions. The cardiopulmonary support system has been previously utilized in the management of critically ill patients.[8] We have termed this technique supported angioplasty or valvuloplasty. Patient descriptions, technique, and outcomes for the first seven patients managed by this approach are described in this chapter.

PATIENT POPULATION

From December 21, 1987 to February 17, 1988 three patients underwent supported angioplasty and four patients underwent supported valvuloplasty at the University of Maryland Hospital. Patients were selected for supported angioplasty based on the following criteria:

1. Presence of severe angina pectoris, unstable angina pectoris, or acute infarction with shock syndrome
2. At least one technically ideal dilatable coronary stenosis
3. Presence of severe left ventricular dysfunction and/or a large amount of myocardium perfused by the index vessel

Brief descriptions of the three patients undergoing supported angioplasty during this period are as follows:

Patient 1: A 68-year-old man was diagnosed with anterior non–Q wave myocardial infarction followed by unstable angina. He had a 10-year history of congestive heart failure recently requiring diuretics, vasodilators, and digitalis. Coronary arteriography revealed high-grade proximal stenosis of a large ramus medianus branch, and radionuclide angiography demonstrated a left ventricular ejection fraction of 26%.

Patient 2: A 53-year-old man had severe angina pectoris 6½ years following saphenous vein bypass graft surgery. Coronary arteriography revealed high-grade stenosis of the distal left main coronary artery; severe diffuse disease of the left anterior descending, left circumflex, and right coronary arteries; and patent grafts to the circumflex marginal and posterior descending vessels. Left ventriculography demonstrated an ejection fraction of 32%.

Patient 3: A 40-year-old man was diagnosed with unstable angina 1 week following an acute inferior myocardial infarction. Coronary arteriography revealed total occlusion of the right coronary artery, which filled by collaterals from the left anterior descending coronary artery, and high-grade stenoses of the proximal left anterior descending coronary artery and distal left circumflex coronary artery. Left ventriculography revealed an ejection fraction of 60%. The patient related a strong preference for coronary angioplasty over bypass surgery.

During the same period, four patients underwent aortic valvuloplasty. The ages of these patients ranged from 68 to 92 years, peak-to-peak aortic valve gradients ranged from 50 to 115 mm Hg and aortic valve areas ranged from 0.3 to 0.5 cm^2. All patients were highly symptomatic and in frail health.

PROCEDURE

All procedures were done in the cardiac catheterization laboratory by a team composed of two cardiologists, a cardiothoracic surgeon, an anesthesiologist, and a perfusionist. Standard premedication and local anesthesia were used and a cardiothoracic operating suite was available on a standby basis. Angioplasty or valvuloplasty arterial sheets were placed in the left femoral artery using Judkins' technique in six patients, and one coronary angioplasty was performed by way of the right antecubital fossa using Sones' technique in the seventh patient. Surgical exposure of the right femoral artery and vein was performed under local anesthesia, following which heparin was administered intravenously (300 units per kg body weight). A guidewire was then inserted into the right femoral vein and advanced under fluoroscopic control to the right atrium. A 20F multihole catheter (C.R. Bard, Inc., Billerica, Mass.) was passed over the guidewire and advanced to the right atrium. An 18 to 20F catheter was inserted over a guidewire into the right femoral artery and passed to the distal aorta. These cannulas were connected to the cardiopulmonary support system (C.R. Bard, Inc., Billerica, Mass.), which consists of a Biomedicus pump proximal in series to an oxygenator. Cardiopulmonary support was performed by pumping 3 to 5 L/min of blood from the femoral vein to the femoral artery. Following establishment of satisfactory cardiopulmonary support, angioplasty or valvuloplasty was performed in the usual manner. Inflation times ranged from 90 to 180 seconds for both types of interventions. In two of three angioplasty patients, oxygenated blood was pumped through the dilatation catheter to provide distal coronary perfusion. Arterial pressure, capillary wedge pressure, and oxygen saturation were followed during cardiopulmonary support, which lasted from 30 to 90 minutes. At the end of each intervention, circulatory support was tapered and the catheters were removed. The femoral vein and artery were closed by suture. Reversal of heparin by protamine administration was performed in the valvuloplasty but not the angioplasty patients.

RESULTS

Dilatation of the ramus medianus branch, left main coronary artery, and left anterior descending and midcircumflex coronary arteries were performed successfully in patients 1 through 3 respectively. Residual stenoses were less than 40% and residual translesional gradients were less than 20 mm Hg in all instances. Aortic valve areas at least doubled in all patients undergoing valvuloplasty. No significant problems were encountered during the supported procedures. Hypotension, responding to fluid load, occurred during one supported angioplasty and self-terminating, 10-second duration ventricular tachycardia occurred during two valvuloplasties.

During cardiopulmonary support, filling pressures dropped substantially and were managed by fluid administration. At the end of cardiopulmonary bypass, approximately 1.5 L of blood remain in the support system, which cannot be pumped directly back into the patient. All patients required blood transfusions of 3 to 8 units following the intervention. Surgical reanastomosis of one right femoral artery perfusion site and of two left femoral artery valvuloplasty insertion sites were required following evidence of ischemia. In one patient a significant hematoma developed in the right thigh that did not require reexploration.

Five of the seven patients had symptomatic relief following the intervention. One angioplasty patient (patient 1) continued to have atypical chest pain unassociated with enzymatic or electrocardiographic evidence of ischemia or infarction. This gradually subsided after medical therapy. The 92-year-old patient undergoing aortic valvuloplasty died 12 hours after the procedure following sudden onset of ventricular fibrillation. All other patients were discharged or returned to referring hospitals within 2 to 5 days.

DISCUSSION

Cardiopulmonary support appears to be a valuable addition to high-risk coronary angioplasty and aortic valvuloplasty performed in the catheterization laboratory. Coronary angioplasty can be performed in patients with large areas of jeopardized myocardium and/or substantially reduced ventricular function. Such patients might otherwise have to undergo high-risk unsupported angioplasty or bypass surgery. In patients with multiple prior surgical interventions, no other revascularization procedure seems possible.

Circulatory support can be maintained irrespective of cardiac rhythm or pump function. Femoral vein–femoral artery technique is a well-established approach and has been widely utilized during open heart surgery. If coronary angioplasty resulted in vessel occlusion, patients could be transported to the operating room in hemodynamically stable condition. Because cardiopulmonary support accomplishes substantial cardiac unloading, myocardial infarction following coronary occlusion would be minimized. Patients going to surgery following failed angioplasty would also have a greater potential for undergoing internal mammary artery grafting, since the urgency for revascularization would be lessened during this more time-consuming but desirable procedure. Additionally, circulatory support permits long balloon inflation times that may improve results for both coronary artery and valvular intervention.

One of seven patients required surgical revision of the arterial perfusion catheter site. This complication may be reducible following greater clinical experience. At present, the greatest problem appears to be the need for blood replacement, although it is likely that the use of cell savers and autotransfusion will reduce this need in the future.

Supported angioplasty and valvuloplasty clearly foster a sense of cooperation between the cardiology and cardiothoracic surgical teams. Operator concern for arrhythmias, hemodynamic instability, and vessel occlusion are clearly reduced. Circulatory support provides a therapeutic bridge between surgical intervention and unsupported angioplasty in terms of decision making. It should also provide less urgency and more optimal bypass procedures following failed angioplasty. Although our experience demonstrates that this new technique is clinically feasible, considerably more experience is required to determine whether it is truly efficacious.

REFERENCES

1. Detre, K., et al.: Percutaneous transluminal coronary angioplasty in 1985-1986 and 1977-1981. The National Heart, Lung, and Blood Institute Registry, N. Engl. J. Med. **318:**265, 1988.
2. McKay, R.G., Safian, R.D., et al.: Balloon dilatation of calcific aortic stenosis in elderly patients: Post-mortem intraoperative and percutaneous studies, Circulation **74:**119, 1986.
3. Cowley, M.J., Dorros, G., Kelsey, S.F., et al.: Acute coronary events associated with percutaneous transluminal coronary angioplasty, Am. J. Cardiol. **53:**12C, 1984.
4. Cowley, M.J., Dorros, G., Kelsey, S.F., et al.: Emergency coronary bypass surgery after coronary angioplasty: The National Heart, Lung, and Blood Institute's percutaneous transluminal coronary angioplasty registry experience, Am. J. Cardiol. **53:**22C, 1984.
5. Margolis, J.R.: The role of the percutaneous intra-aortic balloon in emergency situations following percutaneous transluminal coronary angioplasty. In Kaltenbach, M., Gruentzig, A., Rentrop, K., Bussman, W.-D., editors: Transluminal coronary angioplasty and intracoronary thrombolysis, Berlin, 1982, Springer-Verlag.
6. Alcan, K.E., Stertzer, S.H., Walsh, J.E., et al.: The role of intra-aortic balloon counterpulsation in patients undergoing percutaneous transluminal coronary angioplasty, Am. Heart. J. **105:**527, 1983.
7. Jones E.L., King, S.B.: Intraoperative balloon-catheter dilatation in the treatment of coronary artery disease. Am. Heart. J. **107:**836, 1984.
8. Phillips, S.J.: Percutaneous initiation of cardiopulmonary bypass. Ann. Thorac. Surg. **36:**2, 1983.

Chapter 24

Advances in Percutaneous Transluminal Coronary Angioplasty:
Observations with the Hartzler Micro-Bore Balloon Catheter

Geoffrey O. Hartzler, MD, FACC

The Hartzler Micro balloon catheter ("Micro"), manufactured by Advanced Cardiovascular Systems, Inc., is one of several newer generation angioplasty catheters. This device was developed as a variation of the Hartzler LPS catheter and in response to at least some of the limitations of that device. The Micro is a low-profile, relatively high-pressure, over-the-wire, flexible balloon catheter with a self-venting mechanism for preparation.

MECHANISM OF ACTION

Industry's refinement of the extrusion process has allowed creation of this unique polyethylene balloon catheter with inflated dimensions of 1.5, 2.0, 2.5, 3.0, and 3.5 mm. The deflated Micro balloon dimension averages 2/1000th to 3/1000th of an inch smaller than the Simpson ultra low profile catheter (American Cardiovascular Systems, Inc.) and 3/1000th of an inch larger than the LPS catheter. Independent testing has been performed to measure deflated profiles defined as the ability to pass prepared balloons through prebored holes in an acrylic plastic (Plexiglas) block. Deflated dimensions with 95% confidence limits were 0.038 to 0.039 inch for the 1.5 mm balloon, 0.039 to 0.040 inch for the 2.0 mm balloon, 0.045 to 0.048 inch for the 2.5 mm balloon, and 0.049 to 0.053 for the 3.0 mm balloon.

The Micro balloon incorporates a self-venting mechanism. This simplifies and speeds catheter preparation and has allowed removal of the vent tube from previous catheter designs. When filled with a contrast agent and inflated to 60 to 75 psi, air is gradually expelled from the balloon through a "pore" at the distal balloon tip.

Catheter Shaft

The Micro balloon catheter shaft is significantly smaller than standard angioplasty balloon catheters. The shaft of the 1.5 and 2.0 mm Micro catheter measures 3.2F correlating

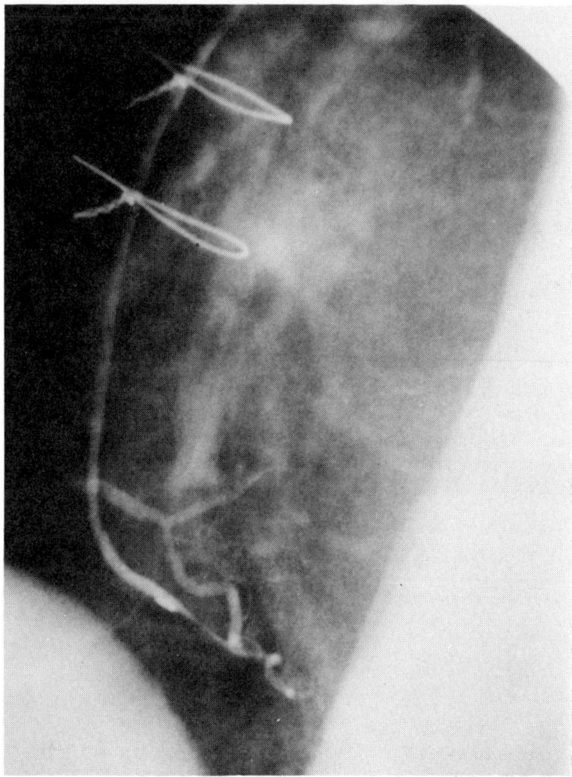

Fig. 24-1. First sequence of cineangiographic frames illustrating many properties of the Micro balloon catheter. There is a high-grade tubular stenosis in the distal aspect of a vein graft that inserts on the midposterior descending branch as visualized in this left anterior oblique (LAO) projection.

with a 63% increase in unobstructed internal guiding catheter area in an 8F, 0.072-inch guiding catheter relative to standard balloon catheters with a 4.3F shaft. The 2.5, 3.0, and 3.5 mm Micro catheters have 3.4F, 3.7F, and 4.1F catheter shafts correlating with 44%, 25%, and 13% increases in unobstructed guiding catheter area relative to standard balloon catheters. The small shaft diameter of the Micro catheter allows for improved guiding catheter pressure measurements and improved guiding catheter contrast injections.

Guidewire

The Micro guidewire is a hybrid structure combining a 0.007- to 0.008-inch core wire attached to a 2 or 3 cm, 0.014-inch platinum coil tip that incorporates a shaping ribbon. The 3-cm-tip Micro catheter utilizes a single flat-core wire design extending 2 cm within the platinum coil. The 2-cm-tip Micro catheter utilizes a double flat-core wire design extending 1 cm within the platinum coil. The guidewire itself moves through a 0.010-inch distal catheter lumen, so that it is movable

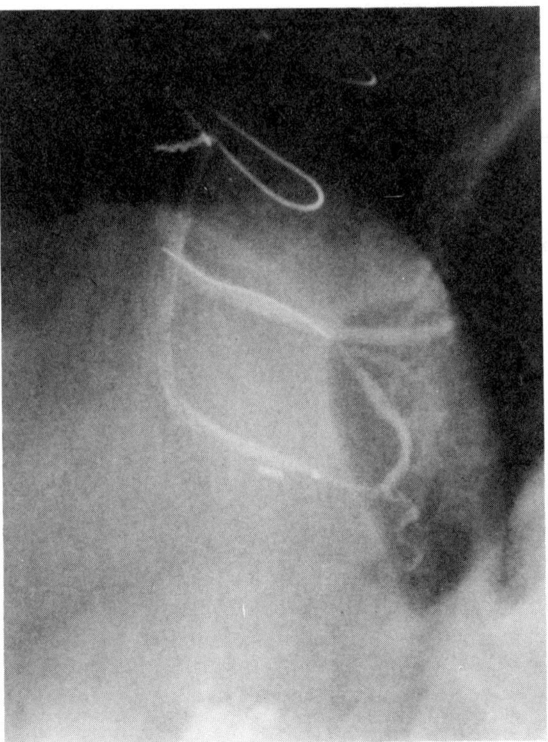

Fig. 24-2. A 2.5 mm Micro balloon catheter has been passed into the graft stenosis with the guidewire tip steered retrogradely into the distal right coronary artery. This injection performed over the balloon catheter itself also shows significant narrowing at the origin of the posterior descending branch.

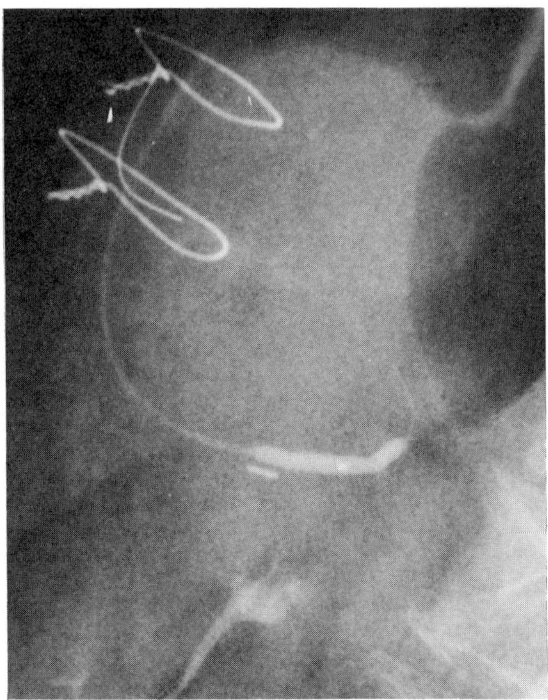

Fig. 24-3. Balloon inflation in the distal vein graft with the tip of the balloon in the posterior descending branch shows the tendency toward conformity to angles and bends by the Micro balloon catheter.

and steerable but not removable from the balloon catheter itself.

CLINICAL INVESTIGATION

Clinical investigation of the Micro catheter under an investigational device exemption by the Federal Drug Administration (FDA) was commenced in October 1985. Fourteen investigators from 10 institutions used the Micro catheter in 229 patients attempting to dilate 424 stenoses. The primary success rate utilizing this device in its early stages was 88%. Failure modes included the inability to select an artery in only 1.2% of patients, the inability to cross the stenosis with the wire in 4.9% of patients, and the inability to cross the stenosis with the balloon segment in 4.9% of patients. Procedural complications occurred in only 2.2% of patients.

From October 1985 through January 1987, 858 Micro catheters were utilized in attempts to dilate 1344 stenoses in 550 patients at the Mid America Heart Institute. Primary success rates ranged from 90 to 96% for all coronary segments with the exception of the posterolateral branch of the right coronary artery, acute

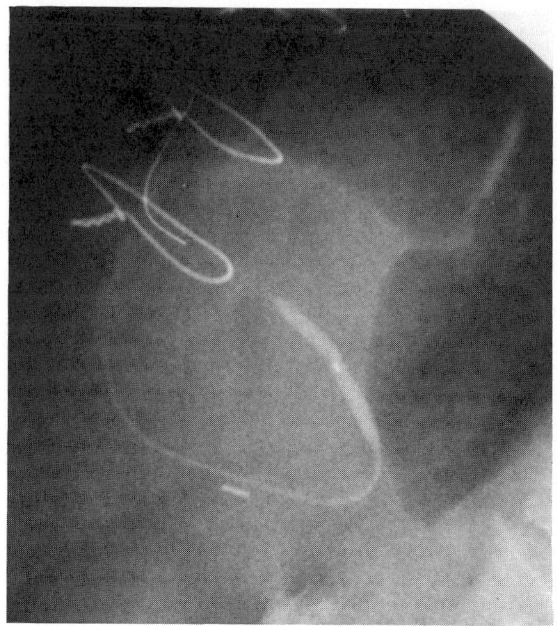

Fig. 24-4. The balloon has been steered retrogradely into the lesion at the origin of the posterior descending branch.

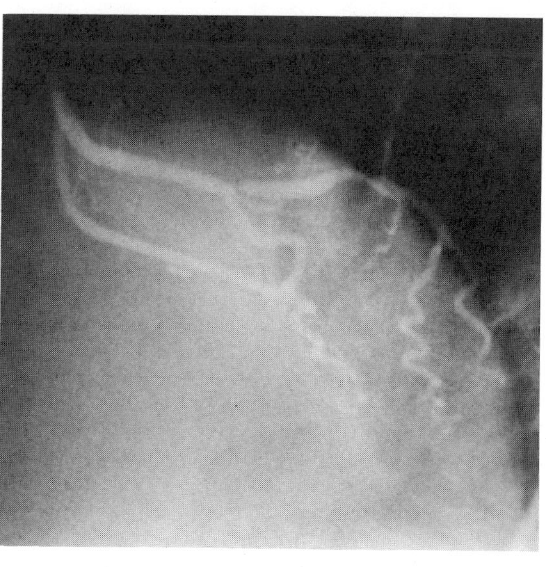

Fig. 24-5. Following withdrawal of the Micro balloon catheter, the guide catheter injections demonstrated a lesion at the origin of the posterolateral segment followed approximately 2 cm more distally by a significant tubular zone of narrowing.

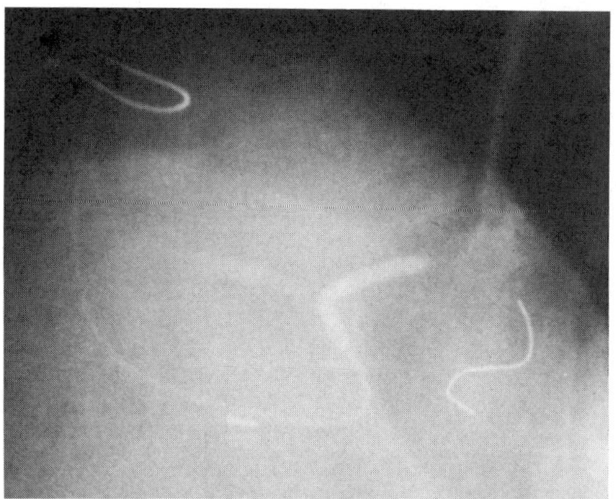

Fig. 24-6. The 2.5 mm Micro balloon catheter was directed back into and across the first lesion of the posterolateral segment, again demonstrating conformity to angles and bends during balloon expansion, in addition to excellent steerability and trackability.

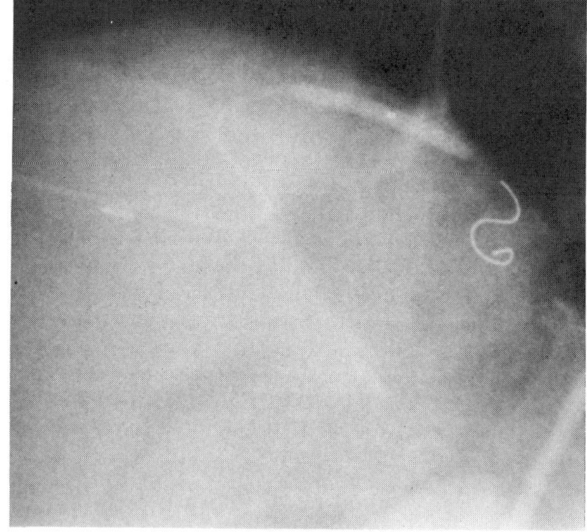

Fig. 24-7. The balloon was further advanced into the second posterolateral segment lesion for dilatation.

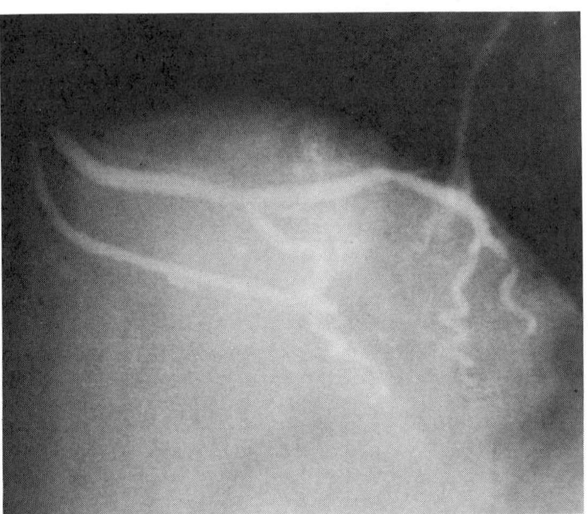

Fig. 24-8. Final injections show wide patency of all dilated sites.

marginal branch of the right coronary artery, and left main coronary stenoses, in which success rates of 86%, 88%, and 85%, respectively were demonstrated.

OBSERVATIONS

The relatively low profile of the Micro catheter clinically translates into an improved ability to cross stenoses compared with standard catheters. Distal visualization is enhanced because of low balloon profile combined with low catheter shaft diameter, both resulting in increased unobstructed guiding catheter area allowing greater dye injections through the guide catheter itself. The hybrid guidewire has proved to be relatively atraumatic and safe, as well as sturdy and responsive. The wire advances, withdraws, and torques with little resistance. The ability of this catheter to flex, bend, and conform to curved segments during expansion is notable to the extent that it has become a catheter of choice for dilatation within tortuous and angled coronary segments. The relatively low profile and small balloon sizes further support its use in patients with intrinsically small coronary arteries and in those with diffuse disease. As for the LPS catheter, we have used the Micro repeatedly and successfully for internal mammary dilatation and the performance of multiple wire techniques.

The flexible tip segment precludes successful use of the Micro for opening chronic total occlusions. It is less "pushable" than standard catheters because of the smaller and more flexible shaft. No distal dye injections or pressure measurements are obtainable with the Micro, and it also cannot be used with an exchange wire. A second-generation Micro catheter with a stiffer shaft (Micro XT; Advanced Cardiovascular Systems, Inc.) can be used for greater pushability. Clinical trials are underway to develop a Micro catheter suitable for use with exchange techniques.

Chapter 25

Balloon-on-Wire Probe System for Coronary Angioplasty

Spencer B. King III, MD, FACC

The application of angioplasty in coronary artery disease first employed 10 years ago has proved to be an effective alternative therapy.[1,2] Gruntzig's original catheters were accompanied by a fixed guidewire on the end of the balloon. Simpson developed a system for placing the balloon catheter over a movable guidewire.[3] In 1982 Gruntzig introduced the first steerable guidewires, which could be rotated and directed selectively into distal coronary segments.[4] Since that time a great deal of effort has been put into reducing the diameter of balloon catheters so that the method can be expanded. This technologic development has resulted in a dramatic expansion of angioplasty beyond its early indications for discrete, proximal, noncalcified lesions.[5] The percentage of patients with such ideal lesions has shrunk dramatically, and angioplasty is now employed frequently to address distal, heavily calcified, eccentric lesions in areas beyond severe tortuosity and frequently in settings of multiple vessel involvement. Although low-profile steerable systems have enabled many of these lesions to be successfully dilated, there remains a large number of lesions that are too severe, too hard, too distal, or located in positions where backup of the catheter is impossible, so that even though a wire can be passed the balloon catheter cannot be advanced across the lesion. These situations were the impetus for the development of the probe system.

MECHANISM OF ACTION

The probe (USCI Division of C.R. Bard, Inc., Billerica, Mass.) consists of a proximal portion of Teflon-coated stainless steel monotubing measuring 0.022-inch in diameter, a midportion 0.013-inch in diameter, and a core wire attached to this intermediate shaft tapering over a 30 cm length ending 2 cm from the tip (Fig. 25-1). The final 2 cm of the coil has no core wire and is constructed similar to the 0.014-inch flexible guidewire manufactured by USCI. Extending from the intermediate shaft and covering the 30 cm guidewire is a thin, polyethylene tetraphthalate covering that terminates in a balloon of the same material and ends just proximal to the 2 cm wire tip.

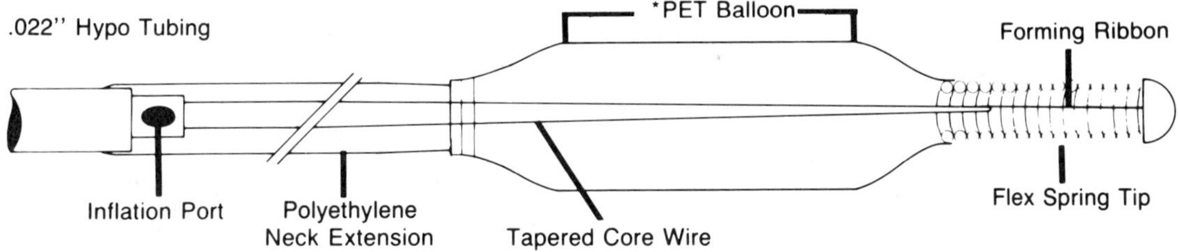

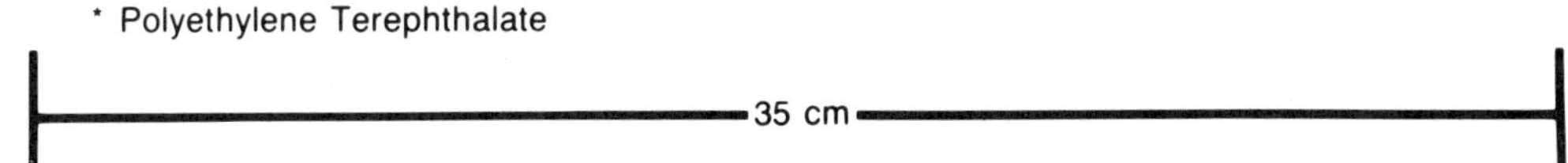

Fig. 25-1. Diagrammatic representation of the structure of the probe catheter.

The only size approved for general use is a 2 mm balloon that has a deflated profile of 0.020 inch (Fig. 25-2). This profile compares very favorably to the smallest available over-the-wire, low-profile system, which measures 0.32 inch. The distal 2 cm flexible guidewire portion is radiopaque; the remainder of the guidewire portion of the catheter system is not. There is no lumen for pressure or dye injection, and balloon inflation is achieved by applying pressure to the contrast media at the proximal end of the monofilament tubing that is transmitted through the monofilament tube to the polyethylene tetraphthalate and ultimately ends at the tip. Filling the balloon is accomplished by injecting and withdrawing a contrast media mix in a similar fashion employed in other conventional over-the-wire systems. Steerability is achieved by placing a custom-design curve on the tip that suits the operator's needs and rotating the entire catheter system up to 180 degrees in either direction.

CLINICAL EXPERIENCE

Clinical trials with the catheter have been concluded and this catheter has now been released. A portion of the clinical experience was obtained at Emory University Hospital and Rhode Island Hospital from January through September of 1987.[6] During this trial the probe catheter was selected for patients with small arteries with a special emphasis on distal lesions in which backup would be a problem and in some lesions in which conventional over-the-wire systems were unsuc-

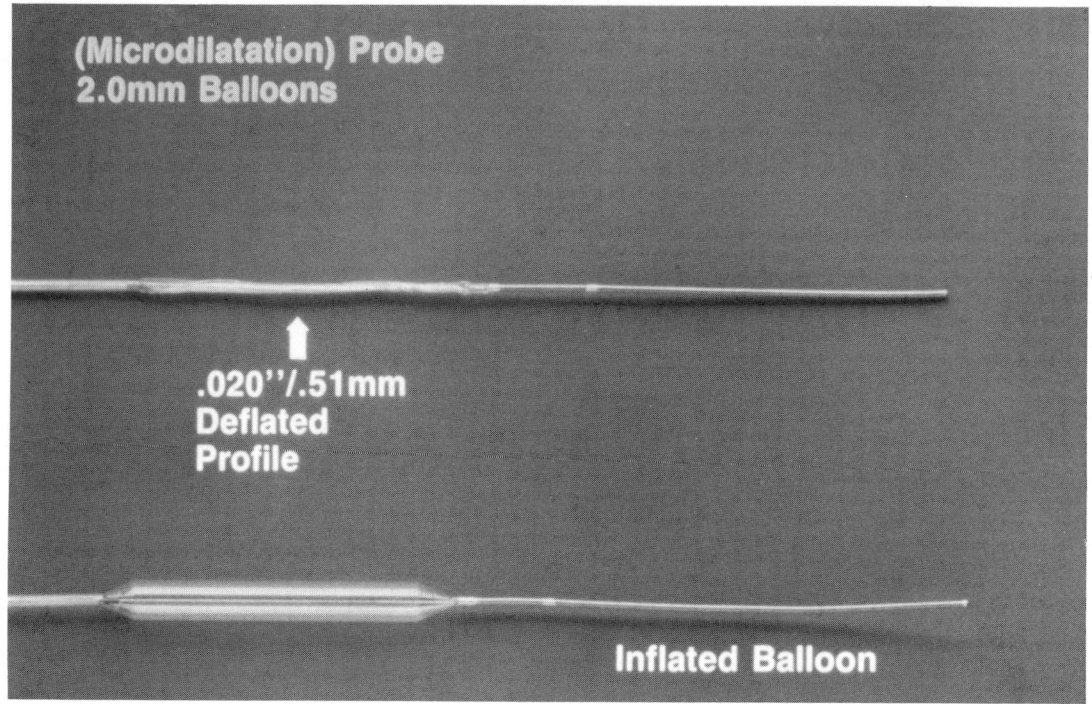

Fig. 25-2. The probe catheter in its deflated state approximates the size of the guidewire. Below, the inflated balloon achieves a 2 mm, 2.5 mm, or 3 mm size.

cessful. The probe was selected in 33 patients as the initial dilatation catheter in circumstances felt to be quite unfavorable for conventional over-the-wire systems and in an additional 20 patients in whom conventional low-profile catheters were unable to cross the lesion (Fig. 25-3). In eight patients the catheter was used even though a conventional system could have been selected.

When the probe was used as the primary catheter without trying over-the-wire systems, the lesions were crossed in 47 of 56 patients (84%). Forty-four of these 47 lesions were successfully dilated and 6 were improved further with conventional over-the-wire systems of a larger dimension. In the nine lesions that could not be crossed, a subsequent conventional dilating system was successful in only one lesion. In 21 lesions, the probe was selected after one or more conventional catheter systems had failed. In most of these circumstances the very lowest profile, commercially available systems were tried. Seventeen of the 21 lesions were crossed with the probe system and 16 of the 17 lesions were successfully dilated. In the four patients in whom the lesion could not be crossed, a second conventional catheter system finally succeeded in one patient. During this trial phase, some 2.5 and 3 mm catheters were available and functioned in a similar manner to the 2 mm probe.

COMPLICATIONS

Several complications were encountered during clinical trials. First of all it should be stressed that this catheter system, because of its hypotubing design, cannot be treated exactly as most flexible catheter systems. The hypotubing segment is rigid and must be kept

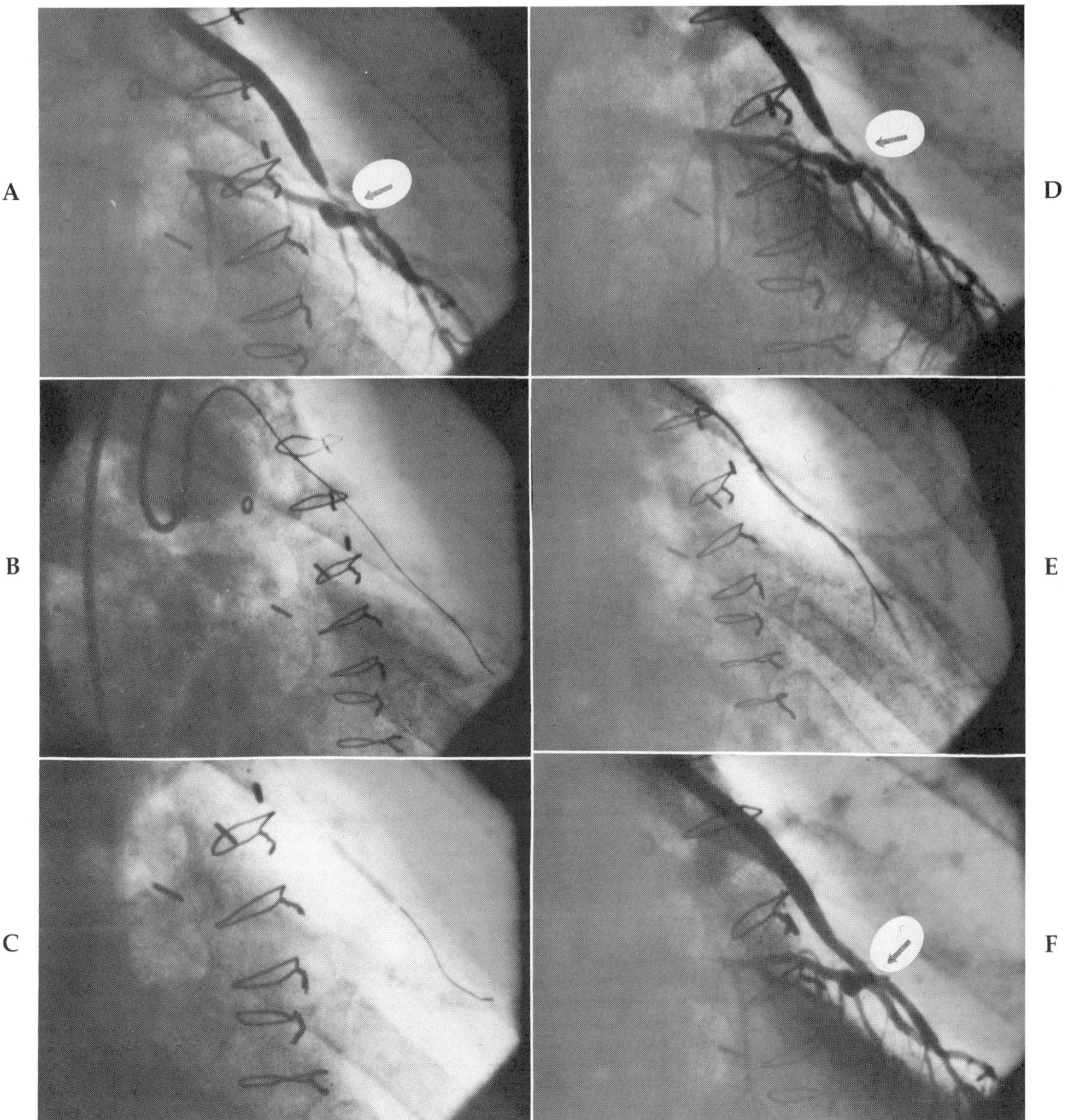

Fig. 25-3. A case in which the over-the-wire low-profile system would not cross. **A,** RAO view of a vein graft to the LAD coronary artery with an old, tight distal lesion. **B,** Guide catheter in strong position located 2 cm inside vein graft with the guidewire well across the lesion; however, the low-profile balloon catheter would not cross the lesion. **C,** A probe catheter easily crosses the lesion and is inflated to 2 mm size. **D,** Angiogram of the mildly improved lumen following probe dilatation. **E,** Follow-up dilatation with an over-the-wire balloon of larger diameter. **F,** Final result following PTCA.

straight. We have found that use of the catheter without attached inflation devices facilitates the movement of the catheter as it is held straight and moved forward and back with a rotating motion to facilitate balloon crossing. Second, the presence of balloon material on the wire means that the catheter cannot be rotated continually in one direction. To do so will invite twisting of the balloon at the tip. In one of the cases in this trial and in two cases subsequent to the trial, excessive rotation of the catheter resulted in twisting of the balloon so that proper inflation and deflation could not be accomplished. In all cases the balloon was ultimately deflated and removed without sequelae. Because of the extraordinarily thin balloon material, balloon rupture has been encountered. Although the balloons are rated to 12 atm, we have experienced rupture in one balloon at 6 atm and in another at 8 atm. It is possible that external impingement on the balloon by rough, extremely calcified spicules may produce balloon rupture. There has been no incidence of fragmentation of the balloon, and all ruptured balloons have been satisfactorily removed. In one case, rupture of the balloon resulted in staining of the artery although recrossing and dilatation with another balloon was accomplished in this case.

ADVANTAGES

This balloon-on-a-wire catheter system offers certain important advantages. Because of the extremely low profile of the catheter, it can be easily placed through 8F guide catheters or 7F angiographic catheters. The ability to pass the probe through a 7F angiographic catheter has been a great advantage when dilating internal mammary artery grafts. The guiding internal mammary artery catheters are frequently too stiff and difficult to manipulate, whereas the 7F angiographic catheters enter the mammary artery easily. Since backup is not a problem with the probe, it is possible to place it through a 7F angiographic catheter into a mammary artery and distally to cross the stenotic lesion. Because the probe is almost as small as a guidewire, it is possible to inject contrast media through the guide catheter to achieve excellent angiographic opacification of the artery during crossing maneuvers. This is possible even when using the 7F angiographic catheter.

Some arterial lesions have been located extremely distal in the coronary circulation, for example, at the apex of the left ventricle where the anterior descending artery curves around to serve a portion of the inferior wall. In these situations, there is not much room for distal wire position. We have found that wires can be placed into extraordinarily small arteries and even crimped to some degree distally in order to allow the balloon to enter the lesion. We have been able to employ this technique without complication.

The small diameter also allows for placing two probes in one guiding catheter system. We have utilized this technique for performing kissing balloon angioplasty on several occasions.[7] The probes can be placed into each side branch and inflated serially or simultaneously as needed. By using two catheter systems, we have been able to dilate trifurcating systems placing either three probes or two probes in one over-the-wire system.

An important concern was the trackability of the balloon system and how it would compare with standard wire systems. We have had the opportunity to pass the balloon through extraordinarily tortuous arterial segments and have seen that the trackability and steerability of the wire is comparable to that of guidewires.

Although no pressure measurements can be obtained with this system, excellent angiographic visualization can be obtained by injecting through the guiding catheter with the probe in place. By obtaining these angiograms in multiple projections, a high level of confidence in the angiographic result may be obtained before removing the probe, thereby minimizing the chance for abrupt closure after the probe has been removed.

CONCLUSION

Our initial experience with the probe balloon on a wire device has convinced us that this is a significant addition to the armamentarium in complex percutaneous transluminal coronary angioplasty (PTCA). As more and more difficult cases are encountered, it is important that new devices of this type are developed to match the complexity of the problem. As we obtain experience with the larger balloon sizes, it may be found that the device can be used more and more for lesions that would otherwise be attempted with over-the-wire systems. Certainly the simplicity of the system is unexcelled. At the present time, however, we continue to feel more comfortable utilizing an over-the-wire system in large important coronary beds. The availability of an exchange wire that allows positioning of bailout or perfusion catheters or the placement of intracoronary stents provides an element of safety that at present is not available with the probe. Currently efforts are underway to provide the possibility for exchanging other systems over the probe. If these efforts are successful, then the probe may become a much more commonly used item in angioplasty of severe proximal lesions. There is no question of its value in distal lesions that are not dilatable by conventional systems.

REFERENCES

1. Gruntzig, A.R., Senning, A., and Siegenthaler, W.: Nonoperative dilatation of coronary artery stenosis, N. Engl. J. Med. **301:**61, 1979.
2. Gruntzig, A.R., King, S.B., III, Schlumpf, M., and Siegenthaler, W.: Long-term follow-up after percutaneous transluminal coronary angioplasty: the early Zurich experience, N. Engl. J. Med. **316:**1127-1132, 1987.
3. Simpson, J.B., Baim, D.S., Robert, E.W., and Harrison, D.C.: A new catheter system for coronary angioplasty, Am. J. Cardiol. **49:**1216-1222, 1982.
4. Anderson, H.V., Roubin, G.S., Leimgruber, P.P., Douglas, J.S., King, S.B., and Gruntzig, A.R.: Primary angiographic success rates of percutaneous transluminal coronary angioplasty, Am. J. Cardiol. **56:**712-717, 1985.
5. Detre, K., Costigan, T., Kelsey, S., et al.: PCTA in 1985: NHLBI PTCA Registry (abstract), J. Am. Coll. Cardiol. **9:**19A, 1987.
6. Thomas, E.S., Neiderman, A.L., King, S.B., III, Douglas, J.S., and Williams, D.O.: Efficacy of a new angioplasty catheter for severely narrowed coronary lesions, J. Am. Coll. Cardiol. **12:**694-702, 1988.
7. Meier, B.: Kissing balloon coronary angioplasty, Am. J. Cardiol. **54:**918-920, 1984.

Chapter 26

Role of the Long Wire Technique in Percutaneous Transluminal Coronary Angioplasty: The Frankfurt Experience

Gisbert Kober, MD
Christian Vallbracht, MD
Martin Kaltenbach, MD

Since 1982, percutaneous transluminal coronary angioplasty (PTCA) has been performed nearly exclusively with the aid of wire-guided steerable balloon catheters, a technical development that had originally been promoted by John Simpson.[1] With this technique, a movable guidewire passing through the balloon catheter and coming out at its tip is introduced together with the balloon catheter into the guiding catheter and the respective coronary vessel.

DISADVANTAGES OF THE CONVENTIONAL STEERABLE TECHNIQUE

When balloon catheters are introduced into the commonly used 8F guiding catheter, sufficient vessel opacification is rarely achieved, and thus probing is impeded, especially in the case of lesions extremely difficult to access. This results in a marked reduction in the degree of safety. Once the tip of the wire has passed the lesion, no further exchange of the balloon catheter for a smaller or larger sized balloon is possible. An exchange can only be achieved by withdrawing the existing equipment and subsequently reprobing the lesion with the exchanged instruments, which involves further procedural risks. Emergency measures undertaken when dissection and subsequent vessel occlusion occur, such as redilatation of the occluded segment or perfusion of the ischemic area to bridge waiting times before emergency bypass operation, are clearly limited since probing of the occlusion through a dissected area can be difficult, not always possible, and possibly risky.

LONG WIRE TECHNIQUE

Further technical improvement was desirable to facilitate the PTCA procedure and to reduce the risk of complications. For this purpose, the long wire technique was introduced in March 1983[2] and has been applied virtually exclusively in 1340 interventions since June 1984. Fig. 26-1 shows statistics for angioplasties performed over the past 10 years in Frankfurt. Commencing in 1977, the frequency of interventions (shown by the dashed line) rose steadily until reaching a capacity of approximately 450 cases per year. The success rate (open circles) rose to nearly 90%, whereas the percentage of emergency operations (dashed-dotted line) decreased to 1 to 3%.

In most cases we start the PTCA procedure with a Cook guiding catheter with side holes, a Schneider 3-m-long wire (available now also in high-torque, superfloppy quality), and a Schneider-Gruntzig or Edwards balloon catheter.*

With the long wire technique, the arterial stenosis is initially passed with a special wire only. This 3-m, Teflon-coated wire with a diameter of 0.012 inch (rarely 0.014 or 0.010 inch) is introduced into the guiding catheter through a valve and advanced through the stenosis into the distal segment of the diseased coronary vessel (Fig. 26-2). To reduce the danger of intimal injuries, the wire is tipped with a 0.45 mm hemisphere. The larger outer part of the wire is protected in a cochleate plastic tube. A small plastic torquer

**Guiding catheters and long wires available from Cook, Angiomed, ACS, and Schneider.*

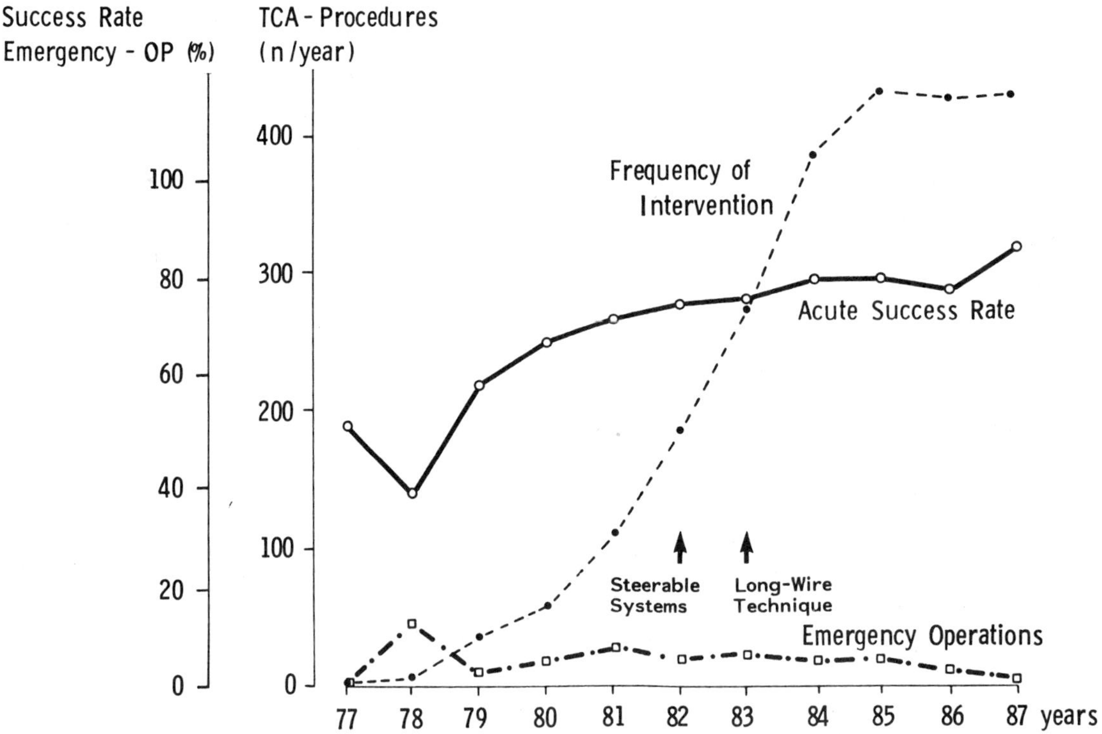

Fig. 26-1. Statistics for angioplasty interventions over 10 years in Frankfurt. Success rates and major complications requiring emergency bypass operations are shown.

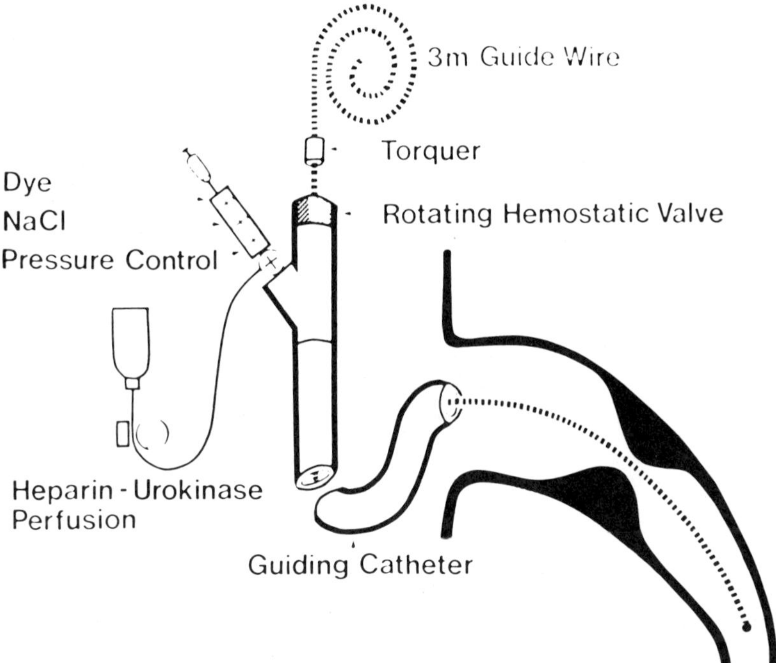

Fig. 26-2. Schematic diagram of the long wire technique. The wire is advanced via a hemostatic valve through the guiding catheter and lesion into the poststenotic coronary vessel. The balloon catheter is then introduced through the valve into the stenosis under fluoroscopic control.

clipped onto the wire sideways enables rotating, longitudinal maneuvering of the wire, thus excluding damage to the Teflon coating and allowing it to be removed without having to pull the entire wire out of its tube. After positioning the guidewire, the selected balloon catheter is threaded across the exterior part of the wire and then advanced through the hemostatic valve into the guiding catheter and stenosis, respectively. The wire tip has to be consistently followed fluoroscopically and held in place while gradually retracting the wire back into the tubing and simultaneously advancing the balloon catheter. Using a 0.012-inch wire, almost all balloon catheters currently available can be applied, even low-profile ones. After dilatation, the balloon catheter is entirely pulled back out of the guiding catheter consequently allowing optimum angiographic visualization of the results of angioplasty. The guidewire is held in place for some minutes until good procedural results are confirmed.

To prevent thrombus formation, especially at the site of the dilated coronary segment, as well as inside the guiding catheter and on the surface of the Teflon-coated guidewire, 100 units per kg body weight of heparin were administered as a bolus at the beginning of the procedure followed by a constant infusion of 2000 units/hour of heparin and 100,000 units/hour of urokinase diluted in a 200 ml saline solution. On account of this treatment, minimization of fibrin deposits and thrombus formations was evident through microscopic evaluation of the wire surface.[3]

In addition, patients were treated with salicylates (1.5 g/day), calcium antagonists (vera-

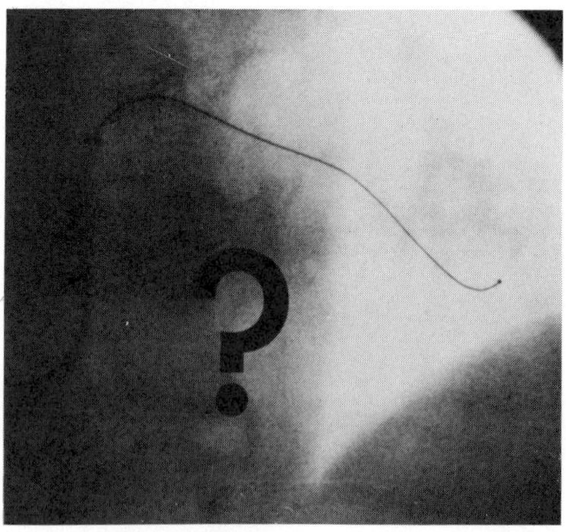

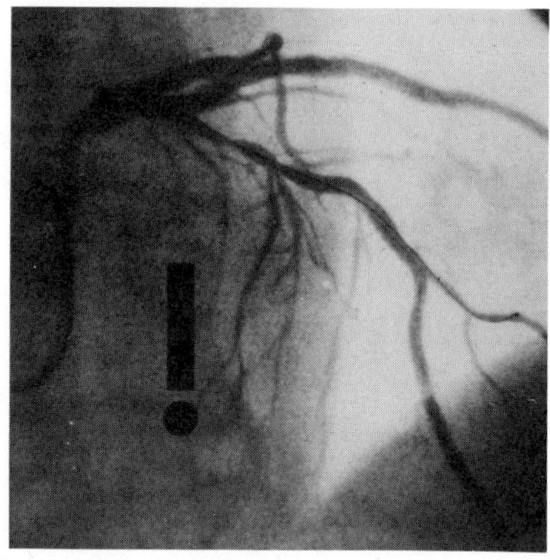

Fig. 26-3. Guidewire with tip in the periphery of the coronary system *(left)*. Optimum opacification *(right)* enables safe confirmation of its position.

pamil, 80 mg t.i.d., or gallopamil, 50 mg b.i.d.), and isosorbide dinitrate (20 mg t.i.d.) at least 24 hours before commencement of the procedure. This treatment was continued over the next 4 months following successful intervention.

Optimum Stenosis Opacification During Probing and Judgment of Dilatation Results

The sole introduction of the guidewire into the guiding catheter does not create any resistance to contrast material flow. Thus opacification of the large coronary vessels and all their side branches, the shape of the stenosis, and the position of the guidewire tip can be achieved optimally (Fig. 26-3).

After dilatation an angiogram permits the observation of not only the runoff of the contrast medium into the distal vessel but also dilatation results regarding stenosis reduction, residual stenosis, dissections, or the sudden occurrence of an occlusion. Further therapeutic consequences can also be derived from this angiogram. Fig. 26-4 shows a left anterior descending (LAD) coronary artery stenosis not yet adequately dilated after using a 2.5 mm balloon and reveals good results after the successive use of 3.7 mm balloons. Both angiograms were taken after dilatation with the wire still in place.

Exchange of Balloon Catheters

With the wire placed in the distal coronary segment, it is often not possible to pass the stenosis using the selected balloon catheter on account of the balloon diameter or catheter stiffness. In this case, changing to a lower-sized balloon catheter presents no problems. Following unsatisfactory dilatation results, wider balloon catheters can be easily introduced with the guidewire still in place without having to reprobe the stenotic area, thus saving time and diminishing procedural risks (Fig. 26-4). Exchanging balloon catheters for smaller or larger sized ones proved necessary in about 20% of the procedures performed.

TREATMENT OF BRANCHING STENOSES

The dilatation of a large vessel bears a certain risk of sudden occlusion of the side branches originating within the stenosis.[4]

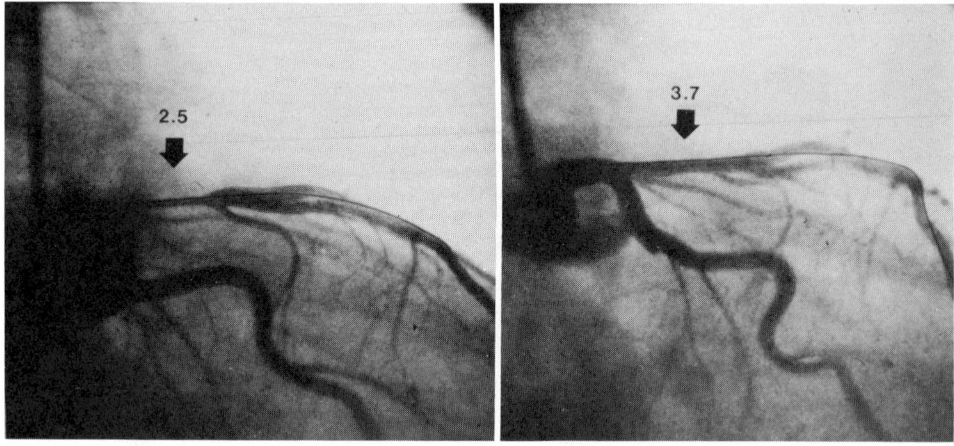

Fig. 26-4. Angiograms obtained with the wire still in place confirming the results of proximal LAD coronary artery angioplasty after successive use of 2.5 and 3.7 mm balloons (*left panel* and *right panel,* respectively).

Thus dilatation of the main vessel and side-branch origin or the protection of the side branch may prove desirable in the case of branching stenoses with larger perfusion areas of the side branches. Usually, probing of the side branch is only feasible before main vessel dilatation. Thus wires have to be placed into both vessels before the first dilatation. Two long wires can be advanced simultaneously into both vessels through the same 8.5F large-lumen guiding catheter, once again under optimum opacification of the anatomy. As a result, it is no longer necessary with this technique to introduce two guiding catheters through two different peripheral arteries. Stenosis dilatation is subsequently performed by changing the balloon catheter from one wire to the other (Fig. 26-5).[5]

It is neither possible nor essential to simultaneously dilate both stenoses as is done with the kissing balloon technique.[6] In many cases, the placement of the wire in the side branch is merely a precaution and dilatation is rendered unnecessary if the flow into the branching vessel is not impeded after dilating the mainstem stenosis. To avoid the impending risk of side-branch occlusions, this technique has been applied in 1.5% of the interventions performed.

TREATMENT OF ACUTE CORONARY OCCLUSIONS FOLLOWING ANGIOPLASTY

In the event of an occlusion of the dilated vessel mainly attributable to a large dissection at the site of the stenosis, an emergency bypass operation may become necessary. The need for emergency operations recently dropped from 5% to 2 to 3%. It is sometimes possible to avoid such an intervention through repeat introduction of balloon catheters through the already inserted guidewire. It may, however, be inevitable to refer the patient for bypass surgery if redilatation of the occluded segment does not result in a stable reopening of the vessel to satisfactorily perfuse the myocardium.

The period of ischemia before operative revascularization of the endangered myocardium is one of the most important determi-

Text continued on p. 316.

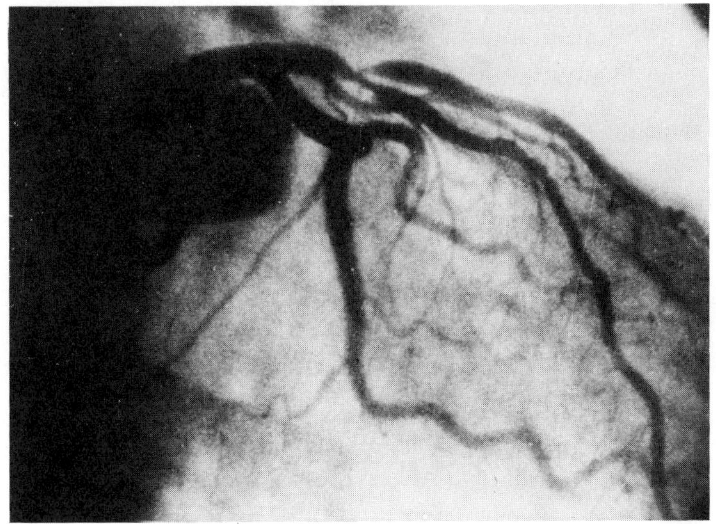

A

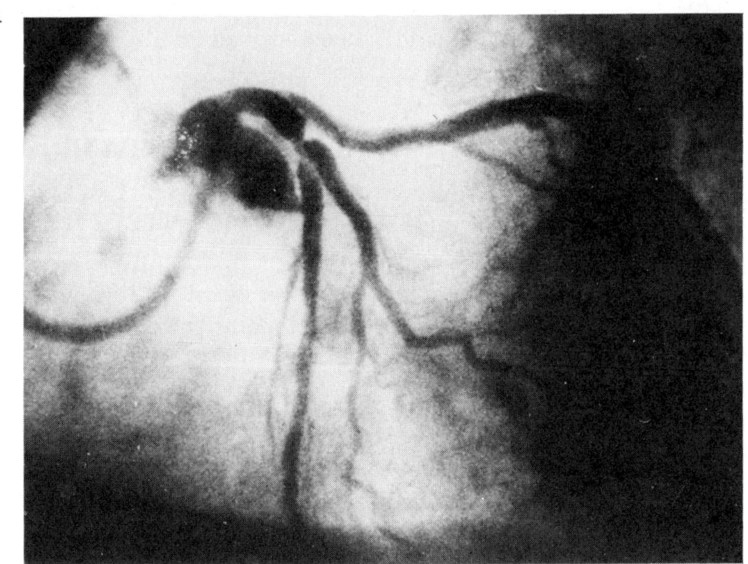

Fig. 26-5. Treatment of a branching stenosis with the double wire technique. **A,** After positioning both wires, the balloon catheter is successively introduced into each vessel and inflated **(B, C).** The control angiogram shows the success achieved acutely **(D).**

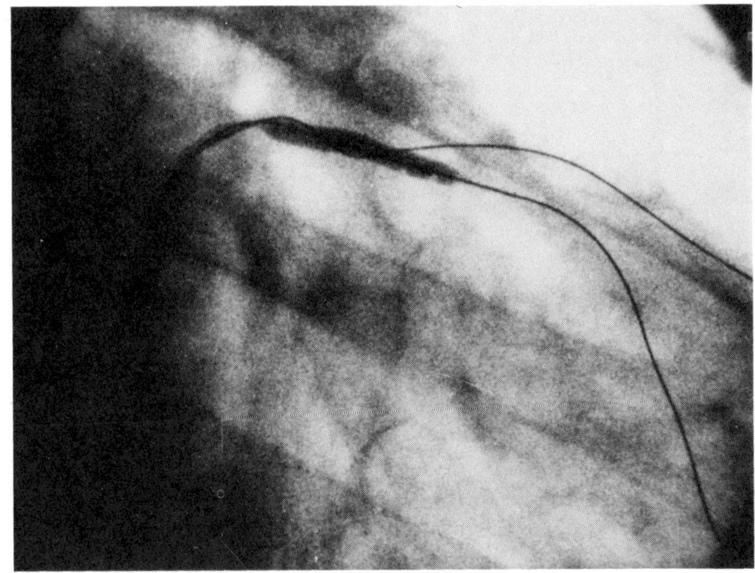

B

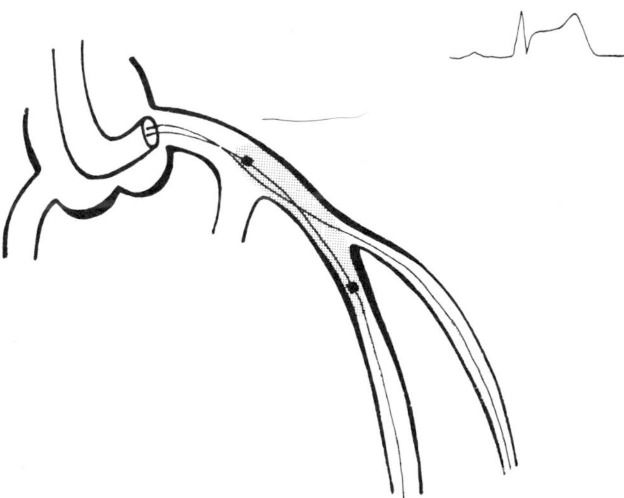

Fig. 26-5, cont'd. For legend see p. 312.

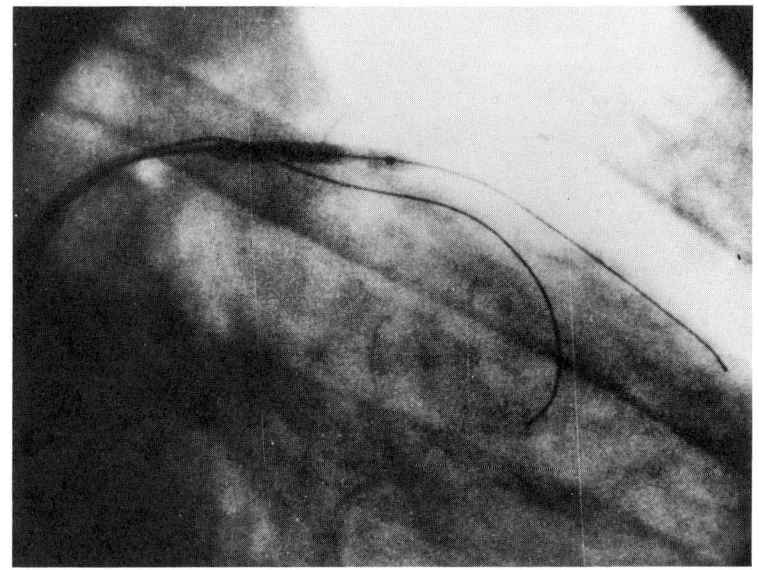

C

Dilatation 3

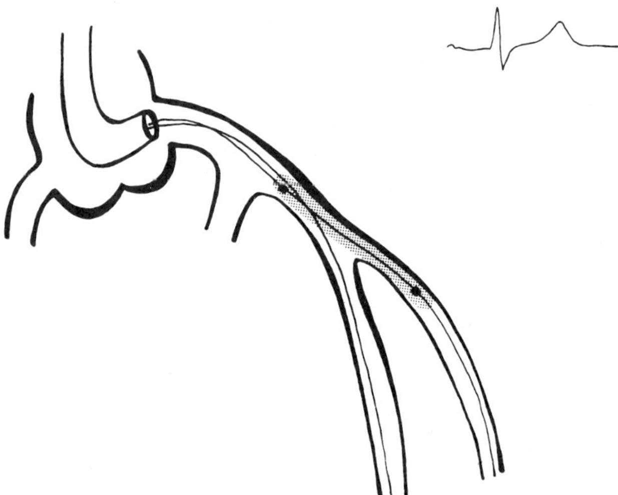

Fig. 26-5, cont'd. For legend see p. 312.

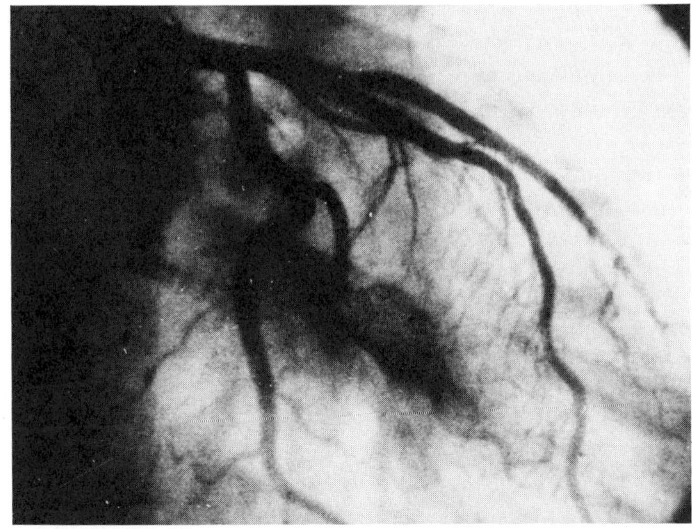

D

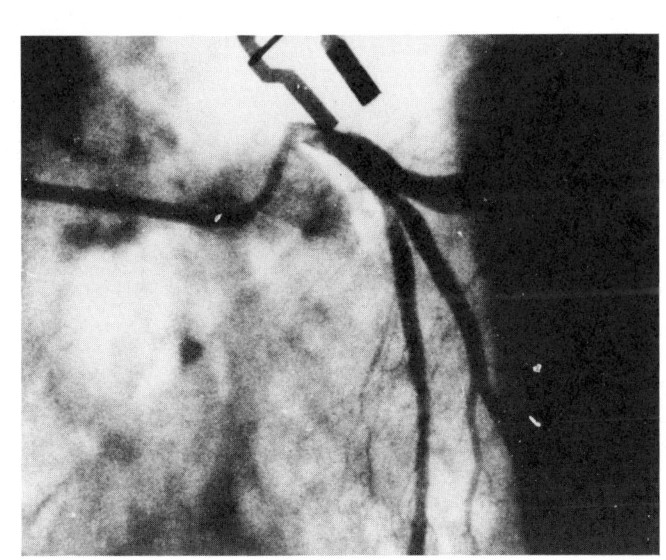

Fig. 26-5, cont'd. For legend see p. 312.

nants of the degree of irreversible damage to the heart muscle.[7] The severity and duration of ischemia can be reduced by perfusing the ischemic area with a 5F perfusion catheter (catheter and 3 m wires available from Schneider-Medintag, Zurich, Switzerland) easily introduced with the aid of the long wire still in place (Fig. 26-6). Oxygenated blood from the femoral artery is then injected manually.[8] Model experiments[9] demonstrated the possibility of appropriate perfusion of the ischemic myocardium using perfusion catheters at a rather low perfusion pressure (Fig. 26-7). The above-mentioned perfusion technique was used in 10 cases. Its clinical value can easily be seen from the favorable response of anginal symptoms and the effect on ischemic changes in the electrocardiogram.

MEASUREMENT OF PERIPHERAL CORONARY PRESSURES

Peripheral pressures can be easily measured by means of the longwire technique. Whereas it is known that intracoronary pressure gradient measurements provide no reli-

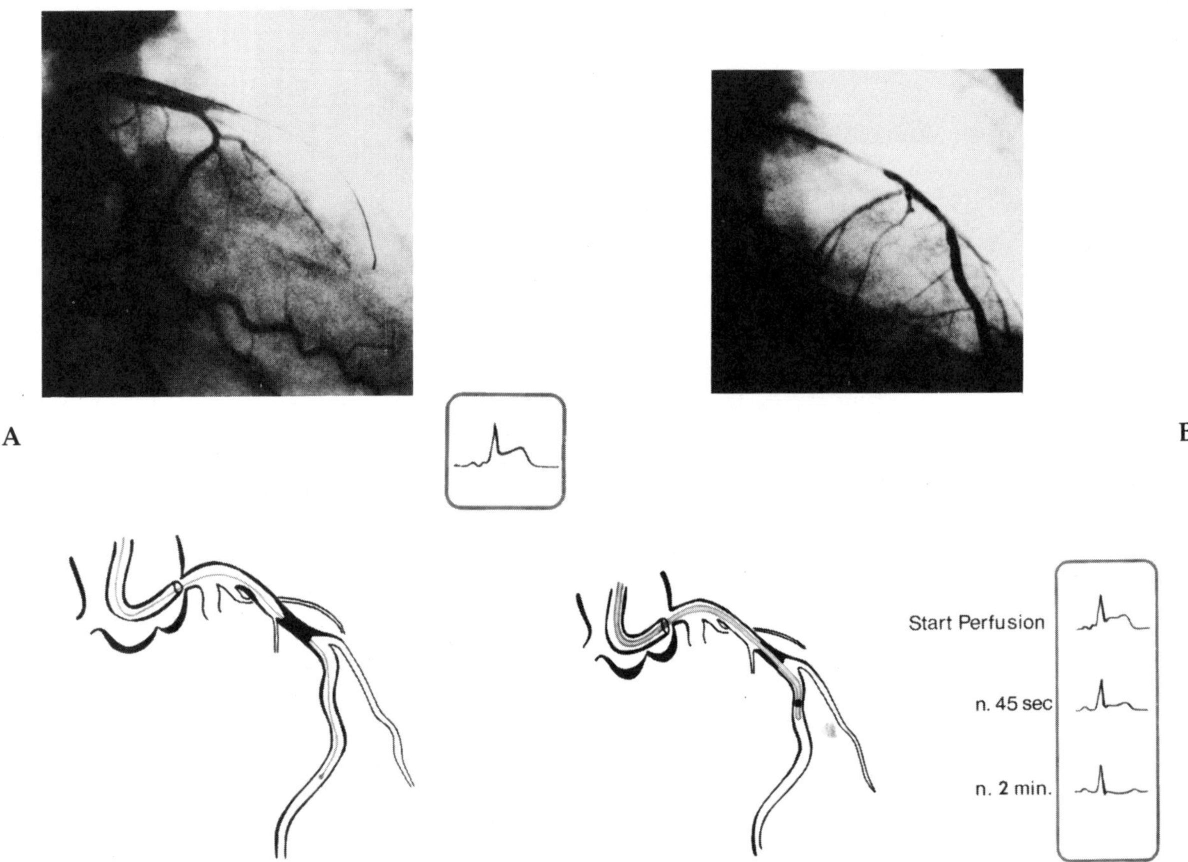

Fig. 26-6. A, Long wire still in place with occlusion of the LAD coronary artery after PTCA causing angina and ischemic ECG changes. **B,** Distal perfusion using a 5F perfusion catheter by means of the long wire immediately minimized symptoms of ECG changes.

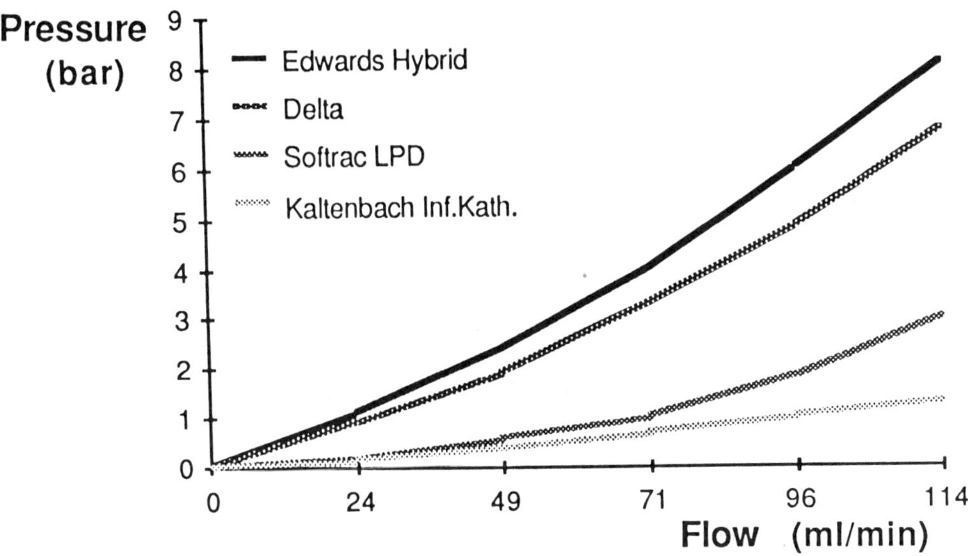

Fig. 26-7. Pressures necessary for establishing equal flow values vary depending on the respective catheter used. (From Simpson, J., et al: Am. J. Cardiol. **49:**1216-1222, 1982.)

able diagnostic indications either of the severity of stenoses or of the results of angioplasty,[10] measurements of the occlusion pressure, on the other hand, are of some diagnostic and prognostic value. Patients with high occlusion pressures (greater than 20 mm Hg) are less prone to severe ischemia or ischemic damage of the myocardium in the event of acute occlusion of the treated vessel. Restenosis, however, tends to occur less often in patients with low occlusion pressures (less than 20 mm Hg).[11]

CONCLUSION

The long wire technique, first introduced in 1983 and applied virtually exclusively in 1340 interventions since June 1984, has effected a slight additional increase in the acute success rate of coronary angioplasty and has reduced the number of emergency operations despite the treatment of more and more complicated cases.

One of the most important advantages of this technique compared with the conventional steerable technique is optimum visualization of the coronary vessels (including side branches and stenoses) during lesion probing and in repeat angiography following angioplasty. Balloon catheters can, if necessary, be exchanged for those of smaller or larger diameter without having to recross the stenosis with the wire, thus improving the procedural safety factor. Branching stenoses can also be treated using two wires introduced with the same 8.5F large-lumen guiding catheter. In emergency cases, distal coronary perfusion can be easily achieved by inserting a perfusion catheter through the wire that is still in place.

Maneuvering the long wire, 170 cm of which is encased in a plastic, cochleate tubing outside the patient, becomes familiar after only a few interventions. The extra fluoroscopy time for introducing the catheter into the lesion from outside and removing it after the procedure is relatively short in comparison with the total fluoroscopy time and is compensated for in many interventions by faster and safer probing of the coronary vessels and stenoses. Thus the long wire technique makes angioplasty easier and more successful and improves the safety both with routine interventions and in the event of complications.

REFERENCES

1. Simpson, J., Balm, D., Robert, T., and Harrison, D.: A new catheter system for coronary angioplasty, Am. J. Cardiol. **49:**1216-1222, 1982.
2. Kaltenbach, M.: The long wire technique: a new technique for steerable balloon catheter dilatation of coronary artery stenoses, Eur. Heart J. **5:**1004-1009, 1984.
3. Kadel, C., Jonczyk, C., and Kaltenbach, M.: Thrombotic deposits on angioplasty guide wires, Eur. Heart J. **8**(suppl. 2):248, 1987.
4. Meier, B., Gruntzig, A.R., King, S.B., Douglas, J.S., Hollman, J., Ischinger, T., Aueron, F., and Galan, K.: Risk of side branch occlusion during coronary angioplasty, Am. J. Cardiol. **53:**10, 1984.
5. Vallbracht, C., Kaltenbach, M., and Kober, G.: Doppel-Langdrahttechnik zur Ballondilatation von Verzweigungsstenosen, Herz/Kreisl. **8:**378-382, 1986.
6. Gruntzig, A.R.: The technique of percutaneous transluminal coronary angioplasty. In Hurst, J.W., Hogue, R.B., Rackley, C.E., et al., editors: The heart, New York, 1904, McGraw-Hill Book Co.
7. Klepzig, H. Jr., Schraub, J., Huber, H., Hör, G., Kober, G., Satter, P., Aortokoronare Bypass-Operation als Notfalleingriff nach transluminaler koronarer Angioplastik: Welche Faktoren verhindern das Auftreten eines groβen Infarktes?, Dtsch. Med. Wochenschr. **111:**737-741, 1986.
8. Hopf, R., Kunkel, B., Schneider, M., and Kaltenbach, M.: Koronarperfusion bei akutem Gefäβverschulβ im Rahmen der transluminalen Koronarangioplastik (TCA), Z. Kardiol. **74:**580-584, 1985.
9. Busch, U.W.: Selective coronary perfusion via angioplasty catheters: technical and physiological aspects. In Höfling, B., editor: Current problems in PTCA, New York, 1986, Springer-Verlag.
10. Sievert, H., and Kaltenbach, M.: Intrakoronare Druckgradientenmessung: Wert und methodische Grenzen, Z. Kardiol. **76:**323-325, 1987.
11. Sievert, H., Kober, G., and Kaltenbach, M.: Pressure measurements during coronary angioplasty, Eur. Heart J. **8**(suppl. 2):245, 1987.

Chapter 27

The Sliding Rail (Monorail) Principle

Description of a New Technique and Its Application for Coronary Angioplasty

Tassilo R. Bonzel, MD
Helmut Wollschläger, MD
Thomas Meinertz, MD
Wolfgang Kasper, MD
Hanjörg Just, MD

With the establishment of percutaneous transluminal angioplasty (PTCA) it has been generally accepted that hemodynamically significant stenoses can be effectively treated in the cardiac laboratory. The result for the patient is relief of symptoms and increase in exercise capacity. In spite of several imperfections the method can now be performed by experienced cardiologists in most hospitals if surgical standby is provided (the provision of which is not universally met in PTCA procedures). Two main reasons may be named for the rapidly increasing application of PTCA: first, the accumulation of knowledge and investigator experience and second, the improvements of intracoronary catheter technology. The following advances in instrumentation have been made since Gruntzig's first intracoronary balloon catheterization:[1] The steerable catheter "system" was introduced by Simpson,[2] a catheter with high trackability was designed by Hartzler, and Kaltenbach advocated the long wire technique for the exchange of intracoronary balloons.[3] We published the first description of the sliding rail principle and the sliding rail (or monorail) balloon catheter in 1986.[4]

It is the purpose of this chapter to give a detailed description of this new system and a report on our own clinical experience with more than 400 procedures. It is our opinion that this system may overcome some of the remaining imperfections of PTCA and may serve as a basic tool for the application of various current or future intracoronary (or intravascular) diagnostic or therapeutic devices. We expect that our system will result in a more effective PTCA procedure than other systems in terms of success rates and patient safety, as well as improved laboratory logistics and staff hours.

DESCRIPTION OF THE SYSTEM

The system consists of two parts: a stationary part, or the guidewire, and an exchangeable part, which holds the diagnostic or therapeutic device (Fig. 27-1). The functional unit formed by the two parts may be called a sliding rail system. The system was first realized as an intracoronary dilatation catheter for PTCA, for which Bernhard Meier of Geneva, Switzerland coined the term "monorail" balloon catheter. Meanwhile this name has been generally accepted and its use expanded to the system (monorail system) and to the technique (monorail technique). The following description is limited to the monorail balloon catheter system.

The guidewire used may be any available standard-length guidewire of appropriate diameter, but guidewires with properties adjusted to the monorail technique may be preferred. The balloon catheter consists of two main parts, the shaft and the balloon. The shaft is made of elastic material of sufficient strength and contains a single lumen to be filled with fluid. The shaft serves to impart axial load to the distal balloon tip for axial pushability and to transmit pressure to the balloon interior, the balloon member, and to the vessel wall. The diameter of the longest

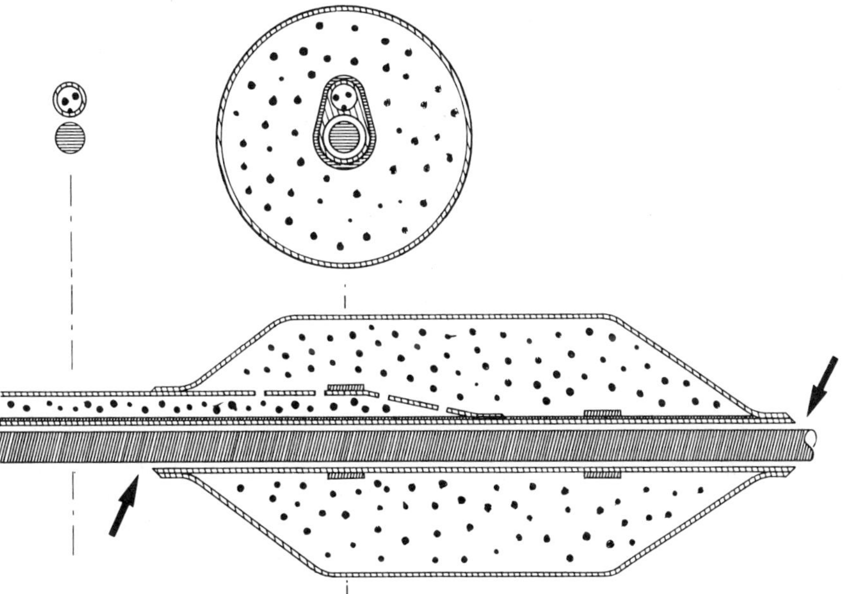

Fig. 27-1. Axial section (below) and cross-sections (above) of the monorail catheter balloon part. Note central coaxial tube *(arrows)* fitting the guidewire. Over most of the shaft distance, the shaft and the guidewire are running parallel to each other. Once the guidewire has passed the stenosis it remains stationary for the rest of the procedure, and the balloon can be moved independently of the guidewire over the whole of the distance or can be exchanged.

part of the shaft is size 3F. With 0.79 mm^2 the shaft cross-sectional area is significantly smaller than that of conventional 3.6F and 4.3F shafts with areas of 1.1 mm^2 and 1.6 mm^2, respectively. When using an 8F guiding catheter with an internal diameter of 1.83 mm, this luminal cross-sectional area is 2.63 mm^2. With an enclosed 3F monorail shaft, the opening available for contrast medium is only reduced to 1.8 mm^2, but is reduced to 1.5 mm^2 and to 1.0 mm^2 with 3.6F and 4.3F shafts, respectively (Table 27-1).

The proximal end of the shaft remaining outside the guiding catheter is reinforced to size 3.6F to control balloon motion within the coronary system. The shaft tube terminates within the balloon.

The most characteristic feature of the monorail catheter is an additional central coaxial tube within the distal balloon part fitting the guidewire. The tube is delimited by an end hole forming the balloon tip (as in conventional catheters) and by a more or less eccentrically placed side hole proximal to the balloon. The length of the tube is between 4 and 11 cm and may be as long as the distal part of the balloon catheter entering the coronary system. The balloon material used until now is polyvinylchloride. When the guidewire is fitted into the central tube, the catheter is suspended with its distal end on the wire and can be pushed forward and backward on the guidewire as on a sliding rail. Distal pressure measurement is not provided in standard models to maintain a low catheter shaft profile.

An additional device to overcome acute ischemia in acute coronary occlusion is a large diameter intracoronary transfusion catheter. This catheter has a 4.3F thin-walled shaft, a 1 cm soft distal tip with a radiopaque marker, and two side holes approximately 1 cm from the tip. The catheter serves to transfuse arterialized blood into the coronary segment distal to the occlusion. The device is not intended for longer treatment periods but only to prevent ischemia during transfer to the operating room.

DESCRIPTION OF THE PROCEDURE

In using the monorail system the PTCA procedure is essentially modified as compared

Table 27-1. Relation of Shaft Diameters of Balloon Catheters and Luminal Space Within Standard 8F Guiding Catheters Remaining for Contrast Flow

		Balloon Catheter Shaft		*Space for Contrast Flow within Guiding Catheter Cross-Sectional Area**	
		Diameter (mm)	*Cross-sectional Area (mm^2)*	*(mm^2)*	*(%)*
Monorail	3.0F	1.0	0.79	1.8	73
Conventional steerable	3.6F	1.19	1.1	1.5	57
	4.2F	1.43	1.6	1.0	38

**The internal luminal cross-sectional area of an 8F guiding catheter (2.6 mm^2 = 100%) is significantly reduced by large shafts of conventional balloon catheters compromising contrast flow. Contrast flow is not impaired with the use of 3Fr monorail catheters.*

with using conventional systems. First, the guidewire alone without the balloon catheter is advanced through the Y-connector, the guiding catheter, and across the stenosis. The large remaining space within the guiding catheter has two consequences: motion of the wire is hardly impeded by friction and contrast flow is unimpaired. These two factors allow for optimal steerability of the guidewire through the fully visualized coronary pathway and stenosis. If necessary, guidewires with different properties in stiffness or tip shape can be rapidly exchanged. After passing the stenosis the guidewire becomes the stationary part for the entire procedure. The proper balloon catheter is selected, pushed up onto the guidewire and, sliding on the guidewire, is advanced through the guiding catheter and across the stenosis. Selection and unwrapping of the balloon can be delayed until placement of the guidewire. While the balloon is pushed forward or drawn backward the guidewire is fixed at the outside. The exchange of a balloon catheter for larger balloon sizes is performed in the same way. Fluoroscopic control is only necessary during the coronary passage of the balloon, but not during the long passage through the guiding catheter. This can contribute to the reduction of fluoroscopy time, especially in exchange procedures. A sufficient flow of dye ensures optimal visualization of the coronary stenosis and the dilatation result even with the use of nondiluted contrast media of standard viscosities and with the balloon tip in the coronary system.

In case of acute coronary occlusion a balloon catheter may be exchanged in favor of a large-diameter 4.3F monorail transfusion catheter. When the side holes and end holes are placed into the coronary segment distal to the occlusion arterialized blood can be transfused into the myocardial area at risk thus reverting ischemia until emergency bypass surgery. The blood can be taken from the contralateral femoral artery and is transfused by hand by means of a three-way stopcock system. The process is a manually controlled femoro-coronary autotransfusion and is regarded as a bailout technique.

PATIENT EXPERIENCE

Routine PTCA with the monorail balloon catheter system was performed in our institution (University of Freiburg Medical Clinic) since the beginning of 1986 and in 1987, for a total of more than 400 PTCA procedures. All PTCAs were performed with biplane multidirectional x-ray systems attempting for optimal triple orthogonal projections of the stenoses. Drugs administered were 600 mg of the night before, and at the beginning of the procedure 10,000 units of heparin, isosorbide dinitrate 5 mg sublingually, and nifedipine 10 mg sublingually were administered. During the procedure urokinase up to 100,000 units (maximum 200,000 units) was given intermittently by intracoronary injection.

Monorail catheters were used in the first consecutive 150 patients in 1986 and in about 90% of the remaining patients. To compare yearly results from 1980 through 1987 statistical analysis was performed as a test of trend. The detailed analysis of the clinical data will be published in the future; in the following we summarize data referring mostly to the comparison between our results up to 1985 and during 1986–1987.

The overall success rate was stable, being more than 90% for subtotal stenoses and 70 to 80% for complete obstructions. The death rate was 0% with monorail catheters, and 0.9% as an average between 1980 and 1985. Myocardial infarction and emergency operation rates were not changed and remained in the range of 3% and 2%. However, there was a statistically significant increase in the percentage of stenosis diameter improvement from 46% in 1985 to 59%. Since 1985 there was also a statistically significant decrease of fluoroscopy time from 22 to 16 minutes and of investigation time (patient in laboratory time) from 94 to 85 minutes. This results in a reduction of radiation exposure by about 27% and in a reduction of staff hours by 10%. With a staff of four this is a gain of 36 minutes or more than ½ hour for one PTCA procedure (Table 27-2).

Monorail procedures were performed by one investigator in the first 150 patients and by four investigators in the rest of the patients. All investigators were senior cardiologists but with different levels of experience in PTCA ranging between 50 and several hundred procedures. The monorail technique was generally judged more simple and easy to perform than conventional techniques. Nevertheless adjustment to the new technique was significantly enhanced by personal training.

In none of the procedures were adverse effects related to the monorail technique observed. Notably, there were no systemic or coronary embolizations. This complication, conceivable by clot formation after backbleeding into the guiding catheter, was also not observed in patients treated by the long wire technique.

Practical experience with steerability led to the conclusion that the steerability of monorail catheters is as good as the steerability of the guidewire itself. This means that steerability is not limited by any balloon catheter property but is dependent only on guidewire properties. No balloon device is more steerable than a well-constructed guidewire.

Visualization of the coronary tree and stenosis was as good as expected from the small monorail shaft diameter. Adequate contrast flow was always available at any time point during the procedure, even with the tip of the catheter within the coronary system. This proved to be especially important in the observation period after stenosis dilatation for the judgment of the result or the discovery of stenosis dissection.

Balloon exchange was performed in about one third of patients. The reason for exchange was usually the intention to use a larger balloon in an angiographically unsatisfactory result. Less frequently the reason was failure to

Table 27-2. Relevant Clinical and Logistic Results of PTCA Procedures Before 1986 Using Conventional Steerable Devices and in 1987 Using Monorail Catheters*

	Clinical Data					*Logistic Data*	
	No. Patients	*Primary Success Rate (%)*	*Stenosis Diameter Increase (delta %)*	*Emergency Operation (%)*	*Death (%)*	*Fluoroscopy Time (min)*	*Laboratory Investigation Time (min)*
1985	94	92	46	2.1	1.0	22	94
1987	276	91	59	1.3	0	16	85
Significance		NS	S	NS	NS	S	S

**Significance relates to differences according to yearly trend analysis for the years 1980 to 1987 ($p <$ or $<<0.05$). The improved stenosis diameter increase is felt to be due to the simplified catheter exchange procedure and thus more frequent use of larger balloons to optimize the PTCA result. Improvement of time factors is caused by the overall simplified and more precise handling of guidewires and monorail balloon catheters.*

NS, Not significant; S, significant.

pass the stenoses and the consequent selection of a smaller balloon. Balloon exchange was usually performed within less than 2 minutes and without technical difficulties.

A transfusion catheter was used in four patients undergoing emergency bypass surgery (in another patient, the transfusion catheter was not yet available). All patients had acute left anterior descending (LAD) artery occlusion with severe ischemia following extended intimal dissection during PTCA. Flow rates maintained with intermittent manually controlled femoro-coronary autotransfusion were between 40 and 60 ml/min over time periods between 60 and 120 minutes starting in the cardiac laboratory and finishing with the institution of cardiocirculatory bypass. In all patients ischemia was at least temporarily reversed during the transfer to the operating room within the same building. In one patient ischemia reappeared after about 30 minutes of transfusion. In this patient with a large LAD artery and diagonal branch distal to the occlusion, transmural myocardial infarction could not be prevented. In the other three patients Q-wave infarction could be ruled out and control left ventricular angiogram showed normal anterior wall motion. One problem was that the initiation of anesthesia and also surgical action was slowed down when the apparently stable and asymptomatic patient appeared at the operating room.

DISCUSSION

With increasing experience and advanced catheter technology primary PTCA success rates have reached a standard level of more than 80% and of more than 90% in outstanding centers. Thus it is difficult to demonstrate increasing success rates with new types of catheters.

In our patients treated with monorail catheters the success rate was also 90% or higher. This result was achieved not only by the main investigator but was also verified by less experienced investigators. They preferred the monorail system for most of their patients, not only because of the simplicity but also because of the safety of the procedure. The transfusion catheter is felt to be especially useful to reduce the risk when dilating proximal stenoses of large vessels. In our opinion the possibility of rapid and safe catheter exchange even in critical situations may in fact reduce mortality to less than 1% or to rates known from early diagnostic coronary angiography.

Another result of catheter exchangeability is the average increase in stenosis diameter by nearly 60% (of the normal vessel diameter). Thus the goal of less than 20 or 30% residual stenosis in routine PTCA seems realistic.

With increasing numbers of PTCA patients logistic data are getting more and more important. The reduction in fluoroscopy time by about 27% and of patient laboratory time by 10% may protect the investigator and reduce overall PTCA costs quite significantly. In our opinion there are three essential reasons for the logistic advantages relating directly to monorail properties: the excellent steerability, the contrast flow yielding uncompromised coronary and stenosis image information at any time during the procedure, and again the rapid exchangeability of catheters. Clinical practice in more than 400 patients undergoing monorail PTCA procedures has confirmed the theoretically conceived advantages of the system without observation of essential disadvantages.

Transstenotic pressure gradient measurements are in our opinion of secondary value. The absence of transstenotic pressure gradient measurement during routine PTCA was never an essential disadvantage. This underlines the superiority of the information derived from optimal coronary imaging. The superiority can be well explained: the information derived from transstenotic pressure gradients is limited. A persisting pressure gradient after dilatation signals a nonsatisfying result but gives no information on the cause of the problem. A pressure gradient across a stenosis of a large vessel of 3 or 4 mm diameter has certainly another meaning than a gradient in a small distal vessel of 2 mm or less. For example, in a 4 mm vessel a residual stenosis of 50% or 2 mm will not show a gradient and thus will remain undetected unless angiographically visualized. On the other hand, in a small 2 mm vessel a 25% or 0.5 mm residual stenosis may still demonstrate a significant gradient suggesting the untoward use of a larger balloon. Furthermore, the pressure gradient is only available as long as the balloon remains within the stenosis. In contrast, optimal angiographic imaging, preferably biplane, delineates the coronary pathway for the guidewire and the pathway through complicated stenoses, ensures the correct balloon position, and generates a complete picture of the dilatation result. This information includes residual stenosis and the detection of intimal tears or dissection, thrombus, and spasm. Thus in our opinion, because of the superiority of the image information, pressure gradients are no longer an essential part in monitoring PTCA and can be easily dispensed with if optimized angiographic images are available.

Future developments in monorail catheters are aiming for increased safety by the use of stabilizing devices such as hot balloons or wall stents, and for diagnostic accuracy by the use of Doppler and other intracoronary catheters. The ease of catheter exchange will favor the monorail technique in these developments.

CONCLUSION

Percutaneous transluminal coronary angioplasty is in increasing numbers performed as a routine procedure with a high success rate for two main reasons: accumulation of available information or experience and continuing progress in dilatation catheter technology. However, properties of catheters are still imperfect in terms of PTCA safety and ease and simplicity of the procedure. A new system according to the sliding rail (monorail) principle and experience with 400 patients are described. The characteristic part of the system is a short coaxial tube within the distal balloon part fitting the guidewire. Thus the balloon is suspended and can slide on the guidewire as on a rail. Distal pressure measurement is not provided in standard models. Advantages are rapid exchangeability of balloons, improved contrast flow resulting from a low shaft profile, and improved contrast flow resulting from a low shaft profile, and improved steerability. A transfusion catheter serves to control ischemia in acute stenosis occlusion.

Clinical experience confirmed a high safety with no mortality and a reduced fluoroscopy and investigation time. The success rate was stable above 90%, and adverse effects related to the technique were not observed. Improved imaging by unimpaired contrast flow was felt to be an advantage compared with distal pressure measurement. It is concluded that the theoretically conceived advantages of the monorail system can be verified by extensive clinical evaluation.

REFERENCES

1. Gruntzig, A., Senning, A., and Siegenthaler, W.E.: Nonoperative dilatation of coronary artery stenosis: percutaneous transluminal coronary angioplasty, N. Engl. J. Med. **301:**61-68, 1979.
2. Simpson, J.B., Baim, D.S., Robert, E.W., and Harrison, D.L.: A new catheter system for coronary angioplasty, Am. J. Cardiol. **49:**1216-1221, 1982.
3. Kaltenbach, M.: Neue Technik zur steuerbaren Ballondilatation von Kranzgefäßverengungen, Z. Kardiol. **73:**669-673, 1984.
4. Bonzel, T., Wollschläger, H., and Just, H.: Ein neues Kathetersystem zur mechanischen Dilatation von Koronarstenosen mit austauschbaren intrakoronaren Kathetern, höherem Kontrastmittelfluß und verbesserter Steuerbarkeit, Biomed. Tech. **31:**195-200, 1986.

Chapter 28

Nonsurgical Implantation of a New Intravascular Stent Prosthesis

Ulrich Sigwart, MD, FACC

EXPERIMENTAL AND CLINICAL EXPERIENCE

Despite the considerable improvements that have been made to angioplasty equipment and the developments made in clinical technique, the procedure of angioplasty is still associated with a traumatic assault on the integrity of both the arteriosclerotic and native vessel walls. The fluid dynamics of the acute postdilatation situation and the long-term healing of the traumatized surfaces remain continuing problems to the extent that acute occlusion occurs in 5% of cases and the restenosis rate may be as high as 35% within the first few months of recovery. The fact that these statistics have remained relatively constant despite the experience and progress attained with angioplasty leads one to propose that a logical approach to both preventing acute occlusion and chronic restenosis may be the use of an intraluminal scaffolding device or stent to support and smooth the traumatized lumen.

Of fundamental importance in early research work with different types of stent prostheses is the consistent finding that cell proliferation occurs over the metal surface, thereby encapsulating the prosthesis into the vessel wall and protecting it from further contact with blood.[1-3] None of today's design concepts, however, come reasonably close to the ideal intravascular stent especially in respect to homogeneous force distribution, ease of access, conformability, and stability. Therefore, a new system was developed comprising a stainless steel, multifilament, self-expanding, macroporous prosthesis and an innovative instrument for prostheses delivery (Medinvent SA, Lausanne, Switzerland).

Methods

The stent is woven from a surgical-grade stainless steel alloy formulated to International Standards Organization prescriptions. Because of its design (Fig. 28-1) and process of fabrication the prostheses can be made geometrically stable, compliant, and self-expanding. The elastic and compliant properties of the prosthesis geometry are such that by moderate longitudinal elongation, the pros-

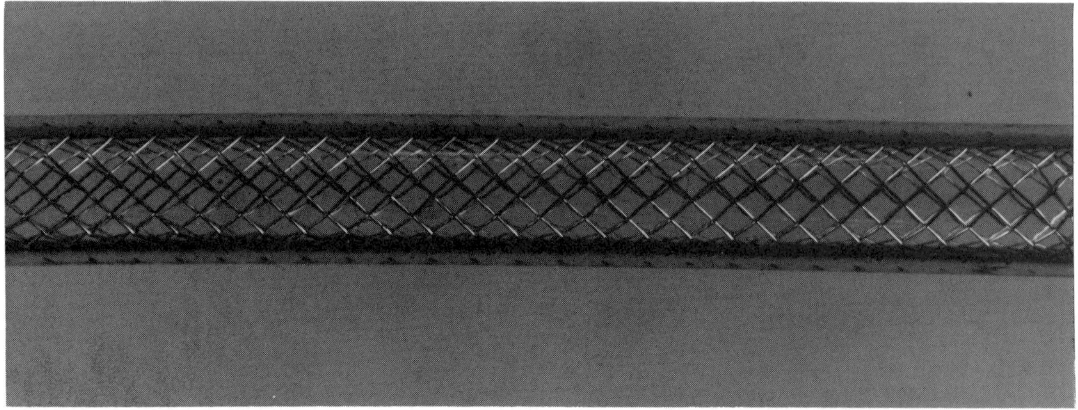

Fig. 28-1. The self-expanding, elastic, macroporous tubular prosthesis, which is woven from stainless steel. The lower part depicts the stent in the unconstrained state.

thesis diameter may be significantly reduced. It can thus be constrained on a small-diameter delivery catheter and as the constraining membrane is progressively removed, the device will elastically try to return to its original unconstrained large diameter. When implanted in a vessel whose caliber is less than that of the unconstrained diameter of the prosthesis, there will be a residual elastic radial force in the prosthesis that will try to dilate the artery until an equilibrium is attained between the circumferential elastic resistance of the arterial wall and the dilating force of the prosthesis.

The constrained wire-mesh prosthesis is retained at the distal end of the delivery catheter by a double-layer membrane that can be progressively withdrawn by virtue of a fluid film between the layers; low friction during the deployment process is maintained by filling of the intermediate space with contrast medium at approximately 3 bars of pressure. Two or three radiopaque metal markers on the delivery catheter permit the better identification of the extremities of the prosthesis at the time of deployment. The outer diameter of the loaded catheter system is 1.57 mm; prostheses up to 6.5 mm nominal diameter can be mounted on such a delivery device. Larger diameter prostheses for peripheral use have correspondingly larger delivery systems.

Animal Experimentation

Prostheses up to 6.5 mm in diameter when mounted on the delivery catheter could be passed through conventional guiding catheters to the femoral, popliteal, and coronary arteries.

Under pentobarbital anesthesia and fluoroscopic control, 15 stents were implanted in the vessels of 25 to 35 kg mongrel dogs, who received no anticoagulants or antiplatelet agents before or after implantation. In general during catheterization the animals were given an intravenous heparin infusion of 25 units per kg body weight per hour. One dog received only 12.5 units of heparin per kg body weight; this led to an acute thrombosis of the prosthesis, which was spontaneously recanalized during the first 3 weeks of follow-up.

In three dogs, eight transluminal implants under adequate heparinization were placed into branches of the femoral arteries at the level of the knee by way of the common femoral artery (Fig. 28-2). The prostheses varied from 2 to 6.5 mm in diameter and between 20 to 70 mm in length. The prostheses were

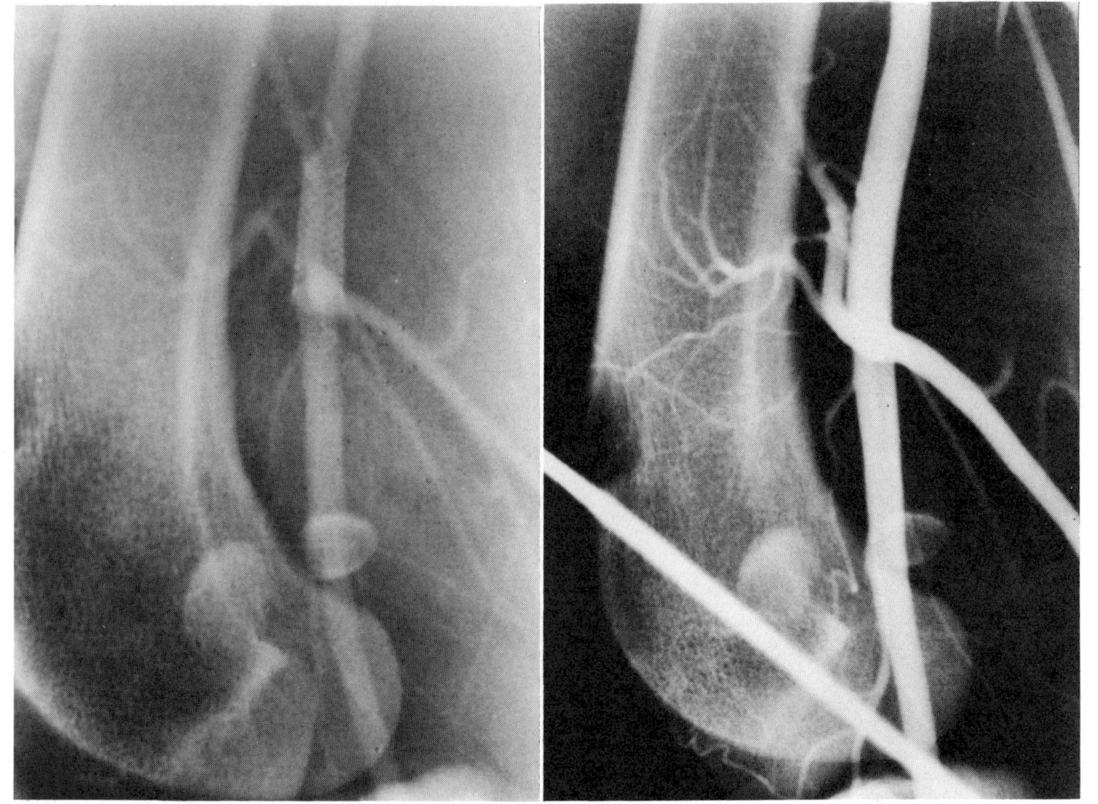

Fig. 28-2. The endoluminal stent prothesis after implantation in a canine femoral artery. The faint contrast injection (2a) allows for better identification of the stent and the side branch leaving the stented segment.

patent immediately after implantation and remained patent after successive angiographic controls at 3-month intervals up to 1 year. Weekly Doppler flow monitoring also indicated equally positive results. Two dogs were electively sacrificed after 6 and 9 months' survival; three stents were perfectly patent, one demonstrating a mural thrombus and one recanalization of a stent perfused retrograde in an artery that had been proximally ligated.

The prostheses remained free from intimal hyperplasia and, moreover, side branches leaving the stented segments of the main vessel remained clearly patent (Figs. 28-2 and 28-3). In seven dogs, seven coronary prostheses were implanted by femoral artery access and 8F coronary guiding catheters.

Under fluoroscopy one stent was placed in the right coronary artery, one stent was placed in the first marginal branch of the right coronary artery, and five prostheses were placed in the proximal left anterior descending coronary artery. Prosthesis dimensions varied between 2.5 and 3.5 mm in diameter and 15 and 20 mm in length. Again, no anticoagulants were given after implantation, but an intraoperative heparinized perfusion was given. On control angiography at 3 and 6 months after implantation, no signs of obstruction either from thrombus or hyperplasia

Text continues on page 333.

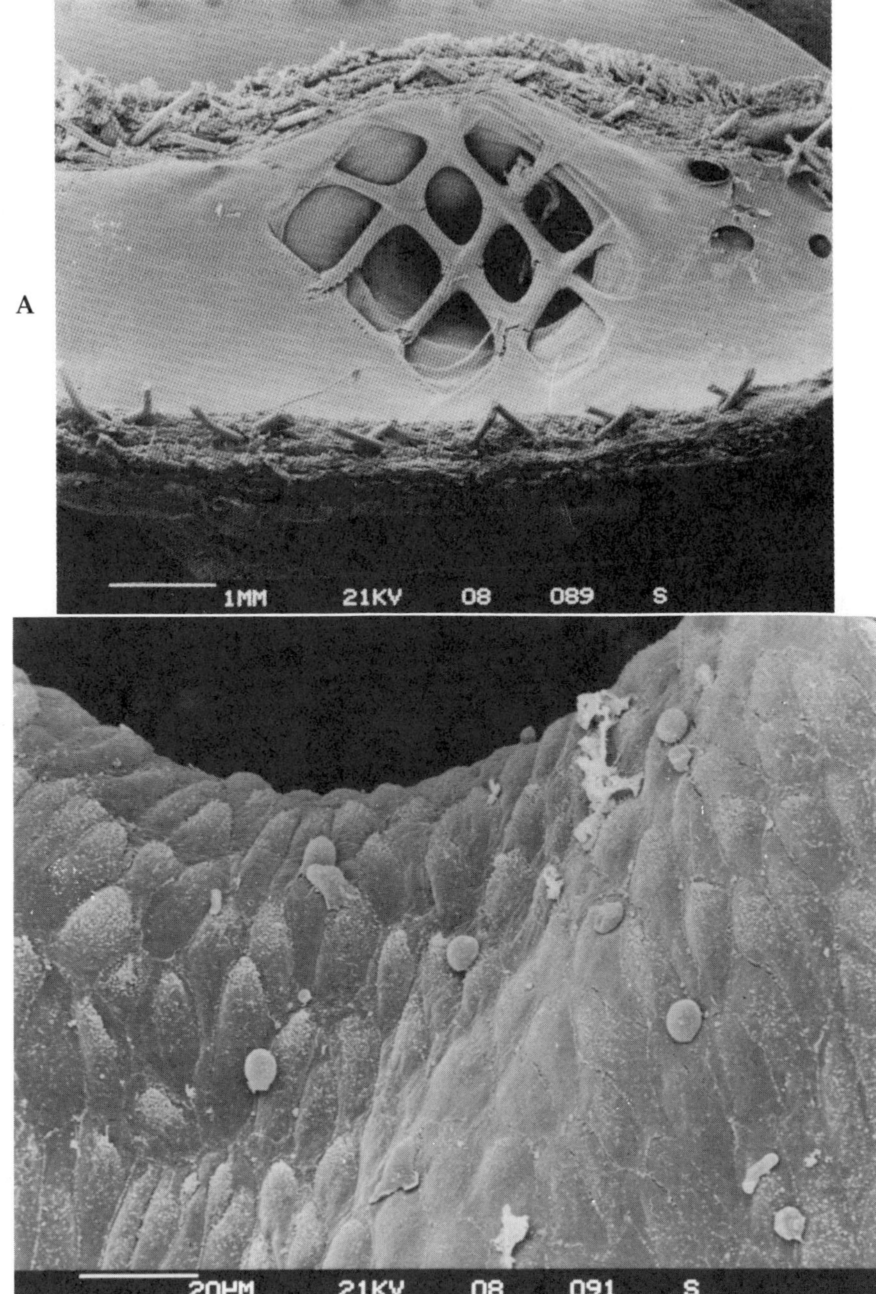

Fig. 28-3. A, Scanning electron micrograph of a stent covering the orifice of a departing side branch of a canine femoral artery (see Fig. 28-2). Nine months after implantation the metal wires are totally coated with a smooth neointimal lining that does not interfere with blood flow to the branch artery. **B,** A high-magnification view of the neoendothelial surface of the junction between stent and branch vessel.

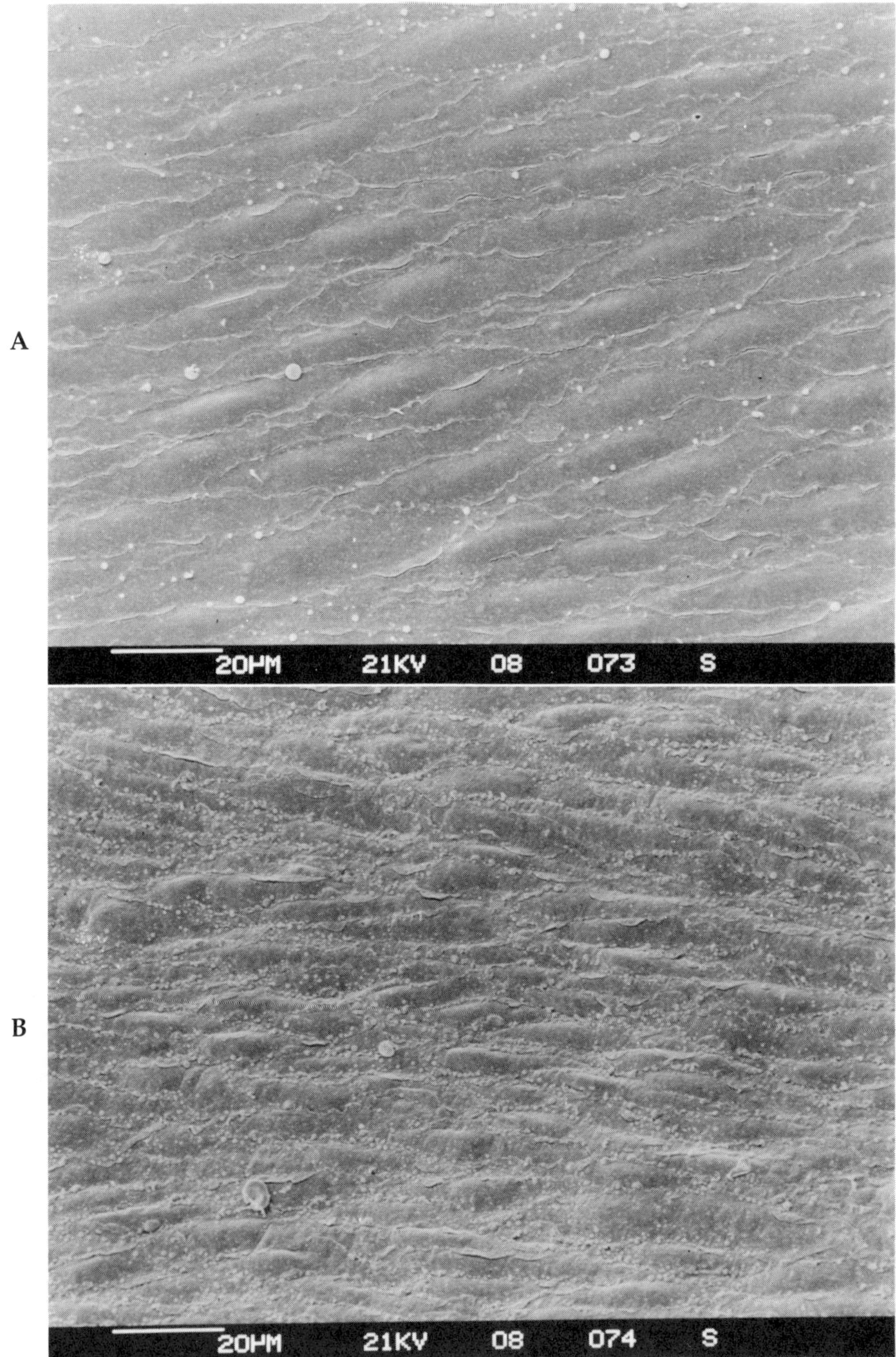

Fig. 28-4. A, Scanning electron microscopy of the endothelial surface covering the prosthesis. **B,** For comparison the endothelium of the adjacent, nonstented artery is shown. The specimen was recovered from a canine femoral artery 9 months after implantation.

were seen; however, at sacrifice at 9 months one case of nonobstructive mural thrombus caused by diameter mismatch between artery and stent was seen.

Two additional animals were electively sacrificed at 3 months and at 6 months respectively for histologic analysis, and the rest of this series of animals continues in perfect health.

Histologic Analysis

From previous trials with an early prosthesis design, histologic analyses at 24 hours, 4 weeks, 3 months, and 6 months demonstrated the mechanism of prosthesis–vessel wall interaction.[2]

The major steps were as follows:

1. An initial abrasion of the endothelial lining.
2. Within a period of 1 month the intima thickens, filling the spaces between the metal filaments of the prosthesis and smoothly covering the entire prosthesis.
3. After 3 months the intimal covering is stabilized and no further evolution occurs.
4. No perforation of the internal elastic lamina is seen and no damage to the media is apparent as evidenced by a lack of vacuolization.

Fig. 28-3 gives an example of a prosthesis firmly embedded in the arterial wall. This specimen was recovered from a branch of the femoral artery at the level of the left knee 9 months after implantation. Scanning electron microscopy shows the neointima filling the pores between the stent filaments in a rather smooth fashion. The thickness of the neointimal layer is about 450 μm and no signs of necrosis caused by the continuous mural pressure of the metal filaments is seen. The endothelial surface (Fig. 28-4A) is very similar to the original arterial endothelium (Fig. 28-4B). All side branches within the stented segments remained open. The stents were covered with smooth intimal lining when the arteries were removed for analysis after 9 months (Fig. 28-5).

First Clinical Experience

Following the encouraging results from animal trials a protocol for human implants was submitted for hospital ethics committee review. The protocol defined indications, methods, and monitoring for stent implants in peripheral and coronary arteries of patients.

For *peripheral implants* highly symptomatic patients were selected for:

1. Recanalization of the iliac or femoral artery with long and complex stenoses and in whom balloon angioplasty either failed or suggested poor prognosis.
2. Iliac or femoral restenosis after previous angioplasty.

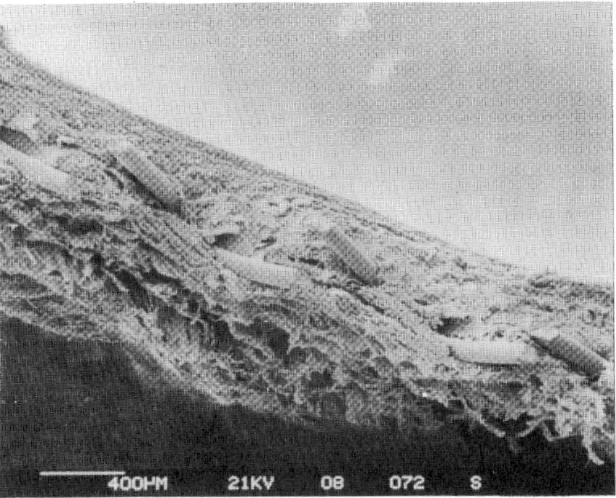

Fig. 28-5. Scanning electron microscopy of a prosthesis firmly embedded in femoral artery of a dog at the level of the left knee 9 months after implantation (see text for details.)

For *coronary implants* three conditions were considered indications for endoluminal stents:

1. Restenosis of a major coronary artery after previous coronary angioplasty.
2. Stenosis of aortocoronary bypass grafts suggesting poor overall graft quality.
3. Acute occlusion secondary to intimal dissection following balloon angioplasty.

The protocol was accepted and the informed patient consent (in accordance with the Helsinki Declaration) was obtained from each patient before the intervention.

Peripheral Implants

Implantation Technique

Fourteen peripheral stent prostheses were implanted in nine patients in femoral and iliac arteries. Stent diameters varied between 6 and 12 mm, and stent length measured from 30 to 80 mm. Prostheses up to 6.5 mm nominal diameter were delivered through an 8F coronary guiding catheter. Larger stents were deployed using an 8F delivery system introduced directly through an ordinary 9F arterial introducing sheath. Drug therapy consisted of 500 mg of acetylsalicylic acid the day before the intervention, a bolus injection of 15,000 units of heparin during the implantation, and a fixed combination of 330 mg of aspirin plus 75 mg of dipyridamole once daily, in addition to oral anticoagulation with sodium warfarin (Coumadin) for the first 3 months of follow-up.

Results

In two patients totally occluded arteries were recanalized and stented. One patient had a left superficial femoral artery occlusion of 30 cm length that failed to remain patent despite adequate balloon angioplasty followed by local urokinase infusion. Two consecutive prostheses of 6 mm diameter and 8 cm length (Fig. 28-6) were implanted, resulting in adequate blood flow and disappearance of severe claudication. Symptoms reappeared after 3 months caused by high-grade stenoses of the nonstented femoral artery segments proximal to and between the stents. These stenoses were then dilated and reinforced by three additional stents, one over the first two prostheses and two upstream to the first implants. There was again very significant clinical amelioration, suppression of pressure gra-

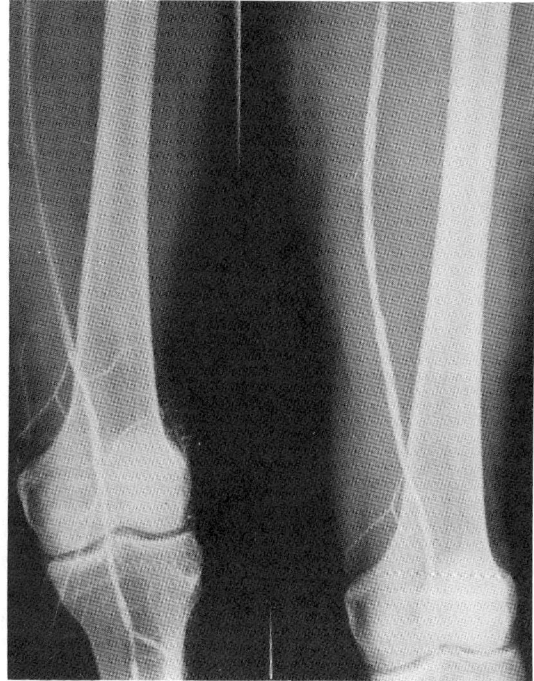

Fig. 28-6. Superficial femoral artery after mechanical recanalization of a 30 cm long total occlusion followed by catheter implantation of 2 consecutive endoprostheses. For better visualization of the stent prostheses the right part of this figure shows injection of contrast medium distal to the two prostheses through a 4F angiography catheter. Note the nonstented lesion 4 cm below the knee. Three more prostheses were implanted 3 months later to treat severe lesions within nonstented segments.

dient, and improvement in peripheral flow as demonstrated by Doppler evaluation. Some endothelial thickening within the stents was noted at the time of control angiography; this intimal hyperplasia, however, was not important enough to produce a significant pressure gradient or significant modification of the Doppler flow signal. Significant focal restenosis, however, developed 1 year later. The most important lesions were transluminally removed with the help of an atherectomy device (Devices for Vascular Interventions, Stanford, Calif.).

The second patient had a long-standing, 8 cm occlusion of the left external iliac artery that was mechanically recanalized, dilated and, since no adequate flow was attained, stented with a prosthesis of 8 cm length and 12 mm diameter. No recurrence of symptoms has been observed over 19 months' follow-up. All other prostheses were placed into subocculded arteries not responding satisfactorily to conventional balloon angioplasty. There was no case of recurrence as judged from reappearance of symptoms or decrease of peripheral flow after Doppler measurements or digital subtraction angiography. No side effects were reported.

Coronary Implants

Implantation Technique

More than 70 coronary stents were implanted following transluminal balloon angioplasty in patients. The same standard drug regimen, including platelet aggregation inhibitors and intraoperative heparin therapy, was used. Intravenous heparin was continued for the first 24 hours postoperatively. Oral anti–vitamin K+ (warfarin) anticoagulation was given postoperatively together with aspirin 100 mg and dypyridamole 150 to 200 mg b.i.d., as well as sulfinpyrazone 200 mg b.i.d. for 3 months. All patients also received calcium antagonists.

After successful angioplasty, the balloon was exchanged for the stent delivery system over a 0.014 or 0.018-inch exchange guidewire. The delivery device was sufficiently supple to permit passage through tortuous vessels. Placement was undertaken under high-resolution fluoroscopy at the site of the previously dilated lesion. The stent diameter was chosen in accordance with that of the native artery. Stents of 15 to 23 mm in length depending on the size of the lesion were used.

In 65 operative sessions implantation attempts were carried out in 59 patients. In one case the deployment of the stent in the left anterior descending (LAD) coronary artery failed because of initial problems with the delivery catheter; since no reserve device was available, implantation was abandoned without complications. Stents were placed 29 times in the LAD coronary artery, 19 times in the right coronary artery (RCA), 4 times in the circumflex artery (Cx), and 18 times in a coronary artery bypass graft (CABG).[7] Seven patients received a second prosthesis at a later date, in each case for a new lesion. There were 12 emergency implantations for acute occlusion after transluminal angioplasty. An example is given in Fig. 28-7, which shows the stented artery 2 months after implantation of a prosthesis of 3.5 mm maximal diameter and 20 mm length. The same patient underwent stenting of the right coronary artery for restenosis (Fig. 28-8).

Occlusion of the stent occurred seven times during the hospital stay; however, the prosthesis remained permanently patent in five patients after redilatation and local infusion of 100,000 units of urokinase. Thrombolytic therapy was refused in one patient.

Results

Three patients of this series have died: one following elective bypass surgery for new left main artery disease and one died suddenly at home. One implantation deserves further comment. This patient had a 90% proximal

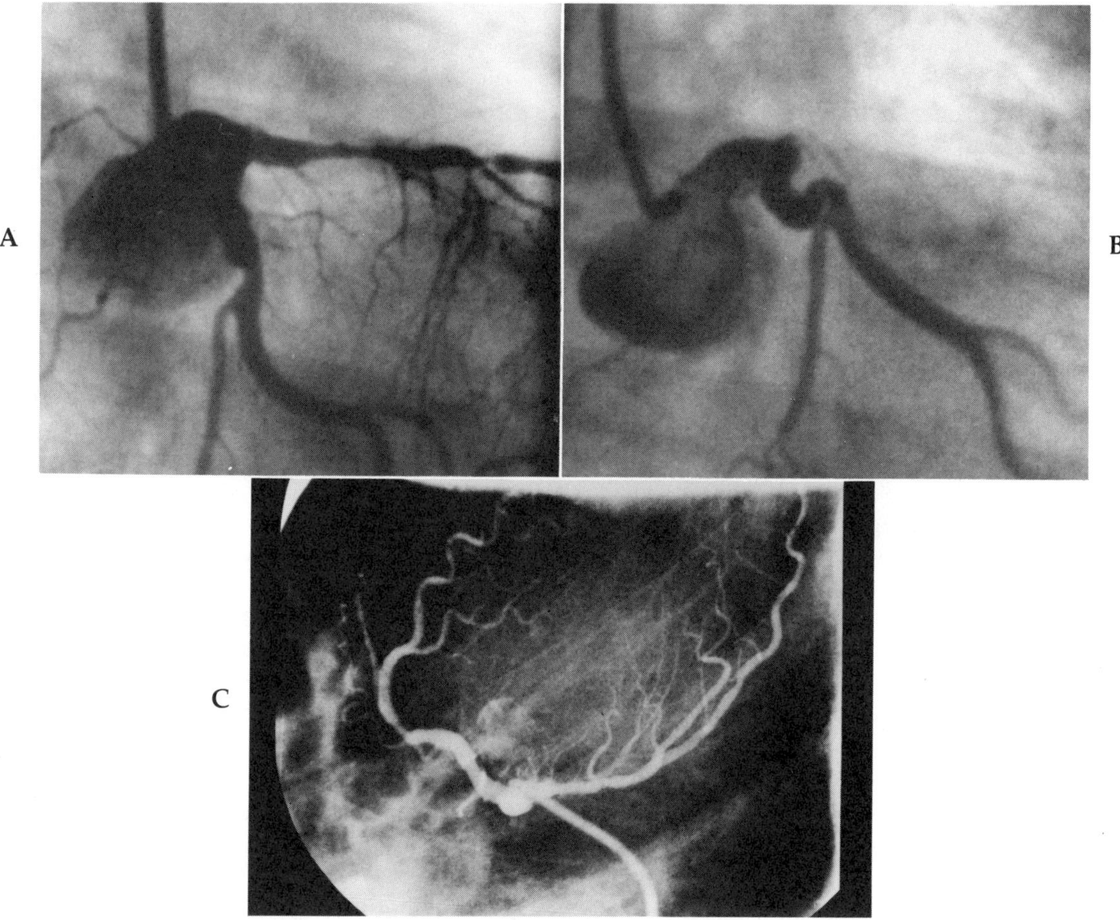

Fig. 28-7. Left coronary artery before angioplasty **(A)**, after angioplasty **(B)**, and 6 months after emergency recanalization and stent implantation of the LAD coronary artery **(C)**. The stent is invisible because of high contrast.

stenosis of the LAD coronary artery causing residual angina 1 week after a limited anteroapical infarction. After angioplasty symptomatic restenosis occurred within 2 months (Fig. 28-9A). The lesion was redilated and stented (Fig. 28-9B) giving a perfect result (Fig. 28-9C). Two days later the patient underwent maximal stress testing without any evidence of ischemia. Shortly afterward he developed a strong vagal reaction with electrocardiographic signs of anterolateral ischemia. In the absence of immediately available angiographic facilities the patient was transferred for bypass surgery (internal mammary implant), at which time the signs of ischemia had disappeared and the prosthesis was found to be fully patent. Immediate postoperative recovery was uneventful except for problems with hemostasis and some signs of cardiac tamponade. The following day the patient went into unexplained hypoxia and subsequently died. Postmorten examination revealed signs of cardiac tamponade, a patent bypass graft, and some traces of recent (less

Text continues on page 339.

A

B

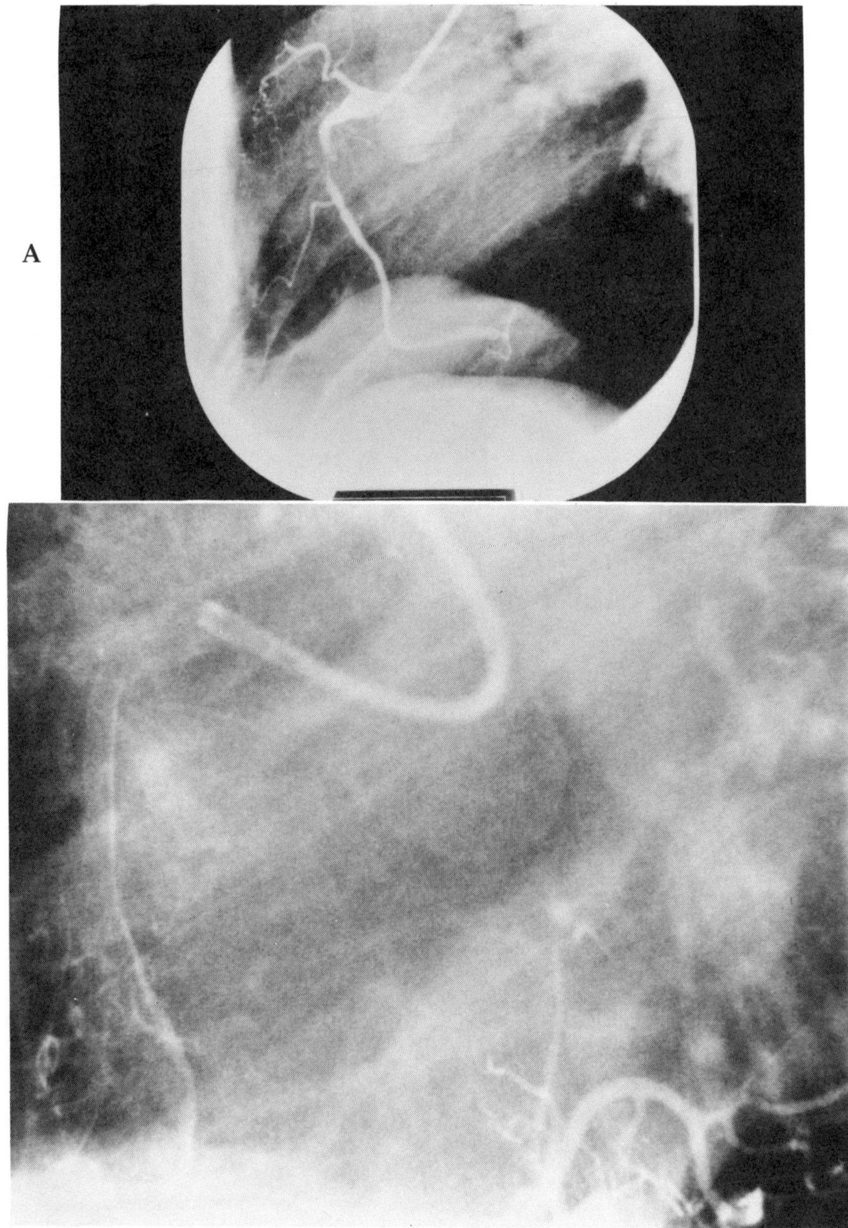

Fig. 28-8. Same patient as in Fig. 28-7. **A,** Restenosis 8 weeks after PTCA of the right coronary artery. **B,** Stenting of the redilated artery using an endoprosthesis of 20 mm length, and 3.5 mm nominal diameter. **C,** A regular contrast injection fails to depict the implanted prosthesis but reveals absence of residual stenosis. **D,** shows the result 6 months later.

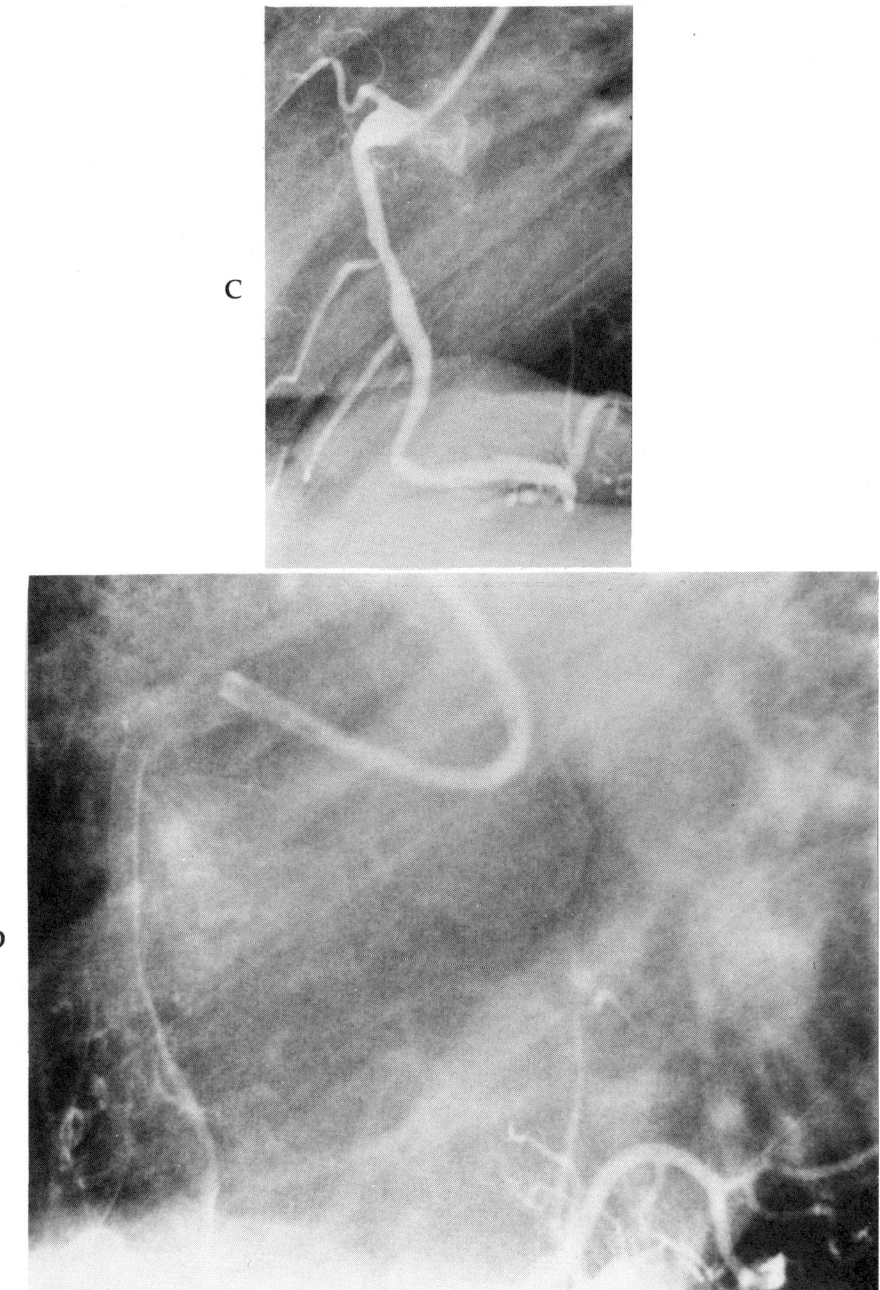

Fig. 28-8, cont'd. For legend see p. 337.

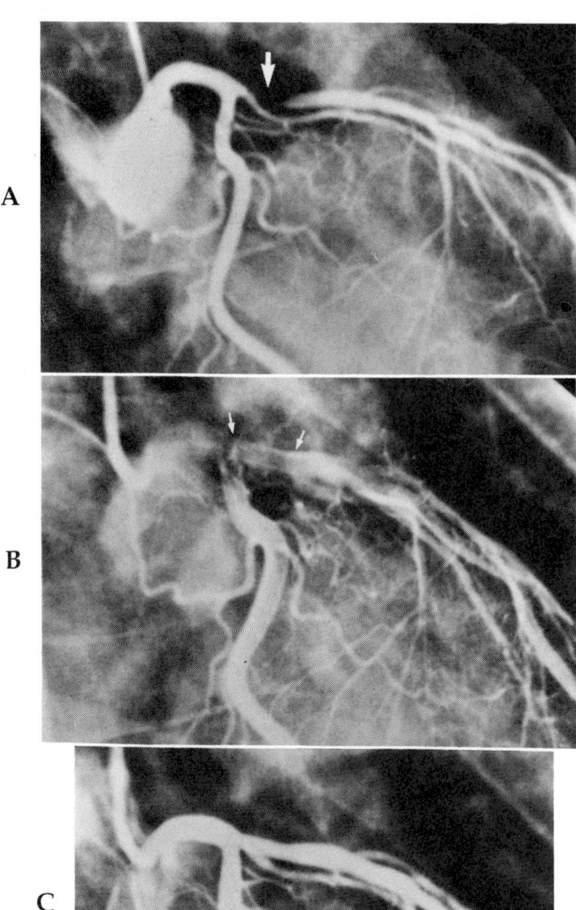

Fig. 28-9. Restenosis of the LAD coronary artery 6 weeks after first angioplasty. **A,** There is a greater than 90% proximal LAD stenosis after implantation of the self-expanding endoprosthesis **(B).** A regular contrast injection reveals a perfect result **(C).**

than 1 hour old) thrombus in the prosthesis. No clear link between death and the prosthesis could be established.

All other patients had essentially normal recovery and left the hospital within 5 days after the procedure. Follow-up consisted of weekly and then monthly clinical examination, stress tests at 2-month intervals, and control coronary angiography within 3 to 6 months following the intervention. There were two patients with clinical signs of restenosis as judged by history and exercise electrocardiogram. Control coronary angiography showed the endoluminal stent embedded in smooth-looking tissue creating 90% luminal narrowing and suggesting intimal hyperplasia within the device segment. Both patients could successfully be redilated; one patient, however, underwent elective surgery for a second recurrence and a new lesion in another vessel. There were three left occlusions.

DISCUSSION

Restenosis and acute occlusion following transluminal angioplasty of coronary and peripheral arterial disease is one of the most challenging issues in cardiovascular medicine. With restenosis rates as high as 33% after coronary angioplasty and even higher (68%) in multivessel angioplasty,[8] the overall value of balloon angioplasty is significantly reduced even when one admits the relatively low morbidity of such a procedure, which is frequently repeated not once but several times. The socioeconomic implications of repeat angioplasty are important and largely counterbalance the initially low comparative cost of the intervention. Experience has shown that the acute and chronic reocclusion rates after peripheral and coronary angioplasty are independent of operator skills and the quality of the materials employed. Longer inflation times calling for sophisticated devices to ensure distal perfusion, high-dose slow-channel-calcium blockers, steroids, and other drug regimens have thus far failed to provide a major contribution to the prevention of this problem. The arterial occlusion rate—acute or chronic—is probably inherent in the composition and structure of the plaque and the nature of the trauma applied to the vessel wall.

Many clinicians have therefore come to the conclusion that there is a need for a suitable endoluminal support of the diseased vessel wall.[1-7] Several designs for supports have been proposed, notably elastically self-expanding types (spirals),[2,3] memory metal types (thermally expandable and relatively inelastic),[5,6] and balloon-deformable (quasi-rigid) models.[1,7] Endothelization with uniform and consistent intimal thickening and collateral vessel patency as we described has also been found by others,[1-3] but with some minor distinctions. It appears that the rate of canine intimal thickening is relatively constant and thus the time for covering of the stent surface depends on the metal element thickness. Thus Wright and associates[3] report only 30% covering at 1 month for 0.46-mm-thick wire, while we found total covering of 0.09 mm filaments within 3 weeks. The relative porosity of the structure also appears to play a determining role in that memory metal grafts of very low porosity tended to induce fibrin deposition, and hence luminal narrowing rather than the intimalization we have seen with an approximately 80% "pore density." Similarly, other groups who report intimal thickening and endothelial cell covering of their prostheses have used high percentage pore density.

We believe that self-expanding prostheses will lead to greater clinical acceptability than balloon-distendable or nonelastic devices for a number of reasons. Primarily, long prostheses of the distendable type have an inherent longitudinal rigidity so that when deployed in a vessel bend, even of relatively large radius, the straightening effect of prosthesis implantation could lead to kinking or abrupt flow path deviation at the prosthesis extremities. Second, Palmaz and co-workers when using an early prototype noted two patients with intimal proliferation leading to about 30% lumen reduction at 2 months in 11 implants. They felt that the radial compliance mismatch between the soft healthy vessel and the rather rigid structure of the stented segment might be responsible for unpredictable intimal proliferation of this type. Whether this is likely to be of significance in the clinical situation, in which the plaque has of itself a certain rigidity, is not clear. However, we feel that the compliant self-expanding stent offers not so abrupt a step in compliance that will be more favorably tolerated. Third, a longitudinal flexible stent, which is also flexible even when mounted on its guiding catheter, as is the situation with our device, permits easier access through tortuous vessels to the target site.

Our experiments in healthy animals have shown that the endoprosthesis is perfectly tolerated for at least up to 1 year. Animal experience not only demonstrated the mechanism of this tolerance, but also permitted valuable improvements in prosthesis and delivery system design to the extent that they now have a very high degree of safety in use and reproducibility in operation. Given the absence of a meaningful animal model of the artherosclerotic human artery, the potentially misleading information that poor models can give and the unanimity of peer opinion that the state of development justified clinical trial, we felt firmly confident in undertaking our clinical evaluation. In our series relating to the prevention of restenosis in peripheral and coronary implants, restenosis has been rare at follow-up ranging from 3 months up to 2 years, whereas the statistical probability of such an event is quite high. We have also found it possible to reopen occluded arteries, resistant to previous angioplasty with favorable medium-term results. The feasibility of this approach has recently been confirmed on a few occasions using the Roubin stent.

Little is known of possible long-term side effects and although the prosthesis is totally intimalized, infection could conceivably be a future pitfall. We have specifically avoided traversing major branch vessels, not only because of uncertainty about long-term patency but also because such a placement would prevent later angioplasty access should it be required. We also specifically avoided sudden changes in vessel caliber, since we feel these constitute an elevated risk of thrombogenesis. Similarly, poor distal bed runoff and competing flow situations must constitute a higher thrombogenesis risk and until such time as an optimized pharmaceutic regimen is defined for stenting we prefer to exercise a high degree of prudence in this respect. Further studies will determine with greater precision the benefits of this new approach, but we have the strong sentiment, even from our still relatively early experience, that stenting represents an important and valuable adjunct to angioplasty and has great potential for wider and more extensive applications.

CONCLUSION

Balloon angioplasty fails to provide acceptable long-term results for a significant proportion of patients. An intravascular mechanical support was therefore developed with the aim of preventing restenosis and acute closure of diseased arteries after transluminal angioplasty. The endoprosthesis consists of a self-expandable, stainless-steel mesh that can be implanted nonsurgically by means of its specially designed percutaneous delivery system by means of conventional angioplasty guiding catheters or introducers into the coronary or peripheral arteries. Animal experiments showed complete intimal coverage within weeks and no late thrombosis during a follow-up period of up to 1 year. The stent proved to be well tolerated in patients with implants for iliac and femoral artery disease. More than 70 stents were implanted in patients who had coronary artery restenoses, abrupt closure after transluminal angioplasty, and deterioration of bypass grafts. As to date, the longest observation in humans extends to 2 years' follow-up. Intravascular stents may present a rational approach to the unresolved problems of transluminal angioplasty.

REFERENCES

1. Palmaz, J.C., Sibbett, R.R., Reuter, S.R., et al.: Expandable intraluminal graft: a preliminary study, Radiology **156:**73-77, 1985.
2. Maass, D., Kropf, L., Egloff, L., et al.: Transluminal implantations of intravascular "Double Helix" spiral prostheses: technical and biological considerations, ESAO Proc. **9:**252-256, 1982.
3. Wright, K.C., Wallace, S., Charnsangavi, C., et al.: Percutaneous endovascular stents: an experimental evaluation, Radiology **156:**69-72, 1985.
4. Dotter, C.T.: Transluminally placed coil spring and arterial tube grafts: long term patency in the canine popliteal artery, Invest. Radiol. **4:**329-332, 1969.
5. Cragg, A., Lund, G., Rysavy, J., et al.: Non-surgical placement of arterial endoprostheses: a new technique using nitinol wire, Radiology **147:**261-263, 1983.
6. Dotter, C.T., Buschmann, R.W., McKinney, M.K., et al.: Transluminal expandable nitinol coil graft stenting: preliminary report, Radiology **147:**259-260, 1983.
7. Palmaz, J.C., Windeler, S.A., Gareia, F., et al.: Atherosclerotic rabbit aortas: expandable intraluminal grafting, Radiology **160:**723-726, 1986.
8. Leimgruber, P.P., Roubin, G.S., Hollman, J., Cotsonis, G.A., Meier, B., Douglas, J.S., Gruentzig, A., and King, S.B., III: Restenosis after successful coronary angioplasty in patients with single-vessel disease, Circulation **73:**710-717, 1986.

Chapter 29

Preliminary Observations with the Wire Coil Endovascular Coronary Stent Prosthesis

Spencer B. King III, MD, FACC
Gary S. Roubin, MB, PhD
John S. Douglas, Jr., MD
Keith A. Robinson, PhD

Patients who undergo coronary angioplasty face two as yet unresolved problems. The first is that of acute vessel closure, and the second is restenosis of the dilated segment over the months following angioplasty.[1] Both of these problems have been vigorously attacked during the past 10 years since Gruntzig's development of angioplasty, but neither has yielded to significant improvement.[2] New radical approaches have been undertaken in an attempt to cope with them more aggressively. The latest of these is the use of the endovascular stent prosthesis. While the wire-mesh self-expanding stent[3,4] has been used primarily in Europe for the purpose of attempting to reduce the restenosis rate, another stent design, the wire coil stent, has undergone extensive testing and is now being evaluated in a clinical trial to determine its suitability for treatment of the acute closure phenomenon.[5]

Acute closure of the coronary artery, thought initially to be due to coronary spasm, has proved most often to be associated with coronary dissection with or without expanding intramural hematoma and secondary thrombosis. It has been shown experimentally that the extent of intimal dissection relates directly to platelet deposition and the potential for flap closure or acute thrombosis. Bredlau and associates[6] showed that the presence of angiographically visible coronary dissection following angioplasty correlated with a sixfold increase in the incidence of coronary occlusion syndrome. Once patients undergo total occlusion of the coronary artery that cannot be solved with the balloon catheter and therefore have to be taken to emergency bypass surgery, some myocardial infarction occurs in approximately 50%, and 25% will develop new Q waves.[7] In turn, myocardial infarction following failed angioplasty and emergency bypass surgery is a significant predictor of late mortality from the procedure.[8] Any technique that can minimize the possibility of myocardial necrosis in patients who have to undergo bypass surgery would be of obvious value.

CURRENT APPROACH TO ABRUPT OCCLUSION

Approaches dealing with abrupt occlusion so far have included redilatation with more prolonged periods of balloon inflation and occasionally exchange to larger balloons if undersizing was a problem. Indeed these efforts have frequently been successful. If the disrupted plaque and intimal lining cannot be remolded to form an adequate flow channel, then bypass surgery is usually required. The coronary perfusion catheter was developed in an attempt to provide some myocardial perfusion in the ischemic zone during the inevitable time delay between acute closure and restoration of flow through the bypass grafts. Ferguson and associates[9] reported that use of such a device eliminated abnormal electrocardiographic (ECG) changes and stabilized approximately 50% of the patients adequately for insertion of mammary grafts. In a larger series from our center, the device was also helpful. Others have noted some limitation, including restricted flow, inadequate perfusion in situations of decreased systemic pressure, and thrombosis of the perfusion catheter. Clearly the perfusion catheter is capable of providing only a partial solution to the acute ischemia induced by coronary occlusion because of its small lumen and restricted flow. Other approaches to coping with acute occlusion syndrome have been the infusion of either arterial blood or oxygenated venous blood obtained from the area of the renal vein through the central lumen of the standard angioplasty catheter. Oxygenated fluosol has also been used to decrease myocardial ischemia during prolonged balloon inflation and may also be helpful in circumstances of acute vessel closure. None of these methods, however, is expected to restore normal perfusion in the setting of acute occlusion. The wire endovascular coronary stent, by restoring coronary architecture, does have the potential for restoring normal perfusion pressure in the previously occluded coronary artery.

DESCRIPTION OF THE STENT

The stent is manufactured from .006-inch stainless steel suture material that has been used in surgical procedures for many years. The wire is formed into a coil that, rather than circling in one direction throughout its length, is reversed every 360 degrees to travel in the opposite direction so that the loops can be interdigitated and pulled tightly around a deflated balloon catheter. Because of this design, which is similar to that used in some spiral notebooks, the expanding balloon can easily deform the stent to assume the diameter determined by the size of the expanding balloon (Fig. 29-1).

Basic Research

Following extensive testing of metal fatigue and other physical properties of the device, a series of canine experiments were performed by Drs. Gary Roubin and Keith Robinson in our laboratories. The experiments were designed to test the ability to place the stent correctly and to examine the immediate and delayed angiographic and histologic results. As reported previously,[5] 39 dogs had stents placed. Stent placement proved to be relatively easy utilizing a multipurpose-type guiding catheter design. The arteries were first instrumented with a standard guidewire placed into the segment of artery to be tested. An appropriately sized balloon catheter was then inserted and inflated so as to induce endothelial damage and was then withdrawn. The second balloon catheter with the stent

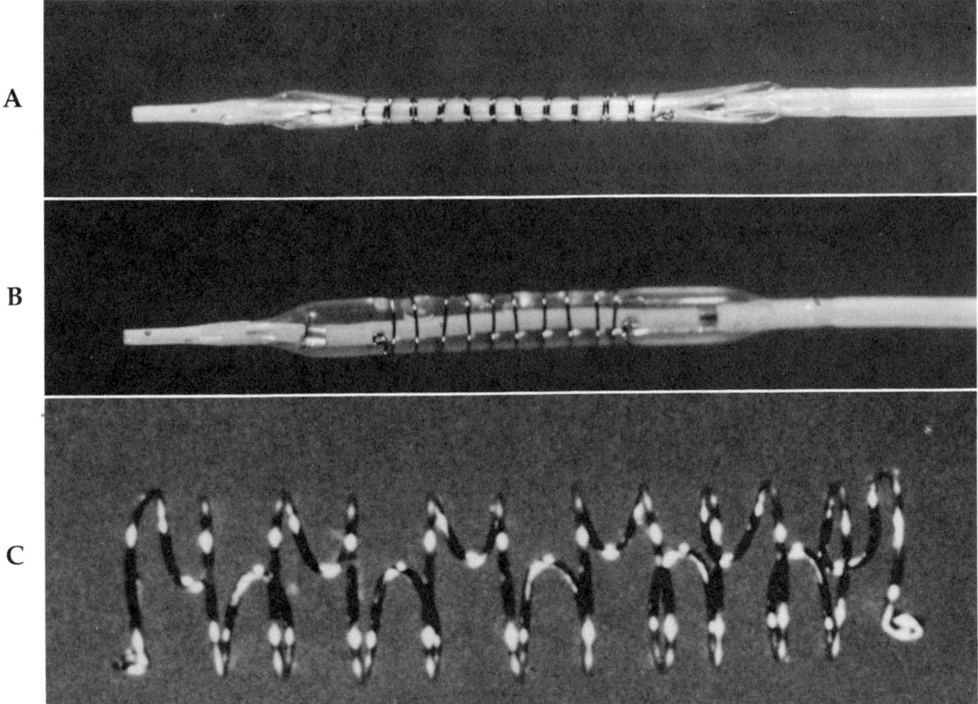

Fig. 29-1. **A,** Deflated balloon delivery system with coil stent wrapped tightly around deflated balloon. **B,** Inflated balloon showing deployment of the stent. **C,** Enlarged photograph of the expanded coil stent showing the reversing interdigitating coils.

mounted on it was then passed over the guidewire into the area previously dilated, and the stent was deployed by inflating the balloon, deflating it and removing the balloon catheter. The stent was thus left in place as demonstrated by fluoroscopy and confirmed by angiography.

All of these dogs had normal coronary arteries in the beginning and the degree of arterial damage was not sufficient to induce angiographically visible dissection in any of the animals. All animals were pretreated with 10,000 units of heparin administered during the course of the procedure. Chronic therapy included warfarin sodium anticoagulation in 13 animals, and aspirin and dipyridamole therapy in the remaining 26. Animals underwent angiography and were sacrificed acutely and at varying intervals following stent implantation in order to document the angiographic patency and the histologic effect of the stent placement. A number of samples underwent scanning electron microscopy testing in addition to the routine histologic examinations.

Result of Stent Placement in the Canine Model

All but three of the stents were correctly placed by varying operators with relative ease and no real evidence of a learning curve. Three stents were incorrectly placed, one because of failure to deflate the balloon fully before withdrawal and two because of significant undersizing of the stent resulting in migration of the device to a more distal segment. Both fluoroscopy and immediate angiography demonstrated that the remaining stents were positioned properly and that the arterial lumen was not compromised. Angiographic examination done from 2 months to 1 year following implantation showed that the diameter stenosis was less than 10% at 2 months and did not increase in dogs examined over time periods up to 1 year. The side branches incorporated within the area of the stent placement all remained patent.

The histologic examination of these animals showed that the stent wires had embedded themselves into the wall of the artery in small trenches and rested on the media of the artery internal to the internal elastic membrane. (Fig. 29-2). Endothelial cell migration and attachment to the wires was noted by 3 days and endothelial cell covering of the wires was complete by 2 weeks (Fig. 29-3). Arteries examined 2 to 18 months following implantation showed the stent to be embedded in the neointimal layer (Fig. 29-4). The neointimal layer was thickest over the stent wires but there was also mild thickening in the area between the wires. The endothelial covering averaged 270 μm in depth and was again maximum in the area over the stent wires. Endothelial cell development along the course of the stent was quite normal in appearance with orientation of endothelial cells in the direction of flow, although at the ends of the stent wires where some flow turbulence could be expected there was disordered endothelial cell orientation.

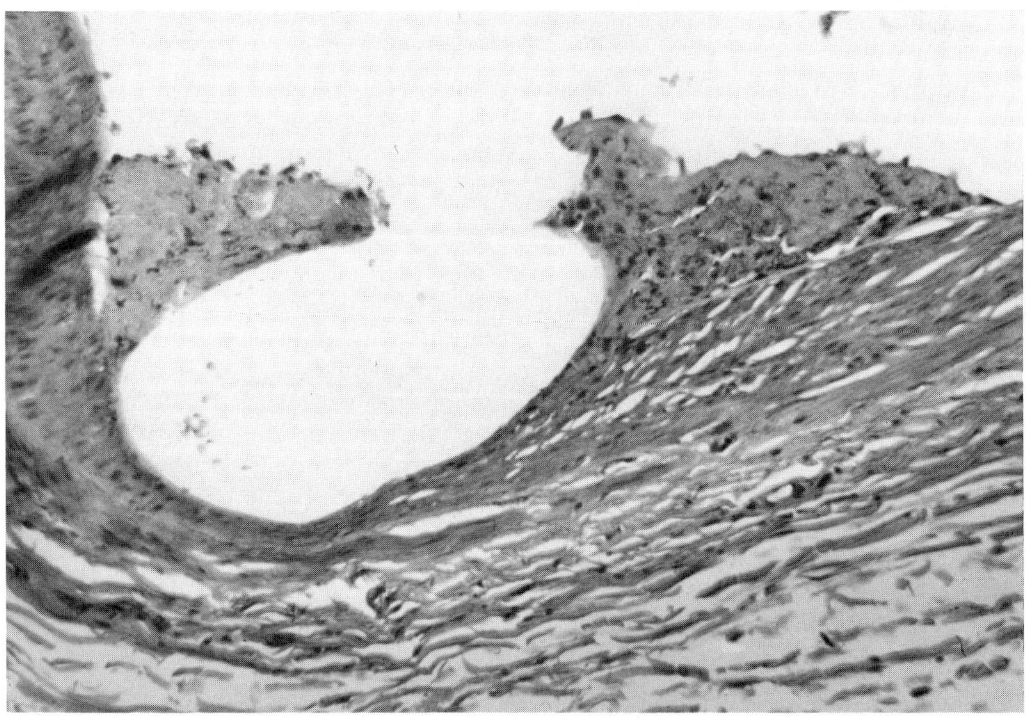

Fig. 29-2. Histologic section through site of stent wire. Note that the wire is resting in a trench just external to the elastic membrane and is being covered by thrombotic material.

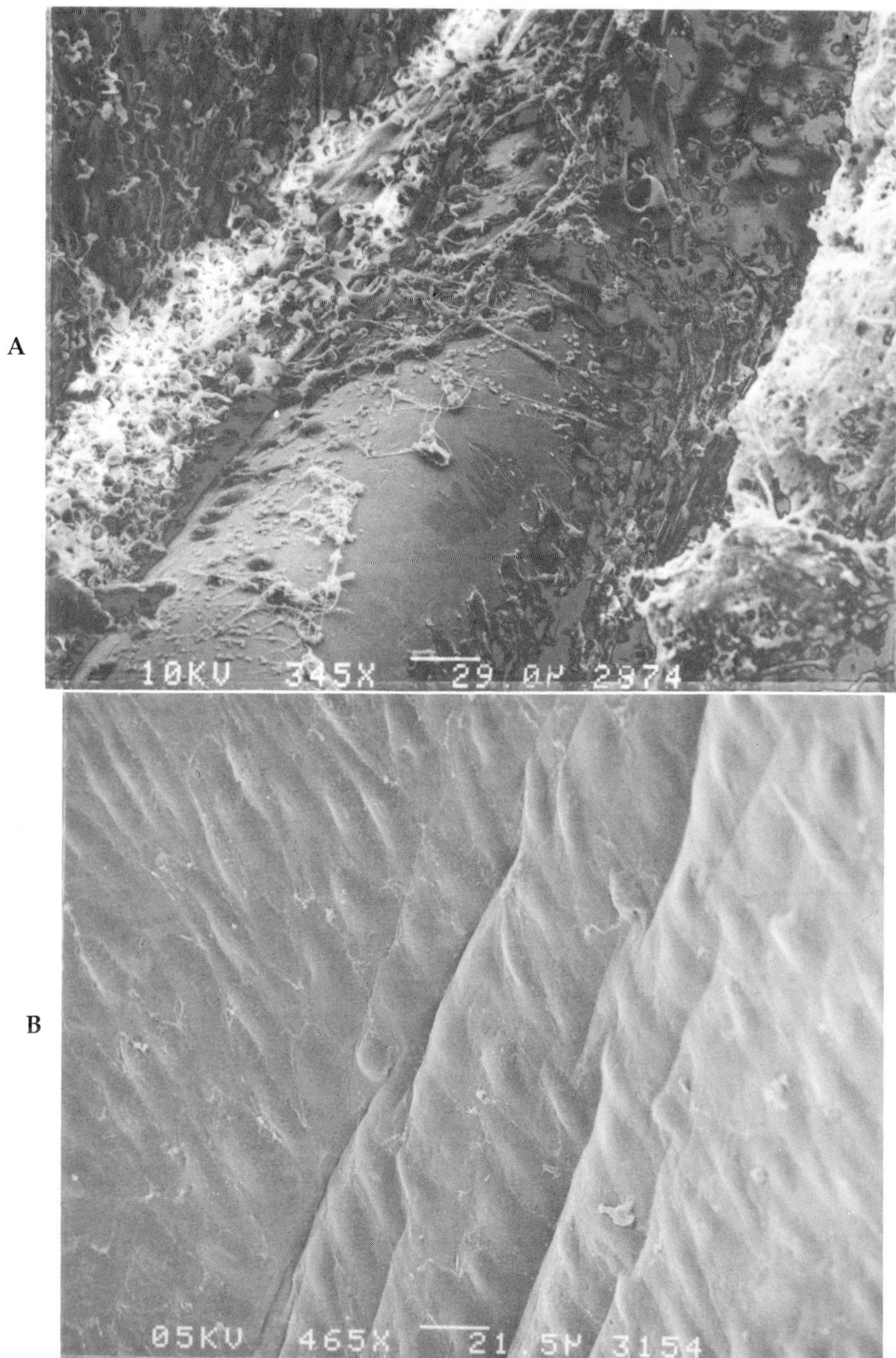

Fig. 29-3. A, Scanning electron micrograph of stent 3 days following implantation. There is a thin fibrin layer with formation of filamentous strands and the beginning of endothelial cell attachment. **B,** Endothelial cell covering of stent wires at 2 weeks after implantation.

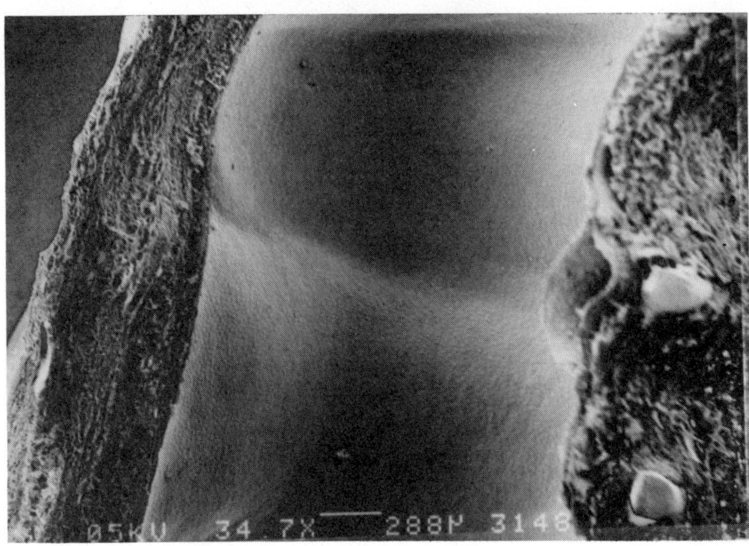

Fig. 29-4. Scanning electron micrograph of longitudinal section of artery 18 months after implantation showing the deep embedding of the stent wires into the arterial wall.

Among the initial cohort of animals treated with sodium warfarin (Coumadin) anticoagulation, there were four deaths. At least two of these were related to thrombosis, and one dog had a mediastinal hemorrhage. It is of note that one dog died several days following discontinuation of the sodium warfarin. On the other hand, all 26 dogs pretreated and continued on aspirin 325 mg and dipyridamole 75 mg three times daily remained free of thrombosis or hemorrhagic problems. Delayed angiographic and histologic results were not different in the surviving dogs in either group.

Experience in the Atherosclerotic Rabbit Model

To assess the effects of stenting in atherosclerotic blood vessels, the cholesterol-fed rabbit model was used.[10] Bilateral angioplasty of induced iliac arterial stenoses was performed 7 weeks after an initial balloon injury and cholesterol feeding. One artery was randomly selected for stent placement. Nine rabbits received only heparin at the time of the procedure (non-aspirin-treated group), while a subsequent group (aspirin-treated) received heparin plus aspirin 60 mg and were continued on aspirin every 3 days until the time of sacrifice (4 weeks after stenting).

The arteriographically measured lumen diameter of stented arteries was significantly greater than control (dilated only) in both groups immediately after stenting. In the non-aspirin-treated group, there was no significant difference in wall thickness of stented arteries compared with control arteries. Lumen diameter of the stented artery remained significantly greater than the control artery. In aspirin-treated rabbits, lumen diameter was significantly greater and wall thickness was slightly but significantly less for stented arteries compared with control arteries. Intraarterial stenting in this model may therefore inhibit restenosis by preservation of a larger functional lumen and in aspirin-treated animals by a modest inhibition of the hyperplastic cellular response to arterial injury.

Scanning electron microscopy of a series of atherosclerotic rabbit aortas was also performed to determine luminal cellular re-

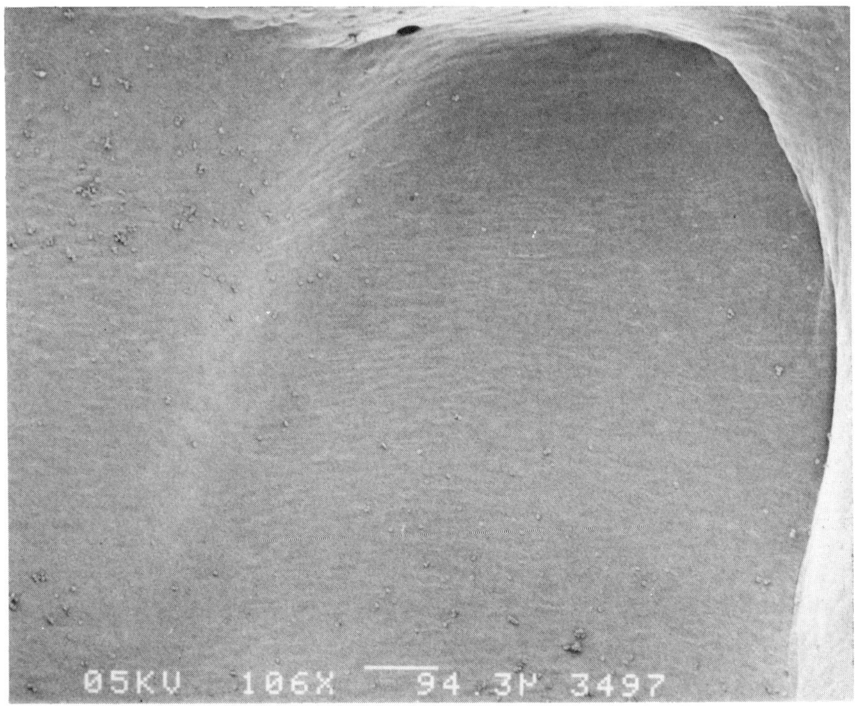

Fig. 29-5. Scanning electron micrograph of the rabbit iliac artery 3 weeks following implantation showing the smooth endothelial coverage.

sponses to stenting. Immediately after stenting, trenches were seen extending into the intima in which the stent wire was embedded; associated with these trenches were small adherent thrombi. One day after stenting, endothelial and/or pseudoendothelial cells were observed attached by pseudopodia to the stainless steel stent wire. By 1 week poststent procedure the luminal cell layer was extensive, and by 2 weeks this layer was nearly confluent. By 3 weeks after stenting the stent wire was incorporated into the arterial wall and covered by a confluent, flow-directed, nonthrombogenic endothelium (Fig. 29-5).

CLINICAL TRIAL

Following these encouraging results from animal experiments, similar positive results from the group of Palmaz and Schatz,[11] and the early human experience with the self-expanding mesh stent in Europe, Federal Drug Administration (FDA) approval was granted for a limited trial of the stent to be used as a bailout device in the event of acute coronary occlusion, which could not be solved by currently available clinical methods. This protocol calls for all usual attempts to open the occluded artery but if the artery cannot be maintained in a satisfactory state and coronary bypass surgery is planned, then the intracoronary stent can be placed in patients who have given prior informed consent in order to attempt to alleviate myocardial ischemia before attempting bypass surgery. At present, four such patients have been instrumented with the stent; all successfully. Three patients experienced dissection during routine coronary angioplasty of the right coronary artery, and one during dilatation of the left anterior descending (LAD) coronary artery. Following unsuccessful attempts at prolonged balloon reinflation, the stent was placed resulting in a completely restored arterial lumen and disappearance of angina and abnormal ECG changes except in one patient with side-branch occlusion related to the intimal dissection. At the time of surgery, there was maintained flow in the distal coronary artery segments beyond the stent. Bypass surgery was accomplished without myocardial infarction in the distribution of the stenotic artery, and restudy done 1 week following the stent implantation was surprising in that all bypass grafts, as well as two of the four stented segments, remained patent.

DISCUSSION

Although there are theoretic reasons why stenting coronary arteries may be helpful in reducing restenosis following coronary angioplasty, our direction thus far has been aimed at establishing the feasibility of using the intracoronary stent in the event of acute coronary occlusion while continuing basic research on the long-term effects of stents. We are looking forward to the opportunity of leaving the stent safely in place without the need for emergency surgery, and perhaps utilizing the stent for other applications such as attempting to reduce the rate of restenosis following angioplasty. The previous animal experimentation done by Palmaz and Schatz[11] demonstrated that acute occlusion in a large number of animal models was not a problem in stent implantation. This experience has not held up as well with the use of wire mesh stents in humans in Europe. This stent has been associated with a significant incidence of acute thrombosis that limits its use at this point. It is not clear whether stents of a different design will have less thrombosis or whether current efforts at coating the stents will be effective. Attempts are underway to change the surface charge on the stainless steel wire, to coat it with various substances, to bond heparin to the wire to prevent thrombosis during the early phase following stent implantation, and to design stents made of other materials. Additional problems with all stents relate to the ease of implantation. Since experience is limited in atherosclerotic human patients, it is unclear how difficult correct stent implantation will be when applied to a broad spectrum of patients. Although the architecture of the artery dissected will undoubtedly be improved by stent implantation, the possibility of irregular areas of high turbulence at the extremities of the stent remain a potential problem. Since the wires are deeply embedded into the wall of the artery and show no signs of migration or rupture, the long-term effect of the stent is likely to be benign.

The beneficial effect of stents is likely due to two mechanisms. First of all, by rearranging the architecture of the dissected artery and disrupted plaque, a smoother and more tubular structure can be created that will improve laminar flow. Laminar flow has been shown by Chesebro and associates[12] to be important in minimizing acute platelet deposition. Endothelial cell growth seems also to be influenced by the flow pattern, assuming its normal appearance in areas where laminar flow is present and growing in a disordered pattern in areas of altered shear stress. The other potential benefit of the stent may be from an entirely different direction, that is, the development of a controlled neointimal fibrous cap on the atherosclerotic process. Once a fibrous neoendothelium has been developed, it may act as a protective barrier against further intrusion on the lumen by the atherosclerotic process. This remains a somewhat hypothetic explanation for the observed decreased late restenosis rate in patients treated with the expanding wire-mesh stent.

This technology is in its infancy and it is unlikely that the ultimate stent design has been achieved. Important characteristics of the stent must be ease and accuracy of implantation in all varieties of human coronary atherosclerotic disease; the ability to maintain an adequate lumen even in the face of elastic recoil of fibrotic, densely clacified, and sometimes incompletely dilated arterial segments; flexibility to accommodate to the uncommonly mobile arterial segments; nonthrombogenicity so that acute thrombosis will not be a problem, thereby allowing chronic use of stents without the need for bypass surgery; and the absence of any late complication from the stent implantation.

The flexible wire stent now undergoing clinical trials moves us in the direction of a satisfactory device that may help overcome the two major problems of angioplasty, acute reclosure and restenosis.

REFERENCES

1. Leimgruber, P.P., Roubin, G.S., Hollman, J., Cotsonis, G.A., Douglas, J.S., King, S.B., and Gruentzig, A.R.: Restenosis after successful coronary angioplasty in patients with single vessel disease, Circulation **73:**710-717, 1986.
2. King, S.B., III: A symposium: restenosis after percutaneous transluminal coronary angioplasty, Am. J. Cardiol. **60:**1B-2B, 1987.
3. Sigwart, U., Puel, J., Mirkovitch, V., Joffre, F., and Kappenberger, L.: Intravascular stents to prevent occlusion and restenosis after transluminal angioplasty, N. Engl. J. Med. **316:**701-706, 1987.
4. Serruys, P.W., Juilliere, Y., Bertrand, M.W., Rickards, A.F., and Puel, J.: Additional improvement in stenosis geometry by stenting human coronary arteries after angioplasty, Circulation **76**(suppl. 4):IV-232, 1987.
5. Roubin, G.S., Robinson, K.A., King, S.B., Gianturco, C., Black, A.J., Brown, J.E., Siegel, R.J., and Douglas, J.S.: Acute and late results of intracoronary arterial stenting after coronary angioplasty in dogs, Circulation **76:**891-897, 1987.
6. Bredlau, C., Gruentzig, A., Douglas, J., Jr., and King, S., III: Acute complications of percutaneous transluminal coronary angioplasty (PTCA): initial experience in 3000 consecutive patient attempts (abstract), Circulation **70:**424, 1984.
7. Roubin, G.S., Talley, J.D., Anderson, H.V., Murphy, D.A., Guyton, R.A., Jones, E.L., Craver, J.M., Lembo, N., Douglas, J.S., Jr., and King, S.B., III: Morbidity and mortality associated with emergency bypass graft surgery following elective coronary angioplasty, J. Am. Coll. Cardiol. **9:**124A, 1987.
8. Talley, J.D., Weintraub, W.S., Anderson, H.V., Jones, E.L., King, S.B., III, Douglas, J.S., Jr., Murphy, D.A., Craver, J.M., Liberman, A., Morris, D.C., Guyton, R.A., and Hatcher, C.R.: Late clinical outcome of coronary bypass surgery after failed elective PTCA, Circulation **76:**IV-352, 1987.
9. Ferguson, T.B., Jr., Hinohara, T., Simpson, J., Stack, R.S., and Wechsler, A.S.: Catheter reperfusion to allow optimal coronary bypass grafting following failed transluminal coronary angioplasty, Ann. Thorac. Surg. **42:**399-405, 1986.
10. Robinson, K.A., Roubin, G.S., Siegel, R.J., Black, A.J., Apkarian, R.P., and King, S.B., III: Intra-arterial stenting in the atherosclerotic rabbit, Circulation. (In press.)
11. Palmaz, J.C., Windeler, S.A., Garcia, F., Tio, F.O., Sibbitt, R.S., and Reuter, S.R.: Atherosclerotic rabbit aortas: expandable intraluminal grafting, Radiology **160:**723-726, 1986.
12. Chesebro, J.H., Lam, J.Y.T., Badimon, L., and Fuster, V.: Restenosis after arterial angioplasty: a hemorrheologic response to injury, Am. J. Cardiol. **60:**10B-16B, 1987.

Chapter 30

New Possibilities for Adjunctive Therapy to Prevent Restenosis After Arterial Angioplasty

James H. Chesebro, MD
William J. Penny, MD
Magdalena Heras, MD
Lina Badimon, PhD
Valentin Fuster, MD

Restenosis following arterial angioplasty continues to cause the greatest morbidity and remains the greatest obstacle to an otherwise successful technical procedure. Experimental studies have led to greater understanding of the acute occlusive process, as well as of the probable mechanisms of the slower evolution of restenosis. Greater understanding of the mechanisms of restenosis are critical for the rational design of intervention trials. Successful angioplasty appears to involve compression and splitting of the obstructive lesion and probably expansion of the external diameter of the artery.[1-3] Major factors that appear to contribute to acute occlusion and restenosis involve both extremely thrombogenic *substrate* within the arterial wall and plaque and the *rheology* of blood flow; both factors contribute to activate the clotting system and platelets with the acute formation of mural thrombus. The animal model and ex-vivo perfusion chamber that we have used to study these mechanisms, as well as the results of these studies, are discussed in this chapter.

METHODS

The pigs used for the study of arterial angioplasty were obtained from local farmers and were normal pigs weighing 30 to 40 kg and of the Babcock four-way cross-stock (mixture of Landrace, Yorkshire, Hampshire, and Duroc breeds). All pigs were fed a normal chow diet.

Experimental Procedures and Angioplasty Technique

The pigs were sedated with ketamine (Ketaject), 300 mg injected intramuscularly (IM), intubated after inhalation of a small amount of ether or halothane (Fluothane), and mechanically ventilated with room air (Harvard respirator) mixed with 0.5% halothane to maintain anesthesia. Continuous electrocardiographic (ECG) and arterial pressure monitoring was performed with a Honeywell multichannel recorder. All pigs were heparinized with 100 units per kg body weight of heparin as a bolus immediately after the insertion of the arterial catheter. In pigs that were followed longer term and awakened after the procedure, heparin was not reversed, and no further doses of heparin were administered beyond the initial bolus during the catheterization.

The angioplasty catheter (Meditech 8 mm × 3 cm, polyethylene balloon) was advanced by way of a right femoral cutdown into the left and right common carotid arteries under fluoroscopic visualization. The balloon was inflated to 6 atm (Meditech pressure manometer; Meditech Inc., Watertown, Mass.) for 30 seconds. Five inflations were performed at 60-second intervals on both common carotid arteries. The average diameter of the common carotid artery was 5 to 6 mm. Selective spot films of the carotid artery were obtained before and immediately after the dilatation procedure by the manual injection of 6 ml of diatrizoate meglumine and diatrizoate sodium (Renografin-76); plain spot films were obtained during dilatation. Measurements from the spot films taken before, during, and after balloon inflation demonstrated that the diameter of the balloon inflated within the artery was only 10 ± 6% (mean ± SD) more than the diameter of the artery on the films obtained before dilatation.

In the initial natural history study angioplasty was performed on 38 pigs that were sacrificed at variable time intervals after the procedure including 1 hour, 24 hours, and 4, 7, 14, 30, and 60 days later. Pigs that received platelet inhibitor therapy by either the intravenous (IV) or oral route were sacrificed at the completion of the angioplasty procedure.

Quantitation of Vasoconstriction

To quantitate the severity of localized vasoconstriction immediately proximal and distal to the dilatation site, angiograms of the common carotid arteries before and after the dilatation procedure were obtained with selective intraarterial injection of 6 ml of Renografin-76 diluted with 6 ml of saline (Fig. 30-1) and with exposure factors of 90 kV, 200 mA, and 20 ms.[4] The degree of vasoconstriction was expressed as the mean of the greatest luminal narrowing just proximal and distal to the dilated segment on the postdilatation angiogram (measured with a caliper), and expressed as percentages of the dimension before dilatation.

Histopathology and Electron Microscopy

After postdilatation angiography the pigs were given an overdose of pentobarbital and perfused antegradely with 2% glutaraldehyde and 1% paraformaldehyde and 0.1 M cacodylate (pH 7.25) at a pressure of 100 mm Hg for 15 minutes to allow fixation of the arteries in situ. Next the carotid arteries were removed and cleaned of all adventitia. The location of the dilated portion of the fixed artery was easily identified because of the in-situ fixation that showed the almost invariable vasospasm proximal and distal to the involved area. This finding was confirmed in vivo by the films taken during and after the angioplasty procedure (Fig. 30-1). The dilated portion was divided into two equal segments of 1.5 cm each; segments were also taken from vasoconstricted regions and from proximal and distal uninvolved segments of artery (Fig. 30-2). From each arterial segment, two or three ring sections were removed and stained with La-

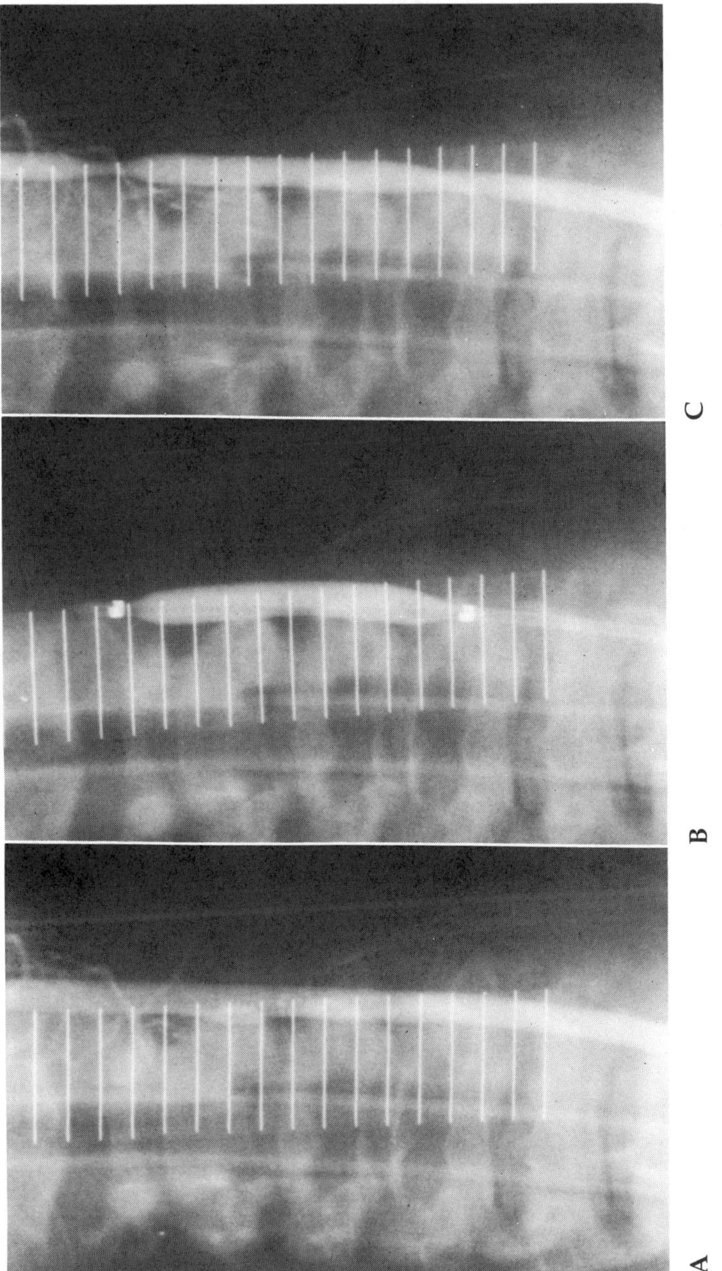

Fig. 30-1. Angiographic films showing the common carotid artery before angiography **(A)**, during angioplasty with the balloon inflated with contrast agent **(B)**, and after angioplasty **(C)** when the vasoconstricted regions (*arrows*) can be clearly seen. (Reproduced with permission from Lam, J.Y.T., et al.: Circulation **75**:243-248, 1987.)

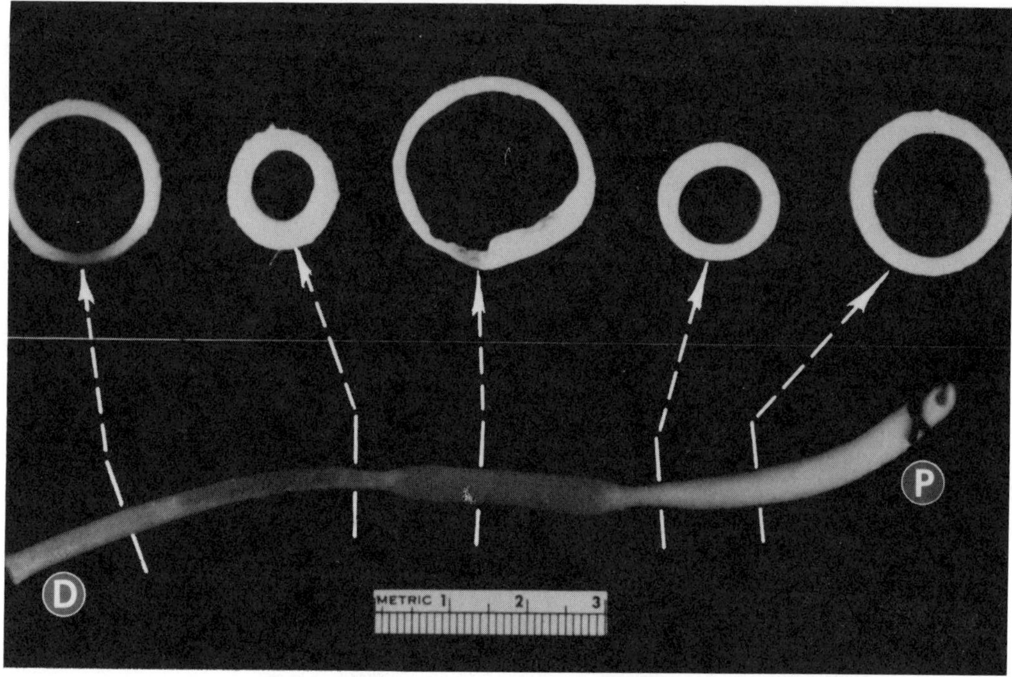

Fig. 30-2. The perfused carotid artery that was fixed in situ shows the length of artery divided into segments with cross-sections removed from the indicated regions. The balloon-injured segment (B, angioplasty), the adjacent vasoconstricted regions (V) with thickened wall consistent with muscular contraction, and the proximal (P) and distal (D) uninvolved regions are shown. (Reproduced with permission from Lam, J.Y.T., et al.: Circulation **75:**243-248, 1987.)

son's elastic–van Gieson stain and with hematoxylin-eosin. Two investigators examined the histologic sections to provide a consensus evaluation of the presence of medial tears. Deep or severe injury was defined as an intimal tear extending through the internal elastic lamina into the media of the arterial wall. Mild injury or subendothelial denudation was defined as endothelial denudation without a tear through the internal elastic lamina. Scanning electron microscopy was used to document the presence or absence of endothelial denudation.

Two longitudinal specimens were cut from each segment, coated with carbon and gold-palladium alloy, and examined with a scanning electron microscope (ETEC Autoscan). Representative areas were photographed and evaluated by at least two investigators, and a consensus reading was made.

Selected specimens were thin-sectioned (600 to 700 A), mounted on a 200-mesh copper grid, and stained with uranyl acetate and lead citrate. Sections were examined with a Philips 201 transmission electron microscope.

Identification of Mural Thrombus. The tissue segments were examined under low-power magnification (X2 lens; Sunnex Laboratories) for the presence of mural thrombus formation.

Quantitation of Platelet Deposition. Platelet deposition on the arterial segments was quantitated by the method of Dewanjee and coworkers,[5,6] using autologous ^{111}In-labeled platelets. Three samples of blood were obtained at the time animals were sacrificed for determination of mean radioactivity in counts per minute (cpm) per weight (microbalance) of blood. The radioactivity (cpm) in each arterial segment was measured in a gamma well counter (Beckman, gamma 8,000) and corrected for radionuclide decay and the percentage of free ^{111}In in plasma (not bound to platelets). The spectrometer of the counter was adjusted to include the photopeaks at 174 keV, 247 keV, and 421 keV (sum peak) of ^{111}In radionuclide. With knowledge of the whole blood platelet count (Coulter counter), the number of platelets deposited on an arterial segment was calculated using the following equation:

$$\text{No. deposited platelets} = \frac{(^{111}\text{In cpm in arterial segment}) \times (\text{platelets/ml})}{(^{111}\text{In cpm/ml})}$$

The number of platelets per unit area was calculated by dividing the number of deposited platelets per arterial segment by the surface area of the arterial wall (area $= \pi \times d \times l$, where d = diameter of segment and l = length of the arterial segment).

Initially platelet deposition was calculated only from the dilated segment. After a relationship between platelet deposition and vasoconstriction was observed, the platelet deposition within the actual vasoconstricted regions was subsequently obtained to document the relationship between platelet deposition in the actual vasoconstricted region and the vasoconstrictive response both proximally and distally.

Ex-Vivo Perfusion Chamber. Cylindric acrylic-plastic (Plexiglas) chambers were designed to mimic the tubelike shape of the vascular system. The cylindric channel of the flow chamber through which blood circulates was machined so that a portion of the circumferential

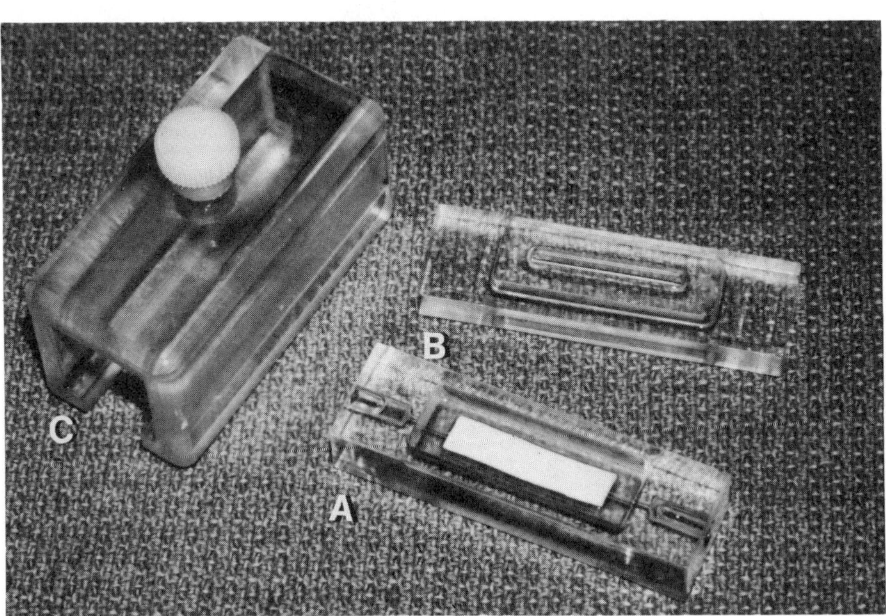

Fig. 30-3. Unassembled Plexiglas perfusion chamber. **A,** Chamber with cylindric channel for blood circulation over which is laid a piece of aortic tissue; **B,** lid of the chamber; **C,** holder of the chamber.

wall (25 mm in length, 1 mm in width) was removed. The resulting "window" permitted direct exposure of the test surface. Different substrates were held in place by the pressure of the upper lid on the lower core. The superfusion chamber was immersed in an outer chamber (water bath) through which water at 37° C was continuously circulated (Fig. 30-3). Three chambers of different internal diameters (1.0 mm, 1.5 mm, or 2.0 mm) were constructed to obtain a broad range of shear rates on the substrate with moderate changes in an average blood flow rate.

Arterial blood from anesthetized pigs flowed directly through polyethylene tubing (20 cm in length, Clay Adams PE200, Cole-Paimer, Chicago, Ill.) to the Plexiglas chamber (Fig. 30-4). The output of the chamber was connected to a peristaltic pump (Masterflex Model 7013). During longer experiments that involved repeated runs at various flow rates and for various time intervals through the ex-vivo perfusion chamber, blood that passed through the chamber was recirculated back into the animal through a contralateral femoral or jugular vein. For these longer experiments pigs were initially heparinized intravenously with 300 units per kg body weight of heparin (Liquemin). When ex-vivo perfusion was done in conjunction with angioplasty, pigs were heparinized according to the experimental protocol, and blood that passed through the chamber was not recirculated back into the animal.

Different substrates may be used in the ex-vivo perfusion chamber including a deendothelized vessel wall, a collagen strip, or a vessel wall torn through the media.

Before initiating ex-vivo perfusion with blood, the specimens were perfused with saline solution, at 37° C for 60 seconds. After the preperfusion period, blood entered the chamber at a preselected flow rate for times ranging from 1 to 30 minutes. At the termina-

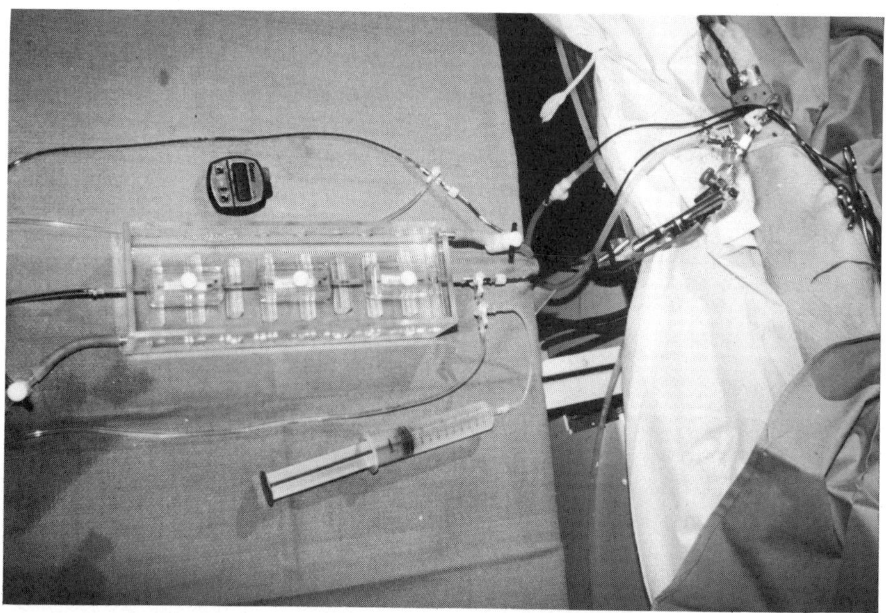

Fig. 30-4. Photograph of the perfusion system. Blood flows directly from the femoral artery through a series of three chambers that are immersed in a water bath at 37° C. The blood flow is regulated by a distal pump (not shown).

tion of blood flow, a buffer was again passed for 30 seconds through the chamber under identical flow conditions. Changes from buffer to blood and vice versa were achieved by a switch valve without the introduction of stasis in the chamber. The selected flow rates ranged from 5 to 20 ml/minute in the different-sized chambers. These blood flows gave theoretically calculated average blood velocities from 2.65 to 42.3 cm/second, and local shear rates from 106 to 3380 sec^{-1}, that is, shear rates ranging from those of large arteries to those of terminal arterial branches and the microcirculation.[7] Within these shear rates blood can be considered as having newtonian fluid properties with constant viscosity.[8,9] Shear conditions at the vessel wall were calculated from the expression for shear rate given for a newtonian fluid in tube flow.[10]

The number of platelets deposited on each specimen was calculated as described above under quantitation of platelet deposition. Results were normalized by area of exposed surface.

Preparation of Deendothelized Vessel Wall. A modification of Fischman's method was used to produce deendothelization.[11] At the end of the experiment in control animals at the time of sacrifice the aorta was exposed, and all branches were ligated. A cannula was inserted in the aortic arch and at the bifurcation of the abdominal aorta. A buffer solution, tromethamine hydrochloride (Tris) 0.01 M, was perfused to clear the vessel of blood; an airstream was then passed through the aorta at a rate of 1000 ml/minute for 10 minutes. The aorta was immediately removed and placed in ice-cold Tris buffer. This procedure induced selective endothelial injury without damage to the basement membrane or deeper structures. The absence of endothelium was demonstrated by staining with silver nitrate. Pieces of aorta 3 cm in length and 2 cm in width were prepared for use in the perfusion chamber. The aortas were stored in Tris buffer with antibiotics (penicillin and streptomycin) at 4° C and were used within 3 weeks of harvesting.

Deeply Injured Vessel Wall. Pig aorta removed from control animals without air injury but by the method described above were stored in Tris buffer and antibiotics as described above. Just before use in the perfusion chamber, the pieces of aorta 3 cm in length and 2 cm in width were torn through the media for immediate use in the perfusion chamber.

Collagen Strips. Collagen strips from pig Achilles tendon, type I collagen bundles,[12] were obtained after the sacrifice of normal pigs. The tendons were dissected, cleaned of surrounding connective tissue, and stored in divalentin-free Tirode's buffer. Immediately before an experiment, strips 3 cm in length were separated for placement in the chamber.

RESULTS AND SIGNIFICANCE

Arterial Response to Injury

Acutely there was denudation of endothelium and immediate deposition of platelets in the dilated and adjacent vasoconstricted region as shown by ^{111}In-labeled platelets deposition and scanning electron microscopy in experimental studies (Fig. 30-5B). There was superficial or mild injury (no damage into or below the internal elastic lamina) over the entire dilated and adjacent vasoconstricted region. Deep injury (damage through the internal elastic lamina and into the media that is exposed to flowing arterial blood) was frequently present in the dilated (but never in the adjacent vasoconstricted region) and led to macroscopic mural thrombus in over 85% of deeply injured arteries within an hour despite an acute bolus of heparin (100 units per kg body weight) that prolonged the activated partial thromboplastin time to four to five

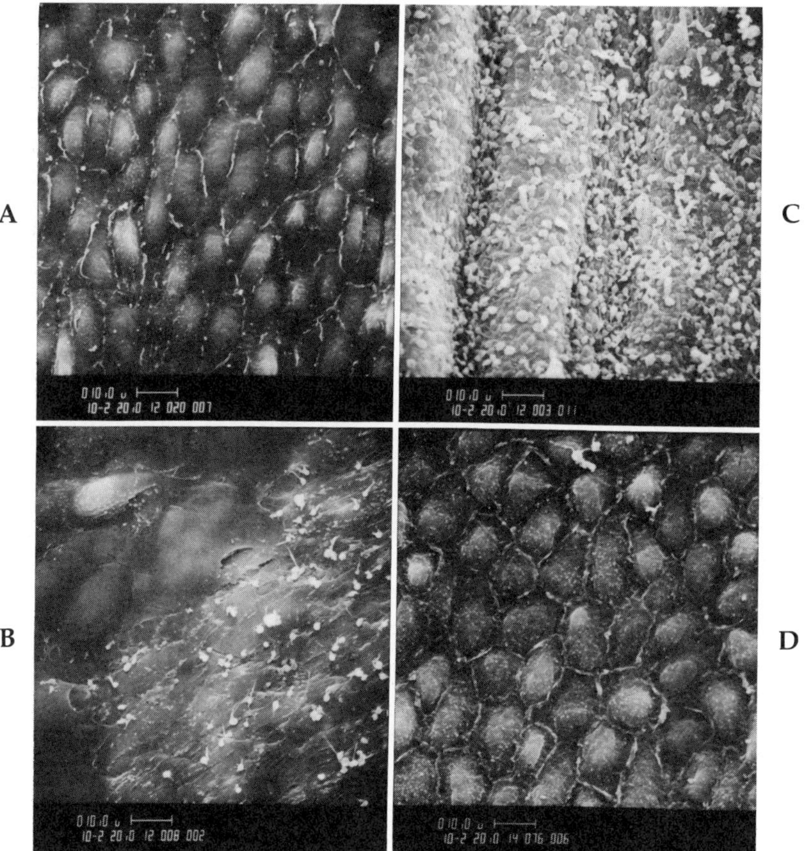

Fig. 30-5. Scanning electron microscopy shows views of the luminal surface of the porcine common carotid artery (×1000). **A,** Normal endothelium. **B,** Completely denuded endothelium replaced by a layer of adherent platelets on the subendothelium 1 hour after angioplasty. **C,** Partial regrowth of endothelium or periluminal lining cells with a few scattered platelets adhering to the uncovered subintima 4 days after angioplasty. **D,** Largely regrown endothelium or periluminal lining cells with no adherent platelets 7 days after angioplasty. (Reproduced with permission from the American Heart Association and Steele, P.M., et al.: Circ. Res. **57:**105-112, 1985.)

times control.[13,14] This marked platelet deposition, if it was greater than 40 × 10^6/cm^2, could usually be imaged in vivo in a peripheral artery with ^{111}In-labeled platelets.[14]

Mild injury with only denudation of the endothelium caused mild platelet deposition (less than 10 × 10^6/cm^2), which is a monolayer of platelets that did not form macroscopic thrombus and could not be imaged in vivo.[13,14] Regrowth of endothelial-like cells was protective against platelet deposition (Fig. 30-5C).

Heparin was only administered acutely as a bolus in our porcine model of angioplasty, was not reversed, and was not continued thereafter; thus platelet deposition remained high at 24 hours (greater than $40 \times 10^6/cm^2$), similar to 1 hour after angioplasty when there was no endothelium lining the lumen. Four days after angioplasty there was partial regrowth of endothelial-like cells and a marked reduction in platelet deposition to a mean of $4.4 \times 10^6/cm^2$ (Fig. 30-5C).[13] At 7 davs after angioplasty when regrowth of the endothelial-like cells was essentially complete, platelet deposition was negligible and similar to baseline or uninjured arteries (Fig. 30-5D).[13] The time course of endothelial regrowth in humans is not known and may also be reduced or incomplete in the presence of risk factors for coronary artery disease.

In this porcine model of arterial angioplasty in which the number of inflations and the inflation pressures were similar to an average dilatation in humans, severe platelet deposition, macroscopic mural thrombus, and acute thrombotic occlusion in 2% of arteries occurred in the absence of any preexisting stenotic lesion.[13,14] This underlines the importance of not performing arterial angioplasty unless the severity of the preexisting stenosis and myocardial ischemia warrant such risks as acute occlusion and restenosis with a severe lesion.

Smooth muscle cell proliferation in the porcine model was mild and patchy 7 days after the procedure and was significantly increased and more uniform 2 weeks to 2 months after angioplasty.[13] Similar smooth muscle cell proliferation can also be seen in human arteries in the few patients who have died at variable times following coronary angioplasty.[15] The relative amount of smooth muscle cell proliferation was small in the porcine model of arterial angioplasty compared with organization of mural thrombus.[13] Greater platelet deposition would theoretically provide greater quantities of platelet-derived growth factor for enhanced smooth muscle cell migration and proliferation. Undoubtedly both processes contribute to restenosis after angioplasty. In addition smooth muscle cell proliferation may be increased in patients with coronary risk factors, since these factors also lead to chronic endothelial injury and chronic low levels of platelet deposition. Thus it might be expected that a greater reduction in platelet deposition and mural thrombus formation would also reduce the amount of smooth muscle cell proliferation. However, this will not totally prevent smooth muscle cell proliferation because only a single layer of platelet deposition, which is not prevented by platelet inhibitor therapy, can stimulate smooth muscle cell proliferation. Significant arterial stenosis developed in one pig a month after angioplasty and was shown by histologic evaluation to be due to organization of mural thrombus (Fig. 30-6). Thus it is likely that major platelet deposition and the formation of mural thrombus with subsequent organization, combined with simultaneous smooth muscle cell proliferation, play a major role in the mechanism of restenosis.

Mural Thrombosis After Arterial Injury

The underlying pathologic substrate and the rheology of blood flow both contribute to the formation of intraluminal mural thrombus. The underlying substrate is initially exposed after endothelial denudation; this denudation eliminates the initial antithrombotic arterial defense which is both a physical separation of flowing blood from the deeper thrombogenic structures and the reduction or elimination of antithrombotic substances such as prostacyclin (PGI_2), heparin-like molecules, and tissue plasminogen activator. Endothelial denudation with exposure of only the subendothelium results in only a monolayer of platelet deposition that does not continuously increase over time even at higher shear rates

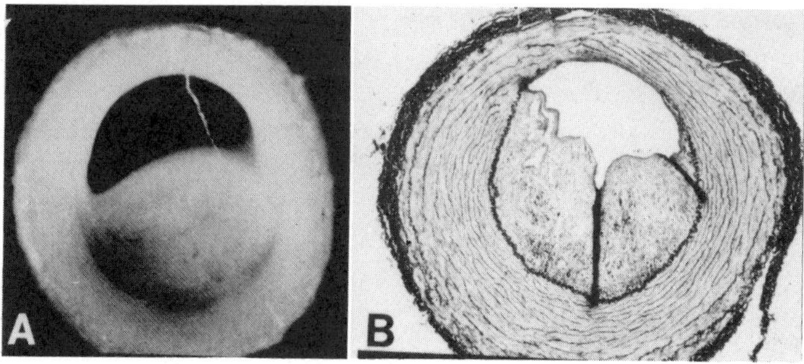

Fig. 30-6. Cross-section of the common carotid artery at the site of balloon dilatation 30 days after angioplasty. **A,** Macroscopic appearance of significant stenotic lesion in an artery that had been normal before angioplasty. **B,** Histologic section of same lesion showing that obstruction is due to organization of mural thrombus (Lason's elastic–van Gieson stain; ×64). (Reproduced with permission from the American Heart Association and Steele, P.M., et al.: Circ. Res. **57:**105-112, 1985.)

(above 800 sec^{-1}, which occur at conditions of higher flow velocity and smaller lumen diameter). Although transient increases in platelet deposition may occur for short time periods, these aggregates appear to be easily washed away and are not anchored in a stable fashion as they are in the presence of deep arterial injury.[16,17] Reasons for this lesser platelet deposition after mild injury include, in part, the underlying substrate, which is composed largely of types IV and V collagen, which are much less thrombogenic and stimulate a much lower platelet deposition than types I and III collagen, found in the arterial media and in plaques.[18-20] In addition, superficial injury results in a lower decrease in the synthesis of prostacyclin than does deeper injury.[21]

On the other hand, exposure of flowing blood to a more thrombogenic substrate such as types I and III collagen and smooth muscle cells results in considerably greater platelet deposition.[18-20] When flowing blood is exposed to arteries torn through the media, there is an increase in platelet deposition that does not plateau but steadily increases exponentially over time without reaching a plateau and not infrequently progresses to total thrombotic occlusion within 30 minutes. The same progressive increase in platelet deposition occurs when flowing blood is exposed to type I collagen.[17] The form of collagen may also contribute to the greater thrombogenicity in the diabetic patient, since diabetic collagen or glycosylated collagen stimulates a significantly greater platelet deposition than does normal collagen.[22] Quantitative ^{111}In-labeled platelet deposition onto both type I collagen and aortic media is shear-rate dependent and is considerably high at high shear rates.[23] Thus deep arterial injury can lead to thrombotic occlusion, especially at high shear rates; therefore incomplete relief of the stenosis after arterial angioplasty increases the likelihood of greater platelet-thrombus deposition and acute occlusion.[24]

The proposed mechanisms of platelet-thrombus deposition after acute and deep arterial injury are outlined in Fig. 30-7.[25] Both

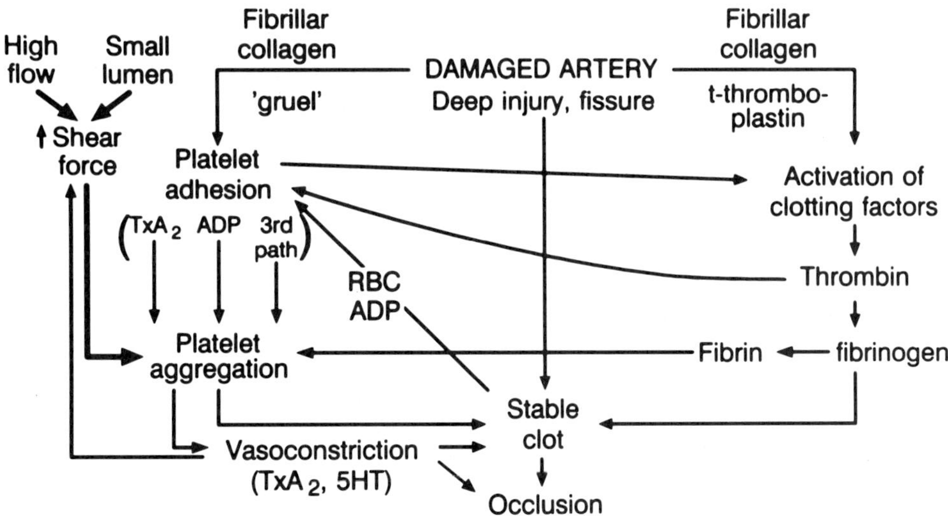

Fig. 30-7. Proposed mechanisms of thrombosis after arterial injury. *Left,* Platelet aggregation by collagen and lipid "gruel" occurs by three pathways: thromboxane A_2 (TxA_2), adenosine diphosphate (ADP), and a pathway that probably involves a platelet activating factor. The degree of acute vasoconstriction is dependent on the severity of platelet deposition (see text), is probably mediated by platelet substances (TxA_2 and serotonin [5HT]), and contributes to occlusion and clot formation. Increased shear forces *(far left)* caused by a small arterial lumen and high flow rates are directly related to increased platelet deposition (see text). *Right,* Collagen and tissue thromboplastin initiate activation of the intrinsic and extrinsic clotting systems. The interaction between platelets and the coagulation system is also depicted by platelet activation of the clotting system, the activation of platelets by thrombin, and the platelet-to-platelet binding by fibrinogen at specific platelet-membrane glycoprotein IIb/IIIa receptors. (5HT, 5-Hydroxytryptamine [serotonin]; RBC, red blood cell.) (From Chesebro, J.H., and Fuster, V.: Circulation **74**[suppl. 3]:1-10, 1986. Modified with permission from the American Heart Association.)

platelets and the intrinsic coagulation cascade are activated by the substrate within the arterial wall, which includes collagen, elastic tissue, smooth muscle cells, and fatty gruel.[26,27] Collagen with its negatively charged molecules appears especially important and probably contributes the major portion to the hemorrheologic response to deep arterial injury.[17-20,22] Deep arterial injury also increases the production of tissue thromboplastin, which activates the extrinsic pathway. In addition, there is mutual facilitation of thrombus formation between the coagulation cascade and platelets.

Soluble Factor V and Xa by binding to specific platelet receptors can produce thrombin 280,000 times faster than soluble Factor Xa alone.[28] The formation of Factor Xa and its binding to platelets is necessary for the activation of prothrombin. Thus the formation of the prothrombinase complex by platelets binding with coagulation factors accelerates the production of thrombin, which is the most potent activator of platelet aggregation (and leads to enhanced platelet deposition) and stimulates the formation of fibrin from fibrinogen.[27,28] Massive and more stable platelet aggregates can be formed when fibrinogen binds to specific glycoprotein IIb/IIIa receptors on the surface of platelets and forms platelet-to-platelet macromolecular bridges.[29]

Platelets are activated by three pathways (Fig. 30-7). Thromboxane A_2 is produced by platelets (during aggregation) from arachidonic acid via platelet cyclooxygenase and thromboxane synthetase. The second pathway involves adenosine diphosphate (ADP), which is released from platelets, red cells, and white cells, stimulates platelet aggregation, acts synergistically with collagen, and increases the exposure of the fibrinogen receptors on the platelet.[29-31] The third pathway of platelet activation appears to involve stimulation of aggregation by a platelet activating factor.

At higher shear rates (greater than 800 sec^{-1}) platelet adherence to collagen and thus to the arterial wall is dependent on both Factor VIII–von Willebrand Factor and fibronectin.[32] Von Willebrand Factor also appears to contribute to platelet-to-platelet attachment [33,34] and is probably more important at higher shear rates. Preliminary studies suggest that there is also shear rate dependence below 800 sec^{-1} when ex-vivo perfusion is done with heparinized blood. The shear force at the arterial wall is related inversely to arterial cross-sectional area (the third power of the lumen diameter) and is directly related to blood flow. Thus, higher blood flow and smaller lumen diameters increase the shear force. For example, the shear rate is 848 sec^{-1} in a 2 mm artery when flow is 40 ml/minute and half that when the flow is 20 ml/minute. The shear rate is 840 sec^{-1}in a 1 mm artery when the flow is 5 ml/minute, double that at 10 ml/minute, and four times that (or 3380 sec^{-1}) at 20 ml/minute. Thus the exposure of collagen with deep arterial injury (whether spontaneous as in unstable angina or acute infarction during plaque rupture, or during a procedure such as arterial angioplasty) leads to severe platelet deposition that is enhanced by an increased shear force. Because of the increased platelet aggregation and deposition with increasing shear force experimentally (Fig. 30-7), it is not surprising that arterial thrombotic events in the presence of spontaneous or procedure-related arterial injury are related to the severity of residual arterial stenosis, which includes the problem of occlusion and restensosis after angioplasty,[35] reocclusion after successful thrombolysis in acute myocardial infarction,[36] and progression to occlusion after plaque rupture in the coronary artery causing unstable angina.[37] These observations are consistent with further hemorrheologic experimental observations that showed that the greatest platelet deposition onto deeply injured arterial tissue is in the region of the stenosis rather than proximal or distal to the stenosis.[38] This suggests that the optimal technique for the prevention of restenosis during the angioplasty procedure is the maximal dilatation of a lesion to the normal lumen size that is proximal and distal to the lesion being dilated.

Thus the interaction among the intrinsic and extrinsic coagulation systems, platelets, and substrates of the deeper arterial wall facilitates platelet activation and aggregation and the growth of mural thrombus. Appropriate changes in any or all three of these factors may reduce platelet-thrombus formation and the incidence of restenosis. Another dynamic characteristic of the arterial wall, vasoconstriction, may also contribute to changes in blood flow, shear rate, and the propensity to restenosis (Fig. 30-7).

Vasoconstriction and Arterial Injury

Endothelial injury appears necessary for the development of arterial vasoconstriction after arterial injury since the loss of endothelium eliminates the diffusion barrier to vasoconstrictive substances and the loss of the so-called endothelial-derived relaxing factor (EDRF).[39-41] When normal endothelium is present in the pig coronary artery, no vasoconstriction results during the infusion of acetylcholine and vasodilation occurs during the infusion of bradykinin.[41] Acute superficial coronary arterial injury with a balloon that only removes the endothelium segmentally but does not damage the medial smooth muscle cells results in segmental vasoconstriction during the infusion of acetylcholine in vivo, in part because of loss of EDRF and in part because of direct effect of acetylcholine on smooth muscle cells. The more distal portion of the coronary artery where the endothelium was not damaged did not vasoconstrict to the infusion of acetylcholine and did vasodilate during the infusion of bradykinin in vivo in the pig. This pharmacologic intervention may be one method for identifying healthy endothelium in vivo.[41]

In acute experimental arterial injury by angioplasty, there is vasoconstriction immediately adjacent to the dilated region both proximally and distally, but never in the dilated region.[4,13] Vasoconstriction cannot and does not occur in the dilated region in this model of angioplasty because of the severe injury to the smooth muscle cells in the media as evidenced by the corkscrew shape to the cell nuclei acutely and the necrosis that is evident by 24 hours after injury.[4,13] In the region of vasoconstriction there is endothelial denudation or mild injury with associated platelet deposition. The severity of vasoconstriction is directly related to the log of the quantitated ^{111}In-labeled platelet deposition.[4] More vasoconstriction occurs distal to the dilated region than proximal, suggesting a normal flow of vasoconstrictor substances from the platelets in the dilated region.

Vasoconstriction can be reduced but not eliminated by reduction of platelet deposition with an effective platelet inhibitor that has no intrinsic vasodilator effects, such as the use of aspirin or ibuprofen.[4,42] Severity of this platelet-dependent vasoconstriction is determined by the severity of platelet deposition and thus the extent and depth of arterial injury, with deeper injury leading to more vasoconstriction in the adjacent regions than mild injury. Reduction of vasoconstriction with receptor inhibitors of the vasoconstricting substances from platelets (ketanserin to block receptors to serotonin and SQ-29,548 to block the receptors of thromboxane A_2 either singly or together) or with an intrinsic vasodilator (prostacyclin) does not reduce platelet deposition.[43,44] Thus vasoconstriction appears to be mediated by vasoconstrictor substances from platelets such as serotonin, thromboxane A_2 and probably the platelet-derived growth factor,[43-45] and effective therapy with a platelet inhibitor not only reduces mural thrombus formation but also reduces the severity of vaso-constriction.[4,42]

Although vasodilation per se does not reduce platelet deposition,[43,44] one drug appears capable of both vasodilating and reducing the severity of platelet deposition. An intravenous infusion of nitroglycerin at a dosage that lowered the mean arterial pressure by 10 mm Hg significantly reduced not only vasoconstriction but also the severity of platelet deposition after deep arterial injury in the pig.[46] Inhibition of whole-blood-platelet aggregation demonstrated at the bedside in blood drawn from patients receiving intravenous nitroglycerin suggests that intravenous nitroglycerin may also be an effective platelet inhibitor in humans,[47] but further studies are required in patients with deep arterial injury.

Mechanisms of Restenosis

The proposed mechanisms of restenosis after arterial angioplasty are summarized in Fig. 30-8.[48] Balloon angioplasty induces arterial injury, which is both mild throughout the region of the artery where the balloon has contacted the arterial wall and deep in the region of the fissure, tear, crack, or split in the arterial wall (usually the plaque) that inevitably

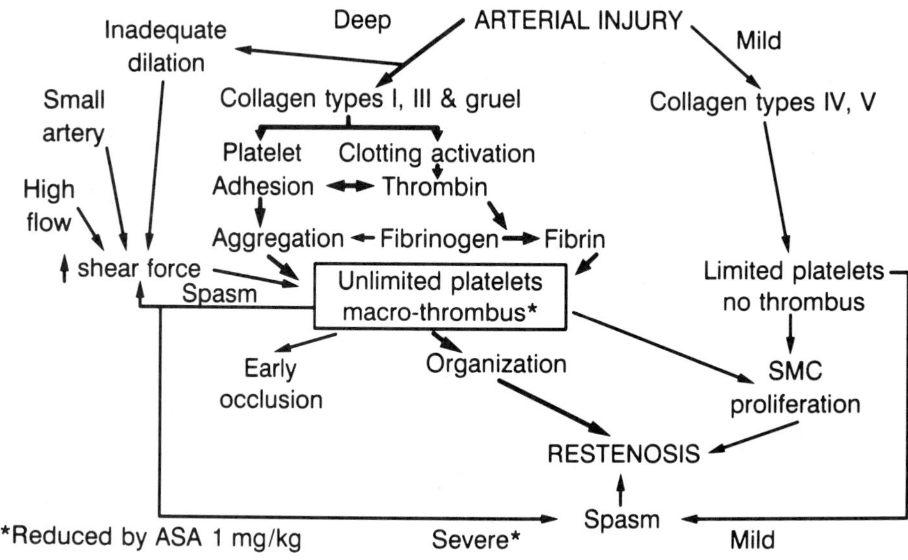

Fig. 30-8. Proposed pathophysiologic mechanisms of restenosis after arterial angioplasty. The major mechanism of restenosis is probably the one indicated by the broad arrows and involves deep arterial injury and activation of both the clotting systems and platelets, which leads to the formation and organization of mural thrombus. Smooth muscle cell (SMC) proliferation owing to the platelet-derived growth factor probably also contributes to restenosis and is likely enhanced by more extensive platelet deposition. Vasoconstriction (spasm) is always present proximal and especially distal to the dilated region after arterial angioplasty in the porcine carotid artery. This vasoconstriction is directly related to the severity of platelet deposition and could further increase shear forces and platelet deposition, but it makes an uncertain contribution to restenosis in patients. Mechanisms with an asterisk (*) after them have been reduced or suppressed by effective platelet inhibitor therapy (see text). (Modified with permission from Chesebro, J.H., et al.: Am. J. Cardiol. **60:**10B-16B, 1987.)

occurs with a successful angioplasty. The deeply injured region is where the type I and type III collagen fibrils are exposed leading to severe platelet deposition and probably inevitable mural thrombus formation. This platelet deposition is enhanced in arteries with high shear forces (small diameter and high flow) that would be present in cases of inadequate dilatation. Our studies in the porcine model suggest that even without a stenosis acute occlusion can occur in 1 to 4% of arteries after angioplasty. Although the major contribution to restenosis appears to be organization of mural thrombus, smooth muscle cell proliferation stimulated by the platelet-derived growth factor also appears to contribute in concert. Previous studies by Baumgartner suggest that regions with less damage to smooth muscle cells have greater proliferation (H.R. Baumgartner, personal communication). Although the role of vasoconstriction and spasm in restenosis is unclear, even subclinical vasoconstriction could enhance shear forces and thus enhance platelet deposition and thrombus formation that could stimulate additional smooth muscle cell proliferation and organization of residual mural thrombus. Vasoconstriction, as well as residual coronary artery risk factors, can lead to chronic and recurrent endothelial damage with continued platelet deposition and release of the platelet-derived growth factor resulting in chronic smooth muscle cell proliferation and a greater propensity for segmental vasoconstriction. This close attention to modifiable risk factors is mandatory.

Intervention Therapy

To minimize the risk of restenosis three factors should be addressed. First, adequate dilatation (with the least amount of deep injury) to maximize the lumen diameter reduces shear forces and the severity of platelet-thrombus deposition by a technical means. Second, there should be adequate anticoagulation with heparin. Third, adequate platelet inhibitor therapy should be combined with anticoagulation.

Although the major action of heparin is to inhibit thrombin, it also acts earlier in the coagulation cascade to inhibit activated Factor X (which is necessary for thrombin formation) by increasing the rate at which antithrombin III combines with Factor Xa.[28,49] Higher doses of heparin (more than 3.1 units/kg body weight/min) especially when administered as a bolus just before acute and deep arterial injury greatly reduced quantitative platelet deposition, quantitative fibrinogen deposition, and mural thrombus formation within the first hour after experimental angioplasty.[50,51] Since thrombin is the most potent activator of platelet adhesion known today, reduction in thrombin generation may be of critical importance in minimizing acute platelet deposition after deep arterial injury. Future platelet inhibitor therapy can be markedly enhanced and should only be tested when added to maximal thrombin inhibition. Thus other medications to inhibit thrombin appear to be a fruitful avenue of future research. The duration of heparin therapy in patients is unclear; it should be at least for 24 hours but probably will evolve to a longer course of therapy in the future and may involve heparin fragments with more specific mechanisms of action. Chronic heparin therapy in the rat has also decreased smooth muscle cell proliferation.[52]

Intervention therapy to minimize platelet deposition and prevent thrombosis should be started before the angioplasty procedure and be at a peak effect at the start of the procedure, since platelet-thrombus deposition begins as soon as blood comes in contact with the injured arterial segment. Thus a large heparin *bolus* should be administered immediately before the start of balloon inflation, and an intravenous *infusion* of heparin should be started immediately to maintain the plasma levels of heparin. The maximally effective platelet inhibitor therapy should be administered before the angioplasty procedure so that the peak effect will be present at the start of the procedure. The value of platelet inhibitor therapy and the optimal choice of therapy is currently under investigation. We have evaluated several platelet inhibitor therapies in our porcine model of angioplasty beginning administration before the procedure in pigs treated with heparin and have evaluated the acute effects by measuring quantitative ^{111}In-labeled platelet deposition and the presence or absence of macroscopic mural thrombus approximately 1 hour after the procedure. Only if such therapy reduced platelet-thrombus deposition acutely after the procedure in the presence of deep arterial injury compared with control animals would we then consider spending the time, effort, and money for a prospective, randomized, double-blind trial to test the effectiveness in reducing the incidence of stenosis after coronary angioplasty in patients. Partially successful platelet inhibitor therapies that were added to heparin and that reduced but did not eliminate platelet-thrombus deposition have included aspirin alone (1 mg/kg/day), dipyridamole (2.5 mg/kg/day) plus aspirin (20 mg/kg/day), anagrelide (an experimental platelet inhibitor drug that was effective with or without the addition of dipyridamole and aspirin), intravenous ibuprofen, and intravenous nitroglycerin.[4,39,43,53] Platelet inhibitor therapy, in addition to heparin, which was ineffective included prostaglandin E_1, prostacyclin (PGI_2) at 10, 50, and 500 ng/kg body weight/min, aspirin alone at 20 mg/kg body weight/day, dipyridamole alone, sulfinpyrazone, ticlopidine at 10 and 20 mg/kg body weight/day initiated 4 days before the procedure, intravenous verapamil, intravenous nifedipine, intravenous ketanserin, and the intravenous thromboxane A_2 receptorblocker SQ-29,548 (administered alone or together).[40,41,53,54]

It is not surprising that platelet inhibitor therapy that showed a beneficial effect in the pig model was only partially successful, since only one of three pathways of platelet activation is blocked by current platelet inhibitor therapy (mainly the prostaglandin pathway involving thromboxane A_2). For example, low-dose aspirin at 1 mg/kg body weight/day reduced the incidence of mural thrombus formation after deep arterial injury from 85% in control animals receiving only a single bolus of heparin (100 units/kg body weight) down to 30% in pigs receiving the same heparin therapy plus low-dose aspirin. It is disturbing that a 30% incidence of mural thrombus remains. This reduction in mural thrombus formation may be insufficient to prevent restenosis when tested in trials in patients. Thus other therapies need evaluation, such as blockade of glycoprotein IIb/IIIa receptors on platelets for fibrinogen binding (which promotes aggregation and platelet-to-platelet bonding), blockade of glycoprotein Ib receptors to Factor VIII–von Willebrand Factor on the platelet and arterial wall, and, especially, blockade of receptors to collagen (critical for platelet adhesion) and receptors to the platelet-derived growth factor (which stimulates smooth muscle cell proliferation). The strategy of blocking platelet membrane glycoprotein receptors appears very promising and will probably offer a much more potent antiplatelet effect as suggested from our preliminary studies in the ex-vivo perfusion chamber in which low-dose aspirin alone only reduced quantitative platelet deposition by 30%, whereas an antibody to the Factor VIII–von Willebrand Factor reduced platelet deposition by 80%.[55]

No controlled trial demonstrating successful therapy for reduction of the incidence of restenosis in patients has been reported. One study suggests no benefit from therapy with low molecular weight dextran.[56] In another study that included patients without occlusion within 48 hours after the angioplasty procedure, there was no significant difference in the incidence of restenosis in a group of patients treated with warfarin compared with a group of patients treated with aspirin (325 mg/day), and restenosis was found in more than 25% of patients in both groups.[57] In another randomized trial comparing groups of patients treated with dipyridamole and aspirin, ticlopidine, or placebo, the trial was stopped prematurely because of an increased incidence of acute occlusion in the placebo group, which received only heparin in dosages that were relatively low but that were also not controlled and defined at each of the centers involved in the study. There was no reduction in the incidence of restenosis in the relatively small number of patients entered into each group.[58,59] Aggressive therapy with heparin (bolus followed immediately by an infusion) appears necessary to minimize mural thrombus formation and acute occlusion.

Current Recommendations

It is important to achieve optimal balloon dilatation to as close to the normal lumen diameter as possible to minimize shear force and thus platelet-thrombus deposition. All patients should receive 5000 units of heparin at the beginning of the procedure in the catheterization laboratory and then another 10000 units as an intravenous bolus just before the first balloon dilatation of the angioplasty procedure. This should be followed immediately by an intravenous infusion of heparin at 18 units/kg body weight/hour for a minimum of 18 to 24 hours after the procedure (or until 7:00 AM the following day when heparin therapy is usually stopped and the arterial sheath removed 3 to 4 hours later). The immediate initiation of an intravenous infusion of heparin helped to maintain the high plasma levels that are protective against acute platelet-thrombus deposition. If the procedure is complicated by a large intimal flap or if thrombus was identified by angiography either before or after the procedure, heparin infusion should be continued for at least 48 hours (and the arterial sheath can be removed 3 to 4 hours after discontinuing the heparin infusion). In some patients in whom we were particularly worried about extensive mural thrombus or those who had acute reocclusion in the laboratory but were successfully redilated, heparin therapy has been continued for as long as 96 hours with the arterial sheath being removed after 24 to 48 hours (after decreasing the heparin infusion to 9 units/kg body weight/hour for 3 to 4 hours and compressing the puncture site for 30 minutes using experienced personnel and a compressive dressing. Thereafter, the heparin infusion was increased to 18 units/kg body weight/hour).

It is uncertain whether any therapy with a platelet inhibitor will be effective in reducing restenosis after coronary angioplasty. Because therapy with dipyridamole and aspirin was effective in reducing the occlusion of aortocoronary bypass grafts and was the first effective platelet inhibitor therapy that reduced quantitative platelet and thrombus deposition after experimental angioplasty in the pig, we are currently conducting a prospective, randomized, double-blind, placebo-controlled trial of dipyridamole (225 mg/day) and aspirin (975 mg/day) in three divided doses starting 1 day before the procedure and continuing for 6 months after the procedure in patients undergoing coronary angioplasty.[60,61] All of our patients receive intravenous heparin for a minimum of 18 to 48 hours as described above and are restudied by angiography 6 months after the procedure or before if symptoms warrant early angiography. This study will test the hypothesis concerning the effectiveness of adjunctive platelet inhibitor therapy for the reduction of restenosis after coronary artery angioplasty.

Our studies in pigs suggest that an equally rational approach would be to start aspirin 325 mg as a loading dose 1 day before angioplasty and continue with 80 mg daily including a dose 1 to 2 hours before the actual procedure. However, this very low dose of aspirin has no clinical basis from actual trials of antithrombotic therapy in arterial thromboembolic disease except for a small study of 46 patients who had aortocoronary bypass graft operation and were randomized to aspirin 100 mg/day or a matching placebo. The researchers noted a very high rate of occlusion in the placebo group and some imbalance in the baseline characteristics, but did observe a significant decrease in occlusion in the aspirin group.[62] New and more effective therapy for inhibiting platelet-thrombus deposition until endothelial regrowth has occurred is needed. These more potent therapies may involve receptor blockers to the glycoprotein receptors on the platelet membrane such as those for fibrinogen, Factor VIII–von Willebrand Factor, or both. If these therapies are effective they will probably only be able to be used on a short-term basis because of the probable higher risk of bleeding. Care will have to be taken in the evaluation of these therapies to be sure that thrombocytopenia does not result.

REFERENCES

1. Castaneda-Zuniga, W.R., Formanek, A., Tadavarthy, M., Vlodaver, Z., Edwards, J.E., Zollikofer, C., and Amplatz, K.: The mechanism of balloon angioplasty, Radiology **135:**565-571, 1980.
2. Block, P.C., Myler, R.K., Stertzer, S., and Fallon, J.T.: Morphology after transluminal angioplasty in human beings, N. Engl. J. Med. **305:**382-385, 1981.
3. Sanborn, T.A., Faxon, D.P., Haudenschild, C., Gottsman, S.B., and Ryan, T.J.: The mechanism of transluminal angioplasty: evidence for formation of aneurysms in experimental atherosclerosis, Circulation **68:**1136-1140, 1983.
4. Lam, J.Y.T., Chesebro, J.H., Steele, P.M., and Fuster, V.: Is vasospasm related to platelet deposition? In vivo relationship in a pig model of arterial injury, Circulation **75:**243-248, 1987.
5. Dewanjee, M.K., Rao, S.A., and Didisheim, P.: Indium-111 tropolene, a new high affinity platelet label: preparation and evaluation of labeling parameters, J. Nucl. Med. **22:**981-987, 1981.
6. Dewanjee, M.K., Tago, M., Jose, M., Fuster, V., and Kaye, M.P.: Quantification of platelet retention in aortocoronary femoral vein bypass graft in dogs treated with dipyridamole and aspirin, Circulation **69:**350-356, 1984.
7. Turitto, V.T., and Baumgartner, H.R.: Platelet-surface interactions. In Coleman, R.H., Hirsh, J., Marder, U.J., and Salzman, E.W., editors: Hemostasis and thrombosis: basic principles and clinical practice, Philadelphia, 1982, J.B. Lippincott Co.
8. Merrill, E.W.: Rheology of blood flow, Physiol. Rev. **49:**863-888, 1969.
9. Copley, A.L.: On biorheology (joint plenary lecture), Biorheology **10:**87-105, 1974.
10. Bird, R.B., Stewart, W.E., and Lightfoot, E.N.: Transport phenomena, New York, 1960, John Wiley & Sons.
11. Fischman, J.A., Ryan, G.B., and Karnovsky, N.J.: Endothelial regeneration in the rat carotid artery and the significance of endothelial denudation in the pathogenesis of myointimal thickening, Lab. Invest. **32:**339-351, 1975.
12. Miller, E.J.: Chemistry of the collagens and their distribution. In Piez, K.D., Reddi, A.H., editors: Extracellular matrix biochemistry, New York, 1984, Elsevier.
13. Steele, P.M., Chesebro, J.H., Stanson, A.W., Holmes, D.R., Dewanjee, M.K., Badimon, L., and Fuster, V.: Balloon angioplasty: natural history of the pathophysiologic response to injury in a pig model, Circ. Res. **57:**105-112, 1985.
14. Lam, J.Y.T., Chesebro, J.H., Steele, P.M., Dewanjee, M.K., Badimon, L., and Fuster, V.: Deep arterial injury during experimental angioplasty: relationship to a positive ^{111}Indium-labeled platelet scintigram, quantitative platelet deposition, and mural thrombus, J. Am. Coll. Cardiol. **8:**1380-1386, 1986.
15. Roberts, W.C.: Pathology of coronary angioplasty, Presented at the First International Workshop on Future Directions in Interventional Cardiology, Santa Barbara, California, September 26, 1987.
16. Baumgartner, H.R., and Sakariassen, K.S.: Factors controlling thrombus formation on arterial lesions, Ann. N.Y. Acad. Sci. **454:**162-177, 1985.
17. Badimon, L., Badimon, J.J., Galvez, A., Chesebro, J.H., and Fuster, V.: Influence of arterial damage and wall shear rate on platelet deposition: ex vivo study in a swine model, Arteriosclerosis **6:**312-320, 1986.

18. Parsons, T.J., Haycraft, D.L., Hoak, J.C., and Sage, H.: Interaction of platelets and purified collagens in a laminar flow model, Thromb. Res. **43**:435-443, 1986.
19. Mayne, R.: Collagenous proteins of blood vessels, Arteriosclerosis **6**:585-593, 1986.
20. Parsons, T.J., Haycraft, D.L., Hoak, J.C., and Sage, H.: Diminished platelet adherence to type V collagen, Arteriosclerosis **3**:589-598, 1983.
21. Moncada, S., Herman, A.G., Higgs, E.A., et al.: Differential formulation of prostacyclin (PGX or PGI_2) by layers of the arterial wall: an explanation for the antithrombotic properties of vascular endothelium, Thromb. Res. **11**:323-344, 1977.
22. Le Pape, A., Guitton, J.D., Gutman, N., Legrand, Y., Fauvel, F., and Muh, J.P.: Nonenzymatic glycosylation of collagen in diabetes: incidence on increased normal platelet aggregation, Haemostasis **13**:36-41, 1983.
23. Lam, J.Y.T., Chesebro, J.H., Heras, M., Penny, W.J., Dewanjee, M.K., Bailey, K.R., and Badimon, L.: Deep and superficial arterial injury: different affinity for thrombus formation at increasing shear rate (abstract), Circulation **76**(suppl. 4):IV-101, 1987.
24. Chesebro, J.H., Lam, J.Y.T., Badimon, L., and Fuster, V.: Restenosis after arterial angioplasty: a hemorrheologic response, Am. J. Cardiol. **60**:10B-16B, 1987.
25. Chesebro, J.H., and Fuster, V.: Antithrombotic therapy for acute myocardial infarction: mechanisms and prevention of deep venous, left ventricular, and coronary artery thromboembolism, Circulation **74**(suppl. 3):1-10, 1986.
26. Fuster, V., Adams, P.C., Badimon, J.J., and Chesebro, J.H.: Platelet-inhibitor drugs' role in coronary artery disease, Prog. Cardiovasc. Dis. **29**:325-346, 1987.
27. Nemerson, Y., and Nossel, H.L.: The biology of thrombosis, Annu. Rev. Med. **33**:479-488, 1982.
28. Mann, K.G., Tracey, P.B., and Nesheim, M.E.: Assembly and function of prothrombinase complex on synthetic and natural membranes. In Oates, J.A., Hawiger, J., and Ross, R., editors: Interaction of platelets with the vessel wall, Am. Physiol. Soc. 47-57, 1985.
29. Peerschke, E.I.B.: The platelet fibrinogen receptor, Semin. Hematol. **22**:241-259, 1985.
30. Adams, G.A., and Feverstein, I.A.: Platelet adhesion and release: interfacial concentration of released materials, Am. J. Physiol. **240**:H99-H108, 1981.
31. Niiya, K., Hodson, E., Bader, R., Byers-Ward, V., Koziol, J.A., Plow, E.F., and Ruggeri, Z.M.: Increased surface expression of the membrane glycoprotein IIb/IIIa complex induced by platelet activation. Relationship to the binding of fibrinogen and platelet aggregation, Blood **70**:475-483, 1987.
32. Houdijk, W.P.M., Sakariassen, K.S., Nievelstein, P.F.E.M., and Sixma, J.J.: Role of factor VIII-von Willebrand factor and fibronectin in the interaction of platelets in flowing blood with monomeric and fibrillar human collagen types I and III, J. Clin. Invest. **75**:531-540, 1985.
33. Turitto, V.T., Weiss, H.J., and Baumgartner, H.R.: Platelet interaction with rabbit subendothelium in von Willebrand's disease: altered thrombus formation distinct from defective platelet adhesion, J. Clin. Invest. **74**:1730-1741, 1984.
34. Nichols, T.C., Bellinger, D.A., Johnson, T.A., Lamb, M.A., and Griggs, T.R.: von Willebrand's disease prevents occlusive thrombosis in stenosed and injured porcine coronary arteries, Circ. Res. **59**:15-26, 1986.
35. Leimgruber, P.P., Roubin, G.S., Hollman, J., Cotsonis, G.A., Meier, B., Douglas, J.S., King, S.B., and Gruentzig, A.R.: Restenosis after successful coronary angioplasty in patients with single-vessel disease, Circulation **73**:710-717, 1987.
36. Harrison, D.G., Ferguson, D.W., Collins, S.M., Skorton, D.J., Ericksen, E.E., Kioschos, J.M., Marcus, M.L., and White, C.W.: Rethrombosis after reperfusion with streptokinase: importance of geometry of residual lesions, Circulation **69**:991-999, 1984.
37. Falk, E.: Plaque rupture with severe preexisting stenosis precipitating coronary thrombosis: characteristics of coronary atherosclerotic plaques underlying fatal occlusive thrombi, Br. Heart J. **50**:127-134, 1983.
38. Badimon, L., Badimon, J.J., Turitto, V.T., Chesebro, J.H., and Fuster, V.: Mechanism of

arterial thrombosis: platelet thrombus deposition in areas of stenosis (abstract), Circulation **76**(suppl. 4):IV-102, 1987.

39. Furchgott, R.F., and Zawadski, J.V.: The obligatory role of endothelial cells in the relaxation of arterial smooth muscle by acetylcholine, Nature **288:**273, 1980.
40. Vanhoutte, P.M., and Houston, D.S.: Platelets, endothelium, and vasospasm, Circulation **72:**728-734, 1985.
41. Penny, W.J., Chesebro, J.H., Heras, M., Badimon, L., and Fuster, V.: In vivo identification of normal and damaged endothelium by quantitative coronary angiography and infusion of acetylcholine and bradykinin in pigs (abstract), J. Am. Coll. Cardiol., 1988. (In press.)
42. Lam, J.Y.T., Chesebro, J.H., Dewanjee, M.K., Badimon, L., and Fuster, V.: Ibuprofen: a potent antithrombotic agent for arterial injury after balloon angioplasty (abstract), J. Am. Coll. Cardiol. **9:**64A, 1987.
43. Lam, J.Y.T., Chesebro, J.H., Badimon, L., and Fuster, V.: Serotonin and thromboxane A_2 receptor blockade decrease vasoconstriction but not platelet deposition after deep arterial injury, Circulation **74**(suppl. 2):II-97, 1986.
44. Lam, J.Y.T., Chesebro, J.H., Badimon, L., and Fuster, V.: The vasoconstrictive response following arterial angioplasty in pigs: evidence for vasoconstriction resulting from rather than causing platelet deposition, J. Am. Coll. Cardiol. **7:**12A, 1986.
45. Berk, B.C., Alexander, R.W., Brock, T.A., Gimbrone, M.A., Jr., and Webb, R.C.: Vasoconstriction: a new activity for platelet-derived growth factor, Science **232:**87-90, 1986.
46. Lam, J.Y.T., Chesebro, J.H., and Fuster, V.: Platelets, vasospasm, and nitroglycerin during angioplasty: a new role for an old drug, Circulation **72**(suppl. 3):III-194, 1985.
47. Diodat, J., Theroux, P., Latour, J.G., Lacoste, L., Pelletier, G.B., Roy, D., and Waters, D.D.: Nitroglycerin at therapeutic doses inhibits platelet aggregation in man, J. Am. Coll. Cardiol., 1988. (In press.)
48. Chesebro, J.H., Lam, J.Y.T., Badimon, L., and Fuster, V.: Restenosis after arterial angioplasty: a hemorrheologic response. Am. J. Cardiol. **60:**10B-16B, 1987.
49. Biggs, R., Denson, K.W.E., Akman, N., Borrett, R., and Hadden, M.: Antithrombin III, antifactor Xa and heparin, Br. J. Haematol. **19:**283-305, 1970.
50. Heras, M., Chesebro, J.H., Penny, W.J., Bailey, K.R., Lam, J.Y.T., Badimon, L., and Fuster, V.: The importance of adequate heparin dosage in arterial angioplasty (abstract), Circulation **76**(suppl. 4)IV-213, 1987.
51. Heras, M., Chesebro, J.H., Bailey, K., Badimon, L., and Fuster, V.: Dose dependent inhibition by heparin of platelet-thrombus deposition during angioplasty (abstract), J. Am. Coll. Cardiol., 1988. (In press.)
52. Guyton, J.R., Rosenberg, R.D., Clowes, A.W., and Karnovsky, M.J.: Inhibition of rat arterial smooth muscle cell proliferation by heparin: in vivo studies with anticoagulant and nonanticoagulant heparin, Circ. Res. **46:**625-634, 1980.
53. Steele, P.M., Chesebro, J.H., and Fuster, V.: The natural history of arterial balloon angioplasty in pigs and intervention with platelet-inhibitor therapy: implications for clinical trials (abstract), Clin. Res. **32:**209A, 1984.
54. Steele, P.M., Chesebro, J.H., Holmes, D.R., Badimon, L., and Fuster, V.: Balloon angioplasty in pigs: comparative effects of platelet-inhibitor drugs (abstract), Circulation **70**(suppl. 2):II-361, 1984.
55. Badimon, L., Badimon, J.J., Chesebro, J.H., and Fuster, V.: Inhibition of thrombus formation: blockage of adhesive glycoprotein mechanisms versus blockage of the cyclooxygenase pathway, J. Am. Coll. Cardiol., 1988. (In press.)
56. Swanson, K.T., Vlietstra, R.E., Holmes, D.R., Smith, H.C., Reeder, G.S., Bresnahan, J.F., and Bove, A.A.: Efficacy of adjunctive dextran during percutaneous transluminal coronary angioplasty, Ann. Intern. Med. **102:**447-448, 1985.
57. Thornton, M.A., Gruentzig, A.R., Hollman, J., King, S.B., and Douglas, J.S.: Coumadin and aspirin in prevention of recurrence after transluminal coronary angioplasty: a randomized study, Circulation **69:**721-727, 1984.
58. White, C.W., Chaitman, B., Lassar, T.A., Marcus, M.L., Chisholm, R.J., Knudson, M., Morton, B., Roy, L., Khaja, F., Vandormael, M., Reitman, M., and the Ticlopidine Study Group: Antiplatelet agents are effective in reducing the immediate complications of PTCA: results from the ticlopidine multi-center trial (abstract), Circulation **76**(suppl. 4):IV-400, 1987.

59. White, C.W., Knudson, M., Schmidt, D., Chisholm, R.J., Vandormael, M., Morton, B., Roy, L., Khaja, F., Reitman, M., and the Ticlopidine Study Group: Neither ticlopidine nor aspirin-dipyridamole prevents restenosis post-PTCA: results from a randomized placebo-controlled multi-center trial (abstract), Circulation 76(suppl. 4):IV-213, 1987.
60. Chesebro, J.H., Clements, I.P., Fuster, V., Elveback, L.R., Smith, H.C., Bardsley, W.T., Frye, R.L., Holmes, D.R., Vlietstra, R.E., Pluth, J.R., Wallace, R.B., Puga, F.J., Orszulak, T.A., Piehler, J.M., Schaff, H.V., and Danielson, G.K.: A platelet-inhibitor-drug trial in coronary-artery bypass operations: benefit of perioperative dipyridamole and aspirin therapy on early postoperative vein-graft patency, N. Engl. J. Med. **307**:73-78, 1982.
61. Chesebro, J.H., Fuster, V., Elveback, L.R., Clements, I.P., Smith, H.C., Holmes, D.R., Bardsley, W.T., Pluth, J.R., Wallace, R.B., Puga, F.J., Orszulak, T.A., Piehler, J.M., Danielson, G.K., Schaff, H.V., and Frye, R.L.: Effect of dipyridamole and aspirin on late vein-graft patency after coronary bypass operations, N. Engl. J. Med. **310**:209-214, 1984.
62. Lorenz, R.L., Weber, M., Kotzur, J., Theisen, K., Schacky, C.V., Meister, W., Reichardt, B., and Weber, D.C.: Improved aortocoronary bypass patency by low-dose aspirin (100 mg daily), Lancet **1**:1261-1264, 1984.

Chapter 31

The Role of Angioplasty in the Treatment of Acute Myocardial Infarction

Allan M. Ross, MD, FACC

The application of PTCA (percutaneous transluminal coronary angioplasty) within the broad scheme of the treatment of acute myocardial infarction (MI) falls into three categories based predominantly on the timing of the intervention. In this discussion, "primary PTCA" is emergency recanalization by interventional techniques; "sequential PTCA" refers to the combination of early administration of intravenous (IV) lytic agents followed very closely by angioplasty; and "adjunctive PTCA" implies angiography and angioplasty delayed by at least several days and possibly reserved for selected patients (as opposed to the nonselective approach implicit in the first two strategies) (Table 31-1).

PTCA as a primary intervention refers to the immediate use of guidewire, balloon catheter, and/or other intracoronary devices to effect disruption of the infarct causing occlusive thrombus. In addition to providing direct and immediate reperfusion, these techniques also allow for reduction of the severe atherosclerotic obstruction that commonly exists at the site of a total interruption of antegrade coronary flow. The successful use of PTCA as primary therapy in acute MI has been reported from numerous centers, Hartzler being among the earliest operators to demonstrate the feasibility of this approach.[1]

In highly experienced hands, primary PTCA without the use of lytic drugs can effect reperfusion with a frequency comparable if not superior to that obtained with the most efficient plasminogen activators, that is, in the range of 75 to 85% of attempts. It has the additional advantages of early definition of the total coronary circulation, which identifies candidates such as those with an obstructed left main artery who would presumably benefit from very early operative intervention, and on the other end of the spectrum identifies those patients with single vessel disease, who are potential candidates for very early discharge.[2] The main conceptual benefit, however, of primary PTCA is the rapid conversion of a total occlusion to a widely patent infarct artery very early in the course of disease. Data from O'Neill and colleagues,[3] and other workers have demonstrated that immediately after reperfusion is accomplished by primary PTCA the infarct-related artery dem-

Table 31-1. Angioplasty in Acute MI

Application	*Definition*	*Advantages*	*Disadvantages*
Primary	Immediate transport to catheterization lab for clot perforation and lesion dilatation without lytic drugs.	High rate of reperfusion; minimizes residual stenosis.	Often prolonged time from infarct to treatment. Requires emergency transport. Therapeutic scheme not available to majority of population.
Sequential	IV lytic therapy is given first then patient is transported for angiography–PTCA within hours.	Avoids initial time to treatment delay. Reduces residual stenosis severity. Identifies lytic failures relatively early.	Emergency transport still required. Not available to significant percentage of population. Randomized trials not encouraging.
Adjunctive	Angiography and angioplasty performed later (1 or 2 days to a week) after lytic therapy. Can be applied routinely or by some selection process.	Avoids initial time to treatment delay. Dilatation performed remote from thrombosis and in patients selected by severity of stenosis and/or other criteria. Transport nonemergent.	Early recurrent ischemia and reocclusion not interdicted. Lytic failure not identified until presumably too late. Severe residual stenosis not relieved until presumably beyond the salvage window.

onstrates a mean residual stenosis of less than 50%, whereas after chemical thrombolysis the former site of occlusion is left initially with a far more severe residual obstruction (83% in O'Neill's series). See comparison of residual stenosis with lytic therapy and PTCA (Table 31-2). While it is now recognized that over time (that is, days to a week) continued clot dissolution after lytic therapy results in an increasingly patent infarct artery (shown with careful quantitative methodology by Serruys, and co-workers,[4] and other researchers), there has been suspicion and some supportive data for the concept that greater early reperfusion flow may effect greater myocardial salvage. Data from Sheehan and colleagues[7] have reported that an infarct-related coronary artery cross-sectional area of 4 mm^2 or greater is associated with improving left ventricular (LV) regional wall motion during follow-up, whereas smaller lumen areas have not been associated with such benefits. Analogous experimental data exist utilizing postocclusion coronary flow control to demonstrate greater salvage with increased blood flow.[8]

Early clinical substantiation of this principle was shown by the Michigan group,[3] who

Table 31-2. Percent Residual Stenosis in the Infarct-Related Artery (Patent Vessels)

Lytic Therapy Alone		
Serruys, et al.[4] (median stenosis)	IV rtPA	80%
O'Neill, et al.[3] (mean stenosis)	IC streptokinase	83%
Erbel, et al.[5] (mean stenosis)	IV streptokinase	73%
PTCA		
Erbel, et al.[5]	After IV streptokinase	47%
Rothbaum, et al.[6]	No lytic therapy	29%
O'Neill, et al.[3]	No lytic therapy	43%

rtPA, recombinant tissue type plasminogen activator; IC, intracoronary.

demonstrated considerably augmented improvement in LV function among infarct patients reperfused by PTCA compared with those in whom reflow was accomplished pharmacologically. Furthermore the augmented benefit correlated directly with the considerably improved infarct artery diameter achieved by PTCA.

Thus there is theoretic, experimental, and clinical support for primary PTCA in acute MI. The limitations of this approach, however, are also clearly evident, and are based on the complexity of required logistics. From a variety of lines of evidence it has become established that for most infarct victims, meaningful myocardial salvage attends reperfusion accomplished within the very first few hours of onset of the clinical syndrome, with a benefit curve steeply declining from 1 or 2 hours after infarction and the range of 4 to 6 hours after an MI. The delays inherent in patient response, triage, and transportation render prompt PTCA within a short time frame (probably) unaccomplishable for most acute MI patients given the currently constituted public awareness and response systems. Furthermore extremely skilled interventionalists in the emergency setting, with laboratories and staffs instantly available on an around-the-clock basis, are required commodities for primary PTCA to work, and are simply not available in most communities. Thus at the present time this mode of therapy can be favored in only very selected environments as a routine approach and more widely for the occasional patient whose infarction begins fortuitously when and where all the resources are locally available.

Because rapidity of reperfusion has been recognized as the most important single variable in producing clinical benefits[9] and since transportation and procedure time preclude the possibility of most infarct victims' receiving early PTCA as effective primary therapy, a larger experience exists adding angioplasty to the management strategy of patients who first are treated with an intravenous thrombolytic agent. From a theoretic basis, this sequence of lysis followed promptly by angiography and angioplasty is highly attractive. It combines the rapidity afforded by initial IV pharmacologic lysis with the additional benefits of angiography and PTCA discussed above. Conceptually it is an ideal algorithm for solving the problems of reocclusion, reinfarction, and recurrent ischemia (see discussion below). Furthermore, from a logistical point of view it affords more orderly transfer of patients after initial therapy to laboratories equipped to receive such patients under slightly less urgent conditions.

The sequence of IV thrombolysis quickly followed by PTCA was also motivated by the dual goals of reperfusing patients who are not perfused adequately on IV lytic drug therapy (20 to 25% with recombinant tissue type plasminogen activator [rtPA], and higher with IV streptokinase) and favorably impacting the reocclusion and recurrent ischemia seen after thrombolytic therapy. The frequency of recurrent coronary occlusion after lysis with IV rtPA or streptokinase has shown considerable variability from study to study, but now with very large numbers of pooled data available it can be reasonably estimated to be between 10 and 15%. Actual reinfarction at the time of reocclusion occurs with a somewhat lower frequency owing to several probable factors, including the reality that not all reperfusion leads to clinically important salvage (thus little myocardium is at risk to reinfarct) and perhaps the development of substantial collateral flow between the first episode of occlusion and the second one.

The setting for reocclusion is the persistence of a severe coronary narrowing and the persistence of some thrombus at the previously occluded site.[10] Logic, therefore, would dictate that conversion of a tight to a mild obstruction by sequential PTCA ought to very favorably influence the rate of reclosure.

Recurrent ischemic events, ascribable to the zone of salvaged myocardium and the severe postlysis stenosis in the infarct-related artery, have also been well documented and are even more frequent than the problem of reocclusion. Again, the occurrence of this phenomenon is dependent on initial salvage of substantial muscle that in turn is dependent on the efficiency of the lytic agent selected and the time delay from symptom onset to reperfusion. The range of reported recurrent ischemia is, therefore, even wider than the reported rates of reocclusion, but with effective early lysis may be estimated to occur in up to 20% of patients during early and intermediate-term follow-up (and in some small series with an even higher incidence). Again the concept that sequential PTCA would reduce the likelihood of recurrent ischemia has been highly attractive.

The careful evaluation of this strategy, that is, intravenous lytic therapy then sequential PTCA has followed the usual progression from sequential observations to more structured randomized trials. Early observations have been published by Uebis and associates[11] who, somewhat surprisingly, found a slightly higher early reocclusion rate (3 days after initial therapy) of 8.8% among 147 patients offered sequential PTCA than the 3.8% reocclusion rate seen in 130 patients with no PTCA (p=NS). By late follow-up in this series (26 weeks) both groups had equivalent total reocclusion rates (14.2 and 16.1% respectively). It is to be noted, however, that this was not a randomized trial. The first formally randomized series on lytic therapy with or without sequential PTCA was published by Erbel and colleagues.[5] PTCA patients in whom the procedure was successful did display a reduced reocclusion rate. However, owing to a significant fraction of procedural failures, in comparing the total group randomized to PTCA versus the total group managed conservatively, the sequential PTCA strategy did not lead to a final reocclusion benefit.

The three most prominent studies of the role of PTCA after lytic therapy to date have been the published Transluminal Angioplasty in Myocardial Infarction (TAMI) trial[12] and the as-yet-unpublished (at the time this chapter is written) Thrombolysis in Myocardial Infarction (TIMI-II) and European Cooperative Group trials. All three study groups selected rtPA as the intravenous lytic agent because of its higher coronary reperfusion rate than streptokinase.

In the TAMI[12] 197 patients were randomized with stenotic and dilatable infarct-related arteries to either immediate PTCA or conservative therapy for a week. The major trial endpoints included reocclusion rate and ventricular function after a week's follow-up. Perhaps, surprisingly, the reocclusion rates of 11% for PTCA versus 13% for conservative therapy (see Table 31-3) and the final LV function (global and regional) were not different based on treatment assignment. More patients in the immediate PTCA group suffered bleeding problems and had emergency coronary artery bypass graft (CABG), whereas

Table 31-3. Reocclusion Rates for PTCA vs. Lytic Therapy

	Lytic Therapy Only	*PTCA*
Uebis, et al.[11*] —3 days	4% (5/130)	9%(13/147)
Uebis, et al.[11*] —6 mo	16% (21/130)	14% (21/147)
Erbel, et al.[5] —Hospital discharge	20% (14/71)	14% (10/69)
Topol, et al.[12] —Hospital discharge	13% (13/98)	11% (11/99)

**Not randomized.*

more of those in the conservatively treated group needed urgent nonprotocol PTCA or CABG between the first and seventh day. Thus at the end of the hospitalization period, early PTCA had shown no particular benefit in terms of preestablished endpoints.

Additional important observations by the TAMI investigators concerned the prognosis of nonrandomized patients in whom lytic therapy failed to produce reperfusion. Finding and mechanically reperfusing this subgroup of approximately 20% of infarct patients given rtPA has been one of the important motivators of the strategy to perform very early angiography and angioplasty. In 95 such patients reported in the TAMI trial, PTCA failed in 15%, resulting in luminal opening but then early or delayed reclosure occurred in more than a third of these patients. Thus about half of the patients in this group had a closed artery at 1 week despite the procedure, and the group's early mortality (10.5%) was twice that of those in whom rtPA had proved beneficial. No group benefit in outcome LV function was observed.

Data available from TIMI II is quite limited and pertains only to 400 patients randomly assigned to PTCA immediately after rtPA infusion versus those undergoing PTCA 18 to 48 hours later. In the early intervention arm persistent total occlusions could be dilated by the protocol used but not for those in the 18- to 48-hour group. The preliminary findings in this comparison include far more frequent procedure-related complications when PTCA is done early, and the absence of a difference between the groups in outcome LV function.

Similarly, preliminary data from the European Cooperative Group included a higher complication rate and mortality for those in whom PTCA immediatley followed rtPA compared with those randomly assigned not to receive the mechanical intervention. Final LV function was actually better and mortality lower in the conservative treatment arm of this trial.

Synthesis of this increasing body of information leads to the conclusion that immediate angioplasty after lytic therapy (sequential treatment) cannot be recommended as a routine treatment strategy, despite what seemed to be the irrefutable logic behind the concept. In separate comparisons, delayed PTCA or a noninterventional approach after tissue plasminogen activator therapy has produced equivalent or preferred results. At this time no information is yet available from the large TIMI-II cohort randomized between delayed angioplasty and no angioplasty. The no-angioplasty group will, in fact, constitute the "adjunctive PTCA" group earlier identified, since these patients do in fact receive angiography and PTCA if signs or symptoms of recurrent ischemic events occur during hospital convalescence or on predischarge exercise testing. The final outcome of the TIMI-II trial should have a truly major impact on the clinical care of acute MI patients.

This synthesis, however, should be considered tentative since much of the supporting data have not been available for scrutiny (unpublished) and because the approach to patient selection in large trials has been randomly assigned treatment to (more or less) all patients. Over time one might hope that more specific patient stratification and possibly other combinations of drugs and mechanical interventions might allow for a more tailored approach than the current generalization that appears to dictate that if sequential PTCA is an all or none choice, one should presently not choose this intervention.

REFERENCES

1. Hartzler, G.O., Rutherford, B.D., McConahay, D.R., et al.: Percutaneous transluminal coronary angioplasty with and without thrombolytic therapy for treatment of acute myocardial infarction, Am. Heart. J. **106**:965-973, 1983.
2. Topol, E.J., Califf, R.M., Kereiakes, D.J., and George, B.S.: Thrombolysis and angioplasty in myocardial infarction (TAMI) trial, J. Am. Coll. Cardiol. **10**:65B-74B, 1987.
3. O'Neill, W.O., Timis, G.C., Bourdillon, P.D., et al.: A prospective randomized clinical trial of intracoronary streptokinase versus coronary angioplasty for acute myocardial infarction, N. Engl. J. Med. **314**:812-818, 1986.
4. Serruys, P.W., Arnold, A.E.R., Brower, R.W., DeBono, D.P., Bokslag, M., Lubsen, J., Reiber, J.H.C., Rutsch, W.R., Uebis, R., Vahanian, A., and Verstraete, M., for the European Co-operative Study Group for Recombinant Tissue Type Plasminogen Activator, Eur. Heart J. **8**:1172-1181, 1987.
5. Erbel, R., Pop, T., Henrichs, K.J., von Olshausen, K., Schuster, C.J., Rupprecht, H.J., Steuernagel, C., and Meyer, J.: Percutaneous transluminal coronary angioplasty after thrombolytic therapy: a prospective controlled randomized trial, J. Am. Coll. Cardiol. **8**:485-495, 1987.
6. Rothbaum, D.A., Linnemeier, T.J., Landin, R.J., Steinmetz, E.F., Hillis, J.S., et al.: Emergency percutaneous transluminary coronary angioplasty in acute myocardial infarction: a 3 year experience, J. Am. Coll. Cardiol. **10**:264-272, 1987.
7. Sheehan, F.H., Mathey, D.G., Schofer, J., Dodge, H.T., and Bolsen, E.L., Factors that determine recovery of the left ventricular function after thrombolysis in patients with acute myocardial infarction, Circulation **71**:1121-1128, 1985.
8. Schmidt, S.B., Varghese, P.J., Bloom, S., Yackee, J.M., and Ross, A.M.: The influence of residual coronary stenosis on size of infarction after reperfusion in a canine preparation, Circulation **73**:1354-1359, 1986.
9. Gruppo Italiano Per Lo Studio Della Streptochinasi Nell'Infarcto Miocardio (GISSI): Effectiveness of intravenous thrombolytic treatment in acute myocardial infarction, Lancet **1**:397-401, 1986.
10. Harrison, D.G., Ferguson, D.W., Collins, S.M., et al.: Rethrombosis after reperfusion with streptokinase: importance of geometry of residual lesions, Circulation **69**:991-999, 1984.
11. Uebis, R., Reynen, K., Dorr, R., Schmidt, W.G., Lambertz, H., Sigmund, M., von Essen, R., Meyer, J., and Effert, S.: Frequency of coronary reocclusion after successful intracoronary thrombolysis in acute myocardial infarction: comparison of immediate PTCA with subsequent medical treatment, J. Am. Coll. Cardiol. **9**:232A, 1987.
12. Topol, E.J., Califf, R.M., George, B.S., et al.: A randomized trial of immediate versus delayed elective angioplasty after intravenous tissue plasminogen activator in acute myocardial infarction, N. Engl. J. Med. **317**:581-588, 1987.

Chapter 32

Thrombolysis in Acute Myocardial Infarction in the Community Hospital

John H.K. Vogel, MD, FACC
Barry J. Coughlin, MD
Ramachandra K. Setty, MD, FACC
Rosa M. Avolio, RN
R. Bruce McFadden, MD, FACC

The major determinate of morbidity and mortality in coronary artery disease is the status of myocardial function[1]. Thus the thrust of our therapy has been directed toward maintenance of normal ventricular function and prevention of loss of heart muscle.[1] Although numerous interventions have been designed to alter the balance of oxygen demand and oxygen supply to favorably affect ventricular performance, nothing has surpassed the restoration of blood flow. In acute myocardial infarction, coronary thrombolysis occurs spontaneously in approximately 20% of patients[2,3] in the early hours after the event, and studies have shown that lytic agents may produce lysis in an additional 40 to 70% of patients. In 1976 Chazov and associates[4] reported successful thrombolysis and in 1978 Rentrop and associates[5] reported their encouraging experience with intracoronary streptokinase. The combination of thrombolytic therapy and spontaneous thrombolysis has achieved an early reperfusion rate of 70 to 90%.[6] However, it is clear that "time means muscle" and strategies that have evolved relate to reducing the time from acute occlusion to thrombolysis. If thrombolysis occurs within 30 minutes of the acute event, there is a high salvage rate of cardiac muscle; if it occurs within 90 minutes of the event, substantial benefits have been demonstrated, but after 3 hours the advantage diminishes.[7-9]

In 1981 and 1983 Schroder and associates[10,11] reported on the use of early, short-time intravenous streptokinase for thrombolysis in acute myocardial infarction. It was their thesis that if the majority of people with acute myocardial infarction were to benefit by thrombolysis it would have to be by the early, short-term, high-dose intravenous route. They reported patency of the infarct-related artery in more than 80% of their patients and emphasized the importance of an early peaking of the creatine kinase (CK)-MB fraction as an indicator of early reperfusion. In veiw of the promising nature of their results, in 1981 we initiated an intravenous streptokinase protocol in Goleta Valley Community Hospital, and Marion Hospital in Santa Maria, Calif. and Lompoc Hospital in Lompoc, Calif. Our experience now extends beyond 6 years' time (Fig. 32-1).

INDICATIONS FOR THROMBOLYSIS

All patients with acute myocardial infarction are candidates for intravenous thrombolytic therapy *if* seen less than 4 hours after the onset of the episode (perhaps longer than 4 hours if severe, continuing pain and ischemia is evident), generally but not necessarily under the age of 75, and with no known potential bleeding problems. We have administered intravenous streptokinase in patients over 75 years, since it is evident that some people above this age are physiologically younger. If the patient is going immedi-

A. Tissue Plasminogen Activator

1. Admit to critical care unit
2. Start two I.V. lines one with #18 gauge catheter with a stopcock to draw blood.
3. PT, PTT, Platelet Count, Chem Panel, CBC, Fibrinogen, Cardiac Enzymes-draw from stopcock
4. Pre-medicate:
   -Nifedipine 10 mg SL now and q 4 hrs SL
   -Heparin 5000 units IVP
   -Procainamide 500 mg po q 4 hrs
5. Check patient for venous or arterial puncture sites. All puncture sites should have pressure dressings.
6. Begin TPA
   A. 10 mg TPA IVP
   B. Follow with 1 mg/kg (less 10 mg IVP dose) To infuse over 60 min. Maximum dose 90 mg First hour.
   C. Then begin TPA infusion 0.5 mg/kg To infuse over three hours.
   D. Maximum dose 150 mg - total TPA
7. After first hour of TPA begin infusion of 500 D5W with 10,000 unit Heparin at 1000u/hr. (50 u/hr. via IMED)
8. EKG before infusion of TPA and 1 hr. after infusion or PRN if sudden change in pain
9. Foley PRN
10. Chest X-Ray
11. CPK and CPK-MB q 2 hrs × 24 hrs. To start from initiation of TPA infusion
12. NTG 1/150 gr SL PRN - chest pain
13. VS q 15 min until infusion completed
14. Avoid venous punctures and arterial punctures; no IM injections
15. For PVC's; Lidocaine 50-100 mg bolus, then Lidocaine infusion at 2-4 mg/min
16. NTG 50 mg/250 D5W titrate to relieve severe chest pain unless hypotensive

Fig. 32-1. A, Protocol for intravenous TPA therapy for acute myocardial infarction.

ately to the catheterization laboratory thrombolytic therapy may be withheld, but this is not recommended. We have utilized intravenous thrombolysis for preinfarction angina, coronary artery thrombosis during cardiac catheterization and in patients with occlusion during angioplasty.

Potential bleeding problems that would serve as a contraindication include active internal bleeding, recent surgery or major trauma, active ulcer disease, recent puncture of noncompressible vessels, severe uncontrolled systemic hypertension, known bleeding diathesis, history of recent cerebrovascular accident (2 months), and recent intracranial surgery or known tumor. In our institutions if cardiopulmonary resuscitation has been of short duration with no obvious trauma, it is not considered a contraindication.

B. Systemic Streptokinase (SK) Therapy for the Acute MI

1. Admit patient to Critical Care Unit - HANDLE GENTLY
2. Start two IV lines - one with #18 gauge cath, one having a 3-way stopcock placed at hub (#18 g on left arm if possible).
3. Obtain these as soon as possible (preferably from the stopcock of the #18 g IV line): PTT, CBC, PT, Cardiac Enzymes, Chem Panel, Platelet Count, Renal Panel, Fibrinogen.
4. Pre-medicate: Nifedipine 10 mg SL now and q 4 hrs SL. Methylpredniolone 250 mg IV; Procainamide 500 mg PO and q 4 hrs, Heparin 5000 units IV (baseline clotting studies should be drawn first).
5. NTG 1/150 gr SL prn chest pain.
6. Check patient for venous or arterial puncture sites. All puncture sites should have pressure dressings applied to them.
7. Begin infusion via #18 g IV line; SK 1.5 million units in 50-100 cc Normal Saline to infuse over 30 minutes via IMED pump. Follow this infusion with 500 cc D5W with 10,000 unit Heparin at 1000u/hr (50cc per hour via IMED).
8. EKG before infusion of SK begun; then 1 hr after infusion, or PRW if sudden change in same.
9. Chest X-Ray.
10. Foley Catheter PRW; HANDLE GENTLY
11. PTT q 2 hrs to start 2 hrs after completion of SK infusion (attempt to draw these, and any other lab work, from stopcock of IV) Call results to MD each time.
12. CPK and CPK-MB q 2 hrs × 24 hrs, to start from completion of SK infusion.
13. Monitor patient's VS and quality of Hemostasis and document q 15″ until SK infusion completed or longer if clinically indicated.
14. Avoid venipunctures and arterial punctures before start of SK and at least 24 hrs after completion of infusion.
    NO IM INJECTIONS.
15. For PVC's; Lidocaine 50-100 mg bolus, then Lidocaine infusion at 2-4 mg/min prn for frequent PVC's.
16. NTG 50 mg in 250 cc D5W titrate to relieve severe chest pain unless hypotensive.
17. 2D Echocardiogram whenever feasible. (Not to interfere with infusion of SK.)

Fig. 32-1, cont'd. B, Protocol for intravenous streptokinase therapy for acute myocardial infarction.

PROCEDURE

Upon entering the emergency room the patient is seen immediately by the physician and if the electrocardiogram indicates the presence of an acute myocardial infarction, the question is asked if the patient is a candidate for thrombolytic therapy. If, based on the preceding indications the answer is yes, intravenous streptokinase or tissue plasminogen activator (TPA) is started. If the catheterization laboratory is immediately available, with the potential for surgical backup, we (Goleta Valley Community Hospital) may consider the possibility of immediate study with percutaneous transluminal coronary angioplasty (PTCA) and/or intracoronary thrombolytic therapy in the patient with a major myocardial infarction and/or shock. Catheterization should be performed by a *very* experienced angiographer, expert in entering and caring for arteries. When the patient is seen in the hospital without a laboratory (Marion Hospital, Lompoc Hospital), thrombolytic therapy is initiated immediately and transport considered if there is evidence of early arterial opening or the patient remains unstable. If the patient is in stable condition, we prefer to wait 24 to 48 hours before study or transport. This has been the protocol followed in our institutions over the past 6 years. In Fig. 32-1 is shown the specific protocol. Streptokinase is given over a 30-minute period utilizing 1.5 million units. As noted, 5000 units of heparin is given intravenously at the beginning and a drip started at a rate of 1000 units/hour after streptokinase is administered. Steroids are utilized, and depending on the clinical situation intravenous nitroglycerin, calcium, and beta blockers may be utilized. There is evidence to suggest that the use of calcium-channel blockers and perhaps beta blockers widen the window of opportunity to preserve muscle with early reopening.[12] Initially we establish two intravenous (IV) lines. Most important is to be *extremely gentle with the patient,* both in moving the patient and with any subsequent interventions. *Intramuscular route medicines are contraindicated* and if IV punctures are performed, pressure bandages should be applied. Arterial sticks are to be avoided. Carelessness in this regard leads to the highest number of complications with thrombolytic therapy. Thus the nurse assumes an extremely important role in this aspect of management of the patient. We do not delay therapy to obtain an echocardiogram. The CK-MB fractions are run at 2-hour intervals for 24 hours. Partial thromboplastin time (PTT) is followed after 4 or 5 hours. We attempt to maintain PTT at 80 seconds. Time is of the essence and *none of the tests should delay the immediate commencement of thrombolytic therapy.* The TPA protocol, utilized in some of our patients since November 1987, is similar to that used for streptokinase and is outlined in Figure 32-1.

RESULTS

From November 1981 to November 1987, 121 patients were treated including 94 men with an average age of 56 (range 35 to 79 years) and 27 women with an average age of 63 (range 43 to 77 years). There were 62 inferior wall myocardial infarctions and 59 anterior wall myocardial infarctions. The regional distribution of patients is seen in Fig. 32-2.

The clinical criteria for luminal opening included an early peaking of the CK-MB fraction within 12 hours; sudden relief of pain in the early minutes (on the average 30 to 60 minutes after starting thrombolytic therapy); sudden emergence of arrhythmias or change in arrhythmia background, accompanied by resolution of ST segment changes; advanced atrioventricular (AV) block; or cardiogenic shock. Serial echocardiograms are useful, but since these changes occur over several days they are of little help early on in indicating early reperfusion. A most useful sign of early reperfusion is *sudden* relief of pain followed by ventricular arrhythmias. This is not an un-

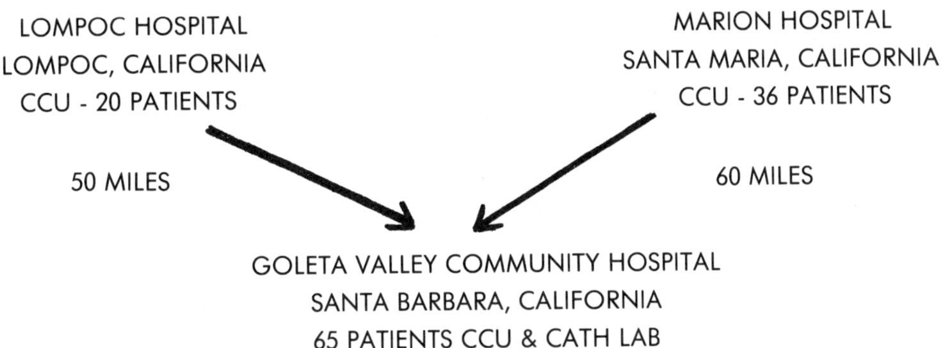

Fig. 32-2. Regional distribution of patients referred to Goleta Valley Community Hospital, including the hospitals involved, the number of patients referred, and distance.

common event. Representative CK-MB curves are shown in Fig. 32-3. The flat curve has been seen in approximately 3% of patients and is associated with early reperfusion and a small or no infarction. The delayed peaking at approximately 20 hours is associated with a failure to reperfuse. Two types of early peaking curves are shown, one with a fairly rapid washout indicating excellent blood flow and early reperfusion, and a somewhat flat curve generally associated with a very tight residual lesion and slow blood flow. In the protocol 107 patients demonstrated clinical signs of early reperfusion. The average time from initiation of streptokinase therapy to their peak CK-MB curve was 7¾ ± 3¾ hours, with a range of 3 to 15 hours. Fourteen patients did not have luminal opening and their average streptokinase to peak CK-MB time was 20 ± 2 hours with a range of 12 to 24 hours. This correlated nicely with the report of Schroder and associates[11] wherein the time to peak CK-MB levels after the start of streptokinase infusion was less than 14 hours in all cases with early reperfusion and more than 16 hours in those patients who remained occluded.

The average time from onset of pain to arriving in the emergency room in our experience was 85 minutes and the time from arrival in the emergency room to beginning of streptokinase therapy averaged 70 minutes. Thirty-five percent of the patients were treated within 30 minutes or less after arrival in the emergency room. The average time from onset of pain to receiving streptokinase in those patients who had early reperfusion averaged 117 ± 90 minutes with a range of 15 to 300 minutes, whereas in those patients who remained occluded the average time to treatment was 228 ± 47 minutes with a range of 75 to 420 minutes. All patients treated within 60 minutes of the onset of their pain were open clinically. The dosage of streptokinase was increased from 250,000 units in one patient to 1.5 million units in the last 109 patients.

Documented arrhythmias of ventricular origin were common after streptokinase therapy, with a similar number of patients experiencing ventricular fibrillation before and after its use (Table 32-1). Complete heart block resolved in six patients after streptokinase therapy. The occurrence of ventricular fibrillation

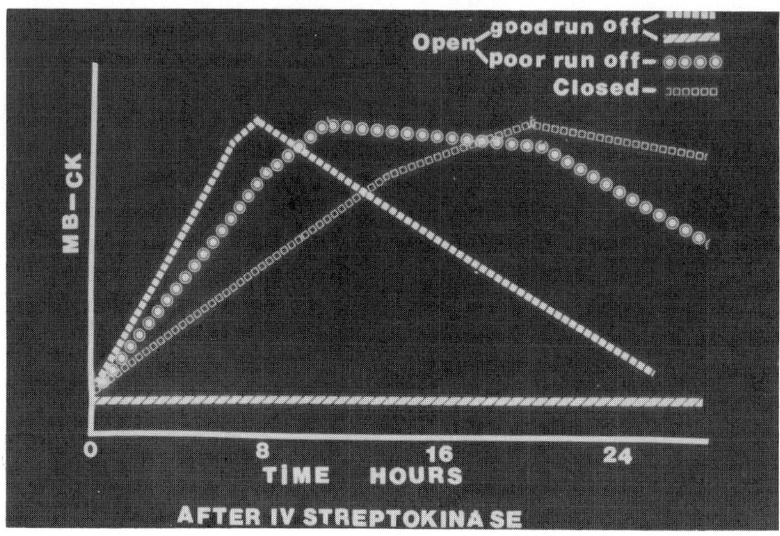

Fig. 32-3. A family of curves are shown, illustrating typical disease courses. The flat curve represents a typical curve for those patients undergoing early reperfusion with no significant infarction. The late peaking curve is typical of those patients who did not have early reperfusion. Two curves are shown with early peaking, one showing a rapid runoff that is typical for those patients who have early luminal opening and good runoff, and a slow curve typical of those who have luminal opening but poor runoff.

after streptokinase use was an excellent indicator of early reperfusion, since all those patients had luminal opening at catheterization. It is our thought that ventricular tachycardia and ventricular fibrillation, occurring before treatment, represent intermittent reperfusion. Spontaneous reperfusion may account for late-onset ventricular fibrillation, since it has been shown that there is continued spontaneous luminal opening several hours after the acute event.[2] If one remains at the patient's bedside during thrombolytic therapy, the changes in pain, arrhythmias, and hemodynamic status are generally obvious with reperfusion.

As shown in Fig. 32-4, of the 107 patients open clinically, 97 underwent cardiac catheterization. The relationship of time from treatment with streptokinase to study and percent studied is shown in Table 32-2. During the first 2 years of our experience not all patients underwent catheterization. If they were stable following early reperfusion, they were treated conservatively. However, it became apparent that it was not clear what the potential dangers were after early reperfusion. Thus in order to effectively treat the patient we thought it was important to assess the coronary anatomy. Since 1983 virtually all patients with evidence of early reperfusion have undergone catheterization prior to discharge. As noted, 89 of the 97 patients (92%) studied had luminal opening. Subsequently 26 of these patients underwent coronary artery bypass surgery and 22 patients were treated by percutaneous transluminal coronary artery angioplasty. The remainder of the patients have been treated medically. Of note is that 11

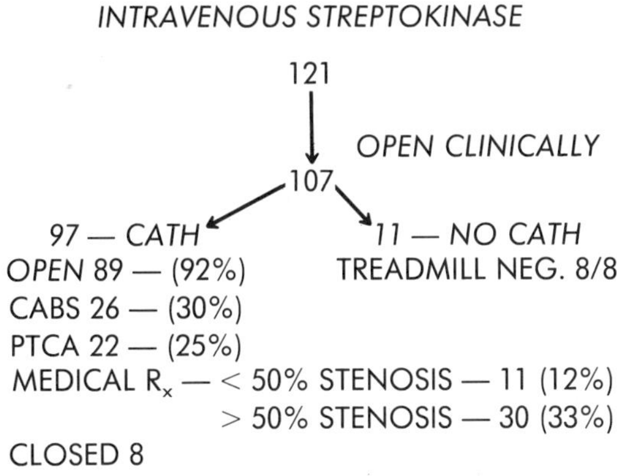

INTRAVENOUS STREPTOKINASE

121

↓ OPEN CLINICALLY

107

97 — CATH | 11 — NO CATH

OPEN 89 — (92%) | TREADMILL NEG. 8/8

CABS 26 — (30%)

PTCA 22 — (25%)

MEDICAL R_x — < 50% STENOSIS — 11 (12%)

> 50% STENOSIS — 30 (33%)

CLOSED 8

Fig. 32-4. Illustration of the number of patients who had luminal opening and underwent catheterization and the subsequent results. (CABS, coronary artery bypass surgery; PTCA, percutaneous transluminal coronary angioplasty.)

Table 32-1. Ventricular Arrhythmias Common After Streptokinase Therapy

	Pre-SK	*Post-SK*
Premature ventricular contraction	21*	36
Ventricular fibrillation	12	10
Congestive heart block	7	3
Sinus bradycardia	6	4
Junctional rhythm	0	2
Wenckebach phenomenon	0	3
Ventricular tachycardia	1	3

**No. of patients.*

(12%) of patients had less than 50% stenosis. These patients have remained stable. Of the 11 patients who did not undergo catheterization, the majority had negative treadmill stress tests and this is one reason they did not undergo further study. In those that were open clinically, but closed at catheterization (9 patients), heparin had not been given in three patients and was inadequate or discontinued early in the remainder. Late reclosure was generally evident clinically. The early reclosing rate in our experience was approximately 8%.

Table 32-2. IV Streptokinase Therapy in 120 Patients (Goleta Valley Community Hospital)

No. of Patients	*% Studied*	*% 1–48 hr*
0–40	55	50
41–80	90	47
81–120	100	58

Of the 14 patients who were closed clinically, 11 underwent catheterization. All were closed. One patient had luminal opening with intracoronary streptokinase and another patient had luminal opening using PTCA.

CASE EXAMPLES

In Fig. 32-5 is shown the electrocardiogram from our first patient, a 65-year-old man, receiving intravenous streptokinase 500,000 units at 2 hours. The control tracing shows acute anterior wall myocardial infarction. When luminal opening had not occurred within 20 minutes, he was taken to the catheterization laboratory where the right anterior oblique (RAO) angiogram showed an occluded left anterior descending (LAD) coronary artery (Fig. 32-6), which spontaneously opened within minutes with no further therapy. This was associated with spontaneous ventricular fibrillation, readily converted with shock treatment. The vessel then reoccluded and intracoronary streptokinase was given with subsequent luminal reopening in 15 minutes. In Fig. 32-7 is shown the cineangiogram

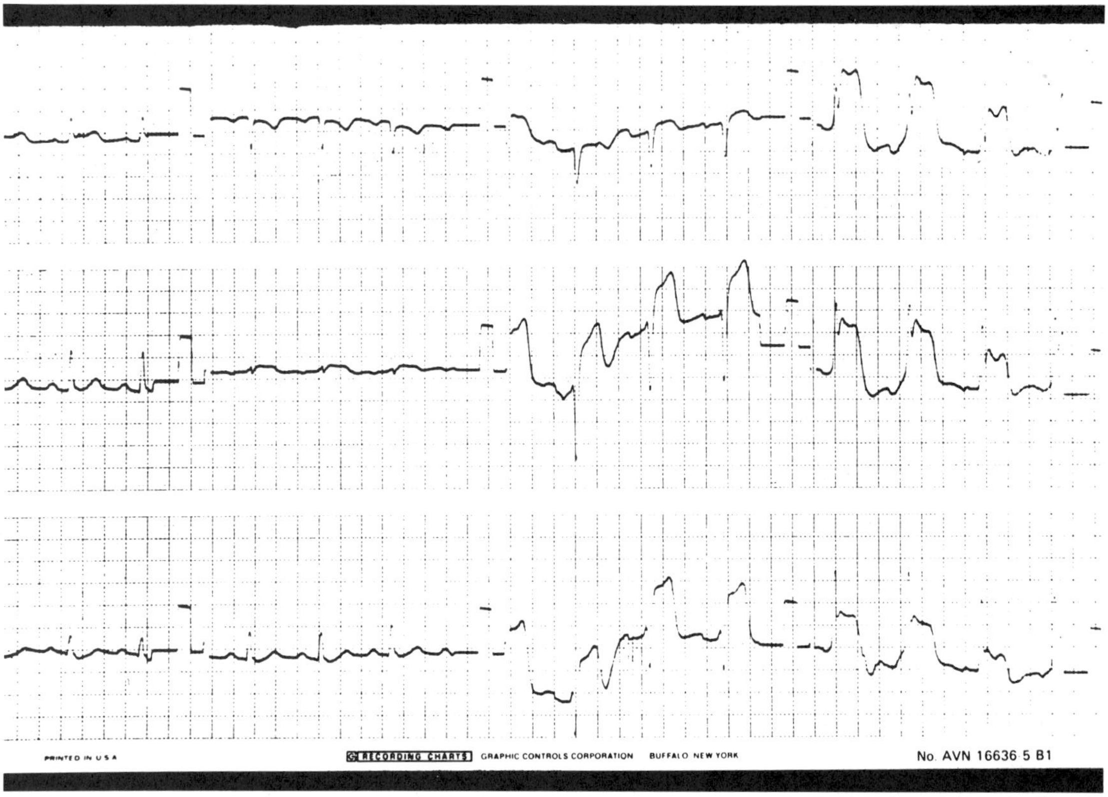

Fig. 32-5. Control electrocardiogram immediately preceding intravenous streptokinase administration, showing acute anterior wall myocardial infarction.

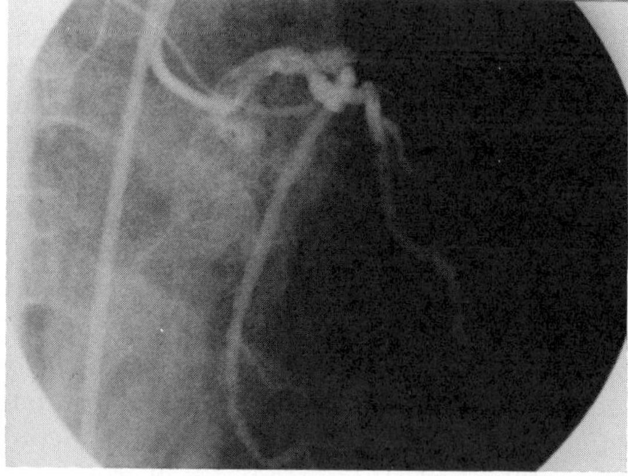

Fig. 32-6. Selective RAO coronary artery cineangiogram showing occlusion of LAD coronary artery.

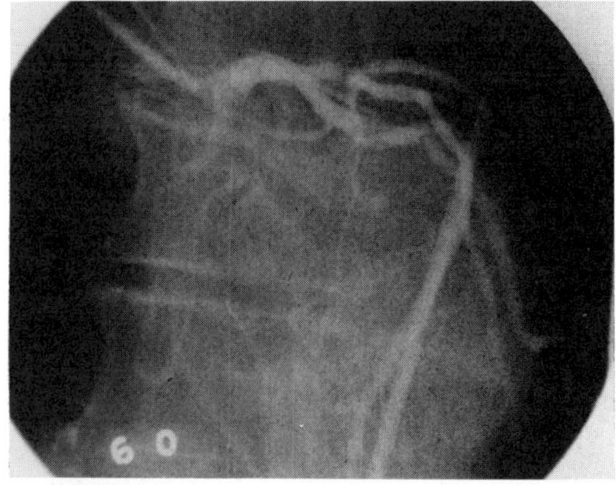

Fig. 32-7. RAO cineangiogram showing perfusion of LAD coronary artery with residual proximal obstruction, at 60 minutes after intracoronary streptokinase infusion.

at 60 minutes, demonstrating the open LAD coronary artery. An 80% diameter stenosis appears to be present. No collaterals were present. No further intervention was performed and this patient remains asymptomatic with a negative, maximal treadmill stress test 6 years later.

In Fig. 32-8 is shown the electrocardiogram from a 59-year-old man with an acute inferior wall myocardial infarction, complicated by hypotension and advanced AV block. One hour after the onset of pain he received 1.5 million units of intravenous streptokinase. Thirty minutes later there was spontaneous relief of pain, resolution of the AV block, and normalization of the blood pressure. The CK-MB fraction peaked at 8 hours. The electrocardiogram showed considerable resolution (Fig. 32-9). Because of the patient's instability before early reperfusion, it was deemed reasonable to study him and he was transferred from Lompoc Hospital to Goleta Valley Community Hospital for study the following morning. In Fig. 32-10 can be seen a significant lesion in a large circumflex artery with crater and clot, disease in the main left coronary artery, and involvement of the LAD coronary artery system. He subsequently underwent internal mammary artery bypass into the LAD coronary artery and saphenous vein

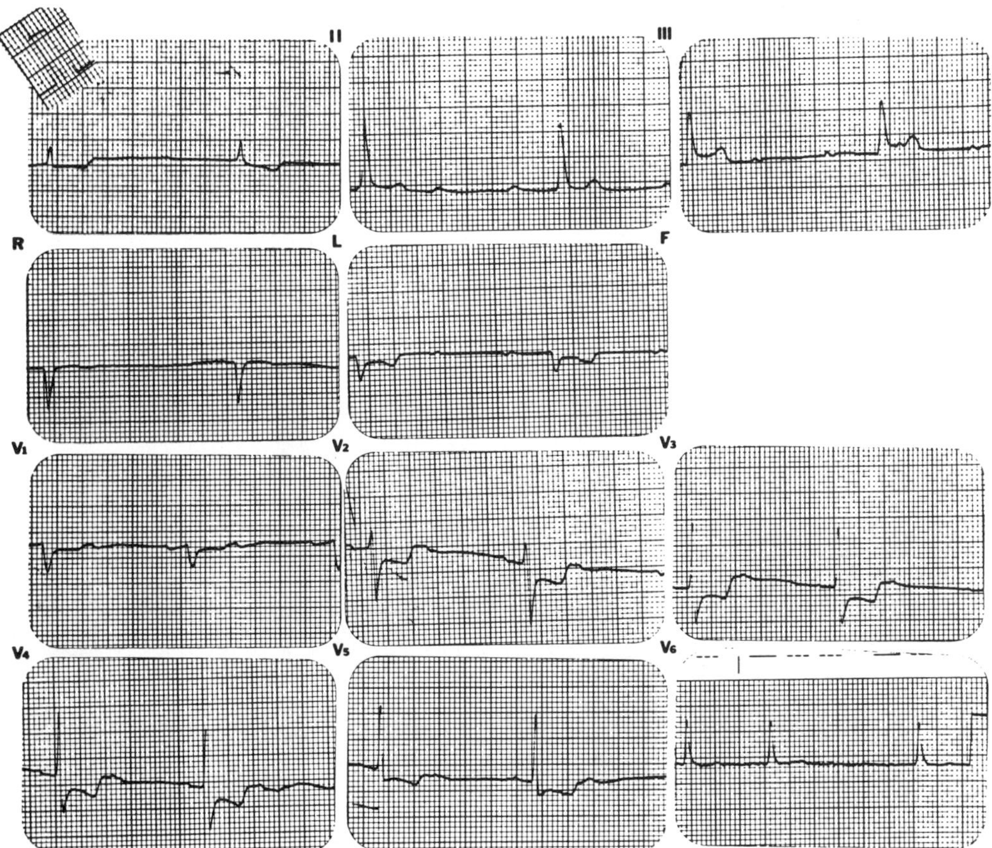

Fig. 32-8. Control electrocardiogram obtained immediately before streptokinase therapy showing acute inferior wall myocardial infarction and complete heart block.

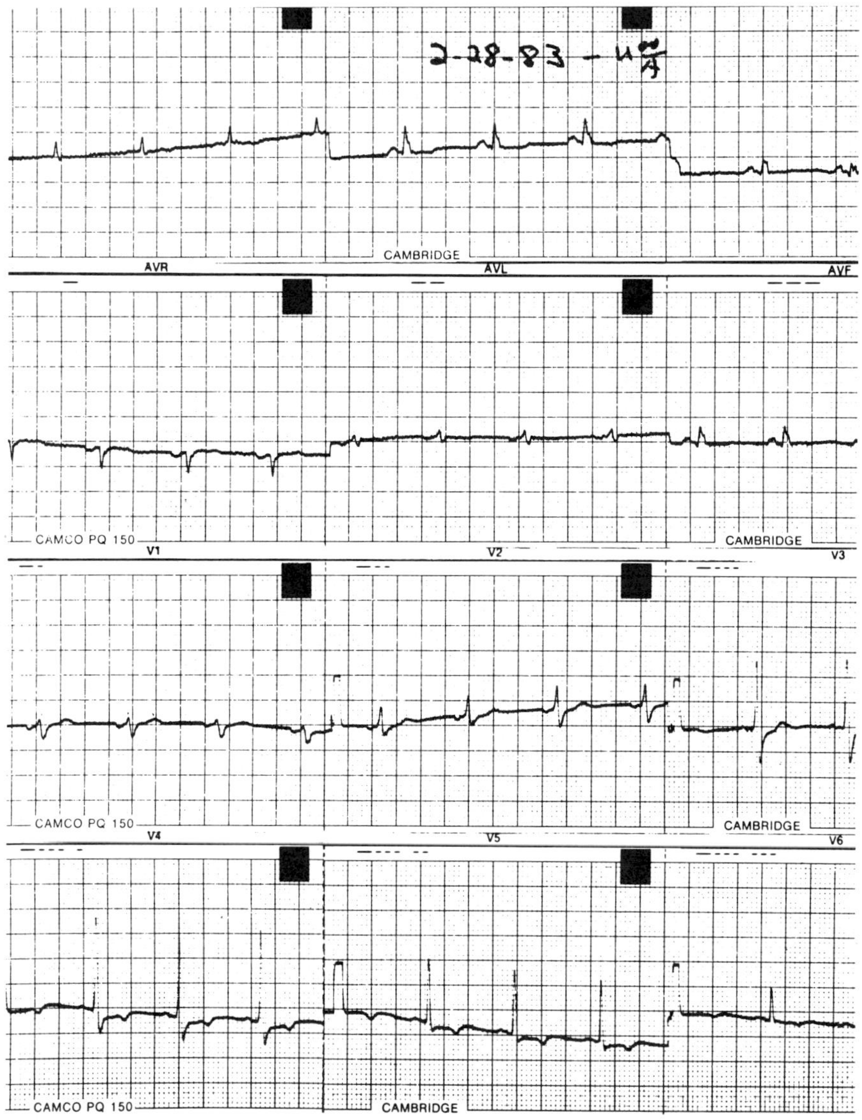

Fig. 32-9. Electrocardiogram obtained immediately following intravenous streptokinase administration showing significant normalization and return of sinus rhythm.

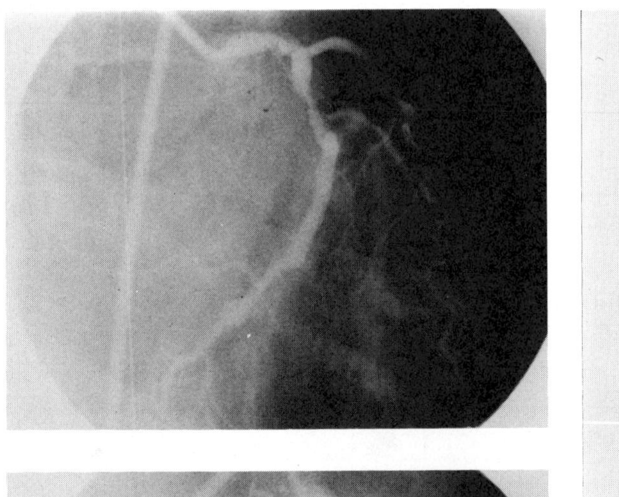

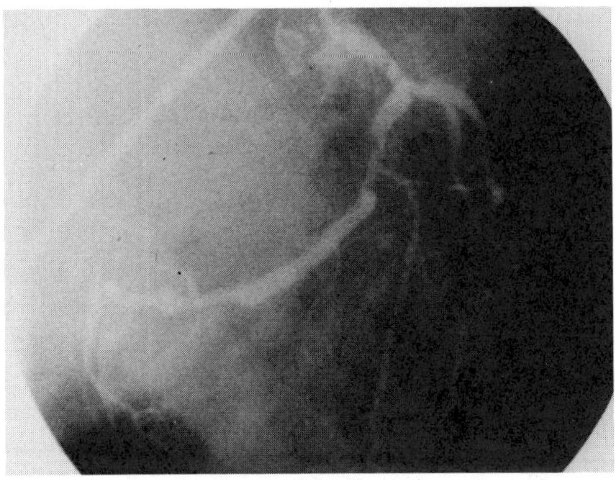

Fig. 32-10. Selective coronary cineangiograms show significant lesion in circumflex artery with involvement of the main left and LAD coronary arteries.

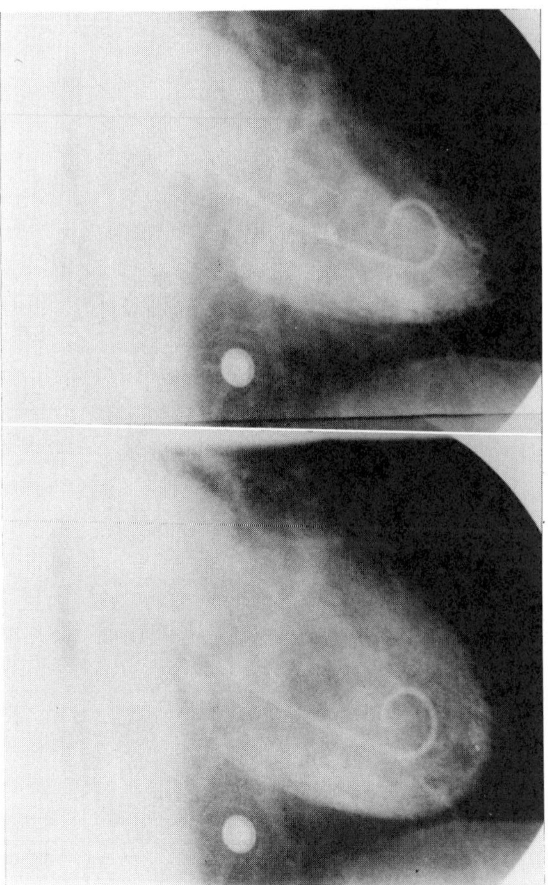

Fig. 32-11. Systolic and diastolic views of the left ventricular cineangiogram revealing inferior wall akinesis.

bypass into the circumflex artery. Fig. 32-11 shows the inferior wall akinesis. Electrocardiogram on discharge showed minor residual ST–T wave changes in the inferior and lateral leads (Fig. 32-12). He remains asymptomatic with a normal treadmill 4 years later.

In Fig. 32-13 is shown the electrocardiogram from a 50-year-old man with acute anterior wall myocardial infarction. He received 1.5 million units of intravenous streptokinase within 30 minutes of the onset of pain with relief of pain within 30 minutes. His subsequent electrocardiogram showed normalization (Fig. 32-14). Because he had normalization, having had an acute anterior wall myocardial infarction in progress, and no enzyme rise, it was deemed reasonable to study him. The study done the following morning revealed 80% diameter stenosis of the LAD coronary artery (Fig. 32-15). Figure 32-16 represents diastolic and systolic frames from the left ventricle cineangiogram showing normal function. Because of continued rest angina and ventricular arrhythmias, revascularization was performed (IMA to LAD). The treadmill remains negative after 3 years.

Another 46-year-old man with acute infe-

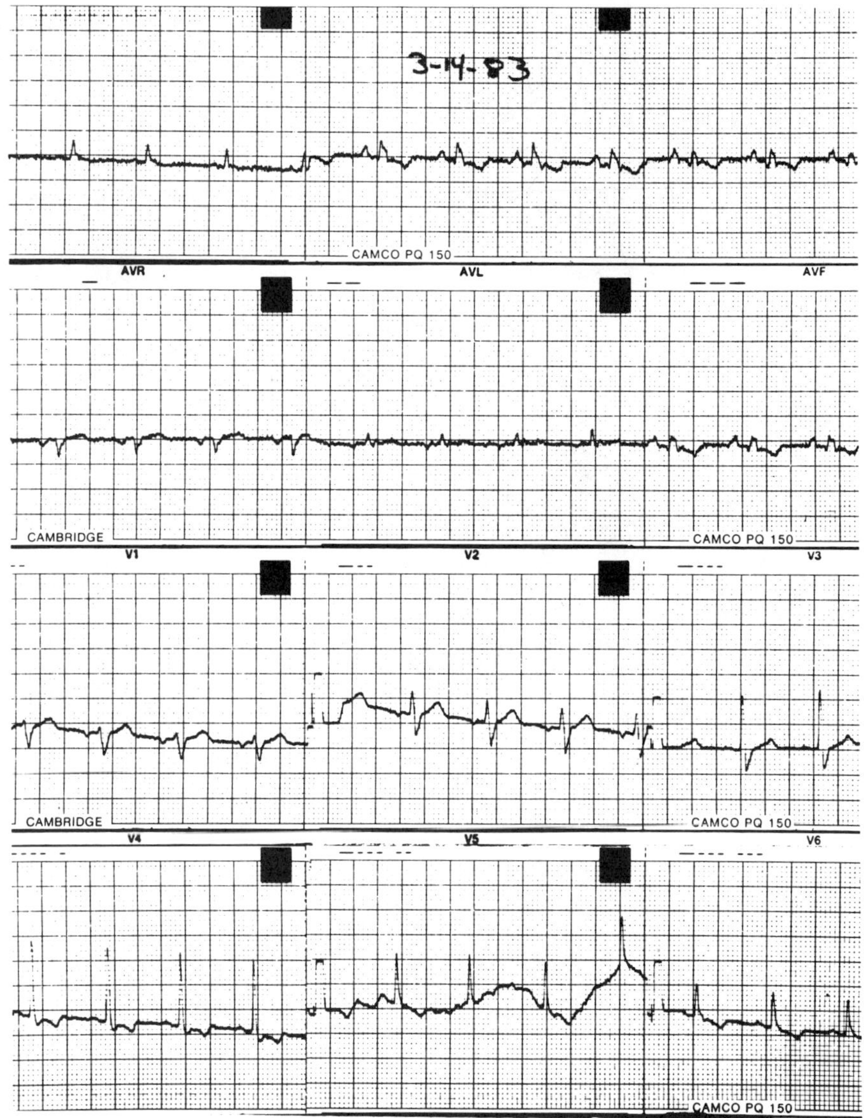

Fig. 32-12. Electrocardiogram at discharge shows nonspecific residual ST–T wave changes, and sinus rhythm.

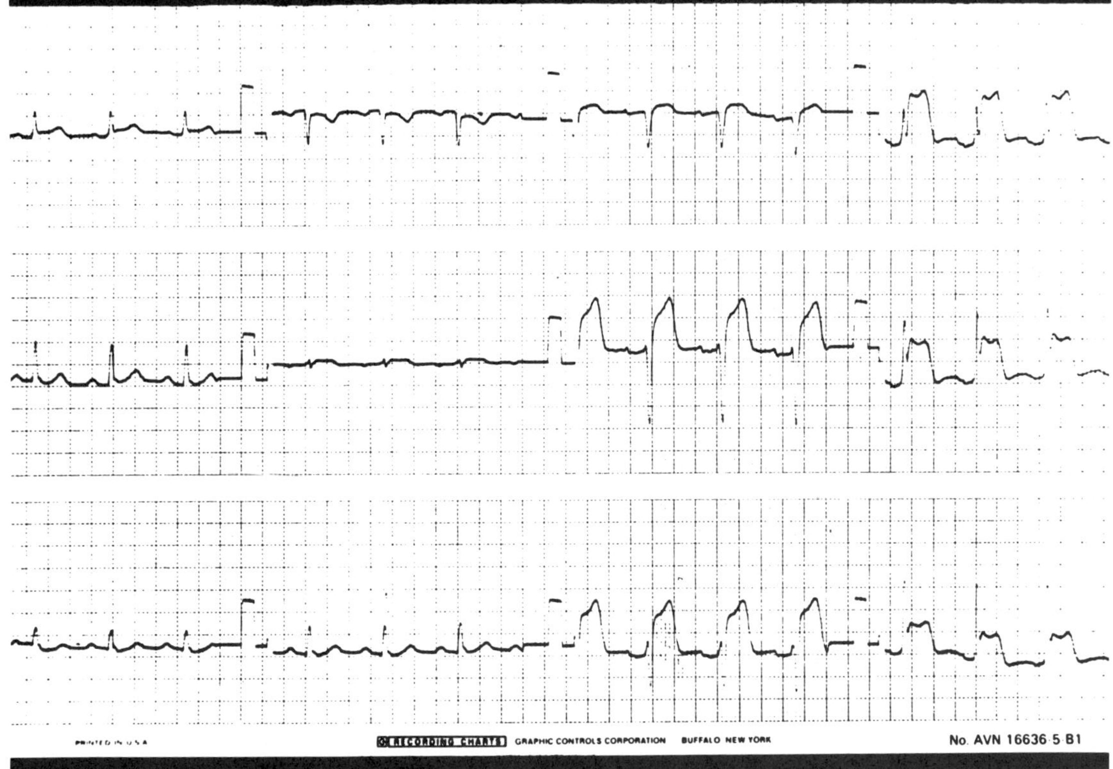

Fig. 32-13. Control electrocardiogram immediately before intravenous streptokinase infusion showing extensive anterior wall myocardial infarction.

rior wall myocardial infarction received 1.5 million units of intravenous streptokinase within 90 minutes of onset of pain. Resolution of chest pain and ventricular arrhythmias occurred at 30 minutes. A subsequent electrocardiogram showed near normalization of the electrocardiogram. Sixty-eight hours later he underwent study and in Fig. 32-17 biplane views show a 45% diameter stenosis of the right coronary artery. No collaterals were seen. The ventriculogram (Fig. 32-18) shows slight akinesis of the inferior wall. Thus the patient was treated medically and recently had a negative maximal exercise treadmill stress test. This case serves to emphasize how a vessel may develop non-critical stenosis over a short period of time. Indeed in the TAMI trial[13] those patients directed to the elective "late" PTCA group had a 14% incidence of less than 50% stenosis on follow-up.

In Fig. 32-19A and B are shown serial strips from a 79-year-old man with marked ischemic lability. Because the patient was alternating between ST segment depression and elevation, as shown in the top two strips, he was given intravenous streptokinase. Approximately 15 minutes into the infusion, his pain intensified with recurrent ST segment elevation as shown in the fourth strip. The remainder of the streptokinase was infused within a few minutes. As the ST segments rose, blood pressure became unobtainable and the patient was unresponsive. At this point, intravenous nitroglycerin was given and the patient received 1 mg of nifedipine (Procardia) sublingually. Atropine was given intravenously.

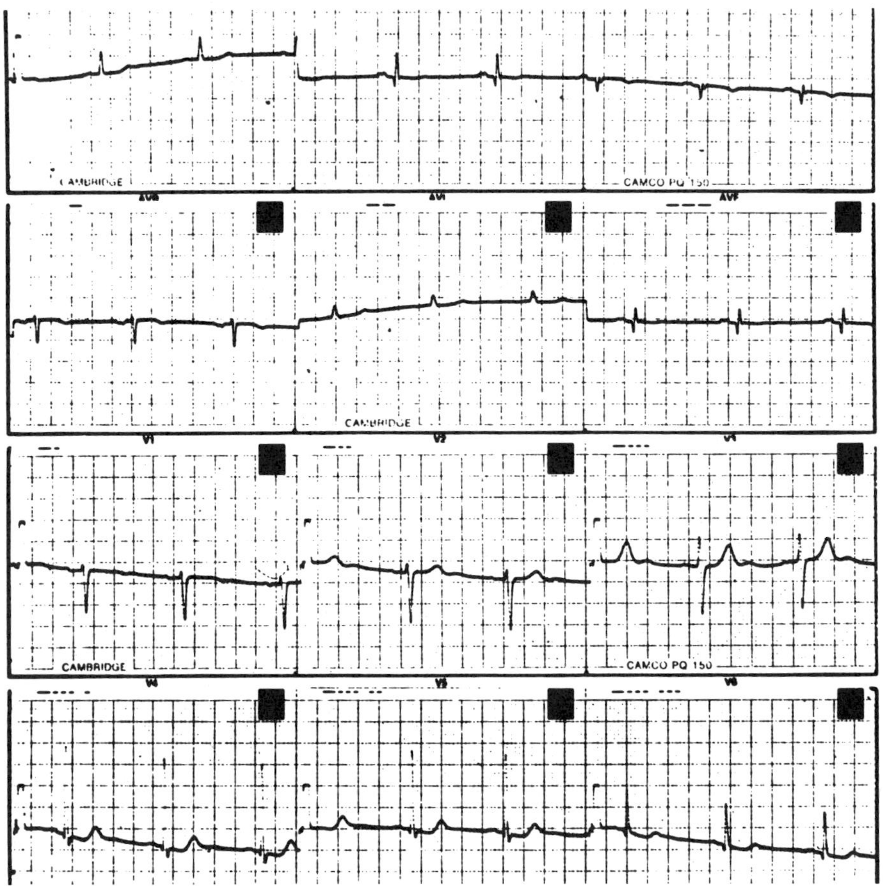

Fig. 32-14. Electrocardiogram obtained immediately after the infusion of intravenous streptokinase showing normalization of the electrocardiogram.

Within 2 minutes the ST segments began to come down, oscillating slightly as shown in the second and third panels, and then tending to become negative at 5 minutes. At this point, blood pressure returned to normal, the patient became alert, and his pain resolved. Fig. 32-20 shows the electrocardiogram associated with severe pain and loss of blood pressure, and Fig. 32-21 shows the subsequent tracing after the pain had resolved. This sequence suggests vasospasm plus clot as recently reported by Hackett and associates.[14] It was apparent that when occluded the patient could not survive, and that a very severe underlying lesion was present. The CK-MB fraction peaked at 6 hours. Therefore the following morning he underwent study. As shown in Fig. 32-22, there was near-total occlusion of a giant right coronary artery and 90% narrowing of the LAD coronary artery. Thus he underwent internal mammary artery to LAD coronary artery bypass, and saphenous vein to right coronary artery bypass without complication. He was discharged 6 days later from the hospital. A treadmill stress test was negative 3 months postoperatively.

In Fig. 32-23 is shown the electrocardiogram of a 66-year-old man with an acute ante-

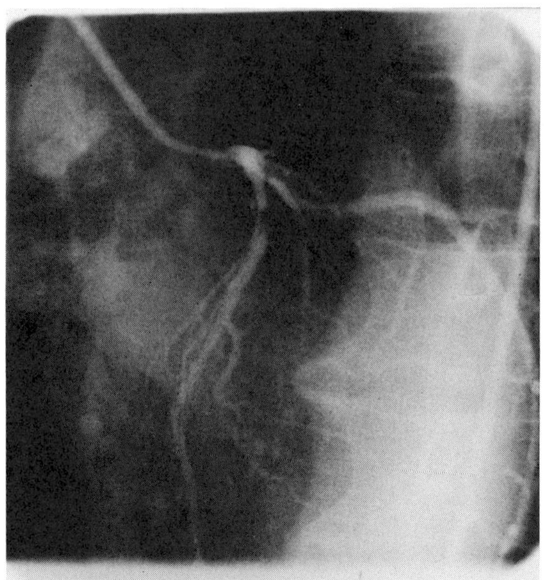

Fig. 32-15. Selective left anterior oblique (LAO) cineangiogram revealing 80% diameter stenosis of the proximal LAD coronary artery.

rior wall myocardial infarction. He received intravenous streptokinase within 60 minutes of onset of acute chest pain. Within 30 minutes of beginning the infusion there was resolution of pain and a burst of ventricular tachycardia. The subsequent electrocardiogram 1 hour after showed considerable normalization (Fig. 32-24). The patient continued to have recurrent rest pain and ventricular arrhythmias and thus underwent study the following day, having been transported to Goleta Valley Community Hospital. The CK-MB fraction peaked at 8 hours. In Fig. 32-25 is shown a high-grade lesion in the proximal LAD coronary artery. The gradient was 60 mm Hg. In Fig. 32-26 is shown the vessel after PTCA, being widely patent with no gradient. This patient remained asymptomatic for one year; then developed pre-infarction syndrome. Studies showed a 90% stenosis of the circumflex and old anterior wall infarction. Percutaneous-supported angioplasty was performed with an excellent result.

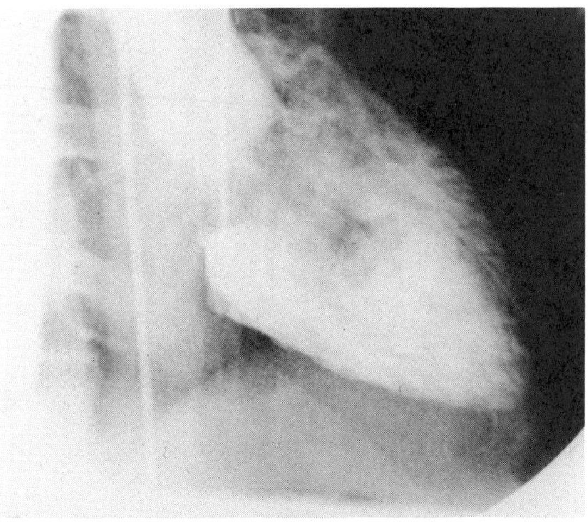

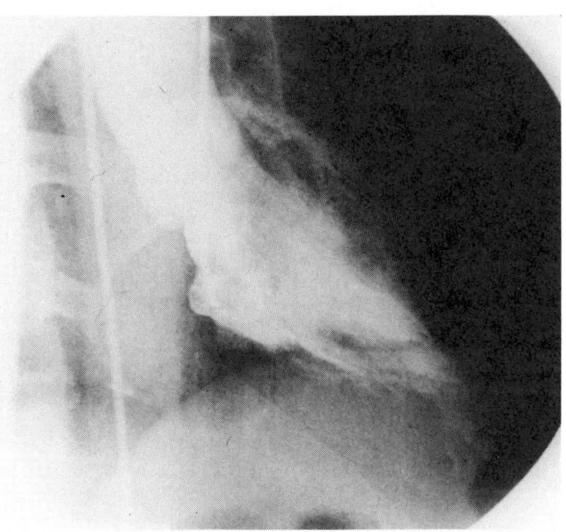

Fig. 32-16. Systolic and diastolic frames from the left ventricular cineangiogram show normal function.

Our overall results are summarized in Table 32-3. All patients have been followed up at least 1 month and up to 6 years. At the time of last follow-up, 118 of the 121 patients were known to be living, with a range of 1 month to 72 months. There was one early hospital death, caused by a cerebrovascular accident 2 days after catheterization (thrombosis), one late death caused by carcinoma of the lung, and one late death resulting from myocardial infarction. Three major morbidity problems

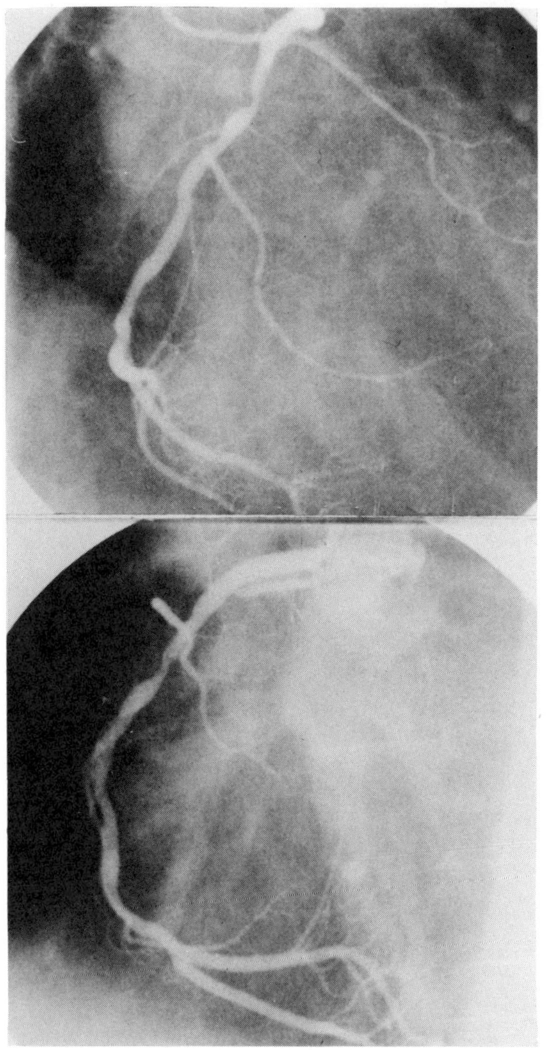

Fig. 32-17. Selective biplane coronary artery cineangiograms showing 45% diameter stenosis of the proximal right coronary artery.

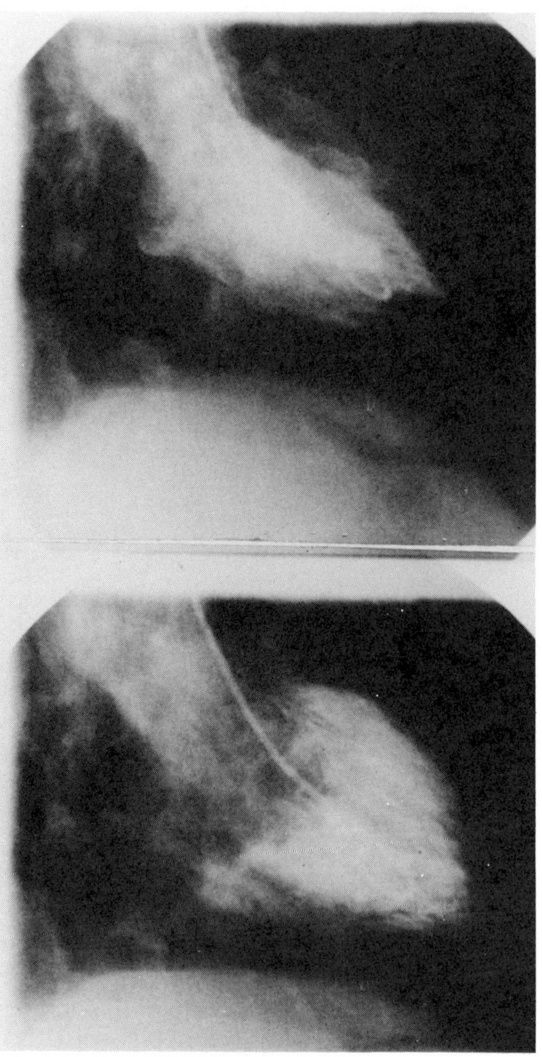

Fig. 32-18. Systolic and diastolic views of the left ventricular cineangiogram reveal minor akinesis of the inferior wall.

have resulted from arterial and venous IV lines. Nausea has been a common complaint, occurring in 50% of patients and transient hypotension is not uncommon. Clinically, 107 out of 121 patients (88%) have had luminal opening, and at catheterization 89 of 97 patients (92%) have had luminal opening.

MANAGEMENT AFTER THROMBOLYTIC THERAPY

Who should be catheterized after thrombolytic therapy? In our institutions all patients receiving streptokinase who have luminal opening clinically undergo study before dis-

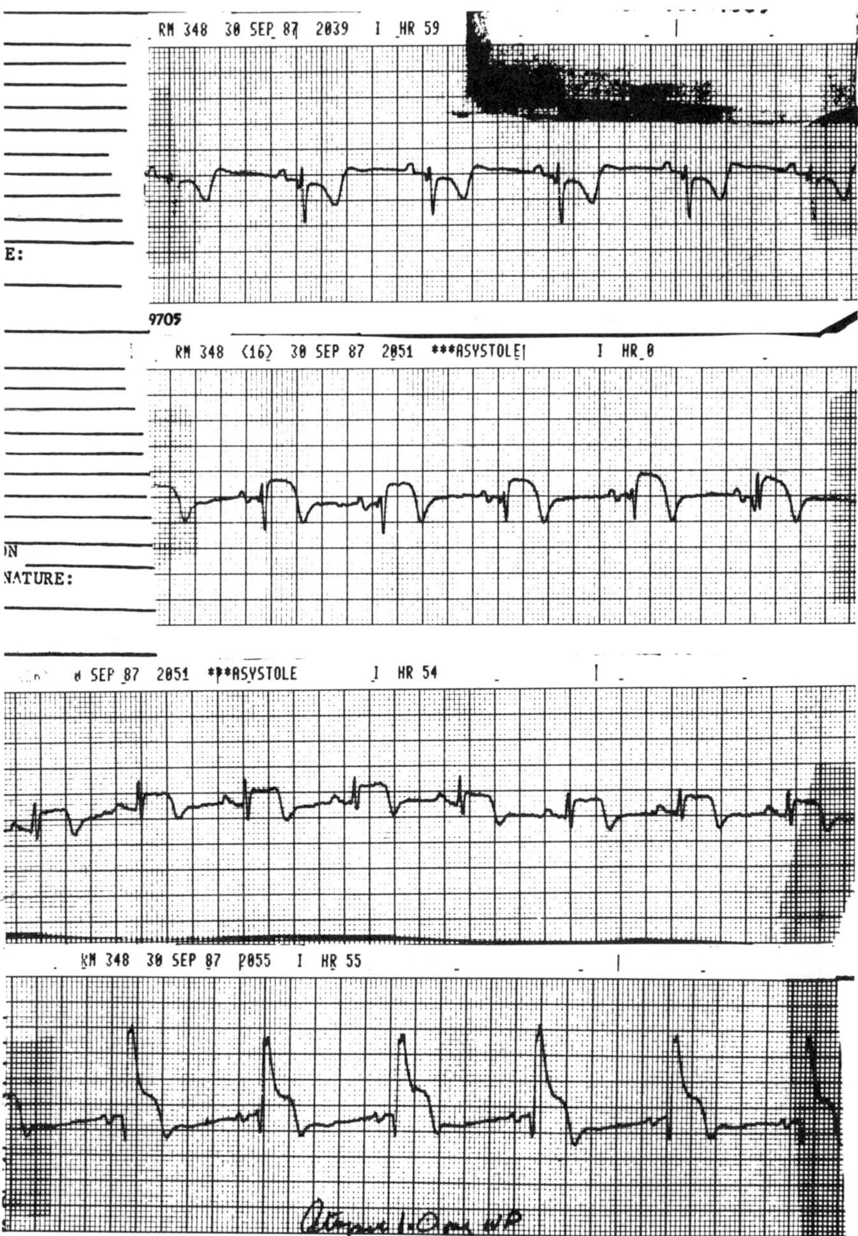

Fig. 32-19. A, Serial rhythm strips revealing variable ST segment displacement. Top strip shows ST–T wave depression with slight elevation of the ST segments in strip 2 and then marked ST-segment elevation in strip 4.

Continued.

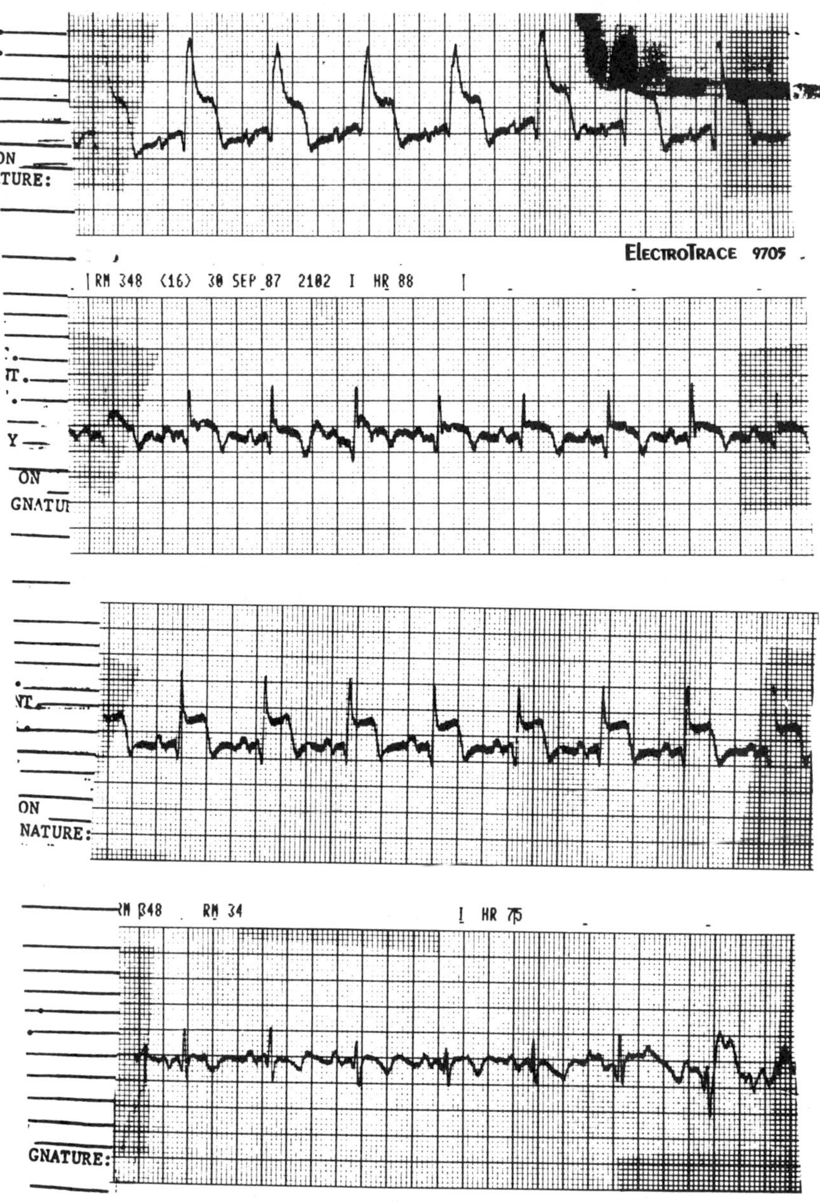

Fig. 32-19, cont'd. B, Further rhythm strips are shown illustrating subsequent reduction in ST segment elevation in the second strip and then recurrent elevation in the third strip, and finally in the fourth strip normalization of the ST segment with T-wave inversion.

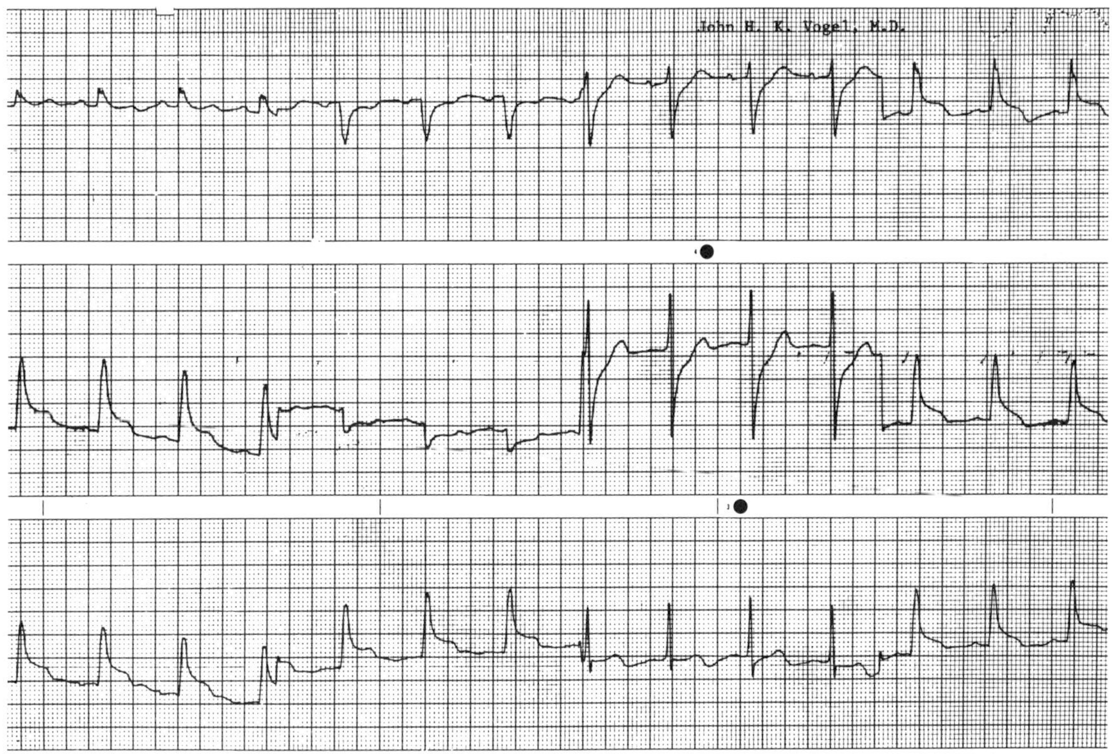

Fig. 32-20. Twelve-lead electrocardiogram obtained from patient during maximal ST-segment change, shown on the rhythm strips revealing acute inferior lateral wall current of injury.

charge. Also patients who remain unstable without early luminal opening undergo catheterization. Other patients who remain stable but who do not have luminal opening should be studied depending on their clinical course, for example, recurrent angina and results of stress testing. *When* to catheterize depends on the clinical situation. Early study should be considered within hours if the initial presentation was critical, for example, the patient was in shock, or had complete heart block and symptoms were then reversed with streptokinase therapy; early study is feasible also in the patient who has early reperfusion and no significant infarction, truly representing an opportunity to salvage muscle, and in those patients with threatened extension. Study is delayed for a few days before discharge in those patients who have no complications or remain without complications but then have late recurrence of pain. This allows further "clean up" to occur. This is the strategy we have evolved over the past 6 years.

It is important to consider *all* myocardial infarctions to be *dangerous*. When early reperfusion has been achieved one does not know what might have happened, and it is important to ascertain what the coronary anatomy is.

DISCUSSION

The 6 year experience involving our three community hospitals has illustrated the effectiveness of intravenous thrombolytic therapy

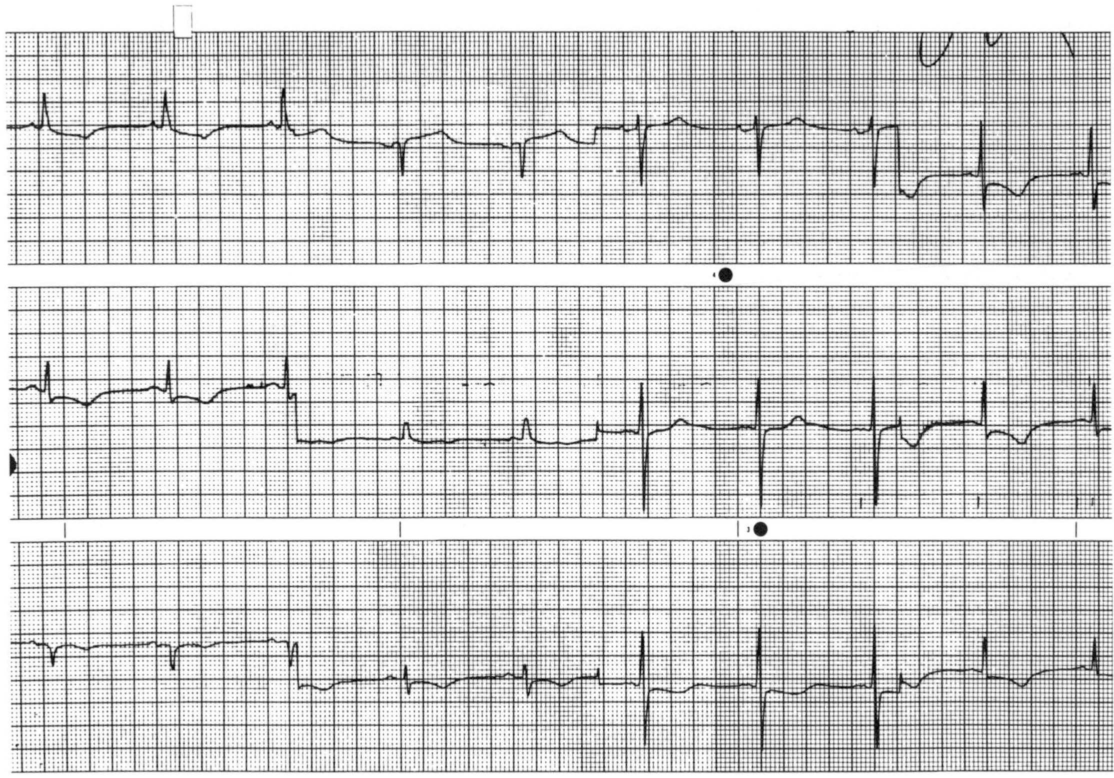

Fig. 32-21. Electrocardiogram obtained immediately following intravenous streptokinase infusion showing reversion from current of injury to marked ST-segment depression, somewhat generalized.

and the feasibility of initiating such therapy in the community hospital without a catheterization laboratory. The morbidity, mortality, and subsequent results in our patients are consistent with this approach. Recently Topol and associates[15] have reported on their experience with the community hospital relationship and have noted excellent results. Although ours was not a randomized study, the occurrence of but one hospital death in our patients indicates the usefulness of intravenous thrombolytic therapy. In Table 32-4 are noted results from recent trials. It is clear that with thrombolytic therapy, whether it consists of streptokinase or tissue plasminogen activator, mortality has decreased into the 6% range. In addition, with *early* therapy there may be very little difference between intravenous streptokinase and tissue plasminogen activator. Clearly in patients who are treated with some delay, such as in the TIMI-I trial,[16] in which the average time to treatment was nearly 4.8 hours, an advantage of tissue plasminogen activator was shown over streptokinase with recanalization rates of 62% versus 31%. However, in the TIMI trial,[16] no patient received streptokinase under 90 minutes, whereas in our study 63% were treated within the first 2 hours with a 96% luminal opening rate clinically. All our patients treated within 1 hour were open clinically. Also Miller and associates[17] had a 100% luminal opening rate with IV streptokinase given within 1 hour. Interestingly, in the TIMI trial there was *no* differ-

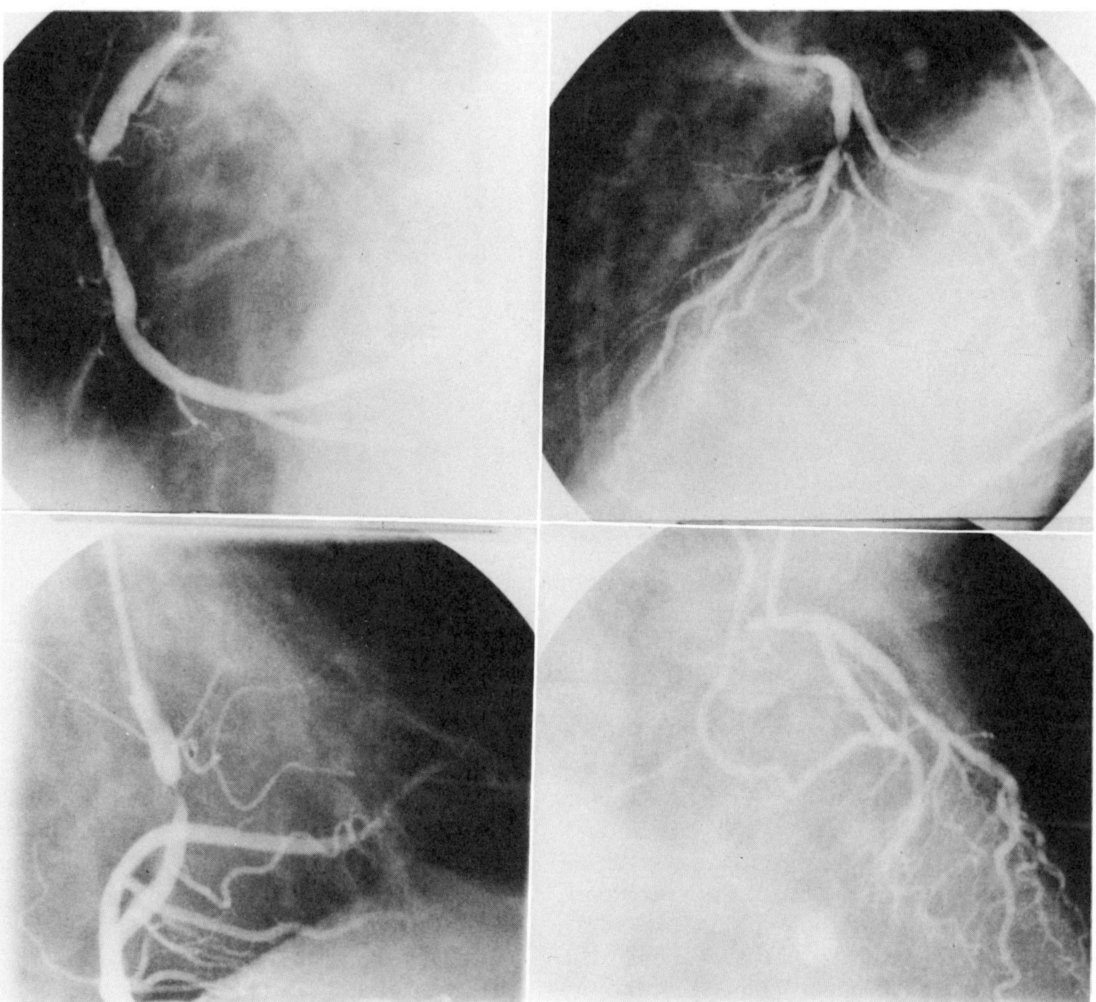

Fig. 32-22. A, Selective biplane right coronary artery cineangiogram showing near-total occlusion of giant right coronary artery and **B,** selective biplane coronary artery angiogram of the left coronary artery showing 90% diameter stenosis of the LAD coronary artery.

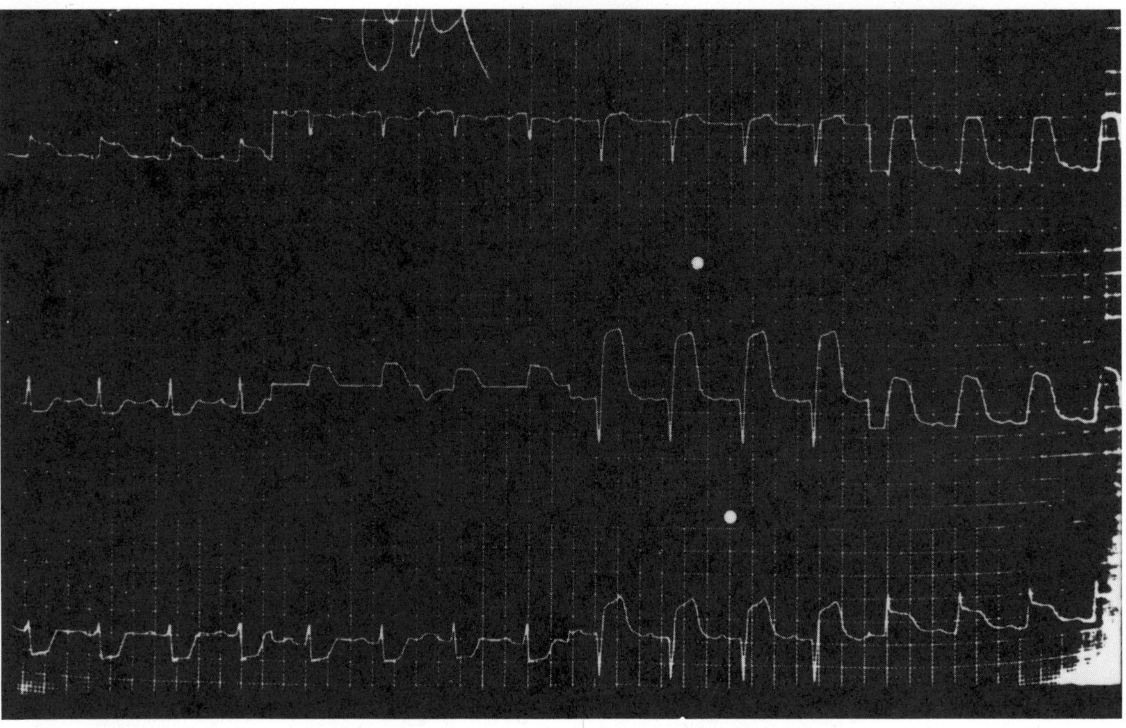

Fig. 32-23. Electrocardiogram obtained immediately before intravenous streptokinase infusion showing acute anterior wall myocardial infarction.

ence in mortality associated with delays in treatment. In fact, the only long-term reduction in mortality has been shown with streptokinase.[18,19]

At the present time streptokinase, tissue plasminogen activator (TPA), and urokinase are available for thrombolytic therapy. Variations of these drugs will be available in the near future. At Goleta Valley Community Hospital the cost to the patient of 1.5 million units of streptokinase plus steroids is $211 and the cost of 100 mg of TPA is $3000. These costs vary from institution to institution. The hospital cost is $2300. Our Disease Related Groups for uncomplicated myocardial infarction reimbursement is $4100. Thus with tissue plasminogen activator a significant markup can result in a major portion of the reimbursement appropriated by the DRG. Therefore, it is important to look at the relative merits of the currently available agents. The ISIS study has shown a dramatic reduction in mortality with streptokinase.[30] If the patient can be treated within the first two hours, the luminal opening rates may be quite similar between streptokinase and TPA (Table 32-5). After 3 hours there is a definite advantage for TPA. However, after 3 hours there is less benefit in terms of improved ventricular function.[9] Indications for TPA, in addition to a somewhat later time of treatment, would include recent administration of streptokinase, and the patient in whom coronary anatomy is known and there is consideration of proceeding to surgery within hours. Bleeding complications have been similar with TPA and streptokinase.[3] However a 1.4% cerebral hemorrhage rate was noted in the European TPA Trial.[22] It

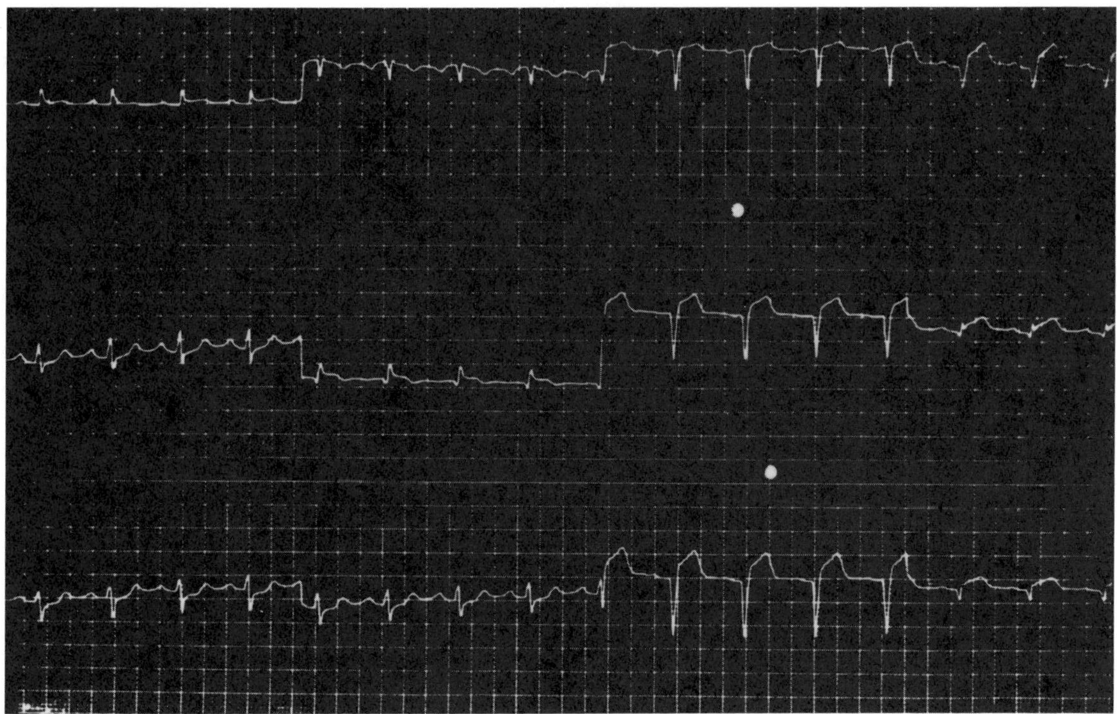

Fig. 32-24. Electrocardiogram obtained immediately after streptokinase infusion showing normalization of the ST segments with a pattern suggestive of "old" anteroseptal wall myocardial infarction.

is not clear at this time what the reocclusion rate will be with these drugs. In our experience the reocclusion rate appears to be 8% with streptokinase and has been over 30% with TPA. This may be a problem requiring further evaluation of the desirable *length* of infusion time and *total* dosage in administering TPA.[27] We now use 1 mg/kg up to 90 mg the first hour with 10% given as a bolus, followed by 1/2 mg/kg over the next 3 hours to a total of 150. In a few cases, after initial luminal opening with streptokinase was followed by reocclusion, tissue plasminogen activator in a 50 mg dose has been successful in luminal reopening. In our experience and from the literature, there is little clinical evidence to support the contention of the superiority of TPA over streptokinase for coronary thrombolysis given under 2 hours. Thus both TPA and streptokinase remain agents for consideration if treatment is instituted within 2 hours. If immediate PTCA is a consideration, streptokinase may be the agent of choice.[28] However, with new variations of TPA it may be possible to achieve similar results with a lower dose, thus maintaining efficacy but reducing cost.

Since the release of TPA on November 13, 1987 we have treated nine patients with TPA and nine patients with streptokinase. All TPA-treated patients had luminal opening clinically (one died). However, four patients had early reocclusion at 3 to 5 hours requiring *additional* TPA beyond the original 100 mg, with all four patients having luminal reopening. Eight of the nine streptokinase-treated patients had luminal opening clinically (no deaths). One patient experienced luminal reocclusion at 72 hours and the lumen was re-

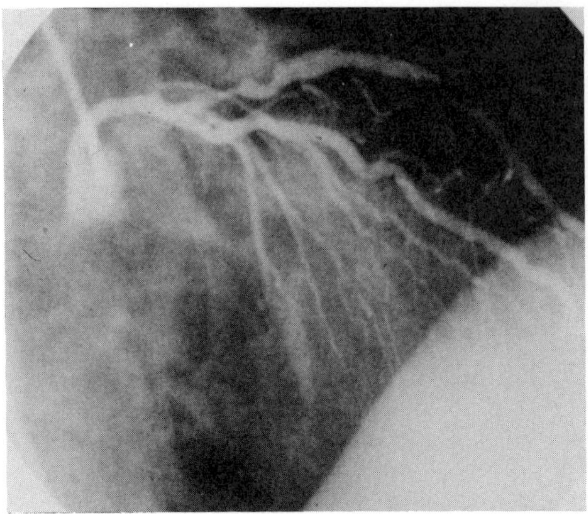

Fig. 32-25. Selective angiogram of the left coronary artery shows a high-grade lesion in the proximal LAD coronary artery.

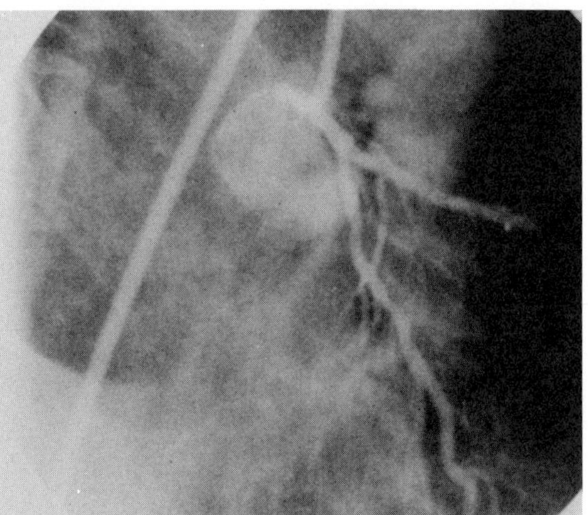

Fig. 32-26. Selective cineangiogram of the left coronary artery following percutaneous transluminal coronary angioplasty demonstrating the vessel to be widely patent. The predilatation gradient was 60 mm Hg and the post dilatation gradient was 0 mm Hg.

opened with 50 mg of TPA. The patient who had no luminal opening had no response to TPA. This experience suggests combined low dose (20–50 mg) TPA and 1.5 million units of streptokinase may be an effective therapy.

Whatever agent is used, it is beneficial to delay study a few days if possible, since there is considerable "clean up" after lysis, so that many patients end up with noncritical lesions (as compared with their appearance immediately after lysis). Thus unnecessary procedures and risk may be avoided, since it appears clear that there is increased hazard with PTCA done urgently, as compared with late (elective) PTCA.[13,23,29] Revascularization procedures are considered if there is continued ischemic instability, such as recurrent angina, arrhythmias, and recurrent electrocardiographic changes in association with significant stenosis. Harrison and associates[32] have shown that residual stenoses of less than 0.4 mm^2 have a 54% rate of rethrombosis. Badger and associates[33] showed that an arterial diameter of 0.6 mm or more was associated with a reduced incidence of reocclusion. In addition Wilson and co-workers[34] have shown normal coronary flow reserve (greater than 3.5) in lesions with less than 70% area stenosis and less than 50% diameter stenosis, or with an area greater than 2.5 $mm.^2$ By using these data, the initial presentation, ongoing clinical findings, and results of thallium stress testing, we then decide on medical and/or revascularization procedures. Also it should be reemphasized that we treat both anterior and inferior wall infarctions. Recent studies suggest benefit to both types of MI with early reperfusion.[35] Moreover the presence of hypotension and heart block in inferior wall infarction is a warning of significant problems: three of our six patients with these findings had main left or equivalent disease.

CONCLUSION

A 6½-year experience with intravenous streptokinase for the treatment of acute myocardial infarction in the small community hos-

Table 32-3. Results of Intravenous Streptokinase Therapy in 121 MI Patients

Living	118/121—1 to 72 months	
Mortality	3/121	
Cerebrovascular accident after catheterization		
lung carcinoma		
Late MI		
Morbidity		
1 Arm: Compartment syndrome—hematoma		
1 Severe nosebleed		
1 Hematoma Arm (Arterial Stick)		
1 Hemoptysis		
Luminal opening clinically	107/121	(88%)
Luminal opening clinically and by catheterization	89/97	(92%)

Table 32-4. Results of Recent Trials Using Intravenous Thrombolytic Therapy

		Mortality	
Early Results	*Type of Therapy*	*Control*	*IV Therapy*
Western Washington[19]	IVSK	9.7%	6.3%
<3 hrs		11.3%	5.2%
>3 hrs		7.5%	7.5%
New Zealand[35]	IVSK	12.9%	2.5%
ISAM[20,21]	IVSK	7.1%	6.3%
GISSI[18]	IVSK		
<1 hr		15.4%	8.2%
<3 hrs		12.2%	9.2%
AIMS(1 month)[25]	IV APSAC	12.2%	6.4%
TICO (100)[24]	IV rtPA	5.5%	5.5%
Hopkins (80)[26]	IV rtPA	7.6%	5.6%
TIMI-IIA (100)[29]	IV rtPA		
PTCA 2 hrs			7.2%
PTCA 33 hrs			5.7%
European (100)[23]	IV rtPA		3.0%
(Patency at 90 min—89%) plus PTCA—at 1 hr (at 3 months)			7.0%
European Coop. Trial rt PA (100)[22]			
at Discharge		6.8%	3.7%
at 3 months		7.9%	5.1%
ISIS-2[30]	IVSK	12.3%	8.2%
<4 hrs	IVSK and ASA	13.1%	6.4%

IVSK, Intravenous streptokinase; rtPA, recombinant tissue type plasminogen activator.

pital, with and without a catheterization laboratory facility, is presented. It has been shown that intravenous streptokinase may be utilized very effectively in the community hospital without a catheterization laboratory when a close relationship exists with another hospital possessing full catheterization and surgical backup. In this study two hospitals located approximately 1 hour's driving time from the third hospital which has a catheterization laboratory, engaged in a highly satisfactory protocol of short-term high-dose intravenous streptokinase. Among the three hospitals, 121 patients were treated and followed from 1 to 72 months. The majority of patients received 1.5 million units of intravenous streptokinase over approximately a 30-minute period. After treatment 118 of the 121 patients were known to be living at least 1 month, with only one death occurring during hospitalization and two known late deaths, one caused by carcinoma of the lung and one

Table 32-5 Estimation of Total Clinical Luminal Opening Rates Between Streptokinase and Tissue Plasminogen Activator Therapy

Time to Treatment	*(%) Early Luminal Opening*	
	TPA	*Streptokinase*
0–1 hr	90	90
1–2 hr	85	80
2–3 hr	80	75
3–4 hr	70	60
>4 hr	65	35

caused by an acute myocardial infarction. Major morbidity was confined to hematomas. There were no instances of cerebral bleeding. In 107 of 121 patients there was evidence of early luminal opening clinically, and at catheterization performed within 2 days in over half of the patients, 89 of 97 patients had open lumens for a 92% patency rate. No problems were encountered in transportation of patients from the two hospitals without a catheterization laboratory to our facility with the laboratory. The results indicate that it is feasible to initiate intravenous streptokinase in the community hospital without a catheterization laboratory. Hartman and associates[31] have had similar excellent results. The patient is followed closely and if there is evidence of luminal opening clinically, further observation is continued. If initially there is evidence of a potentially large infarct, of a very unstable situation, or of total normalization with no evidence of infarction, transfer is initiated the same day for catheterization. In the stable patient with early luminal opening, transfer may be delayed 2 to 4 days, with study done, however, before discharge. In the patient who remains unstable, or has questionable luminal opening, transport is initiated as soon as possible after administering thrombolytic therapy. In view of the tendency for many vessels to clean up over a matter of hours, an effort is made to wait several hours before study to obtain a better picture of what the true appearance is. Patients seen in the facility with a catheterization laboratory are managed in the same way. However, if a very large infarct is present and there is no evidence of luminal opening within an hour, the patient does undergo study immediately, or if the patient is in shock, the patient goes to the laboratory immediately. Of note is that a number of patients seen in the outlying hospitals with hypotension and heart block responded dramatically to intravenous thrombolytic therapy. At the time of catheterization if there is less than 50% stenosis and the patient is asymptomatic, medical therapy is considered, particularly if subsequent thallium stress testing is normal. However, some of these patients have stenosed further and then had PTCA. In those patients with over 70% residual stenosis who are symptomatic and/or who have positive stress testing results, revascularization is considered, the form and type depending on the extent of disease. If the patient is symptomatic but stable, PTCA may be delayed a few days. In the patient with total occlusion and instability, studied early, emergent PTCA should be attempted.

Approximately 25% of our patients ultimately underwent PTCA, and approximately 25% had coronary artery bypass surgery. Fifty percent have been treated medically. These results are consistent with the experiences of other investigators in community hospitals and reflect the excellent results that are possible in such a setting with individualized evaluation and therapy. We believe that all patients with acute myocardial infarction are candidates for intravenous thrombolysis unless specific potential bleeding problems are present, or they are quite elderly, although this is not a definite exclusion. Finally, we believe that all patients who demonstrate luminal opening clinically should undergo study before discharge, earlier study being performed in those patients who are critically unstable before thrombolytic therapy is administered and in those patients who have total resolution without infarction. GISSI II and numerous other studies now in progress comparing TPA, streptokinase, APSAC, urokinase; with or without ASA and heparin; given in the home, ambulance, or emergency room, by various personnel, will help to develop optimal treatment. The most important factor is still *time* and the necessity to educate the patient on the importance of *prompt evaluation* of chest pain.[1]

REFERENCES

1. Vogel, J.H.K.: Coronary thrombolysis: second chance therapy—maximizing the advantage, J. Am. Coll. Cardiol. **8**:1218-1219, 1986.
2. DeWood, M.A., Spores, J., Notske, R., Mouser, L.T., Burrughs, R., Golden, M.S., and Lang, H.T.: Prevalence of total coronary occlusion during the early hours of transmural MI, N. Engl. J. Med. **303**:897, 1980.
3. Chesebro, J.H., et al.: Thrombolysis in myocardial infarction (TIMI) trial, phase I: a comparison between intravenous tissue plasminogen activator and intravenous streptokinase; Circulation **76**:142-154, 1987.
4. Chazov, E.L., Mateeva, L.S., Mazaev, Sargin, K.E., and Sadovskaia, G.V.: Intracoronary administration of fibrinolysis in acute myocardial infarction, Ter. Arkh. **48**:8, 1976.
5. Rentrop, K.P., De Vivie, E.R., Karsch, K.R., and Kreuzer, H.: Acute coronary occlusion with impending infarction as an angiographic complication relieved by a guidewire recanalization, Clin. Cardiol. **1**:101, 1978.
6. Rentrop, K.P.: Thrombolytic therapy in patients with acute myocardial infarction, Circulation **71**:627, 1985.
7. Italian Group for the Study of Streptokinase in Myocardial Infarction (GISSI): Effectiveness of intravenous thrombolytic treatment in acute myocardial infarction, Lancet **1**:397-402, 1986.
8. Koren, G., Weiss, A.T., Hasin, Y., et al.: Prevention of myocardial damage in acute myocardial ischemia by early treatment with intravenous Streptokinase, N. Engl. J. Med. **313**:1384-1389, 1985.
9. Sheehan, F.H.: Determinants of improved left ventricular function after thrombolytic therapy in acute myocardial infarction, J. Am. Coll. Cardiol. **9**:937-944, 1987.
10. Schroder, R., Biamino, G., and Leitner, E.R.: Intravenous short-term thrombolysis in acute myocardial infarction, Circulation **64**(suppl. 4):10, 1981.
11. Schroder, R., Biamino, G., Leitner, E.R., et al.: Intravenous short-term infusion of Streptokinase in acute myocardial infarction, Circulation **67**:536, 1983.
12. Sobel, B.E.: Coronary thrombolysis with tissue-type plasminogen activator: emerging strategies, J. Am. Coll. Cardiol. **8**:1220-1225, 1986.
13. Topol, E.J., Califf, R.M., George, B.S., et al.: A randomized trial of immediate versus delayed elective PTCA after intravenous tissue plasminogen activator in acute myocardial infarction, N. Engl. J. Med. **317**:581-588, 1987.
14. Hackett, D., Davies, G., Chierchia, S., and Maseri, A.: Intermittent coronary occlusion in acute myocardial infarction: value of combined thrombolytic and vasodilator therapy, N. Engl. J. Med. **317**:1055-1059, 1987.
15. Topol, E.J., Bates, E.R., Walton, J.A., Jr., Baumann, G., Wolfe, S., Maino, J., Bayer, L., Gorman, L., Kline, E.M., O'Neill, W.W., and Pitt, B.: Community hospital administration of intravenous tissue plasminogen activator in acute myocardial infarction: improved timing, thrombolytic efficacy and ventricular function, J. Am. Coll. Cardiol. **10**:1173-1177, 1987.
16. The TIMI Study Group: The thrombolysis in myocardial infarction (TIMI) trials, N. Engl. J. Med. **312**:932-936, 1985.
17. Miller, H.I., et al. Early intervention in acute myocardial infarction: significance for myocardial salvage of immediate intravenous Streptokinase therapy followed by coronary angioplasty, J. Am. Coll. Cardiol. **9**:608-614, 1987.

18. Italian Group for the Study of Streptokinase in Myocardial Infarction (GISSI): Long-term effects of intravenous thrombolysis in acute myocardial infarction: Final report of the GISSI study, Lancet **2**:871, 1987.
19. Kennedy, J.W., Martin, G.V., Davis, K.B., Maynard, C., Stadius, M., Sheehan, F.H., and Ritchie, J.L.: The Western Washington intravenous Streptokinase in acute myocardial infarction randomized trial, Circulation **77**:345-352, 1988.
20. The ISAM Study Group: A prospective trial of intravenous Streptokinase in acute myocardial infarction (ISAM): mortality, morbidity, and infarct size at 21 days, N. Engl. J. Med. **314**:1465, 1986.
21. Schroder, R., Neuhaus, K.L., Leizorovicz, A., Linderer, T., Tebbe, U., for the ISAM Study Group: A prospective placebo-controlled double-blind multicenter trial of intravenous Streptokinase in acute myocardial infarction (ISAM): long-term mortality and morbidity, J. Am. Coll. Cardiol. **9**:197, 1987.
22. Van de Werf, F., Arnold, A. E. R. and the European Cooperative Study Group. Effect of Intravenous Tissue Plasminogen Activation on Infarct Size, Left Ventricular function, and Survival in Patients With Acute MI. Presented at American College of Cardiology Meeting 1988.
23. Simoons M.L. and the European Cooperative Study Group. Thrombolysis with Tissue Plasminogen Activation in Acute Myocardial Infarction: No Additional Benefit from Immediate Percutaneous Coronary Angioplasty. Lancet 1988 I: 197-202.
24. O'Rourke, M., Baron, D., Keogh, A., Kelly, R., Welson, G., Barnes, C., Raftos, J., Graham, K., Hillman, K., Newman, H., Heaky, J., Wooldridge,J., Rivers, J., White, H., Whitlock, R., and Norris, R. Limitation of Myocardial Infarction by Early Infusion of Recombinant Tissue-Type Plasminogen Activation. Circulation **77**:1311-15, 1988.
25. Aims Trial Study Group. Effect of Intravenous APSAC on Mortality after Acute Myocardial Infarction: Preliminary Report of a Placebo-Controlled Clinical Trial. Lancet I: 545-49, 1988.
26. Guerci, A.D. and Associates. A Randomized Trial of Intravenous Tissue Plasminogen Activation for Acute Myocardial Infarction with Subsequent Randomization to Elective Coronary Angioplasty, NEJM, **317:** 1613-8, 1987.
27. Topol, E.J. and the TAMI Study Group: Comparison of two dose regimens of intravenous tissue plasminogen activator for acute myocardial infarction, AJC **61**:723-728, 1988.
28. Topol, E.: In discussion. Third Annual Southern California Conference of Society of Interventional Cardiac Angiography, June 1988.
29. TIMI Research Group: Immediate vs. delayed catheterization and angioplasty following thrombolytic therapy for acute myocardial infarction. TIMI A Results. J. Am. Med. Assoc. **260**:2849-58, 1988.
30. Collaborative Group. Second International Study of Infarct Survival (ISIS-2). Lancet **13**:349-360, 1988.
31. Hartman, J., McKeever, L., Bufalino, V., Marek, J., Brown, A., Goodwin, M., and Amirparviz, F.: Intravenous Streptokinase in acute myocardial infarction in community hospitals served by paramedics: A three year experience. In preparation.
32. Harrison, D.G., et al.: Rethrombosis after reperfusion with Streptokinase: importance of geometry of residual lesions, Circulation **69**:991-999, 1984.
33. Badger, R.S., et al.: Usefulness of recanalization to luminal diameter of .6 millimeter or more with intracoronary Streptokinase during acute myocardial infarction in predicting "normal" perfusion status, continued arterial patency and survival at one year, Am. J. Cardiol. **59**:519-522, 1987.
34. Wilson, R.F., Marcus, M.L., and White, C.W.: Prediction of the physiologic significance of coronary arterial lesions by quantitative lesion geometry in patients with limited coronary artery disease, Circulation: **75**:723-732, 1987.
35. White, H.D., et al.: Effect of intravenous streptokinase on left ventricular function and early survival after acute myocardial infarction, N. Engl. J. Med. **317**:850-855, 1987.

Chapter 33

Rotational Approaches to Atherectomy and Thrombectomy

Percutaneous Transluminal Rotational Atherectomy (PTRA) and Percutaneous Rotational Thrombectomy (PRT)

Margaret Hall, MD
D. Dennis Hansen, MD
Michael Intlekofer, MD
David Auth, PhD
James L. Ritchie, MD, FACC

Percutaneous transluminal coronary angioplasty (PTCA) has become increasingly popular and effective in the past decade.[1] Additionally a wealth of intravascular techniques and equipment have been developed, so that placement and manipulation of intravascular catheters within the coronary arteries have become highly refined.[2] However, PTCA suffers from several important limitations at present. Patients with total occlusions are generally not successfully treated, and patients with diffuse disease are difficult to treat effectively. In addition, restenosis occurs in up to one third of all such lesions subjected to PTCA. Lastly, the presumed mechanism or mechanisms of therapeutic effect do not involve removal of the offending plaque, but rather appear to stretch, remodel, or rupture plaque. Thus a number of other approaches have been suggested. The approaches discussed herein are mechanical ones similar to PTCA in capitalizing on existing technology and skills for the delivery of the instruments to the appropriate circulation, using an over-the-guidewire technique, but they differ in that plaque and/or thrombus are removed rather than remodeled and left in place.

MECHANICAL ABLATION OR ATHERECTOMY

The basic mechanical principle involved in percutaneous transluminal rotational atherectomy (PTRA) is the rotation of a small elliptically shaped bur or tip over a flexible, helical drive shaft, all centered and advanced over a guidewire. The tip is coated with a diamond abrasive agent. Rotational energy is transmitted through the drive shaft and atherectomy is performed by cleaving or microablation of millions of small divots of plaque as the diamond chips intercept atherosclerotic material. Fig. 33-1 is a schematic that illustrates the device within the artery containing an atherosclerotic plaque.

One feature of this system that differs greatly from traditional PTCA or most laser systems is the differential cutting of hard tissue. The principle involved is differential engagement of hard tissue and is similar to that of a cast-cutting saw in which the hard cast is removed, but soft tissue such as skin beneath is pushed aside. Elastic tissue in the vascular system is more easily deflected away, whereas calcified tissue, because of its harder consistency, is engaged and cut. Microfractures are generated at the point of intersection of the diamond microchips in the hard tissue. This feature is illustrated schematically in Fig. 33-2. Lipid, on the other hand, is quite soft and not as elastic as smooth muscle tissue, and is also scraped away readily. Thus the more elastic or normal tissues in an artery are least likely to be engaged, whereas the calcium and lipid components of plaque are most likely to be affected.

DETAILS OF A PTRA DEVICE

The rotational atherectomy device consists of an elliptically shaped, nickel-plated, stainless steel bur or tip to which small abrading diamond particles have been electroplated (Fig. 33-3). The diamond particle size varies between 30 and 80 μm, and particle size combinations are sometimes employed in the same device. As a general rule, bur "aggressiveness," or depth of cutting, increases with the size of the diamonds. In addition, preliminary studies suggest that the size of athero-

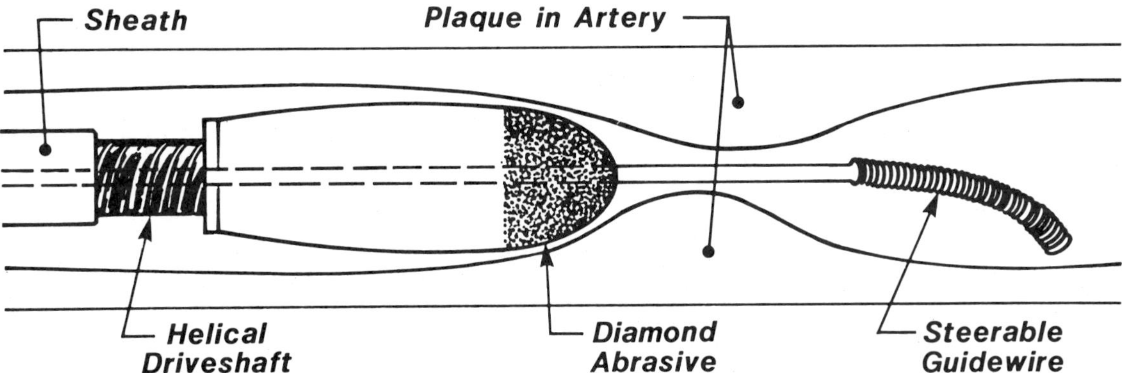

Fig. 33-1. PTRA catheter schematic showing, from left to right, cutaway views of the housing sheath, the helical drive shaft, the tip or bur with its diamond abrasive, and a central rail or guidewire around which the system rotates. Plaque that protrudes into the lumen is engaged by the diamond microchips.

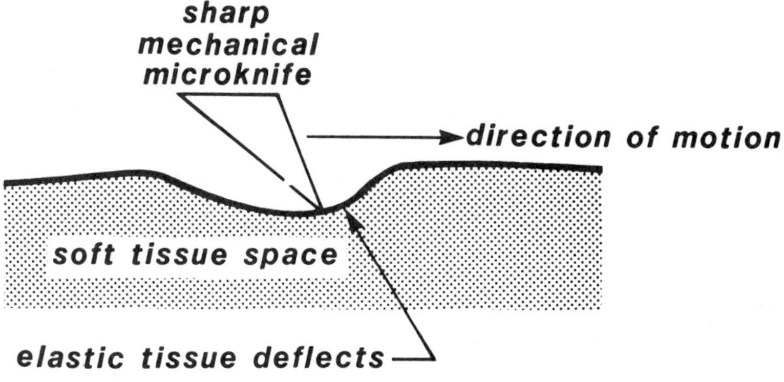

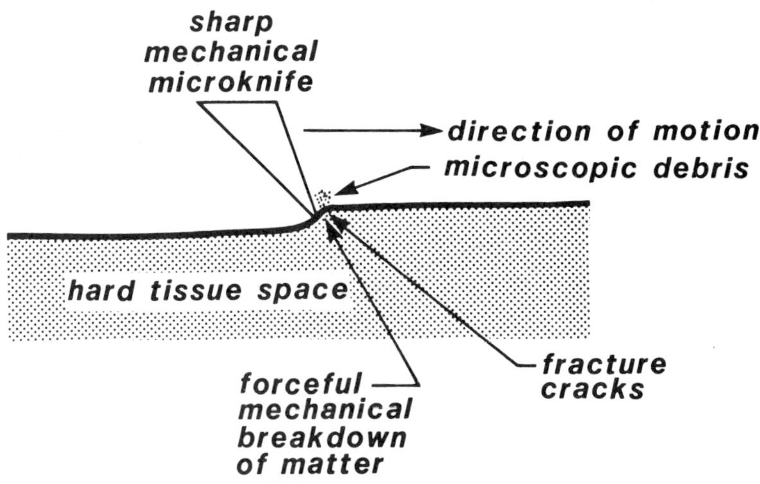

Fig. 33-2. *Top,* Elastic tissue is deflected away by the sharp microknife, whereas hard tissue *(bottom)* is engaged and cut away.

matous debris removed by the device varies with the size of the diamond particles, with small (3 to 8 μm) fragments generated by the small diamonds and larger (8 to 15 μm) fragments generated by the larger diamonds. In the coronary circulation the smaller diamond size is probably a necessity, since significant downstream embolization of material may produce infarction. Particles of up to about 8 μm in diameter should clear the capillary circulation and be taken up by the reticuloendothelial system, as is the case with biodegradeable, radiolabeled particles used in liver-spleen imaging. Tip or bur size can be chosen for the artery and lesion being treated and varies in greatest dimension between 1.25 mm and 4.5 mm (Fig. 33-3).

The bur is mounted on a helical drive shaft that is in turn enclosed with a Teflon sheath through which saline is infused as both cool-

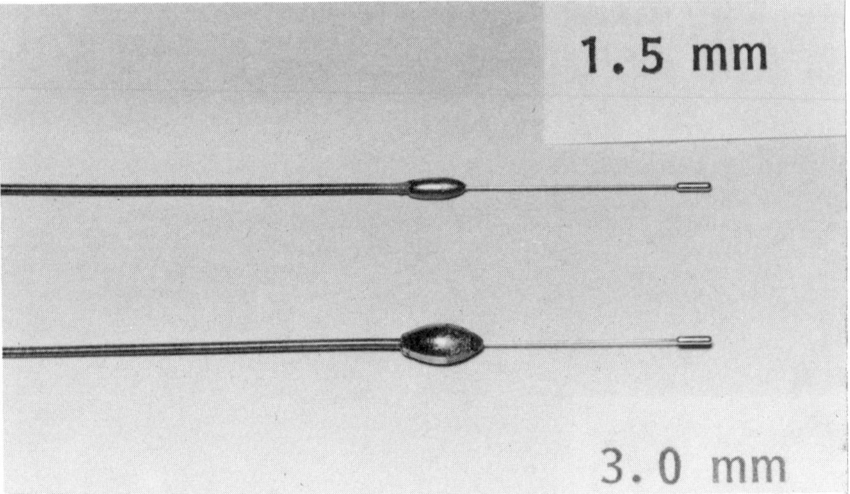

Fig. 33-3. Photographs of a 1.5 mm tip or bur *(above)* and 3 mm tip *(below)*. The helical drive shaft is to the left, the bur is in the center, and the guidewire to the right. These examples have a relatively short and stiff guidewire tip for use in the periphery, as opposed to the coronary spring tip shown in Fig. 33-1.

ant and lubricant. Nominal rotation speed is 150,000 rpm, which produces an average circumferential advance rate of 25 m/second at the bur-tissue interface. This drive is powered by compressed gas (nitrogen or air) supplied through a tank.

The bur, drive shaft, and their advancer (see above) accept a coaxially mounted guidewire that is independently movable and fixable. The distal 3 cm of the guidewire is generally a 0.012-inch shapeable, radiopaque platinum spring tip, similar to commercially available balloon angioplasty guidewires, although other guidewire tip configurations are also available. The proximal wire or rail (currently available in exchange length) is 0.009-inch in diameter and is coated with a biocompatible lubricant. The spring tip will not traverse the bur lumen, thus wire exchanges through the bur cannot be performed. Fig. 33-1 is a schematic of the distal components of the system in an artery, illustrating the sheath, drive shaft, tip or bur, and steerable guidewire.

The entire system is controlled by means of an advancer unit that accepts the gas and activation inputs and provides for fixation of the guidewire during rotation of the bur (Fig. 33-4). Activation occurs by way of a foot pedal accelerator that is controlled by the primary operator. The system is monitored by a tachometer. Visual feedback from the tachometer display and auditory feedback from the unit allow the operator to readily identify decreases in rotational speed, an indicator of increased resistance at the tissue interface. Careful attention to this parameter assists the operator in altering lesion attack strategy (advance-retreat sequence) and in assessing the completeness of stenosis reduction. When a stenosis has been optimally treated with a particular bur, there will be no speed decrease during recrossing of the lesion. The unit "stalls" with precipitous speed decreases, thus preventing continued treatment when resistance is high. The bur is manipulated during rotation by way of the advancer rather than by direct manual advancement. This al-

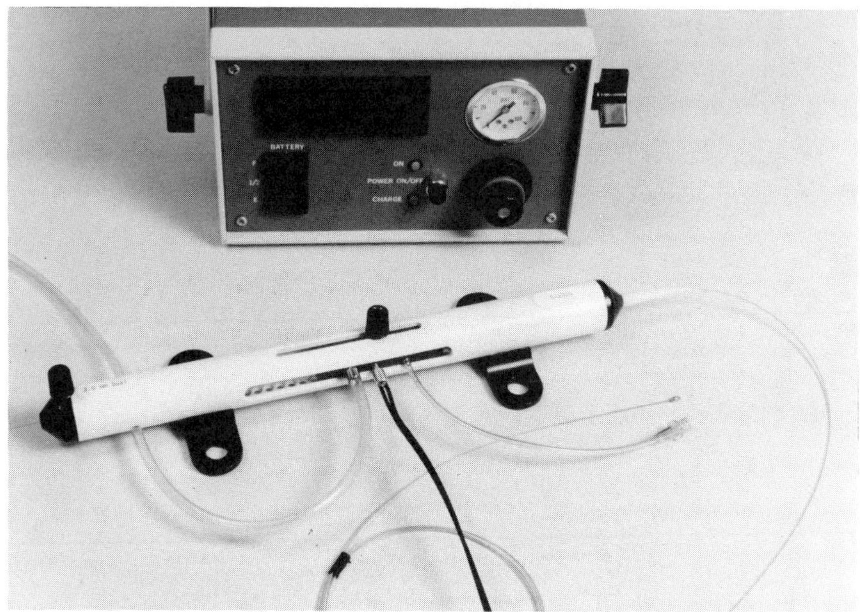

Fig. 33-4. The motor advancer for the PTRA catheter is the tubular device in the center, with air-tank, tachometer, and flush attachments. The box at the back contains the tachometer and air pressure gauge. The PTRA catheter and tip exit from the right-hand side of the motor and can be seen coiled at the bottom of the photo.

lows for easy measurement of the length traversed and greater control of the advance rate. The operator can develop a sense of the "feel" of proper device progress with some experience.

EXPERIMENTAL ANIMAL VASCULAR DISEASE STUDIES

Atherosclerosis of the iliac arteries was induced in New Zealand white rabbits with a diet supplemented by 2% cholesterol for 10 weeks.[3] Following 2 weeks of the diet, the iliac artery was subjected to balloon inflation and endothelial denudation along a 2 cm segment by Fogarty catheter. Following 8 additional weeks on the high cholesterol diet, rabbits underwent arteriography and 13 such arteries with 60% or greater stenosis then had PTRA performed in an antegrade fashion with access by a carotid approach.

The animals were treated with heparin and intraaortic nitroglycerin with manual advancement of the guidewire first, followed by the abrasive tip, under direct fluoroscopic visualization. Once the region of the stenosis was reached, rotation was begun at 150,000 rpm with slow manual advancement at a rate of about 1 mm/second. Atherectomy was repeated until the vessel appeared near normal in size, with progressively larger bur sizes used as needed to achieve this result. Up to four rotations were used in any one artery. The percent diameter stenosis was measured before and following PTRA by calipers from the contrast arteriograms and showed that mean percent diameter stenosis was reduced from more than 80% diameter to less than

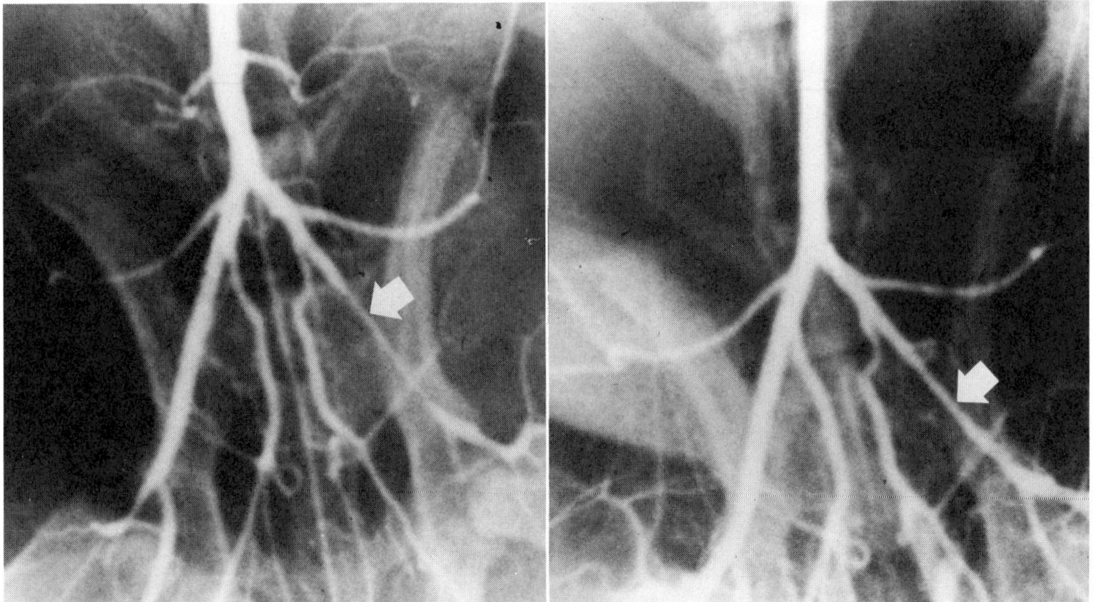

Fig. 33-5. Rabbit iliac vascular disease with greater than 60% stenosis before therapy *(left)* and less than 30% stenosis after PTRA *(right)*.

40%.[3] Fig. 33-5 shows an example. Two complications occurred in this series. One was a perforation from guidewire manipulation in the distal artery, and the second was perforation at the site of rotation, apparently from use of a tip that was relatively oversized. Histologically, dissections and splitting of the media were generally not seen, although the internal elastic lamina was occasionally interrupted. Medial injury, when present, was usually limited to the innermost portions of the media, thus leaving a residual or new lumen that was smooth-walled.

In four of the animals in this series, the atherosclerotic aortas were removed and perfused with saline while the PTRA device was directly applied to an atherosclerotic wall in a manner similar to that used in vivo. The particles generated were collected and passed through a 150 μm filter. Only an occasional particle of macroscopic size was identified by filtering. Of the remaining particles less than 150 μm in diameter, more than 98% were less than 10 μm and the mean particle size averaged under 5 μm. Particles of this size (i.e., less than 7 or 8 μm in diameter) should pass through the circulation and thus not require downstream collection.

Percutaneous Application in Normal Dog Coronary Arteries

The PTRA device was next employed percutaneously through a femoral approach in a series of normal dogs[4] (in the rabbit studies an operative approach was used in a relatively straight vessel). This study was performed to mimic the percutaneous use that might be employed in humans and to demonstrate that the more tortuous and distant coronary arteries could be successfully cannulated with easy advancement to the most distal portion of either the left anterior descending (LAD) or circumflex coronary artery. The device was advanced as described above in the rabbit study into the distal one third of both the circumflex and the LAD coronary artery in normal dogs. In each dog, the LAD coronary artery was approached on day 1, and the dog was then brought back for a repeat study at 1 week and the opposite artery was treated at 1 week. In alternate animals, the opposite artery was approached first. Arteriograms were performed before and after the acute study and at 1 week. Overall, quantitative caliper arteriography showed no significant differences following PTRA and all arteries appeared angiographically entirely normal. No dissections or thrombi were seen. There were no perforations or other complications. Histology demonstrated considerable disruption of endothelium, but showed no dissections or deep medial involvement and again showed histologically smooth lumens.[4]

POSTMORTEM HUMAN ATHEROSCLEROSIS

Based on the animal experiments described above, we have evolved a protocol used in postmortem amputated limbs or postmortem coronary arteries. Postmorten arteries were studied in the fresh or nonpreservative fixed state. A baseline or pretreatment contrast angiogram was performed, and arteries were classed as being either (1) normal or (2) having discrete (2 cm or less in length) stenoses estimated at 50% diameter or more, or (3) diffuse disease with no normal-appearing artery and no discrete stenoses, or (4) being totally occluded. Use of the PTRA catheter was as described above, in which 50% or greater lesions were treated and in which a target endpoint of 70 to 80% of the estimated normal arterial diameter was selected. Overall, in those arteries successfully treated, basal stenoses of greater than 60% diameter were reduced to less than 30%. Perforations occurred in two arteries early in our experience, one in which the catheter tip or bur was incorrectly sized to a diameter larger than the normal artery. In both normal and diffusely diseased arteries, there were no perforations. Total occlusions were not treated, because guidewire penetration of the occlusion was not achieved. Similar preliminary results have been achieved in postmortem coronary arteries.

PERCUTANEOUS ROTATIONAL THROMBECTOMY (PRT)

Thrombosis is another important feature of atherosclerotic vascular disease, both in the coronary arteries and in peripheral arteries. In the periphery, thrombi or emboli may be relatively easily retracted by the use of a Fogarty balloon catheter. However, this is not feasible

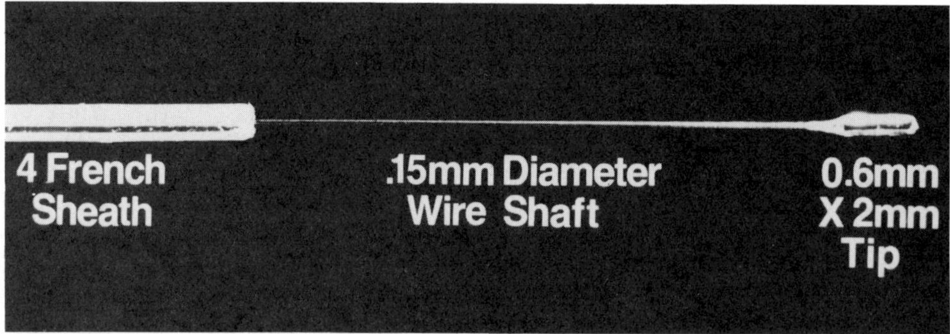

Fig. 33-6. PRT catheter with housing sheath *(left),* and central wire and atraumatic radiopaque tip *(right).*

in the coronary arteries because of the exposure of the vessels of the head and neck and thus, to date, when thrombotic occlusions are approached by balloon catheters following acute myocardial infarction, these thrombi are either remodeled and left in situ or are embolized downstream.

We have employed another rotational device to remove thrombi. It is simpler than our atherectomy device. The catheter is basically a very thin guidewire-like device of 0.006 to 0.008-inch in diameter (Fig. 33-6) that is capped with an atraumatic and easily identifiable radiopaque tip. By rotation of this catheter at a slow speed, two novel results are achieved. First, orthogonal displacement of longitudinal friction reduces the force needed to advance the catheter by a factor of about five-fold, thus allowing more rapid penetration of thrombus with less likelihood of downstream embolization. Second, and more importantly, we have learned that at rotation speeds of 5,000 to 10,000 rpm the elongated and filamentous strands of fibrin, which constitute about 5 to 10% of the mass of fresh thrombus, are selectively extracted and wrapped around the shaft of this rotating catheter. This material adheres tightly to the catheter and is then removed by withdrawal of the entire catheter system. On histologic examination this material appears to be essentially exclusively fibrin and does not contain substantial numbers of red blood cells or normal-appearing thrombus. In-vitro studies have shown that with rotation of the catheter in fresh clot, the clot is liquefied following removal of about 10% of its weight. Thus our approach removes the matrix or scaffold for thrombus and allows the downstream release of red blood cells. The emphasis of this approach is then quite different from the atherectomy catheter in that no abrasive or cutting surface is employed and the rotation speeds are relatively slow.

This percutaneous rotational thrombectomy (PRT) system has been studied in experimentally induced thrombi in canine femoral arter-

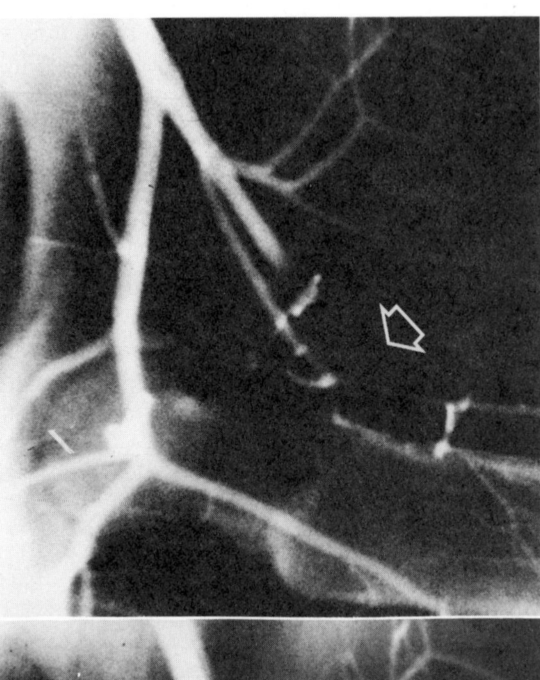

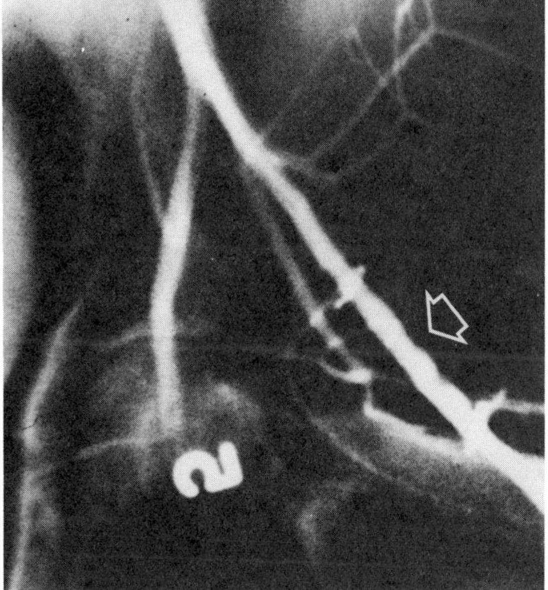

Fig. 33-7. Baseline 100% thrombotic occlusion in the canine femoral artery *(top)* (metal sutures around the artery define the extent of injury) and near-normal arteriogram *(bottom)* after PRT application. (From Ritchie, J.L., et al.: Circulation **73:**1006-1012, 1986. Reproduced with permission of the American Heart Association.)

ies.[5] We were able to restore arterial patency angiographically in 91% of such arteries (Fig. 33-7). A single perforation occurred early in our experience with the PRT device, in which it was rotated in a small branch artery. This approach has similarly been studied in acute coronary thrombi, where it is similarly effective.[6] In a model of older thrombi, ranging from 2 to 7 days old, the rotational thrombectomy device, however, was ineffective. We presume that as older thrombi experience cellular ingrowth, or further cross-linking of fibrin, fibrin can no longer be removed by simple wrapping. However, in this setting the atherectomy device was successful in restoring patency.[7]

DISCUSSION

We have developed and tested new percutaneous transluminal rotational atherectomy (PTRA) and similar percutaneous rotational thrombectomy (PRT) devices in a series of experimental animal studies and in postmortem human peripheral and coronary artery atherosclerosis. The atherectomy device resembles PTCA in the sense that it uses a steerable flexible guidewire that may be left in place. This approach differs from PTCA in that atheromatous material is removed. Diffuse lining plaque that does not intrude into an arterial wall and normal walls are not subjected to cutting. Since there is no outer housing, the device can be manufactured in sizes down to 1 mm in diameter. The distal portion of the system is thus quite steerable and flexible and can be manipulated into small and tortuous arteries of down to slightly more than 1 mm in diameter. The PRT system accomplishes selective wrapping and removal of fibrin with defibrination of fresh thrombus. Thus the matrix for thrombus is removed rather than remodeled or embolized downstream as is the case with PTCA. Both of these rotational approaches directly remove the offending material, that is, atherosclerotic plaque and/or thrombus. Neither approach has as yet been tested in clinical trials in humans, but such trials are now beginning.

Editor's note: PTRA has been performed in both human coronary and peripheral arteries since the preparation of this chapter.

ACKNOWLEDGMENTS

These studies were supported by the Medical Research Service of the Veterans Administration, Washington, D.C., and by a grant from Biophysics International, Bellevue, Washington.

REFERENCES

1. Bredlau, C.E., Roubin, G.S., Leimgruber, P.P., Douglas, J.S., King, S.B., and Gruentzig, A.R.: In hospital morbidity and mortality in patients undergoing elective coronary angioplasty, Circulation **72:**1044, 1985.
2. Vlietstra, R.E., and Holmes, D.R., Jr., editors: PTCA: percutaneous transluminal coronary angioplasty, Philadelphia, 1987, F.A. Davis Co.
3. Hansen, D.D., Auth, D.C., Vracko, R., and Ritchie, J.L.: Rotational atherectomy in atherosclerotic rabbit iliac arteries, Am. Heart J. (In press.)
4. Hansen, D.D., Vracko, R., Auth, D., Ritchie, J.L., and Intlekofer, M.J.: In vivo rotational angioplasty in canine coronary arteries (abstract), International Symposium on Interventional Cardiology, Texas Heart Institute (suppl.)
5. Ritchie, J.L., Hansen, D.D., Vracko, R., and Auth, D.C.: Mechanical thrombolysis: a new rotational catheter approach for acute thrombi, Circulation **73:**1006-1012, 1986.
6. Hansen, D.D., Auth, D.C., Vracko, R., and Ritchie, J.L.: Mechanical thrombolysis in acute canine coronary thrombosis (abstract), Am. J. Cardiol. **7:**207, 1986.
7. Hansen, D.D., Auth, D.C., Vracko, R., and Ritchie, J.L.: In vivo mechanical thrombolysis in subacute canine arterial occlusion, Am. Heart J. (In press.)

Chapter 34

The Theory of Relative Selective Emulsification of Atherosclerotic Tissue by a High-Speed Rotating Cam

Kenneth R. Kensey, MD

Present interventional methods of treating atherosclerotic disease involve bypassing surgically or reshaping with a balloon the offending occlusive material. These two therapeutic approaches have a high incidence of postprocedure reocclusion. Theoretically the reocclusion rate could be reduced if the occlusive material was removed, and therefore great effort and ingenuity have been applied to developing a device that removes the occlusive material (e.g., lasers). No device or method that removes occlusive material is commonly used today. The Kensey catheter does remove occlusive material, and under controlled variables it removes the diseased tissue selectively. A description of the device and the principles involved in how it selectively removes only diseased tissue is the topic of this chapter.

The device is a catheter with a specially shaped cam on the tip. Driven by a cable system, the cam revolves at up to 200,000 rpm. Fluid is forced through the catheter and out the tip near the cam's center of rotation (Fig. 34-1). The device can be made as small as size 2F, in lengths up to several meters, and its flexibility can be made to meet the patient's needs. When passed transluminally through an artery, the cam pulverizes most occlusive material and causes relatively little damage to the artery wall. In addition, the device dilates stenotic areas with its laterally directed fluid jets yielding pathologic results similar to those attainable with balloon angioplasty (Fig. 34-2).

The ability of a rotating cam to selectively pulverize atherosclerotic tissue relies on the premise that the quantity of energy absorbed per mass of material per unit time is inversely proportional to the time that the material remains intact. (This same principle is used in a cast cutter when the operator selectively opens a plaster cast without harming the patient.) Like skin, the normal artery wall is viscoelastic and absorbs far less energy per unit time when exposed to high-frequency vibratory motion than nonviscoelastic material does. This can be seen more closely schematically (Fig. 34-3). As seen here, the tissue yields continually under stress and will return

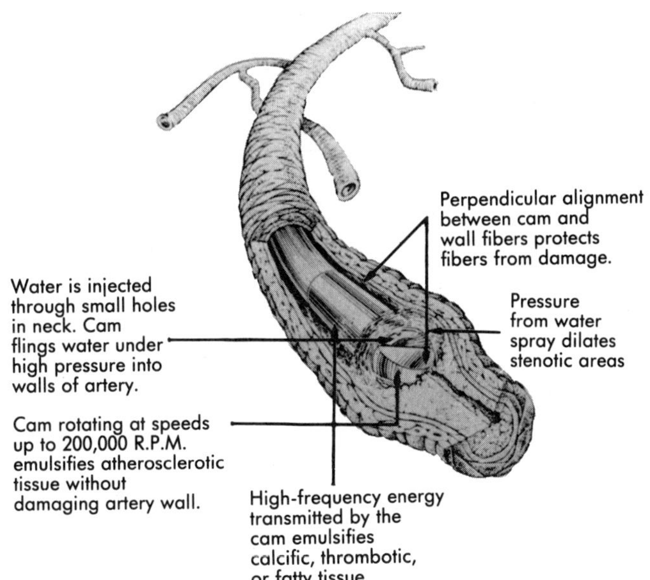

Fig. 34-1. Water is injected through small holes in neck. The cam flings water under pressure into the walls of the artery. Cam rotating at speeds up to 200,000 rpm emulsifies atherosclerotic tissue without damaging artery wall. High-frequency energy transmitted by the cam emulsifies calcific, thrombotic, or fatty tissue. Perpendicular alignment between cam and wall fibers protects fibers from damage. Pressure from water spray dilates stenotic areas.

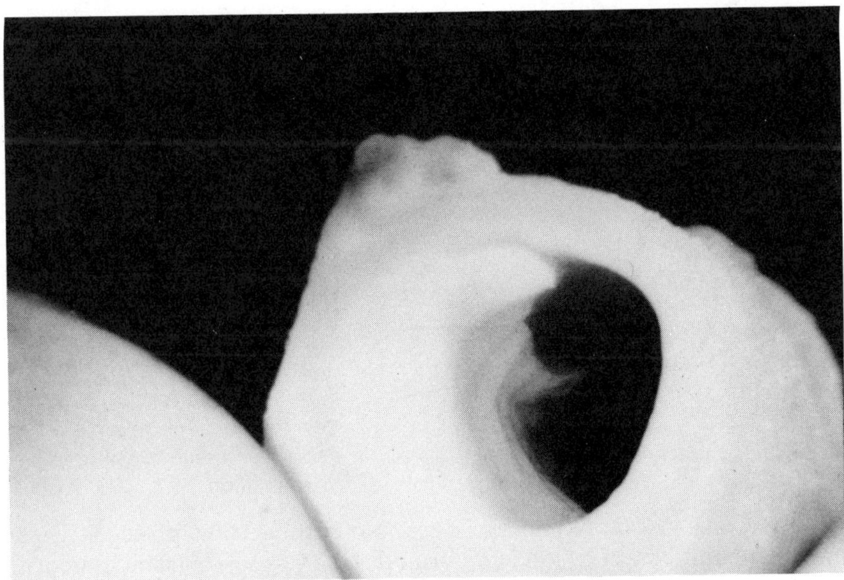

Fig. 34-2. Stereomicroscopic view of a recanalized occluded popliteal artery from a freshly amputated human lower limb. There is a longitudinal intimal tear that winds around into the dense fibrous plaque. The artery wall is stretched and the lumen is dilated.

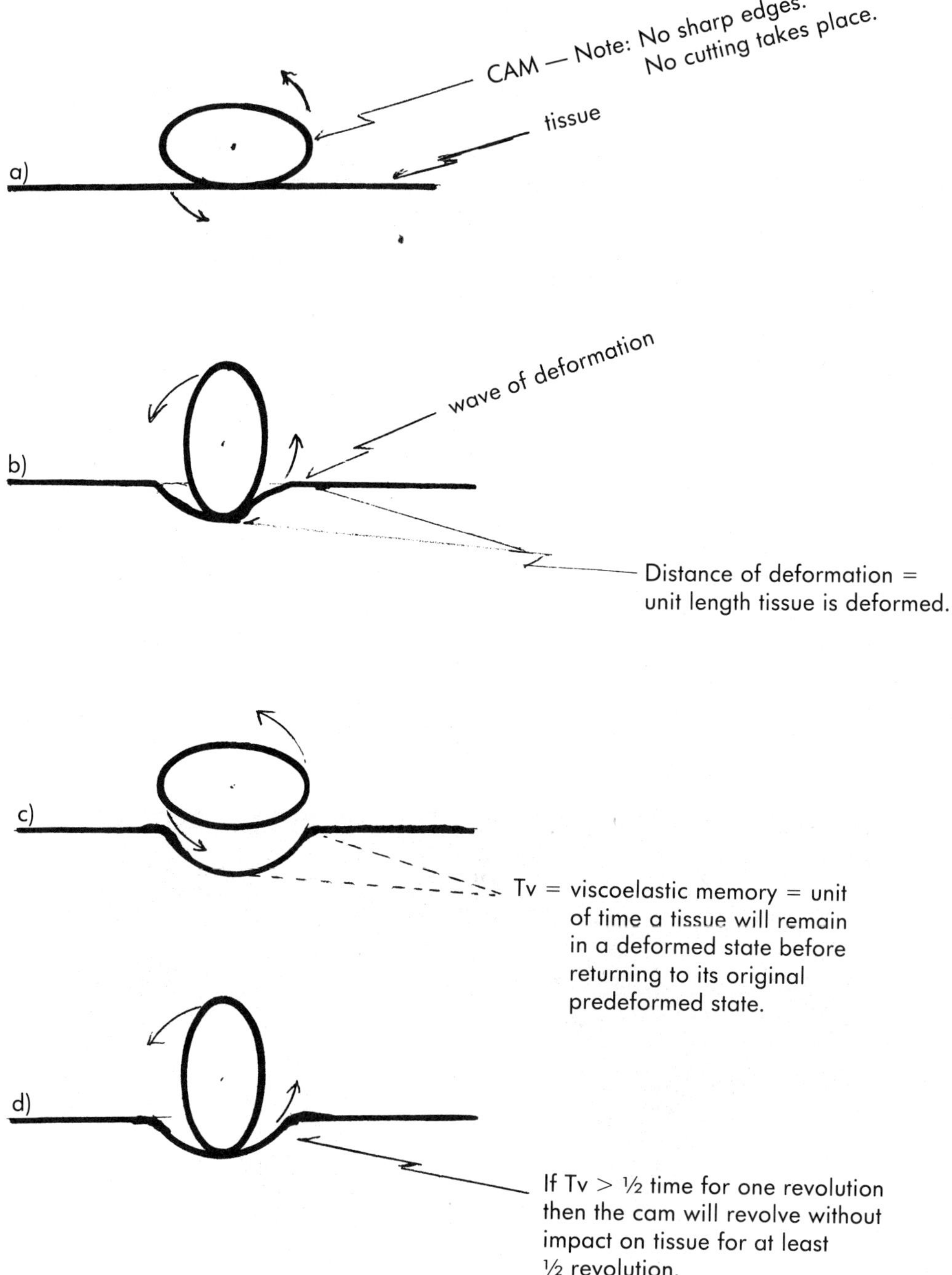

Fig. 34-3. **A,** Cam—Note: No sharp edges. No cutting takes place. **B,** Distance of deformation = unit length tissue is deformed. **C,** Tv = viscoelastic memory = unit of time a tissue will remain in a deformed state before returning to its original predeformed state. **D,** If Tv > ½ time for one revolution then the cam will revolve without impact on tissue for at least ½ revolution.

Continued.

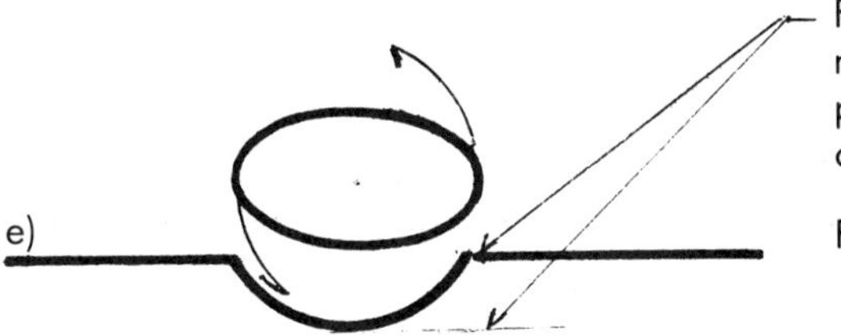

Fig 34-3, cont'd. E, Frequency at deformation = how many times deformation takes place/unit time with RPM at cam held constant. Frequency of deformation α $^1/_{Tv}$. Frequency of deformation α Energy absorber. Energy absorbed α $^1/_{Tv}$ i.e. the longer the viscoelastic memory the less energy that is absorbed by the tissue.

to its original shape only after some delay when the stress is removed. The delay (Tv) is the tissue's viscoelastic memory. As Tv increases, the amount of energy absorbed by that tissue decreases (holding all other variables constant). Simply stated, if the time for one revolution of the cam is $\ll$ Tv, then the cam will revolve many times during Tv before the tissue begins to return to its original shape, but during Tv, the tissue is not moved by the cam and therefore the tissue is not absorbing energy. If (quantity of energy absorbed)/(mass of tissue)/(unit time) = K 1/(unit time tissue will remain intact), and Tv is directly related to the (energy absorbed)/(revolution), then it should require a much greater time for viscoelastic tissue to absorb enough energy to be destroyed (where Tv >0), than if Tv = 0. As Tv approaches 0 the tissue loses its viscoelasticity and becomes more elastic.

The viscoelasticity of tissue varies widely from patient to patient and varies widely within the body itself. Age, disease state, type of disease, and oxygen deprivation are a few of the many variables observed that will change the Tv of tissue and thus the relative selectivity of the spinning cam. In atherosclerotic disease, as long as the disparity between the Tv of the occlusive material and the artery wall remains high, then it is possible to selectively pulverize the occlusive material with a spinning cam.

Exactly how this cam is able to pulverize the varied types of atherosclerotic tissue is beyond the scope of this discussion. Suffice it to say that, besides viscoelasticity, there are other physical properties of tissue that can also be used advantageously to selectively pulverize occlusive material but, in general, diseased tissue is nonviscoelastic. The tissue's viscoelastic memory (Tv) approaches 0. With each revolution of the cam, energy is transmitted to the tissue in the form of kinetic energy, that is, the tissue vibrates to and fro laterally with each rotation of the cam. Little time is necessary to transmit a highly destructive quantity of energy to the tissue. Consistent with this, we find that most occlusive tissue is immediately pulverized on contact with the spinning cam.

Understanding the limitations of a mechanical device such as this will require a great deal of scientific investigation and before any device will be commonly accepted as a treatment for occlusive atherosclerotic disease we will have to know its limitations. It is hoped that this theory will provide a nidus from which future ideas and research can develop.

REFERENCES

1. Kensey, K.R., Nash, J., Abrahams, C., Lake, K., and Zarins, C.K.: Recanalization of obstructed arteries using a rotating tip catheter (abstract), AHA Nov. 1986.
2. Kensey, K.R., Zarins, C.K., Whittemore, A., and Nash, J.: Dynamic angioplasty as a treatment modality in peripheral vascular disease: the first clinical results, Poster, J. Am. Coll. Cardiol., March 1987.
3. Kensey, K., and Nash, J.: Dynamic angioplasty using a flexible rotating tip catheter, Cleveland Clinic Foundation, Oct. 1987.
4. Kensey, K., Nash, J., Abrahams, C., and Zarins, C.K.: Recanalization of obstructed arteries with a flexible, rotating tip catheter, Radiology **165:**387-389, 1987.

Chapter 35

Transvenous Catheter Ablation for Cardiac Arrhythmias

Michael A. Ruder, MD
R. Hardwin Mead, MD
Nellis A. Smith, MD
Roger A. Winkle, MD

In 1982, two separate reports of transvenous catheter ablation of the atrioventricular (AV) junction in a series of patients with severely symptomatic, drug-refractory supraventricular tachyarrhythmias were published.[1,2] Before this, open heart surgery with surgical dissection or cryoablation of the His bundle area was required to create heart block in these patients. Although the number of patients in need of permanent disruption of AV conduction is small compared with the number requiring other interventional techniques such as percutaneous coronary angioplasty, the interest generated among electrophysiologists by these early reports was enormous. Patients with refractory supraventricular tachycardias could now be treated effectively and apparently safely without thoracotomy. With this early promise, transvenous catheter ablation was then applied to accessory pathways and ventricular and atrial tachyarrhythmias of apparent focal origin. Although the results for these other arrhythmias have not approached the success rate of ablation of the AV junction, it is clear that catheter ablation will continue to play a role in the management of patients with a variety of arrhythmias.

TECHNIQUE

The technique used for catheter ablation has been similar for the various cardiac sites. A standard electrode catheter is introduced percutaneously, positioned against the intended area of ablation, and connected to the output of a defibrillator. A chest wall patch or, in some cases, another pole of the same catheter or a separate endocardial catheter is connected to the defibrillator's current sink. The amount of energy to be delivered is set on the defibrillator (typically 50 to 400 J) and one or more shocks, synchronized to the QRS interval, are delivered under general anesthesia.

Until recently, most reports of ablation have involved the use of these high-energy, direct current discharges. This is due to the early success of the technique, as well as the expediency inherent in using readily available catheters and defibrillators. However, energy delivery by means of a defibrillator is by its very nature uncontrolled and future developments in abalation therapy will involve developing a more precise mode of transporting controlled energy. Nevertheless, a great deal has been learned about the potential uses of ablation.

ABLATION OF THE ATRIOVENTRICULAR JUNCTION

Early techniques used to achieve complete AV block involved thoracotomy and surgical division of the AV node–His bundle area under direct vision.[3,4] Subsequent developments included the use of injected formalin,[5] electrocautery,[6,7] or cryoablation,[8] all requiring surgery. In an effort to avoid thoracotomy, several investigators achieved AV block in as many as 60% of animals by injecting formalin into the AV junction by means of a percutaneously positioned needle catheter.[9,10]

The use of high-energy discharges was first described by Beazell and colleagues,[11,12] who modified a transseptal catheterization needle by insulating it with Teflon. With the needle placed against the septum, a direct current discharge was delivered through the catheter using a standard defibrillator. Complete AV block was produced in 45 of 46 dogs. Gonzalez and colleagues[13,14] simplified this approach by making use of a readily available electrode catheter. Complete AV block was produced in a series of nine dogs, and following the sacrifice of the animals there was no evidence of perforation or visible damage to the heart valves or valvular apparatus. Microscopic examination showed marked damage in the AV node, the approaches to the node, the penetrating bundles and, with higher energies, the bundle branches themselves.

Using essentially this same technique, Scheinman and associates[1] and Gallagher and co-workers[2] safely and effectively produced heart block in a series of patients with refractory supraventricular arrhythmias.

Indications

Ablation of the AV junction is primarily indicated for those patients with symptomatic atrial tachyarrhythmias in whom control over the arrhythmia itself or the ventricular response to the arrhythmia is not attainable with drugs. In practice, patients typically have long-term chronic or paroxysmal atrial fibrillation/flutter or ectopic atrial tachycardia with a rapid ventricular response. Although patients are usually left with a supra-Hisian or infra-Hisian escape rate sufficient to prevent complete ventricular asystole, the resultant complete AV block does require implantation of a permanent pacemaker. Theoretically other supraventricular tachycardias incorporating the AV node as an integral part of the tachycardia circuit are also amendable to ablation therapy. Ablation of the AV junction has been used to control AV nodal reentry tachycardia, as well as orthodromic AV reciprocating tachycardia utilizing extranodal Kent or Mahaim accessory pathways.[15,16] However, because of the potential for rapid antegrade conduction over the accessory pathway during atrial fibrillation and because of the high success rate of surgical division of accessory pathways, the applicability of AV junctional ablation in these situations is limited. Similarly, since surgical cure of AV nodal reentry tachycardia can now be achieved in a high proportion of patients with preservation of AV conduction and without the need for a permanent pacemaker,[17-19] AV junctional ablation should be used in only a small percentage of these patients.

Results

In 1982 a worldwide voluntary registry, the Percutaneous Cardiac Mapping and Ablation Registry (PCMAR), was formed to collect data on catheter ablation procedures performed for control of cardiac arrhythmias.[20] PCMAR recently reported the results of 475 patients who underwent ablation of the AV junction.[21] The majority of patients (60%) had atrial fibrillation/flutter, 22% AV nodal reentry tachycardia, 13% ectopic atrial tachycardia, and the remainder had accessory pathways. The patients had failed or proved intolerant to a mean of 3.5 ± 1.2 antiarrhythmic drugs. In long-term follow-up, 63% of the patients remained in complete AV block. Although the remainder resumed conduction, in 10% of patients conduction was modified enough that the patients were asymptomatic without drug therapy and another 12% now responded to AV nodal blocking drugs that were previously ineffective. The ablation was ineffective in 15%. The mean heart rate of the residual escape rhythm was 45 beats/minute.

Complications included ventricular tachyarrhythmias requiring cardioversion in six patients, transient hypotension in six patients, and complications related to the pacemaker in four patients. There were no deaths related to the procedure. Nineteen patients died during long-term follow-up; the deaths were felt to be due to progression of underlying cardiac disease or from other causes unrelated to the ablation in all but one patient, who died suddenly without apparent heart disease.

Our experience has been even more favorable, perhaps related to a "learning curve" involved with the ablation technique. Since 1984, 39 patients have undergone ablation of the AV junction at Sequoia Hospital. The mean age of the patients was 59 ± 11 years (range 38 to 83 years). Their clinical and arrhythmia characteristics are shown in Table 35-1. Thirty-five patients (90%) had atrial fi-

Table 35-1. Clinical Characteristics of 39 Patients Undergoing Ablation of the AV Junction

Arrhythmia (% of Patients)	*Symptoms (% of Patients)*	*Prior Therapy (% of Patients)*	*Cardiac Disease (% of Patients)*
Atrial fibrillation/flutter (90)	Palpitations (72)	Digoxin (97)	None (41)
Ectopic atrial tachycardia (5)	Presyncope (38)	Type IA (97)	Coronary artery disease (26)
AV nodal reentry tachycardia (2)	Syncope (28)	Ca^{2+} channel blocker (90)	Valvular (15)
Junctional ectopic tachycardia (2)	Fatigue (36)	Beta blocker (77)	Others (18)
	Congestive heart failure (33)	Amiodarone (41)	
	Chest pain (26)	Flecainide (38)	
	Cardiac arrest (2)		

brillation/flutter, two (5%) ectopic atrial tachycardia, one (2%) AV nodal reentry tachycardia, and one (2%) junctional ectopic tachycardia. Eleven patients (28%) had previously had syncope associated with their arrhythmia and 15 (38%) presyncope. Thirteen patients (33%) had worsening of baseline congestive heart failure caused by an uncontrolled ventricular response during arrhythmia. One patient suffered a previous cardiac arrest secondary to atrial fibrillation with a very rapid ventricular rate. The patients had failed or proved intolerant of a mean of 3.6 ± 2.1 antiarrhythmic drugs. Eleven patients had arrhythmia recurrence with amiodarone therapy and five patients could not tolerate the drug.

Thirty-two (82%) of the 39 patients had persistent AV block after a single ablation attempt. In 7 of the 39 patients, conduction returned within 4 to 96 hours and these patients underwent a second ablation attempt. Complete, persistent AV block was achieved in four additional patients. Three of the seven patients resumed AV conduction; one is doing well on medication previously ineffective and two are unimproved. One of the unimproved patients underwent successful open heart cryoablation of the AV junction. The mean follow-up on all patients is 14 ± 11 months.

Thus ablation of the AV node was successful in producing persistent AV block in 36 of 39 patients (92%). By increasing the amount of block at the AV node, it improved symptoms in another patient. The failure rate was 5%. The average rate of the escape rhythm with the pacemaker inhibited was 42 ± 13 beats/minute.

Complications developed in seven patients. Four of these seven complications were related to the pacemaker, including pneumothorax in one patient, ventricular lead migration requiring reoperation in one, late lead fracture requiring lead replacement in one, and pacemaker syndrome necessitating an "upgrading" of the pacemaker to a dual-chamber device in one patient with paroxysmal atrial fibrillation. Two of the seven complications were related to delivery of the shock, consisting of hypotension after the discharge requiring transient pressor support in one of the two patients. One patient, who had previously not been known to have ventricular ectopy, had frequent PVCs for 48 hours after the ablation that resolved spontaneously.

There have been five deaths during long-term follow-up. Two patients died of metastatic carcinoma. Three patients died of congestive heart failure after a mean of 6 ± 3 months. Each of these patients had preexisting severe left ventricular dysfunction and the ablation procedure had initially been performed because rapid ventricular rates during chronic atrial fibrillation had exacerbated preexisting heart failure. All three patients did, in fact, benefit clinically from the ablation, but went on to die of progressive left ventricular failure.

In summary, in our experience control over refractory supraventricular tachyarrhythmias can be achieved in nearly 95% of patients with an acceptable rate of complications. The patients have been pleased with the results of the ablation and have become essentially asymptomatic with the single exception being the one patient with pacemaker syndrome whose symptoms of arrhythmias returned when his pacemaker was "upgraded" to a dual-chamber device. When catheter ablation is compared with the results of surgical cryoablation,[22] the success rates were found to be identical with fewer postprocedure complications in those undergoing the percutaneous procedure. Nevertheless, because of the potential induction of pacemaker dependency, the small risk of minor complications, and the question of sudden death several months after the procedure raised by the report of one patient in the PCMAR series,[20] ablation of the AV node should be considered a therapy of "last resort" for symptomatic supraventricular arrhythmias.

ABLATION OF ACCESSORY PATHWAYS

Surgical division of the accessory pathway in patients with the Wolff-Parkinson-White syndrome can be performed with a high success rate and a low operative risk.[23,24] The indications for surgery have broadened to include not only those patients who have not responded to medical management, but also young patients who wish to avoid lifelong therapy with potentially toxic agents or those patients who have previously had life-threatening arrhythmias and prefer not to rely on drug therapy. Like ablation of the AV node–His bundle axis, ablation of accessory pathways was initiated with the intention of achieving cure without major surgery. In general, about 50% of accessory pathways occur along the left free wall, 25% in the posterior septal area, and the remainder along the right free wall or anterior septum.[25]

Left Free Wall Accessory Pathways

Brodman and Fisher[26] delivered high-energy shocks between poles of an electrode catheter inserted percutaneously into the coronary sinus in a canine model. Although transmural injury at the level of the anulus fibrosus was consistently produced, discharges within the thin-walled venous structure occasionally led to rupture of the coronary sinus and subsequent tamponade. Coltorti and coworkers[27] demonstrated that this rupture was likely due to the barotraumatic effects of the high-voltage shock. In addition, damage of the adjacent left circumflex artery was seen with higher energies, perhaps a direct electrical effect. Ablation procedures in a series of eight patients by Fisher and associates[28] led to coronary sinus rupture in one patient with no permanent disruption of anomalous conduction. For these reasons, the use of high-energy discharges within the coronary sinus to ablate left free wall bypass tracts has generally been abandoned.

Posteroseptal Accessory Pathways

Ablation of accessory pathways in the posterior septal area has proved feasible. By delivering high-energy discharges at or immediately outside the coronary sinus os, rupture of the coronary sinus is avoided. There have been a number of reports of permanent disruption of posteroseptal bypass tracts, with success rates as high as 75%.[29-32]

From 1984 to 1986 we attempted transvenous catheter ablation in 12 patients with accessory pathways located in the posteroseptal area.[33] Seven patients had previously been diagnosed with episodes of atrioventricular reciprocating tachycardia only, four patients with both atrioventricular reciprocating tachycardia and atrial fibrillation (with ventricular responses of 220 to 300 beats/minute), and two patients with atrial fibrillation only. The patients had previously failed or proved intolerant to a mean of 1.8 ± 0.9 antiarrhythmic drugs.

By inserting an electrode catheter with a central lumen into the coronary sinus and identifying the location of the os with a contrast injection within the coronary sinus, the location of the earliest atrial activation during reciprocating tachycardia via the accessory pathway was defined within 5 mm. The location of the accessory pathways is shown in Table 35-2. Earliest atrial activation was at or within 5 mm of the coronary sinus os in eight patients, 5 to 15 mm within the coronary sinus in three patients, and 10 mm outside the os along the posterior right atrium in one patient.

A standard 6F quadripolar catheter was then placed in the coronary sinus and the proximal pair of electrodes adjusted to straddle the area of earliest retrograde atrial activation. Because of the known deleterious effects of discharges within the coronary sinus, care was taken not to place the most proximal electrode of the ablating pair within the os. For those accessory pathways located further within the coronary sinus, we hoped that the destructive energy of the shock would diffuse through myocardial tissue sufficiently to disrupt accessory pathway conduction. The proximal pair of electrodes were made electrically common and connected to the cathodal output of the defibrillator with an anterior chest wall patch serving as the current sink. Two synchronized discharges, 300 J followed by 200 or 300 J, were delivered under anesthesia over a period of 30 minutes.

The immediate and late results are shown in Table 35-2.[33] For those eight patients with pathways at or within 5 mm of the os, pathway conduction was abolished in five (63%) and modified in one patient, so that anterograde conduction was abolished and retrograde conduction was slowed. For the other four patients with pathways more than 5 mm from the os, pathway conduction was modified in only two.

There were no complications other than a brief episode of pericarditis in one patient. Five of the patients with unsuccessful ablations subsequently underwent surgical division of the accessory pathway, and minor tissue damage surrounding the area of ablation was seen in two patients. There was no appreciable alteration in AV nodal conduction. The patients with successful ablations are doing well over a follow-up period of 20 ± 7 months.

Despite the minimal gross tissue effects seen at the time of surgery, the alteration in atrial electrograms around the area of ablation was dramatic. The amplitude of the atrial signal was reduced a mean of 80 ± 43% and the signals were typically broad and indiscrete. In view of the marked effect of the shocks on the electrical properties of atrial tissue, even in unsuccessful ablations, the mechanism of a successful ablation may be due to interruption of pathway conduction at the anulus fibrosus or destruction of tissue surrounding the pathway's atrial insertion point rather than direct damage of the acces-

Table 35-2. Ablation of Posteroseptal Accessory Pathways

Patient No.	*Pathway Location*	*Results*
1	CS os	0
2	CS os	+
3	CS os	0
4	CS os	+
5	5 mm in os	0
6	5 mm in os	0
7	10 mm in os	+
8	10 mm in os	+
9	15 mm in os	Modified
10	CS os/15 mm in os*	0/+
11	5 mm outside os	Modified†
12	10 mm outside os	+

From Ruder, M.A., et al.: J. Am. Coll. Cardiol. 1988. (In press.)
**Two separate pathways, one at the os and the other 15 mm within the coronary sinus, were identified.*
†Anterograde conduction was abolished; retrograde conduction was slowed.
CS, Coronary sinus; 0, no pathway conduction; +, pathway conduction.

sory connection itself. Unsuccessful ablation attempts may be due to interpatient variations of the location of the coronary sinus os (where ablation occurs) relative to the point of atrioventricular continuity, so that atrial conduction may occur below the area of ablation but above the atrial insertion of the accessory pathway. In some unsuccessful cases the ablation altered retrograde atrial activation so much that the presence of another low right free wall bypass fiber was falsely suggested.

Based on available data, ablation of posteroseptal accessory pathways is a safe and reasonably effective alternative to surgery for those patients with pathways at or within 5 mm of the os. Surgical division of pathways in this area is associated with a 10% risk of permanent AV block, a complication not reported with posteroseptal ablations.

Right Free Wall Accessory Pathways

Ruder and associates[34] showed in a canine model that high-energy discharges along the tricuspid anulus could consistently produce transmural injury at the anulus that might be expected to disrupt anomalous conduction. Although there were no perforations or obvious hemodynamic deterioration, higher energies (200 to 400 J) occasionally produced inflammation of the adventitia of adjacent right coronary arteries. Lower energies (50 to 100 J) produced transmural necrosis at the anulus but without effects on adjacent coronary arteries.

There have been very few reports of successful right free wall accessory pathway ablations in humans.[35-37] In addition, in one instance right coronary artery spasm occurred immediately after an unsuccessful ablation procedure.[38] We have attempted ablation of a single patient with a right lateral accessory pathway and a diminutive right coronary artery and succeeded in only modifying pathway conduction.

Permanent Junctional Reciprocating Tachycardia

The tachycardia mechanism involved in permanent junctional reciprocating tachycardia (PJRT) consists of conduction anterogradely via the AV node and retrogradely via an accessory pathway with decremental (or "nodelike") conduction properties located immediately posterior to the AV node.[39] There have been several reports of successful ablation of this accessory pathway using discharges delivered just outside the coronary sinus os, similar to the technique described for ablation of posteroseptal accessory pathways.[40-42]

ABLATION OF VENTRICULAR TACHYCARDIA

Because of the prevalence of recurrent ventricular tachycardia and the persistent difficulty in adequate pharmacologic control, it was hoped that catheter ablation of the reentry focus responsible for ventricular tachycardia would come to play a prominent role in its management. Early reports by Hartzler[43] of success in three patients with ventricular tachycardia were encouraging. With further experience, however, ablation of ventricular tachycardia has proved to be at best only modestly effective with a relatively high complication rate.

Technique

The substrate for ventricular tachycardia in patients with prior myocardial infarction is felt to be an area, usually on the border of scar, of altered conduction giving rise to microreentry. This area of focal reentry can be mapped in the electrophysiology laboratory during induced ventricular tachycardia to an accuracy of 4 cm.[44-46] By making use of further, more accurate mapping at the time of aneurysmectomy and endocardial resection and/or cryoablation, surgical control of ventricular tachycardia can be satisfactorily achieved with a success rate of 60 to 85% and an operative mortality of 10%.[47-50] In theory a high-energy discharge applied to the area of reentry by way of a percutaneous electrode catheter could similarly destroy a sufficient amount of tissue to effectively control ventricular tachycardia. The ventricular tachycardias that are suitable for catheter ablation must of necessity be hemodynamically well-tolerated to permit detailed mapping with catheters to localize the origin of the arrhythmia.

A number of investigators have analyzed the effects of high-energy discharges in the canine ventricle.[51-53] Discrete areas of tissue destruction can be reliably produced with ventricular perforations seen only at high energies. Although the induction of malignant ventricular tachyarrhythmias associated with the shock is frequently seen in animals,[51-53] this has proved to be less of a problem in humans.

Results

The reported results of ablation attempts in humans has been variable, in part because of the inherent difficulty of assessing success in any procedure applied to eradicate ventricular tachycardia. Because of the unpredictable and sporadic nature of arrhythmia prevalence, long-term follow-up is necessary. In a patient with arrhythmia occurrence once a year, a postprocedure, arrhythmia-free interval of 2 years may not necessarily indicate success. Patients frequently are diagnosed with multiple clinically occurring tachycardia morphologies; eradication of only one morphologic type may prove, with time, to be of only marginal benefit. Similarly, even in a patient with a single spontaneously occurring morphology, other morphologies may be induced during electrophysiology studies before or after the procedure. These so-called "nonclinical" ventricular tachycardia morphologies may become "clinical" over the long term. Continued tachycardia inducibility of any morphology at the time of follow-up electrophysiology study must be considered ominous. Finally, the use of antiarrhythmic drugs after the procedure that were not used previously or of drugs with long washout periods (amiodarone) given before the procedure often confounds evaluation of long-term success. It appears prudent to use the same rigorous criteria for ablation success that have been applied to surgery for ventricular tachycardia.

Three large series of ablation procedures for ventricular tachycardia have been published.[54-56] The Percutaneous Cardiac Mapping and Ablation Registry (PCMAR) recently reported on 141 patients.[54] One ablative session was used in 78% and the remainder underwent two to four separate sessions. Over a follow-up of 12 ± 10 months, 34 patients (24%) are asymptomatic without drugs, 59 patients (42%) have arrhythmia control with concomitant drug therapy, and 48 patients (34%) failed to respond. Of those 118 patients tested with programmed ventricular stimulation, 43 patients (27%) were not inducible following the procedure.

Seven procedure-related deaths (defined as death occurring within 24 hours) occurred. These were in patients who were moribund at the time of the procedure. Other serious in-hospital complications developed in an additional 23 patients including ventricular fibrillation 5 days after the procedure in 1 patient, hypotension in 12 patients, pericarditis in 4, systemic emboli in 3, myocardial infarction in 2, ventricular perforation in 1, and sepsis in 2 patients. Fourteen patients died suddenly 2 weeks to 23 months after the ablation.

Morady and co-workers[56] reported on 33 patients. Fifteen patients (45%) have had no arrhythmia recurrence over a period of 15.5 ± 10 months. There were no procedure-related deaths and serious in-hospital complications occurred in five patients. Ten patients (33%)

were not inducible at the time of follow-up study. Six patients died suddenly 2 weeks to 18 months after the ablation.

Fontaine and colleagues[55] have consistently reported excellent clinical results. Of 38 patients ablated, 34 patients (89%) were controlled long-term during a follow-up period of 19 ± 13 months (range 0 to 43 months). Of these, 16 patients (42%) have also required antiarrhythmic drug therapy. There were three deaths in the 24 hours following ablation. Sixteen of 24 patients tested (66%) were not inducible at the time of follow-up study. Data interpretation is difficult, however, since 21 patients have been placed on amiodarone therapy after the ablation. Three patients died suddenly 4 to 22 months after the ablation.

A summary of these series is shown in Table 35-3. It should be noted that the data of both Morady and Fontaine may be included in the PCMAR report. However, a separate analysis of the latter two investigators' data points out the wide variability in both success rates and complications.

At Sequoia Hospital we have performed ablation procedures for ventricular tachycardia in nine patients. The origin of the ventricular tachycardia was from the left ventricle in eight of the nine patients. In seven of nine patients the ablation procedures were performed under emergency conditions for incessant or intractable recurrent ventricular tachycardia in patients who had failed amiodarone and were not excellent candidates for endocardial resection. The average energy used was 455 ± 260 J (range 200 to 900 J). The two patients who had the procedure performed electively remained with inducible sustained ventricular tachycardia and were considered failed ablation attempts. Among the seven patients with incessant tachycardia treated under emergent conditions the procedure was a long-term success in three. All three patients remained with inducible ventricular tachycardia and were kept on previously ineffective antiarrhythmic drug therapy. In each of the three patients the incessant tachycardia was controlled at the time of the procedure and has not recurred during the period of follow-up. Our experience with ablation for ventricular tachycardia suggests that it is unlikely to provide complete long-term cures when de-

Table 35-3. Ablation For Ventricular Tachycardia

	Total Patients (No.)	*Arrhythmia Control Without Drugs (% of Patients)*	*Arrhythmia Control with Drugs (% of Patients)*	*Ineffective (% of Patients)*	*Not Inducible (% of Patients)*	*Mean Follow-up (mo)*	*Deaths* (No.)*	*Late Sudden Deaths (No.)*
PCMAR[54]	141	24	42	34	27	12	7	14
Morady, et al.[56]	33	27	27	45	33	16	0	6
Fontaine, et al.[55]	38	50	42	8	66	23	3	3

**Deaths within 24 hours of procedure.*
NA, Not available; PCMAR, Percutaneous Cardiac Mapping and Ablation Registry.

fined as elimination of inducible ventricular tachycardia and long-term absence of tachycardia without antiarrhythmic therapy. It can, however, on occasion be lifesaving in patients with intractable ventricular tachycardia who have failed multiple drug trials and cannot be ideally approached by endocardial resection because of other underlying medical problems or because of extremely poor ventricular function.

In summary, ablation of ventricular tachycardia can be considered, at least in the short term, modestly successful. In most series, patients undergoing ablation procedures were generally not considered candidates for surgery because of the severity of their left ventricular dysfunction and they frequently had incessant ventricular tachycardia. For this reason, even the modest success seen with ablation is remarkable. Nevertheless, we feel that the use of ablation should be restricted to those patients who are not candidates for map-guided electrophysiologic surgery and whose arrhythmia prevalence precludes the use of automatic implantable cardioverter-defibrillators. When more sophisticated defibrillators, which include antitachycardia pacemaking capabilities, become available, the need for ablation for ventricular tachycardia may be less.

ABLATION OF ATRIAL TACHYCARDIA

For patients with incessant ectopic atrial tachycardias refractory to drug management, intraoperative mapping and surgical excision of the tachycardia focus has been used to control the arrhythmia.[57-60] This approach is limited by the tendency of the tachycardia to recur in a different area of what is usually a diffusely diseased atrium. Catheter ablation of ectopic atrial tachycardia has been performed in both children and adults with variable success.[61-63] In the series of patients reported by Davis and co-workers,[63] the procedure appeared to be most successful in the patients with discrete anatomic abnormalities responsible for the tachycardia, with long-term success achieved in one patient with tachycardia arising from a previous atrial septal defect repair and in another patient with tachycardia arising from the site of a previous division of a posteroseptal accessory pathway.

PROBLEMS AND FUTURE DIRECTIONS

For ablation to achieve wider applicability, limitations associated with the present technique must be overcome. Current problems and future directions in energy delivery, as well as problems specific to the different cardiac sites are summarized.

Energy Delivery

To date, most reports in humans on catheter ablation have used high-energy shocks delivered at the endocardial surface. High-speed cinematography has shown a yellow or blue gaseous "fireball" with violent shock waves produced by the sudden creation of gases associated with the vaporization of plasma and possibly by aftershocks generated by the collapse of the initial "fireball."[64-66] The mechanism responsible for tissue destruction in high-energy ablation is currently unknown. There is probably an element of direct *mechanical* damage caused by the shock waves as described by Bardy and associates.[66] Direct *electrical* damage from the massive, abrupt voltage changes associated with the electrical discharge have been demonstrated both in an in-vitro canine epicardial preparation[67] and in cell culture.[68] Finally, *thermal* effects from the heat generated by the explosion may directly injure cells and plasma.[69]

It is probable that the desirable and undesirable effects of ablation are produced by different mechanisms. For example, it appears that barotrauma caused by the shock waves generated by the discharge is responsible for some of the adverse effects of ablation such as coronary sinus rupture or hypotension following intraventricular discharges. On the other hand, the deep tissue destruction necessary for disruption of conduction in the AV junction or accessory pathways is probably not due to barotrauma but rather the electrical or thermal effects of the discharge. Further research will be critical in determining the mechanism responsible for the desirable effects of ablation in order to control these factors more precisely and to eliminate the undesirable effects.

Other forms of energy delivery will play an increasing role in ablations. Because of convenience, standard defibrillators have usually been used. These typically deliver discharges with a dampened sinusoidal waveform of a relatively long duration (35 ms). It is now known that truncated exponential waveform of shorter duration (6 to 10 ms) may deliver similar amounts of current with considerably less barotrauma. "Cathodal" shocks, in which the ablating catheter is connected to the cathode of the defibrillator, are also associated with less barotrauma and less hemolysis than "anodal" shocks, and for this reason are probably preferable.[65]

Laser has been used percutaneously to achieve AV nodal block.[70] Lasers have also been employed in conjunction with endocardial resection and aneurysmectomy to destroy ventricular tachycardia foci at the time of open heart surgery.[71,72] For the laser to gain widespread use in percutaneous ablation procedures the catheter delivery system will require further refinement and the destructive energy will need to be carefully controlled.

In the immediate future, radiofrequency energy appears promising.[73] The energy delivered is in the form of a continuous sinusoidal waveform of high frequency (750 kHz), much like surgical electrocautery. Radiofrequency energy presumably causes tissue destruction by causing a localized area of heat that drives water out of the myocardium and results in coagulation necrosis. The advantages of radiofrequency energy are primarily that it delivers energy in a much more controlled fashion, producing discrete lesions without barotrauma and without the need for anesthesia. Preliminary reports in animals and humans are encouraging.[73,74]

AV Junctional Ablation

Because AV junctional ablation produces complete AV block requiring a permanent pacemaker, the procedure is currently limited to those patients with severely symptomatic, drug-refractory supraventricular tachyarrhythmias. Modification of impulse conduction by means of catheter ablation but leaving AV nodal conduction intact would be preferable in many patients. Attempts to reliably achieve this in both animals and humans using lower energy, more precisely directed discharges have been unsuccessful.[75,76] However, reports of AV conduction modification using cryoablation at the time of surgery and the 10% incidence of resumption of AV conduction but with symptom control reported by PCMAR suggests that it is feasible. More precise control over the amount of tissue destruction and therefore the degree of AV block may be possible using radiofrequency energy.[73]

Accessory Pathway Ablation

It is unlikely that high-energy discharges will have a role in disrupting accessory pathways located along the left free wall because of the risk of coronary sinus rupture. Huang and co-workers[77] and Langberg and associates,[78] using canine models, have reported that radiofrequency energy delivered by the use of catheters placed in the coronary sinus reliably produces transmural necrosis at the anulus without deleterious effects on the coronary sinus or left circumflex coronary artery. Accessory pathways on the left free wall are frequently broad and have divergent atrial and ventricular insertion points. Surgical experience indicates that division of the pathway is most often successful with wide incisions. It is likely that, for many patients, successful ablation of left free wall pathways will require substantial destruction of tissue along the length of the coronary sinus.

Ventricular Tachycardia Ablation

Ablation of ventricular tachycardia presents the greatest challenges. The lack of precise endocardial mapping and incomplete knowledge of the pathophysiology of the arrhythmia are significant limitations. With presently available catheters, the accuracy of locating ventricular tachycardia foci is approximately 4 cm^2. Until more precise mapping catheters are available, improvement in the success rate of ventricular tachycardia ablation is unlikely. The critically ill nature of these patients and the inability to tolerate sustained ventricular tachycardia in many cases further complicate widespread use of ablation. Intraaneurysmal and mural thrombi are frequently encountered on or near the area of endocardium identified as the origin of ventricular tachycardia at the time of surgery. The dissipation of energy of any form of ablation by these thrombi will need to be overcome. Many patients undergoing intraoperative epicardial and endocardial mapping with extensive destruction by endocardial resection and/or cryoablation still fail to have their ventricular tachycardia eliminated. It seems unlikely that these patients would be "cured" by the comparatively limited destruction achieved by catheter ablation.

REFERENCES

1. Scheinman, M.M., Morady, R., Hess, D.S., and Gonzalez, R.: Catheter-induced ablation of the atrioventricular junction to control refractory supraventricular arrhythmias, J. Am. Med. Assoc. **248:**851-855, 1982.
2. Gallagher, J.J., Svenson, R.H., Kasell, J.H., German, L.D., Bardy, G.H., Broughton, A., and Critelli, G.: Catheter technique for closed-chest ablation of the atrioventricular conduction system, N. Engl. J. Med. **306:**194-200, 1982.
3. Starzl, T.E., Gaertner, R.A., and Baher, R.R.: Acute complete heart block in dogs, Circulation **12:**82-86, 1955.
4. Starzl, T.E., and Gaertner, R.A.: Chronic heart block in dogs: a new method of production, Circulation **12:**259-269, 1955.
5. Steiner, C., and Kovalik, A.T.: A simple technique for production of chronic complete heart block in dogs, J. Appl. Physiol. **25:**631-632, 1968.
6. Smyth, N.P., and Magassy, C.L.: Experimental heart block in the dog: an improved method, J. Thorac. Cardiovasc. Surg. **59:**201-205, 1970.
7. Sealy, W.C., Hackel, D.B., and Seaber, A.V.: A study of methods for surgical interruption of the His bundle, J. Thorac. Cardiovasc. Surg. **73:**424-430, 1977.
8. Harrison, L., Gallagher, J.J., Kasell, J., Anderson, R.H., Mikat, E., Hackel, D.B., and Wallace, A.G.: Cryosurgical ablation of the A-V node-His bundle: a new method for producing A-V block, Circulation **55:**463-470, 1977.
9. Fisher, V.J., Lee, R.J., Christianson, L.C., and Kavaler, F.: Production of chronic atrioventricular block in dogs without thoracotomy, J. Appl. Physiol. **21:**1119-1121, 1966.
10. Turina, M., Babotai, I., and Wegmann, W.: Production of chronic atrioventricular block in dogs without thoracotomy, Cardiovasc. Res. **2:**389-393, 1968.
11. Beazell, J.W., Tan, K.S., Fewkes, J.L., Furmanski, M., and Fisher, D.A.: Technique for the production of permanent lesions in the intracardiac conduction system (abstract), Clin. Res. **25:**141, 1977.
12. Beazell, J.W., Adomian, G.E., Furmanski, M., and Tan, K.S.: Experimental production of complete heart block by electrocoagulation in the closed chest dog, Am. Heart J. **104:**1328-1334, 1982.
13. Gonzalez, R., Scheinman, M., Margaretten, W., and Rubinstein, M.: Closed-chest electrode-catheter technique for His bundle ablation in dogs, Am. J. Physiol. **241:**H283-287, 1981.
14. Gonzalez, R., Scheinman, M., Bharati, S., and Lev, M.: Closed chest permanent atrioventricular block in dogs, Am. Heart J. **105:**461, 1983.
15. Eldar, M., Griffin, J.C., Seger, J.J., Abbott, J.A., Ruder, M.A., Davis, J.C., Herre, J.M., Scheinman, M.M.: Catheter atrioventricular junctional ablation in patients with accessory pathways, PACE **9:**810-820, 1986.
16. Bhandari, A., Morady, F., Shen, E.N., Schwartz, A.B., Botnivic, E., and Scheinman, M.M.: Catheter induced His bundle ablation in a patient with reentrant tachycardia associated with a nodoventricular tract, J. Am. Coll. Cardiol. **4:**611-616, 1984.
17. Ross, D.L., Johnson, D.C., Denniss, A.R., Cooper, M.J., Richards, D.A., and Uther, J.B.: Curative surgery for atrioventricular junctional (AV nodal) reentrant tachycardia, J. Am. Coll. Cardiol. **6:**1383-1392, 1985.
18. Cox, J.L., Holman, W.L., and Cain, M.E.: Cry-

osurgical treatment of atrioventricular node reentrant tachycardia, Circulation **76:**1329-1336, 1987.

19. Guiraudon, G., Klein, G.J., Sharma, A.D., and Yee, R.: Pathological insights gained by direct surgical approach to atrioventricular nodal reentrant tachycardias (abstracts), Circulation **76**(suppl. 4):IV-500, 1987.
20. Scheinman, M.M., and Evans-Bell, T.: Catheter ablation of the atrioventricular junction: a report of the Percutaneous Mapping and Ablation Registry, Circulation **70:**1024-1029, 1984.
21. Scheinman, M.M., and Evans, G.T.: Catheter electrical ablation of cardiac arrhythmias: a summary report of the Percutaneous Cardiac Mapping and Ablation Registry. In Brugada, P., and Wellens, H.J.J., editors: Cardiac arrhythmias: where to go from here?, Mount Kisco, N.Y., 1987, Futura Publishing Co., Inc.
22. Marchese, A.C., Pressley, J.C., Sintetos, A.L., Gilbert, M.R., and German, L.D.: Cryosurgical versus catheter ablation of the atrioventricular junction, Am. J. Cardiol. **59:**870-873, 1987.
23. Gallagher, J.J., Sealy, W.C., Cox, J.L., Geman, L.D., Kassell, J.H., Bardy, G.H., and Packer, D.L.: Results of surgery for preexcitation caused by accessory atrioventricular pathways in 267 consecutive cases. In Josephson, M.E., and Wellens, H.J.J., editors: Tachycardias: mechanisms, diagnosis, treatment, Philadelphia, 1984, Lea & Febiger.
24. Cox, J.L., Gallagher, J.J., and Cain, M.E.: Experience with 118 consecutive patients undergoing operation for the Wolff-Parkinson-White syndrome, J. Thorac. Cardiovasc. Surg. **90:**490-501, 1985.
25. Gallagher, J.J., Pritchett, E.L.C., Sealy, W.C., Kasell, J., and Wallace, A.G.: The preexcitation syndromes, Prog. Cardiovasc. Dis. **20:**285-327, 1978.
26. Brodman, R., and Fisher, J.D.: Evaluation of a catheter technique for ablation of accessory pathways near the coronary sinus using a canine model, Circulation **67:**923-929, 1983.
27. Coltorti, F., Bardy, G.H., Reichenbach, D., Greene, H.L., Thomas, R., Breazeale, D.G., Alferness, C., and Ivey, T.D.: Catheter-mediated electrical ablation of the posterior septum via the coronary sinus: electrophysiologic and histologic observations in dogs, Circulation **72:**612-622, 1985.
28. Fisher, J.D., Brodman, R., Kim, S.G., Matos, J.A., Brodman, L.E., Wallerson, D., and Waspe, L.E.: Attempted nonsurgical electrical ablation of accessory pathways via the coronary sinus in the Wolff-Parkinson-White syndrome, J. Am. Coll. Cardiol. **4:**685-694, 1984.
29. Morady, F., and Scheinman, M.M.: Transvenous catheter ablation of a posteroseptal accessory pathway in a patient with the Wolff-Parkinson-White syndrome, N. Engl. J. Med. **310:**705-707, 1984.
30. Bardy, G.H., Poole, J.E., Coltorti, F., Ivey, T.D., Block, T.A., Trobaugh, G.B., Greene, H.L.: Catheter ablation of a concealed accessory pathway, Am. J. Cardiol. **54:**1366-1368, 1984.
31. Morady, F., Scheinman, M.M., Winston, S.A., DiCarlo, L.A., Jr., Davis, J.C., Griffin, J.C., Ruder, M., Abbott, J.A., and Eldar, M.: Ablation of posteroseptal accessory pathways, Circulation **72:**170-177, 1985.
32. Bardy, G.H., Ivey, T.D., Coltorti, F., Stewart, R.B., Johnson, G., and Greene, H.L.: Developments, complications and limitations of catheter mediated electrical ablation of posterior accessory atrioventricular pathways, Am. J. Cardiol. **61:**309-316, 1988.
33. Ruder, M.A., Mead, R.H., Gaudiani, V., Buch, W.S., Smith, N.A., Winkle, R.A.: Transvenous catheter ablation of extranodal accessory pathways, J. Am. Coll. Cardiol., 1988. (In press.)
34. Ruder, M.A., Davis, J.C., Eldar, M., Finbeiner, W., and Scheinman, M.M.: Effects of catheter-delivered electrical discharges near the tricuspid anulus in dogs, J. Am. Coll. Cardiol. **10:**693-701, 1987.
35. Weber, H., and Schmitz, L.: Catheter technique for closed-chest ablation of an accessory atrioventricular pathway (letter), N. Engl. J. Med. **308:**653-654, 1983.
36. Jackman, W.M., Friday, K.J., Scherlag, B.J., Dehning, M.M., Schechter, E., Reynolds, D.W., Olson, E.G., Berbari, E.J., Harrison, L.A., and Lazzara, R.: Direct endocardial recording from an accessory atrioventricular pathway: localization of the site of block, effect of antiarrhythmic drugs, and attempt at nonsurgical ablation, Circulation **68:**906-916, 1983.
37. Ward, D.E., and Camm, A.J.: Treatment of tachycardias associated with the Wolff-Parkinson-White syndrome by transvenous electrical

ablation of accessory pathways, Br. Heart J. **53:**64-68, 1985.

38. Hartzler, G.O., Giorgi, L.V., Diehl, A.M., and Hamaker, W.R.: Right coronary spasm complicating electrode catheter ablation of a right lateral accessory pathway, J. Am. Coll. Cardiol. **6:**250-253, 1985.
39. Critelli, G., Gallagher, J.J., Monda, V., Coltorti, F., Scherillo, M., and Rossi, L.: Anatomic and electrophysiologic substrate of the permanent form of junctional reciprocating tachycardia, J. Am. Coll. Cardiol. **4:**601-610, 1984.
40. Critelli, G., Gallagher, J.J., Perticone, F., Monda, V., Scherillo, M., and Condorelli, M.: Transvenous catheter ablation of the accessory atrioventricular pathway in the permanent form of junctional reciprocating tachycardia, Am. J. Cardiol. **55:**1639-1641, 1985.
41. Critelli, G., Gallagher, J.J., Monda, V., Scherillo, M., and Condorelli, M.: Catheter ablation of accessory pathway in the permanent form of junctional reciprocating tachycardia, Arch. Mal. Coeur **78:**49-55, 1985.
42. Gang, E.S., Oseran, D., Rosenthal, M., Manel, W.J., Deng, Z.W., Meesmann, M., and Peter, T.: Closed chest catheter ablation of an accessory pathway in a patient with permanent junctional reciprocating tachycardia, J. Am. Coll. Cardiol. **6:**1167-1171, 1985.
43. Hartzler, G.O.: Electrode catheter ablation of refractory focal ventricular tachycardia, J. Am. Coll. Cardiol. **2:**1107-1113, 1983.
44. Josephson, M.E., Horowitz, L.N., Spielman, S.R., Waxman, H.L., and Greenspan, A.M.: Role of catheter mapping in the preoperative evaluation of ventricular tachycardia, Am. J. Cardiol. **49:**207-220, 1982.
45. Josephson, M.E., Horowitz, L.N., Spielman, S.R., Greenspan, A.M., VandePol, C., Harken, A.H.: Comparison of endocardial catheter mapping with intraoperative mapping of ventricular tachycardia, Circulation **61:**395-404, 1980.
46. Josephson, M.E., Horowitz, L.N., Farshidi, A., Spear, J.F., Kastor, J.A., and Moore, E.N.: Recurrent sustained ventricular tachycardia. 2. Endocardial mapping, Circulation **57:**440-447, 1978.
47. Harken, A.H., Horowitz, L.N., and Josephson, M.E.: Comparison of standard aneurysmectomy and aneurysmectomy with directed endocardial resection for the treatment of recurrent sustained ventricular tachycardia, J. Thorac. Cardiovasc. Surg. **80:**527-534, 1980.
48. Lawrie, G.M., Wyndham, C.R., Krafchek, J., Luck, J.C., Roberts, R., and DeBakey, M.E.: Progress in the surgical treatment of cardiac arrhythmias: initial experience of 90 patients, J. Am. Med. Assoc. **254:**1464-1468, 1985.
49. Krafchek, J., Lawrie, G.M., Roberts, R., Magro, S.A., and Wyndham, C.R.: Surgical ablation of ventricular tachycardia: improved results with a map-directed regional approach, Circulation **73:**1239-1247, 1986.
50. Haines, D.E., Lerman, B.B., Kron, I.L., and DiMarco, J.P.: Surgical ablation of ventricular tachycardia with sequential map-guided subendocardial resection: electrophysiologic assessment and long-term follow-up, Circulation **77:**131-141, 1988.
51. Lerman, B.B., Weiss, J.L., Bulkley, B.H., Becker, L.C., and Weisfeldt, M.L.: Myocardial injury and induction of arrhythmia by direct current shock delivered via endocardial catheters in dogs, Circulation **69:**1006-1012, 1984.
52. Kempf, F.C., Jr., Falcone, R.A., Iozzo, R.V., and Josephson, M.E.: Anatomic and hemodynamic effects of catheter-delivered ablation energies in the ventricle, Am. J. Cardiol. **56:**373-377, 1985.
53. Davis, J.C., Finkebeiner, W., Ruder, M.A., DiCarlo, L., Jr., Matsubara, T., Chu, W., Winston, S.A., Bharati, S., Scheinman, M.M., and Lev, M.: Histologic changes and arrhythmogenicity after discharged through transseptal catheter electrode, Circulation **74:**637-644, 1986.
54. Scheinman, M.M., and Evans, G.T.: Catheter electrical ablation of cardiac arrhythmias: a summary report of the Percutaneous Cardiac Mapping and Ablation Registry. In Brugada, P., and Wellens, H.J.J., editors: Cardiac arrhythmias: where to go from here?, Mount Kisco, N.Y., 1987, Futura Publishing Co., Inc.
55. Fontaine, G., Tonet, J.L., Frank, R., Gallais, Y., Touzel, I., Kounde, S., Fareng, G., Baraka, M., and Grosgogeat, Y.: Electrode catheter ablation of resistant ventricular tachycardia by endocavitary fulguration associated with antiarrhythmic therapy: experience in 38 patients. In Brugada, P., and Wellens, H.J.J., editors: Cardiac arrhythmias: where to go from here?,

Mount Kisco, N.Y., 1987, Futura Publishing Co., Inc.

56. Morady, F., Scheinman, M.M., DiCarlo, L.A., Jr., Davis, J.C., Herre, J.M., Griffin, J.C., Winston, S.A., de Buitleir, M., Hantler, C.B., and Wahr, J.A.: Catheter ablation of ventricular tachycardia with intracardiac shocks: results in 33 patients, Circulation **75:**1037-1049, 1987.
57. Wyndham, C.R., Arnsdorf, M.F., Levitsky, S., Smith, T.C., Dhingra, R.C., Denes, P., Rosen, K.M.: Successful surgical excision of focal paroxysmal atrial tachycardia: observations in vivo and in vitro, Circulation **62:**1365-1372, 1980.
58. Anderson, K.P., Stinson, E.B., and Mason, J.W.: Surgical exclusion of focal paroxysmal atrial tachycardia, Am. J. Cardiol. **49:**869-874, 1982.
59. Josephson, M.E., Spear, J.F., Harken, A.H., Horowitz, L.N., and D'Orio, R.J.: Surgical excision of automatic atrial tachycardia: anatomic and electrophysiologic correlates, Am. Heart J. **104:**1076-1085, 1982.
60. Gillette, P.C., Garson, A., Jr., Hesslein, P.S., Karpawich, P.P., Tierney, R.C., Cooley, D.A., and McNamara, D.G.: Successful surgical treatment of atrial, junctional and ventricular tachycardia unassociated with accessory connections in infants and children, Am. Heart J. **102:**984-991, 1981.
61. Silka, M.J., Gillette, P.C., Garson, A., Jr., and Zinner, A.: Transvenous catheter ablation of a right atrial automatic ectopic tachycardia, J. Am. Coll. Cardiol. **5:**999-1001, 1985.
62. Gillette, P.C., Wampler, D.G., Garson, A., Jr., Zinner, A., Ott, D., and Cooley, D.: Treatment of atrial automatic tachycardia by ablation procedures, J. Am. Coll. Cardiol. **6:**405-409, 1985.
63. Davis, J., Scheinman, M.M., Ruder, M.A., Griffin, J.C., Herre, J.M., Finkebeiner, W.E., Chin, M.C., and Eldar, M.: Ablation of cardiac tissues by an electrode catheter technique for treatment of ectopic supraventricular tachycardia in adults, Circulation **74:**1044-1053, 1986.
64. Downar, E., Harris, L., Parson, I.D., and Easty, A.: Characterization of catheter ablation with high speed cinematography (abstract), J. Am. Coll. Cardiol. **7:**131A, 1986.
65. Holt, P.M., and Boyd, E.G.: Hematologic effects of the high-energy endocardial ablation technique, Circulation **73:**1029-1036, 1986.
66. Bardy, G.H., Coltorti, F., Ivey, T.D., Alferness, C., Rackson, M., Hansen, K., Stewart, R., and Greene, H.L.: Some factors affecting bubble formation with catheter-mediated defibrillation pulses, Circulation **73:**525-538, 1986.
67. Levin, J.H., Spear, J.F., Weisman, H.F., Kadish, A.H., Prood, C., Siu, C.O., and Moore, E.N.: The cellular electrophysiologic changes induced by high-energy electrical ablation in canine myocardium, Circulation **73:**818-829, 1986.
68. Jones, J.L., Lepeschkin, E., Jones, R.E., and Rush, S.: Response of cultured myocardial cells to countershock-type electric field stimulation, Am. J. Physiol. **235:**H214-222, 1978.
69. Doherty, P.W., McLaughlin, P.R., Billingham, M., Kernoff, R., Goris, M.L., and Harrison, D.C.: Cardiac damage produced by direct current countershock applied to the heart, Am. J. Cardiol. **43:**225-232, 1979.
70. Narula, O.S., Bharati, S., Chan, M.C., Embi, A.A., and Lev, M.: Microtransection of the His bundle with laser radiation through a pervenous catheter: Correlation of histologic and electrophysiologic data, Am. J. Cardiol. **54:**186-192, 1984.
71. Saksena, S., Hussain, S.M., Gielchinski, I., Gadhoke, A., and Pantopoulos, D.: Intraoperative mapping-guided argon laser ablation of malignant ventricular tachycardia, Am. J. Cardiol. **59:**78-83, 1987.
72. Svenson, R.H., Gallagher, J.J., Selle, J.G., Zimmern, S.H., and Fedor, J.M.: Intraoperative laser photoablation of ventricular tachycardia (abstract), Circulation **74**(suppl. 2):II-461, 1986.
73. Huang, S.K., Bharati, S., Graham, A.R., Lev, M., Marcus, F.I., and Odell, R.C.: Closed chest catheter desiccation of the atrioventricular junction using radiofrequency energy—a new method of catheter ablation, J. Am. Coll. Cardiol. **9:**349-358, 1987.
74. Borggrefe, M., Budde, T., Podczeck, A., and Breithardt, G.: High frequency alternating current ablation of an accessory pathway in humans, J. Am. Coll. Cardiol. **10:**576-582, 1987.
75. Scheinman, M.M., Bharati, S., Wang, Y.S., Shapiro, W.A., and Lev, M.: Electrophysiologic and anatomic changes in the atrioventricular junction of dogs after direct-current shocks through tissue fixation catheters, Am. J. Cardiol. **55:**194-198, 1985.

76. McComb, J.M., McGovern, B.A., Garan, H., and Ruskin, J.N.: Modification of atrioventricular conduction using low energy transcatheter shocks (abstract), J. Am. Coll. Cardiol. **5**:454, 1985.

77. Huang, S.K., Graham, A.R., Bharati, S., Lee, M.A., and Gorman, G.: Chronic effect of radiofrequency catheter ablation of the coronary sinus (abstract), Circulation **76**(suppl. 4):IV-406, 1987.

78. Langberg, J., Griffin, J., Bharati, S., Lev, M., Chin, M., and Scheinman, M.: Radiofrequency catheter ablation in the coronary sinus, J. Am. Coll. Cardiol. **9**:99A, 1987.

Chapter 36

Transluminal Atherectomy

Matthew R. Selmon, MD
John B. Simpson, MD, FACC

Since the beginning of interventional vascular procedures by Dotter[1] and Gruentzig,[2] the problems of acute occlusion, vascular dissection, and restenosis have offered a formidable challenge. Acute occlusion within 24 hours following angioplasty occurs in 2 to 6%[3-5] of coronary procedures, presumably as a result of vascular dissection and thrombosis. Reports of restenosis rates range from 20 to 30%[6-8] for coronary arteries. For peripheral arteries, restenosis rates range from 20 to 60% after 1 year.[9-12] Despite increased experience, improved balloon technology, and pharmacologic manipulation, restenosis rates have remained relatively unchanged.

The resultant morbidity and mortality of acute occlusion syndrome, as well as the expense and anxiety of repeat procedures for restenosis, make these statistics unfavorable. In an effort to improve safety, efficacy, and long-term durability of transluminal revascularization, a new approach was devised for the percutaneous removal of atherosclerotic plaque. The term "atherectomy" was coined by Simpson[13] to denote percutaneous catheter-mediated removal of atheroma, applying otherwise standard interventional techniques. An atherectomy catheter has been designed for the percutaneous removal of atheroma, and the initial clinical experience is presented here.

PERIPHERAL TRANSLUMINAL ATHERECTOMY

Description of the Device

The peripheral atherectomy catheter is 70 cm long, with three components (Fig. 36-1). The distal component is a cylindrical housing with a 15- to 30-mm window in one side. Housings range in size from 7F through 11F. Opposite the housing window is a balloon support member that is usually inflated to pressures less than 40 psi to anchor the device in place during cutting. A fixed guidewire is attached distally and can be directed by torquing the catheter. Enclosed within the housing is a rotating cup-shaped cutter, attached to a cable that transverses the length of the cathe-

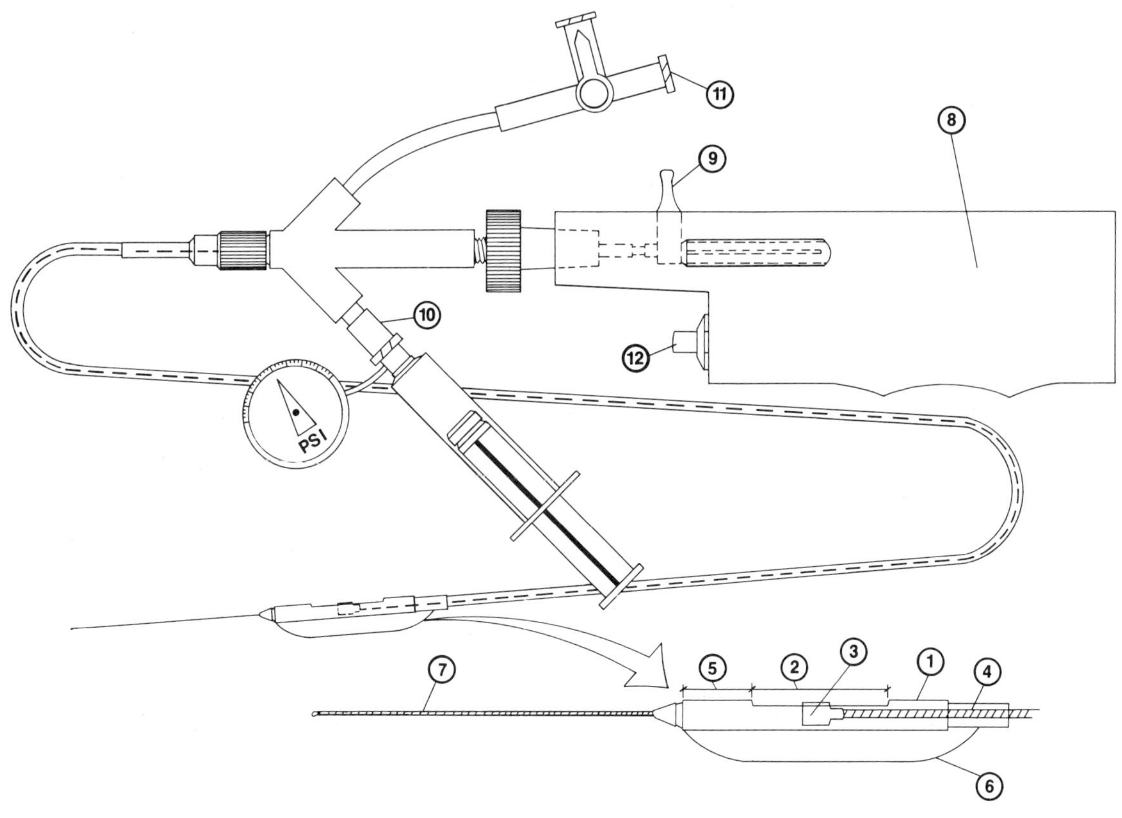

Fig. 36-1. Peripheral atherectomy system: *(1)* housing, *(2)* window, *(3)* cutter, *(4)* cutter drive cable, *(5)* collection area, *(6)* balloon, *(7)* fixed guidewire, *(8)* motor, *(9)* cutter-advancement lever, *(10)* balloon inflation port, *(11)* flush port, *(12)* on-off switch for motor drive unit.

ter and provides high-speed rotation for the cutter at approximately 2000 rpm. The cutter is manually advanced and retracted as needed. The middle component is a braided catheter that houses the cutter torque cable and provides rotational torque for positioning the housing. The proximal component is an assembly with ports for balloon inflation and access to the central lumen for flushing. A motor drive unit (MDU) is attached to the proximal end, and is battery operated, hand-held, and disposable. As seen in Fig. 36-2, the device is positioned across the stenosis, the balloon is inflated, and the cutter is activated and advanced. This shaves any material that protrudes into the housing and collects the material distally in the housing. Multiple cuts are made and removed; the procedure is repeated until the desired angiographic result is obtained.

Preclinical Experience

Early investigation of the atherectomy catheter involved trials with cadaver vessels. Peripheral vessels were used including iliac, superficial femoral, and popliteal as well as carotid arteries. We made 590 passes in 90 cadaver stenoses, retrieving 500 specimens, with only one perforation noted. These studies were felt to confirm the feasibility of a transluminal approach to revascularization, and clinical studies were subsequently begun.

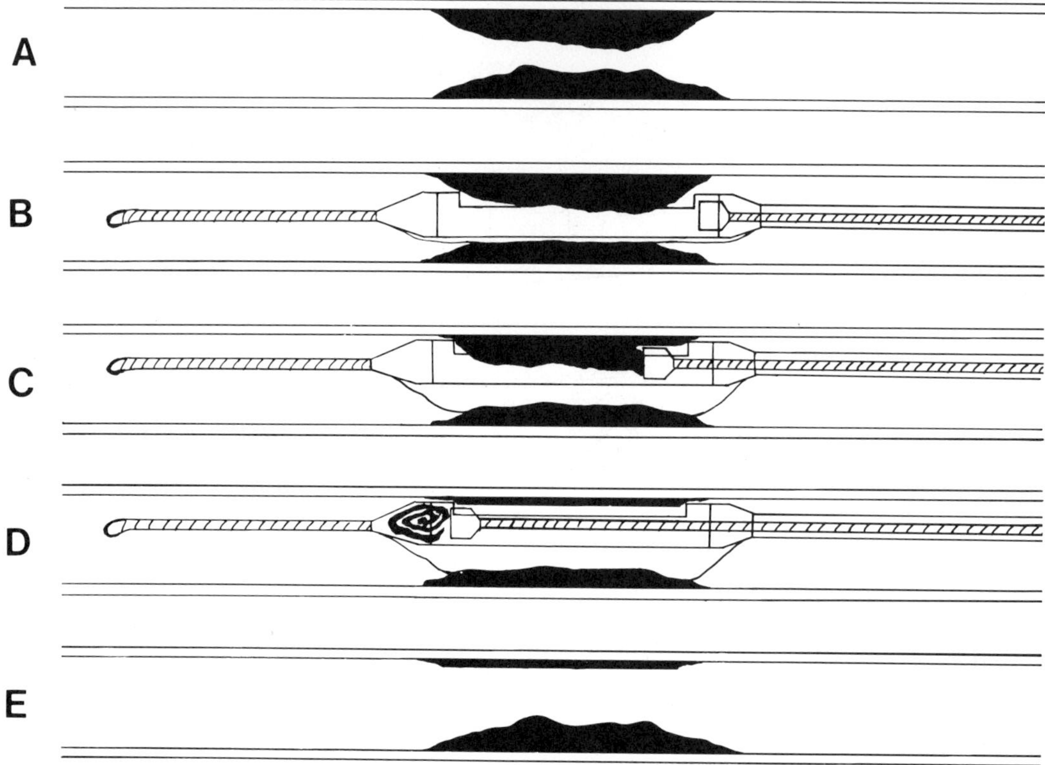

Fig. 36-2. Diagram of the atherectomy procedure. **A,** The lesion before atherectomy. **B,** Atherectomy catheter in position across the lesion. **C,** The balloon inflated and the cutter beginning to advance. **D,** The cutter fully advanced and the specimen trapped in the housing. **E,** The balloon deflated and the catheter removed.

Initial Clinical Experience

Initially, atherectomy was performed intraoperatively at the proximal or distal arteriotomy site. We performed 13 procedures in the operative setting. Angiographic results were favorable in all cases, with specimens retrieved in all cases. One complication of a small suspected calf embolus occurred without clinical sequelae. No acute occlusions or perforations occurred.

Current Clinical Status

Clinical trials for percutaneous atherectomy were begun in 1987 using the same indications as for peripheral angioplasty. These included significant symptoms, abnormal ankle-brachial indices, and angiographic stenoses appearing amenable to atherectomy. Long-segment total occlusions >10 cm were avoided unless recent occlusion was suspected clinically. Location of lesions included iliac, superficial femoral, profunda, popliteal, and anterior tibial arteries. Protocol included Doppler examination before, immediately after, then at 2 weeks, 2 months, and 6 months, with yearly follow-up afterward. Six-month angiography was requested of all patients, with approximately 78% compliance rate.

Patients were treated preatherectomy with aspirin and Dipyridamole, and continued postatherectomy with standard postangioplasty

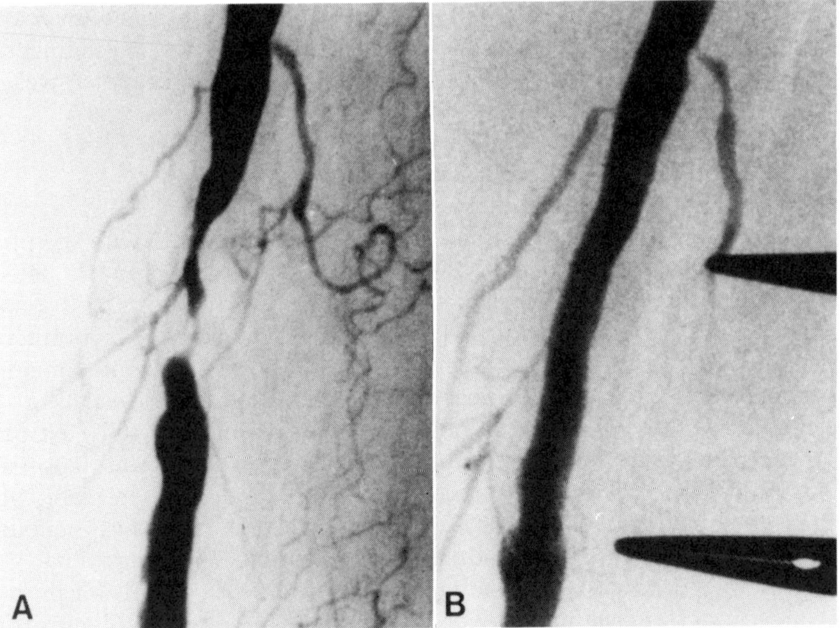

Fig. 36-3. Angiograms before and after atherectomy. **A,** Preatherectomy angiogram of a superficial femoral artery. **B,** Postatherectomy angiogram of the same artery.

therapy. During atherectomy, patients received 10,000 units heparin, which was not reversed with Protamine after the procedure. Most patients were discharged after one night of hospitalization. Examples of typical atherectomy findings can be seen in Fig. 36-3. Of note is the consistent smooth residual lumen postatherectomy.

Results

Between August 1986 and March 1988, 102 patients underwent peripheral atherectomy at Sequoia Hospital in Redwood City, California; 139 procedures were performed in the patient population, addressing 176 lesions. Distribution by location involved the superficial femoral artery (SFA) in 82%, iliac in 9%, and popliteal in 9%. Success was defined by a decrease in luminal narrowing to <50%, increase in ankle-brachial index by 0.1, and symptomatic improvement of at least one Fontaine classification. Of the 139 procedures, 124 were successful (89%). Mean stenosis was reduced from 76% to 24% angiographically, with a mean ankle-brachial index increase of 0.17.

Complications

One of the original goals of atherectomy was to devise a technique that added not only predictability but safety to existing technologies. One acute occlusion out of 132 procedures (0.8%) required bypass surgery. The occlusion occurred 24 hours following popliteal atherectomy and presumably was a result of thrombosis. There were no other serious complications, and specifically there were no perforations or amputations. For the minor complications with no significant hemodynamic consequences, the occurrence rate was 6.6%. Both rates are below the accepted norms for interventional complications.

Follow-up

Follow-up protocol included ankle-brachial indices immediately postatherectomy, then at 2 weeks, 2 months, 6 months, and yearly thereafter, with 6-month follow-up angiography. All stenoses were measured, and restenosis was defined as >50% luminal diameter stenosis, return to preatherectomy clinical status, and deterioration of ankle-brachial indices to preatherectomy state. The compliance rate for follow-up angiography was 74% (asymptomatic patients seem to be less likely to return for repeat angiography). With closer evaluation statistically, the follow-up angiographic group can be divided into two populations. Group A consists of patients in whom a >30% residual remained following atherectomy; Group B patients had <30% residual following atherectomy. When >30% residual stenoses remained, restenosis rates were high, approximately 67%. If a <30% residual remained, restenosis rates were approximately 17%. After this clinical realization, the procedure technique was changed (approximately December 1986) to be relatively more aggressive in atheroma removal. Since that time, restenosis rates of approximately 10% have been achieved in the femoral and popliteal arteries.

CORONARY ATHERECTOMY

Coronary AtheroCath

After considerable experience with peripheral atherectomy, the cut and retrieval technology was applied to the coronary circulation. The catheter had to fulfill additional demands, however, including reduction in size, adaptation to "over-the-wire" technology, ability to go through a guiding catheter, and most important, flexibility. After multiple prototypes, the current design evolved, which is a scaled-down, flexible, over-the-wire version of the peripheral device. The coronary atherectomy catheter is available in 5.5F, 6F, and 7F outer diameters with 7 to 10 mm window lengths. An 11F guiding catheter with various tip configurations was used in all cases.

Clinical Experience

Initial experience with coronary atherectomy involved prototype catheters of various designs. Case selection required circumstances conceptually favoring atherectomy, such as multiple previous angioplasties with recurrent restenosis, ostial or eccentric lesions, or inability to fully expand the dilatation balloon. High-grade stenoses in either ostial or proximal location were chosen. All native vessels, as well as saphenous vein grafts, are accessible if the proximal vessel is relatively straight. Protocols for preprocedure and postprocedure were identical to accepted standards for percutaneous transluminal coronary angioplasty (PTCA), including calcium-channel blockers, nitrates, and aspirin before the procedure, and standard antiplatelet drugs postatherectomy. Patients received 10,000 units of heparin preatherectomy, with additional heparin as needed during prolonged procedures. Follow-up treadmill testing within 1 week and 3 months along with 6-month follow-up angiography are scheduled.

Results

A total of 33 patients have undergone coronary atherectomy as of April 1988. The first nine procedures (group I) were initial study patients using a variety of different catheter designs. The other 24 procedures (group II) were performed using the current design catheter. Of the total group, tissue was obtained from 21 patients, with atherectomy as a definitive procedure in 12. Of the group II patients, 17 had tissue removed, with definitive atherectomy in 65%. Typical findings in coronary atherectomy again show a smooth residual lumen without the dissection or haziness typically seen following PTCA. This is dramatically evident in eccentric stenoses, which usually create large angiographic dissections following balloon angioplasty. An average of five passes per lesion were made with the cutter, with an average of four specimens retrieved per stenosis. Mean diameter stenosis was reduced from 87% to 34% in group II patients. In the patients with atherectomy failure, the mode of failure usually involved inability to place the device across the stenosis owing to tortuosity, severity of the stenosis, or inadequate guiding catheter support. Occasionally the device was positioned but tissue was not removed; all such patients had subsequent balloon angioplasty.

Complications

Only one serious complication occurred in the initial coronary atherectomy group. This was an air embolus into the left anterior descending artery, as a result of catheter failure of an early device design. No myocardial infarction resulted, however. Minor complications included groin hematomas (none requiring repair), transfusion, or prolonged hospitalization.

Histopathology

Atheroma retrieval during percutaneous transluminal atherectomy has provided a biopsy-like tool for studying the ongoing atherosclerotic and restenosis processes. Postmortem examination of angioplasty restenosis lesions has previously suggested myointimal hyperplasia or fibrocellular hyperplasia as the predominant cause of restenosis. Thus far, atherectomy findings, in peripheral as well as coronary arteries have supported this conclusion.

In original atherosclerotic lesions, typical findings are old organized plaque with fibrous cap and lipid core, frequently with components of intraplaque and surface thrombus in varying stages of organization. Ulceration is often evident, with disruption of plaque and hemorrhage into and below the atheroma. In postangioplasty, as well as postatherectomy restenosis lesions, two separate populations of cells exist. This is frequently appreciated grossly as well as microscopically, with old atheroma appearing dense and yellowish and restenosis lesions appearing white and glistening and somewhat translucent. Microscopically in restenosis lesions, old atheroma is seen underlying the proliferative restenosis process above, and is typically devoid of cells and densely collagenous. Overlying the old atheroma is a layer of new growth, densely cellular with only loose collagen. The cells appear to be modified smooth muscle cells or fibrocytes, with irregular nuclear and stellate cytoplasmic configuration, all suggesting metabolic activity. This proliferative myointimal hyperplasia is typically devoid of other characteristics of atherosclerosis such as lipids, calcification, and foam cells. Occasional macrophages and lymphocytes are seen, however. In the more mature restenosis lesions, neovascularization is frequently seen. Occasionally, stenosis removal yields only organized thrombus. This has been seen both in original lesions and in postangioplasty restenosis lesions. This biopsy technique should aid in the future study and understanding of atherogenesis and restenosis.

FUTURE DIRECTIONS

Percutaneous transluminal atherectomy now appears not only feasible but predictable and safe, in both the peripheral and coronary circulations. Future directions include improvements in catheter design to allow larger specimens, extended collection chambers, and increased flexibility to facilitate smaller guiding catheters. These improvements may increase accessibility to tortuous and distal vessels. Potentially, areas previously felt to be poor candidates for PTCA, such as ostial lesions, eccentric lesions, and possibly left main coronary lesions, may be well suited for atherectomy. Further indications await follow-up studies for long-term effects of atherectomy. Other areas of active investigation include modified smooth muscle cultures of retrieved restenosis lesions, in an attempt to further understand and possibly pharmocologically modify the restenosis process. Other promising and exciting new technologies may also be used in combination with atherectomy, such as angioscopy and new intraluminal imaging devices to further improve the predictability of the intervention.

SUMMARY

Interventional technology and experience has progressed rapidly over the past 10 years. The persistent problems of acute occlusion and restenosis, however, limit the effectiveness and long-term durability of conventional balloon angioplasty. Atherectomy has now been shown to be effective, reliable, and safe in the peripheral as well as in the coronary circulations. The technique appears to reduce acute occlusion as well as restenosis rates in peripheral stenoses. The preliminary coronary experience suggests a similar pattern; however, confirmation awaits further follow-up. As with any investigational technique, objective data must be collected and compared with conventional therapy. Atherectomy currently offers an alternative therapy for most patients with angioplasty restenoses and may provide useful therapy for many other patients with eccentric or calcified lesions who previously were thought to be poor candidates for conventional angioplasty techniques.

REFERENCES

1. Dotter, C.T., and Judkins, M.P.: Transluminal treatment of arteriosclerotic obstruction: description of a new technique and a preliminary report of its application, Circulation **30:**654-670, 1964.
2. Gruentzig, A.R., Senning, A., Siegenthaler, W.E.: Nonoperative dilatation of coronary artery stenosis: percutaneous transluminal angioplasty, N. Engl. J. Med. **301:**61-68, 1979.
3. Cowley, M.J., Dorros, G., Kelsey, S.F., Van Raden, M., Detre, K.M.: Emergency coronary bypass surgery after coronary angioplasty: the National Heart, Lung and Blood Institute's Percutaneous Transluminal Coronary Angioplasty Registry Experience, Am. J. Cardiol. **53:**22C-26C, 1984.
4. Bredlau, C.E., Roubin, G.S., Leimgruber, P.P., Douglas, J.S., Jr., King, S.B. III, Gruentzig, A.R.: In-hospital morbidity and mortality in patients undergoing elective coronary angioplasty, Circulation **72:**1044-1052, 1985.
5. Simpfendorfer, C., Belardi, J., Bellamy, G., Galan, K., Franco, I., Hollman, J.: Frequency, management and follow-up of patients with acute coronary occlusions after percutaneous coronary angioplasty, Am. J. Cardiol. **59:**267-269, 1987.
6. Kent, K.M., Bentivoglio, L.G., Block, P.C., Cowley, M.J., Dorros, G., Gosselin, A.J., Gruentzig, A., Myler, R.K., Simpson, J., Stertzer, S.H., Williams, D.O., Fisher, L., Gillespi, M.J., Detre, K., Kelsey, S., Mullin, S.M., Mock, M.B.: Percutaneous transluminal coronary angioplasty: report from the registry of the National Heart, Lung and Blood Institute, Am. J. Cardiol. **49:**2011-2020, 1982.
7. Holmes, D.R., Jr., Vlietstra, R.E., Smith, H.C., Vetrovec, G.W., Kent, K.M., Cowley, M.J., Faxon, D.P., Gruentzig, A.R., Kelsey, S.F., Detre, K.M., Van Raden, M.J., Mock, M.B.: Restenosis after percutaneous transluminal coronary angioplasty (PTCA): a report from the NHLBI registry of the National Heart, Lung and Blood Institute, Am. J. Cardiol. **53:**77C-81C, 1984.
8. Levin, S., Ewels, C.J., Rosing, D.R., Kent, K.M.: Coronary angioplasty: clinical and angiographic follow-up, Am. J. Cardiol. **55:**673-676, 1985.
9. Borozan, P.G., Schuler, J.J., Spigos, D.G., Flainigan, D.P.: Long-term hemodynamic evaluation of lower extremity percutaneous transluminal angioplasty, J. Vasc. Surg. **2:**785-793, 1985.
10. Krepel, V.M., van Andel, G.J., van Erp, W.F.M., Breslau, P.J.: Percutaneous transluminal angioplasty of the femoropopliteal artery: initial and long-term results, Radiology **156:**325-328, 1985.
11. Murray, R.R., Hewes, R.C.H., White, R.I., Jr., et al.: Long-segment femoropopliteal stenoses: is angioplasty a boon or a bust? Radiology **162:**473-476, 1987.
12. Gallino, A., Mahler, F., Probst, P., Nachbur, B.: Percutaneous transluminal angioplasty of the arteries of the lower limbs: a 5 year follow-up, Circulation **70:**619-623, 1984.
13. Simpson, J.B., Selmon, M.R., Robertson, G.C., Cipriano, P.R., Hayden, W.G., Johnson, D.E., Fogarty, T.J.: Transluminal atherectomy for occlusive peripheral vascular disease, Am. J. Cardiol. **61:**96G-101G, 1987.

Chapter 37

Quantitative Analysis of Coronary Arteriograms by Cinevideodensitometry

Allen B. Nichols, MD, FACC

The hemodynamic significance of coronary stenotic lesions is routinely based on visual estimates of the severity of stenosis from projected coronary arteriograms. However, several studies have documented the large interobserver variability of subjective visual analysis of coronary arteriograms.[1-4] Furthermore, pathologic studies have demonstrated a poor correlation between the severity of coronary stenoses estimated from coronary arteriograms and the actual severity of stenotic lesions measured in postmortem hearts.[5-8] Grondin and co-workers[6] demonstrated that patients dying after coronary bypass surgery often had more extensive coronary disease than was appreciated by visual assessment of the coronary arteriogram. Failure to recognize significant lesions occasionally resulted in inadequate surgical revascularization.

The poor accuracy of visual estimates of coronary stenosis can be readily explained. First, coronary atherosclerotic lesions are almost always eccentric[9,10]; thus an eccentric lesion may appear highly stenotic in one radiographic projection and minimally stenotic in another. Second, normal-appearing arterial segments are frequently narrowed by intimal atherosclerosis or are aneurysmally dilated.[11,12] Third, normal arterial segments are often tapered or include branch arteries making it difficult to select a truly normal segment.[13] Fourth, the number of gray levels that can be discerned visually is limited to only approximately 20 gray levels[14]; therefore, visual estimates may fail to detect focally reduced radiopacity reflecting an eccentric lesion. Last, the margins of the intraluminal column of contrast medium are always blurred on the projected arteriogram because of quantum mottle, Compton scatter, absorption unsharpness, focal spot penumbra, and cardiac motion.[15] Quantum mottle is the grainy texture in projected film caused by individual x-ray photons, which inherently limits the resolution of cinearteriograms because the number of x-ray photons is necessarily limited to minimize patient x-ray exposure. Scatter radiation from Compton scattering is an unavoidable cause of radiographic unsharpness that diminishes the quality of the radiographic image significantly. A third cause of indistinct arterial margins on projected coronary arteriograms is absorption unsharpness, which results from the gradual attenuation of the x-ray beam passing through a contrast-filled artery with a circular shape. Penumbra or geometric unsharpness is another inevitable cause of blurred arterial margins, which results from diffuse emission of x-rays from the focal spot rather than from a single-point source. Last, motion of the coronary arteries caused by cardiac contraction contributes to image unsharpness. As a result of these five unavoidable causes of radiographic unsharpness, the borders of contrast-filled arteries always appear blurred on a projected arteriogram when viewed with a magnifying lens.[16]

THEORETIC BASIS OF CINEVIDEODENSITOMETRY

Computer-assisted cinevideodensitometry is a new approach to quantitative analysis of coronary arteriograms, which is suitable for quantitative analysis of eccentric stenotic lesions from projected angiographic images with indistinct margins.[16-20] Cinevideodensitometry quantifies film density and reflects the amount of contrast medium in the arterial lumen, which provides a three-dimensional measurement of the cross-sectional area of the arterial lumen. The cinevideodensity signal recorded across the contrast-filled arterial lumen reflects the cross-sectional area of the column of contrast medium.[18] Since the amount of contrast medium directly reflects the volume of the arterial lumen, this measurement reflects the dimensions of the arterial lumen in three dimensions. As shown schematically in Fig. 37-1, the area under the videodensitometric profile curve is proportional to the amount of contrast medium and thus provides a measurement of the cross-sectional area of irregular stenotic lumens. The area under the videodensity profile curve can be calculated by summing the videodensity values recorded for each pixel and subtracting average background density. As shown in Fig. 37-1, the shape and width of the videodensity profile curve varies for different radiographic projections, but the background-corrected area under the curve remains the same regardless of the radiographic projection used. The summated background-corrected videodensity value for the profile curve can be easily calculated by computer. An important advantage of this approach is that the need for precise localization of indistinct arterial margins is eliminated, because background subtraction, in effect, truncates the base of the curve. Since videodensity values near arterial borders are small compared with videodensity values near the center of the arterial lumen, border videodensity values representing indistinct arterial margins contribute relatively little to the total summated videodensity value for the stenosis.

High-quality video cameras permit precise resolution of optically magnified projected video images with high pixel densities, and widely available analog-to-digital converters make it possible to quantify gray levels in video images with high degrees of precision into 256 or more gray levels (Fig. 37-2). Using these newly available computer-video techniques, precise quantification of film density is readily obtainable with more than 50 pixel measurements for each square millimeter of area of coronary artery.

Cinevideodensitometric analysis is based on the finding that the videodensitometric signal recorded from the projected cine film varies linearly with the concentration of interluminal contrast medium. This finding was demonstrated experimentally from cine radiographs of contrast-filled acrylic plastic (Plexiglas) cylinders.[18] In these experiments, it was also shown that the integrated densitometric signal measured over contrast-filled cylinders correlated linearly with cross-sectional areas of the cylinders over a wide range of contrast concentrations (Fig. 37-3). In experimental models of eccentric stenoses, relative reduction in the videodensitometric signal mea-

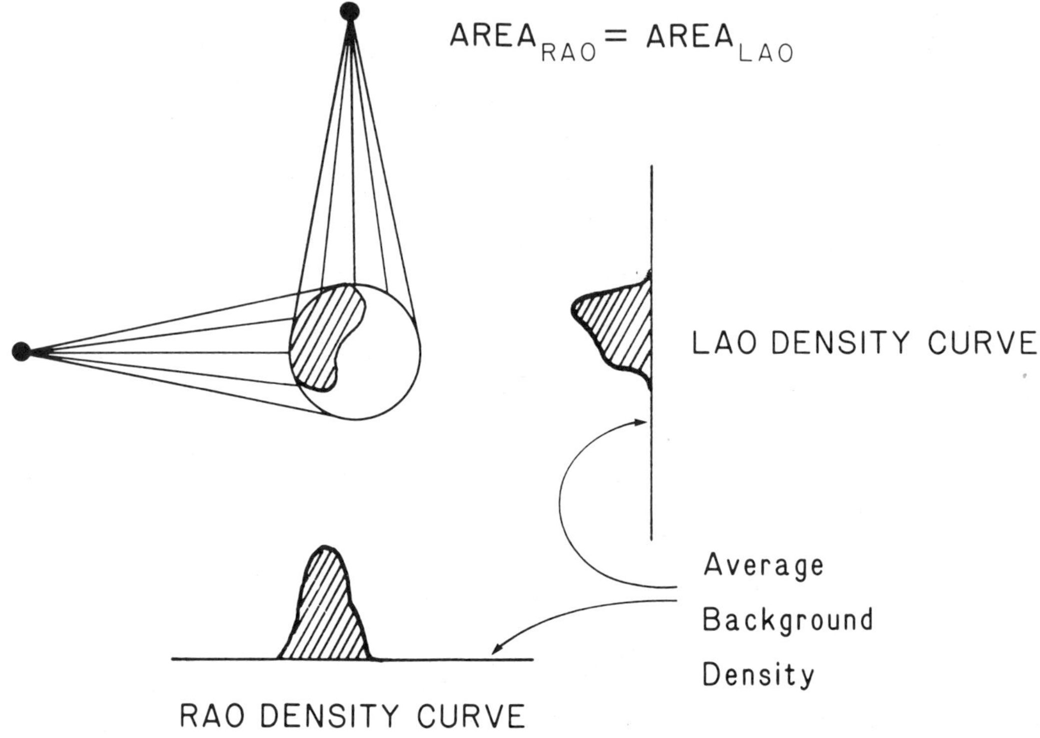

Fig. 37-1. Schematic illustration of the effect of different radiographic projections on cinevideodensitometric profile curves recorded for an eccentric stenotic lesion. Although the shapes of the videodensity curves differ in right anterior oblique (RAO) and left anterior oblique (LAO) projections, the areas under the curves after subtraction of average background density are equivalent.

sured over narrowed contrast-filled cylinders correlated highly with actual reduction in cross-sectional area.[18]

Cinevideodensitometric Measurement of Relative Coronary Stenosis

The theoretic basis for the linear relationship between the amount of intraluminal contrast medium and the summated densitometric signal was provided previously.[18] This linear relationship results from the exponential effects of x-ray attenuation (Lambert-Beer Law), which is reversed by the logarithmic effect of light intensity transmitted from the projector through the film. The absolute densitometric signal is dependent on many factors including the type and concentration of contrast medium, the effective x-ray energy, light gain of the image intensifier, characteristic curve of cine film, film processing methods, light output and lens characteristics of the projector, thickness of the column of contrast medium in the arterial lumen, and recording characteristics of the cinedensity digitizing system. However, for relative measurement of the density across a stenosis compared with the density across a normal segment in a single cine frame, the viedodensity signal is dependent only on the concentration and amount of intraluminal contrast medium.[21] Therefore cinevideodensitometry is ideally suited for measurement of relative

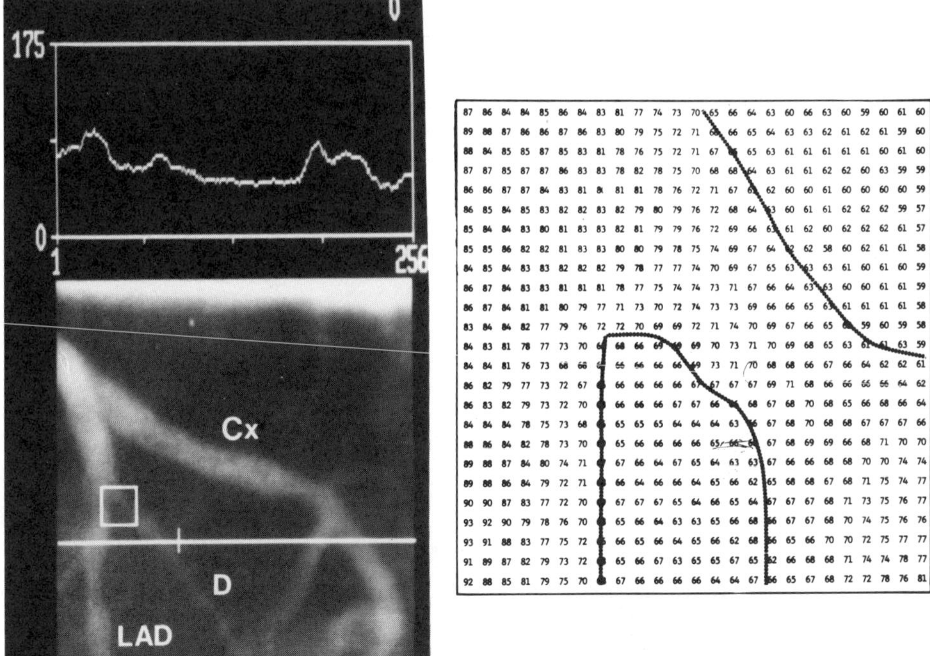

Fig. 37-2. Digitized image of one quarter of a cine frame showing proximal segments of the left anterior descending (LAD) and left circumflex arteries recorded in the LAO projection. The matrix of videodensity values *(right)* represents individual pixel measurements obtained for the small square positioned over the LAD coronary artery and illustrates the high pixel density possible with optically magnified projected images. Shown above is the computer-generated profile density curve recorded for the profile line positioned across the digitized image. (From Nichols, A.B., et al.: Circulation **69:**512, 1984. With permission of the American Heart Association.)

coronary stenosis, since the concentration of contrast medium in the normal arterial segment can be assumed to equal the concentration contrast medium in the stenotic arterial segment. If the stenotic and normal arterial segments are adjacent, this assumption is valid. This approach requires that the normal and stenotic arterial segments be in the same cine frame to ensure that radiographic exposure is uniform for both the stenotic and normal arterial segments. It is also important that radiographic magnification is uniform with little field distortion from the image intensifier. Finally, optical distortion resulting from projection of the cine image into the video camera should be minimized.

A major practical advantage of cinevideodensitometry is that analysis of a stenotic lesion in only one radiographic projection is sufficient for calculating the degree of stenosis. This advantage eliminates the need for multiple angiograms of each coronary stenotic lesion in precisely aligned complementary radiographic projections, as required by methods based on geometric assumptions of lesion shape.[22] Because virtually all stenotic coro-

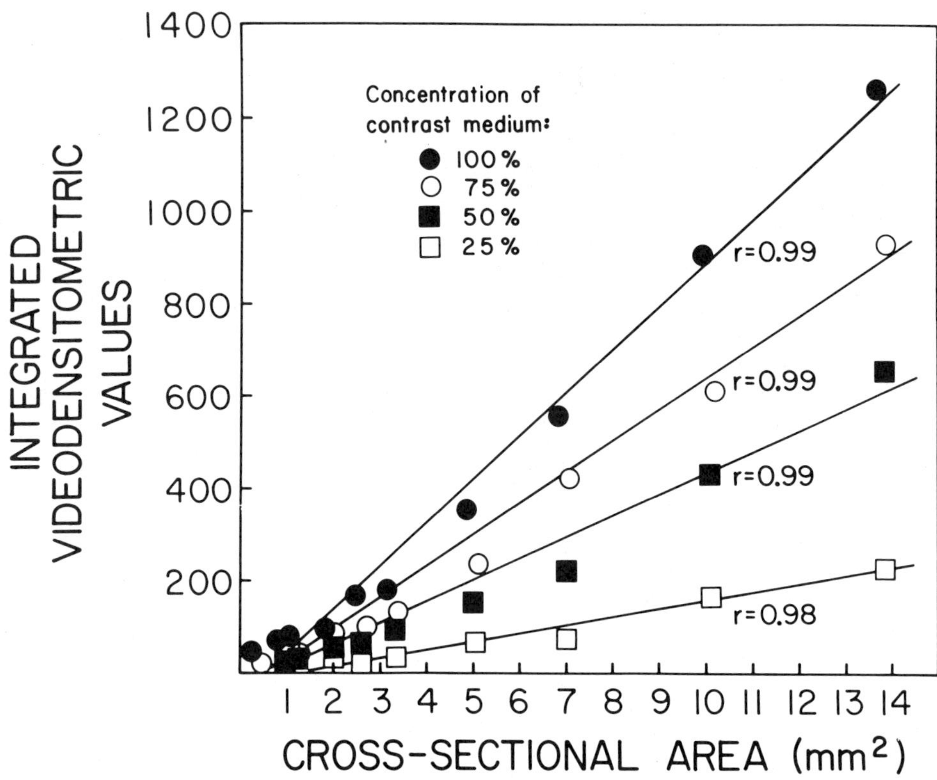

Fig. 37-3. Linear relationship observed between background-corrected videodensity values and actual cross-sectional areas of contrast-filled cylinders over a wide range of concentrations of contrast medium. (From Nichols, A.B., et al.: Circulation **69:**512, 1984. With permission of the American Heart Association.)

nary lesions are visualized well without foreshortening in at least one projection, cinevideodensitometric analysis is applicable to nearly all coronary stenosis. Furthermore, the time required for analysis of a stenotic lesion is shortened significantly, compared with older systems requiring manual tracing of arterial borders.

However, radiographic projections that foreshorten the long axis of the artery are unsuitable for cinevideodensitometric analysis and must be avoided. Furthermore cine frames should be selected that show the stenotic and normal segments of the artery clearly without superimposed branch vessels. Videodensitometric values measured across each arterial segment must be corrected for adjacent background density, because background density is a relatively large component of the total videodensitometric signal caused in part to the wide latitude of the cine fluorographic film. Film densities can be readily subtracted, however, because density is a logarithmic function. Since background density often differs on the two sides of the arterial segment, the average background is subtracted from the videodensitometric value recorded for each pixel. Subtraction of average background values approximately corrects for differences in background density but may be inadequate for radiographic projections that display the left ventricular myocardium on one side of the artery and lung field on the other side of the artery. Further experiments addressing this issue are needed.

The fundamental parameter measured in computer-assisted cinevideodensitometry is film density, and experiments conducted with a calibrated photographic step tablet have revealed a linear relationship between film density and the resulting video signal over a range of light transmittance, which includes the range of regional film densities in a typical coronary arteriogram (Fig. 37-4). However, if the density of cine film analyzed is extremely dark, the relationship between videodensity value and film density becomes nonlinear and erroneous values may result, particularly if the background for one arterial segment is extremely light and the background for the other is extremely dark.

Cinevideodensitometric Measurements of Absolute Coronary Dimensions

This cinevideodensitometric method of analysis provides relative measurements of severity of coronary stenosis expressed as percent reduction in cross-sectional area. The accuracy of these measurements has been validated in experimental models in radiographic phantoms and in a small number of postmortem human hearts studied histologically (Fig.

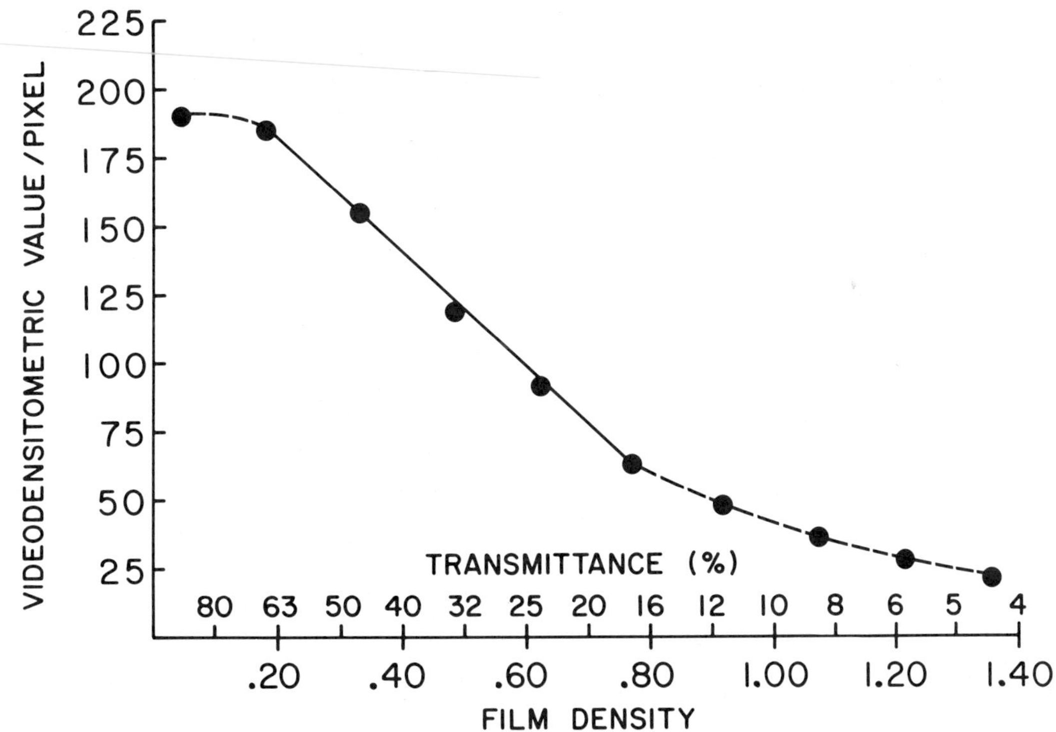

Fig. 37-4. Relationship between videodensity values recorded by cinevideodensitometry and actual film density of a calibrated film strip. Over the range of light transmittance from 70 to 16%, the relationship is linear. This range corresponds to the typical film density of coronary arteriograms. (From Nichols, A.B., et al.: Circulation **69:**512, 1984. With permission of the American Heart Association.)

37-5).[18] Percent area stenosis has been shown in anesthetized animal models to be the best single measurement for characterizing the severity of coronary stenotic lesions in terms of regional myocardial flow reduction.[23] However, in patients with coronary artery disease, percent area stenosis is of limited usefulness because the normally appearing arterial segment is often narrowed by atherosclerotic disease or tapered, making selection of a normal arterial segment difficult. In a study of the interobserver variability of repeat measurements of percent area stenosis, it was found that different observers tended to select similar stenotic sites for focal lesions but different sites for normal arterial segments.[24] As a result, cross-sectional areas for stenotic lesions were reproducible, but percent area stenosis varied considerably owing to the poor reproducibility of measurements of tapered normal arterial segments made in different radiographic projections by different observers.

Because of these limitations of relative measurements of stenosis expressed as percentages, conversion of percent measurements to absolute dimensions is necessary. The tech-

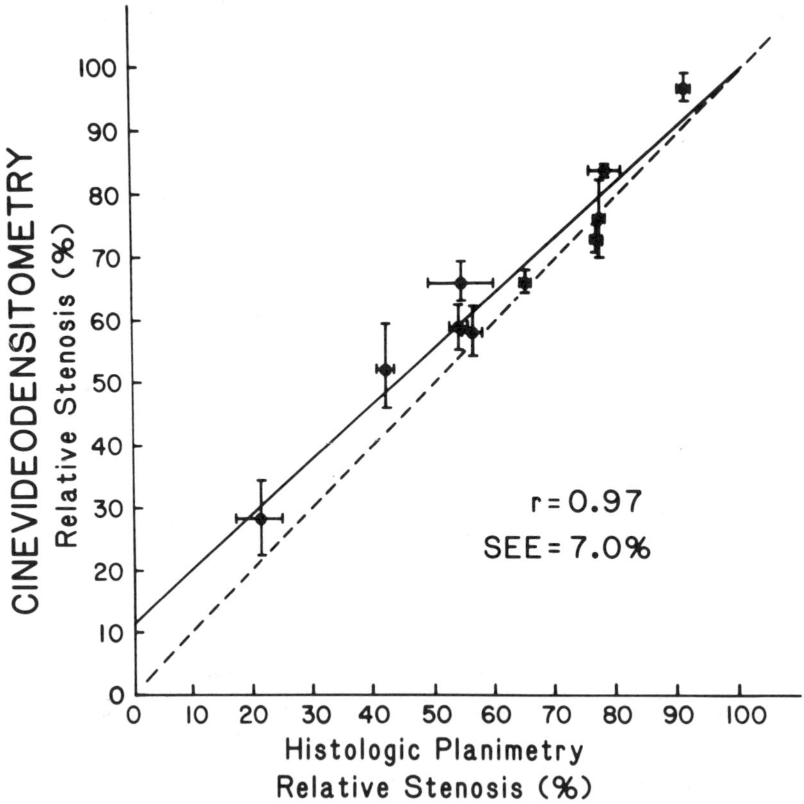

Fig. 37-5. Correlation between percent area stenosis measured by cinevideodensitometric analysis of coronary arteriograms and actual stenotic cross-sectional areas measured by computer-assisted planimetry in four postmortem human hearts. (From Nichols, A.B., et al.: Circulation **69**:512, 1984. With permission of the American Heart Association.)

nique of quantitative videodensitometry developed in our laboratory uses the catheter shaft as a spatial reference for calculation of arterial dimensions (Fig. 37-6). As shown by Reiber and colleagues[25] in videodensitometric experiments, commercially available coronary catheters provide excellent radiopacity and are suitable for videodensitometric measurements, with the exception of nylon catheters. The diameter of extruded coronary catheters are quite uniform and rarely deviate more than 2% from the diameter specified by the manufacturer.

Using the catheter shaft as a basis for measurements of coronary dimensions requires automated edge detection for calculations of catheter diameters. However, the catheter margins on projected arterial cinegrams

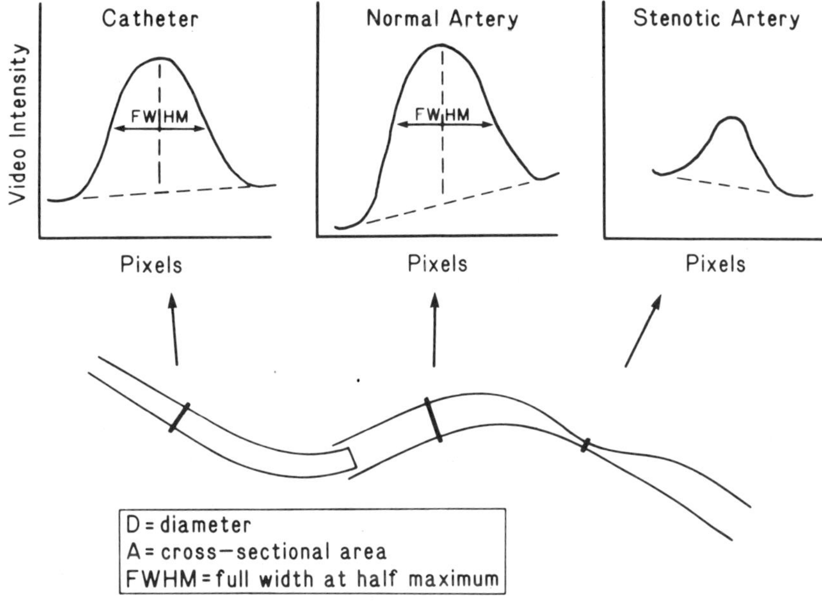

1) $\frac{\text{D artery}}{\text{D catheter}} = \frac{\text{FWHM artery}}{\text{FWHM catheter}}$

2) $\text{A artery} = \pi\left(\frac{\text{D artery}}{2}\right)^2$

3) A stenosis = A artery − (% stenosis)(A artery)/100

Fig. 37-6. Method for calculating dimensions for normal and stenotic arterial segments from cinevideodensitometric profile curves recorded across the full-width-at-half-maximum (FWHM) widths of the density curves for the catheter *(1)* and normal artery, and the known diameter of the catheter. The area of the normal artery *(2)* is calculated from its diameter, and stenotic area *(3)* is calculated from the area of the normal artery and percent area stenosis. (From Nichols, A.B., et al.: Circulation **74:**746, 1986. With permission of the American Heart Association.)

are often indistinct because of absorption unsharpness and quantum mottle. We have found that full-width-at-half-maximum (FWHM) measurements are a useful method for comparing the diameters of catheter shaft and normal arterial segment.[26,27] This approach provides precise measurements of relative diameters because the videodensitometric profile signal is strongest over the central portion of the profile curve, compared with the inflection points of the curve, which represent the indistinct borders where the videodensity value is weakest. Furthermore the FWHM measurement in pixels can be accurately measured by computing interpolated values, which result in a precise measurement of width (Fig. 37-7). Slight errors in measurement of the curve peak or background density alter the width measurement very little because the upstroke and downstroke of the videodensitometric curve are steep. Actual diameters are readily calculated from FWHM ra-

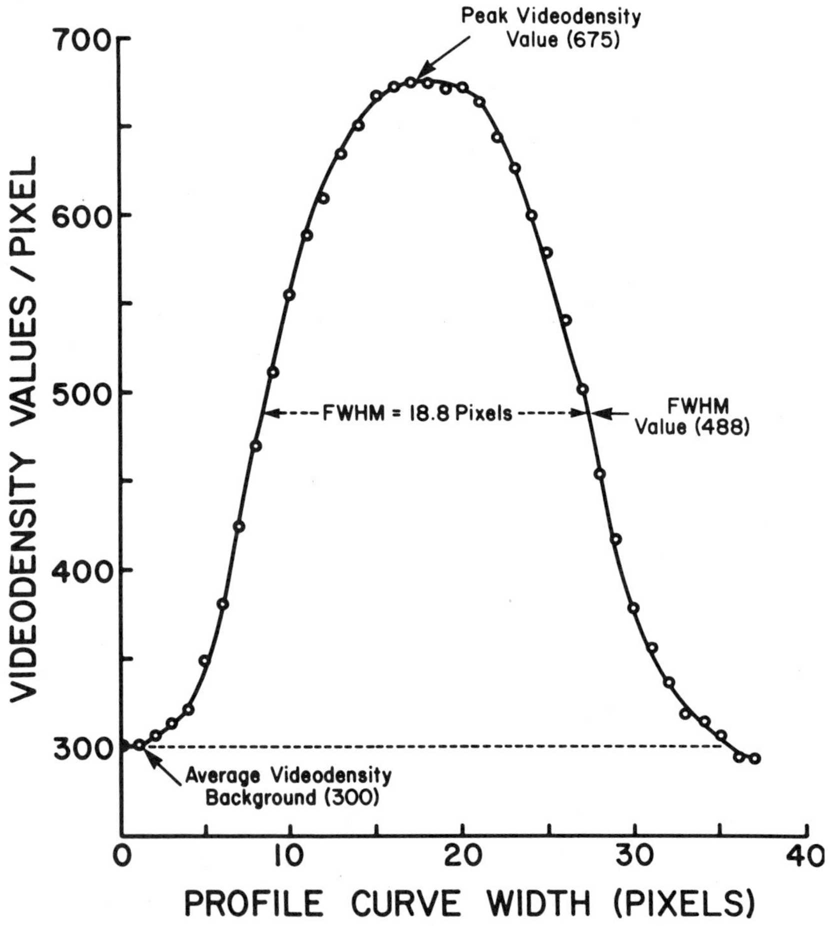

Fig. 37-7. Typical videodensity profile curve recorded from a projected cine frame of a contrast-filled cylinder, showing the full-width-at-half-maximum (FWHM) method for measuring diameters from images with blurred margins. (From Nicoloff, E.L., et al.: Invest. Radiol. **22:**815, 1987. With permission of Investigative Radiology.)

tios for the catheter and normal arterial segment, since the diameter of the catheter shaft is known (see Fig. 37-6). The accuracy of videodensitometric measurements of diameters based on FWHM calculations was validated in radiographic phantom experiments of cineradiographed contrast-filled cylinders (Fig. 37-8). These experiments showed that the method was accurate within 2.7% for cylinder diameters from 1.78 to 4.17 mm, which is the typical range of diameters for normal coronary arteries. The FWHM method is not suitable for measuring the diameter of the stenosis, which is much smaller and eccentric. In experiments with two postmortem hearts of patients dying following cardiac surgery, we found that videodensitometric measurements of normal arterial diameters based on FWHM calculations accurately predicted true lumen diameter measured directly from acrylic casts of the coronary arteries (Fig. 37-9).[28]

Absolute dimensions of coronary stenotic

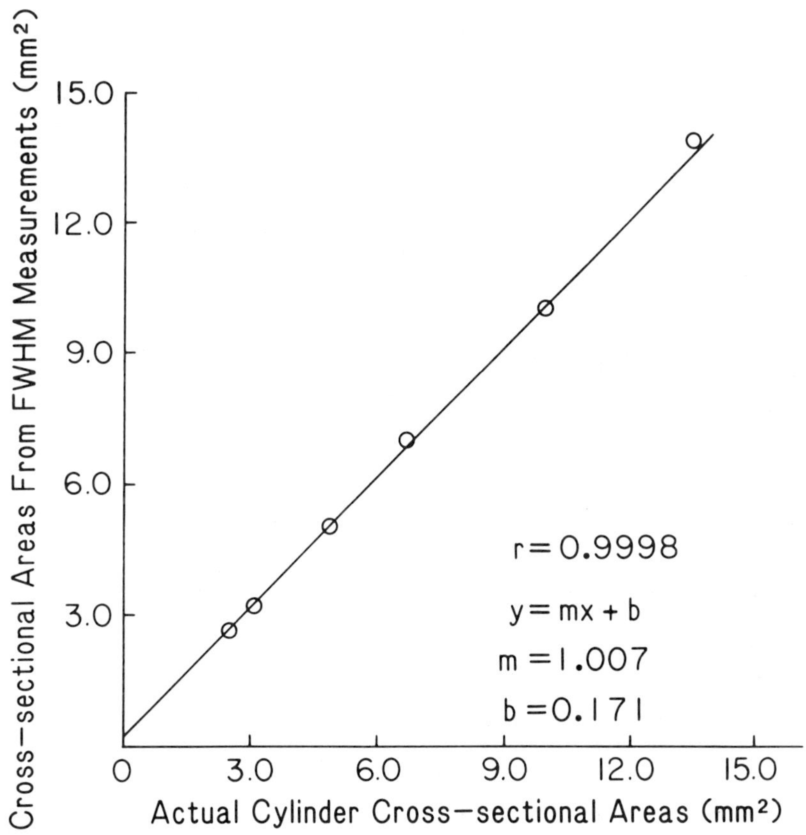

Fig. 37-8. High correlation resulting between cross-sectional areas of contrast-filled cylinder predicted by full-width-at-half-maximum (FWHM) calculations of cinevideodensity profile curves and actual cross-sectional areas of cylinders. (From Nicoloff, E.L., et al.: Invest. Radiol. **22**:815, 1987. With permission of Investigative Radiology.)

lesions can then be readily determined by first calculating the cross-sectional area of the normal arterial segment using the diameter obtained by comparing the FWHM widths of the catheter and the normal arterial segment.[26,28] Since the percent area stenosis was previously determined by comparing the profile curves for the stenotic and normal arterial segments, the absolute cross-sectional area of the stenosis can be readily calculated as shown schematically in Fig. 37-6.

PHYSIOLOGIC BASIS OF QUANTITATIVE CORONARY ARTERIOGRAPHY

Absolute stenotic dimensions are important determinants of the hemodynamic significance of a coronary stenosis, as suggested by recent clinical studies in patients.[26,29] Percent stenosis has been shown to be a relatively poor index of the severity of a coronary stenotic lesion for several reasons. First, nor-

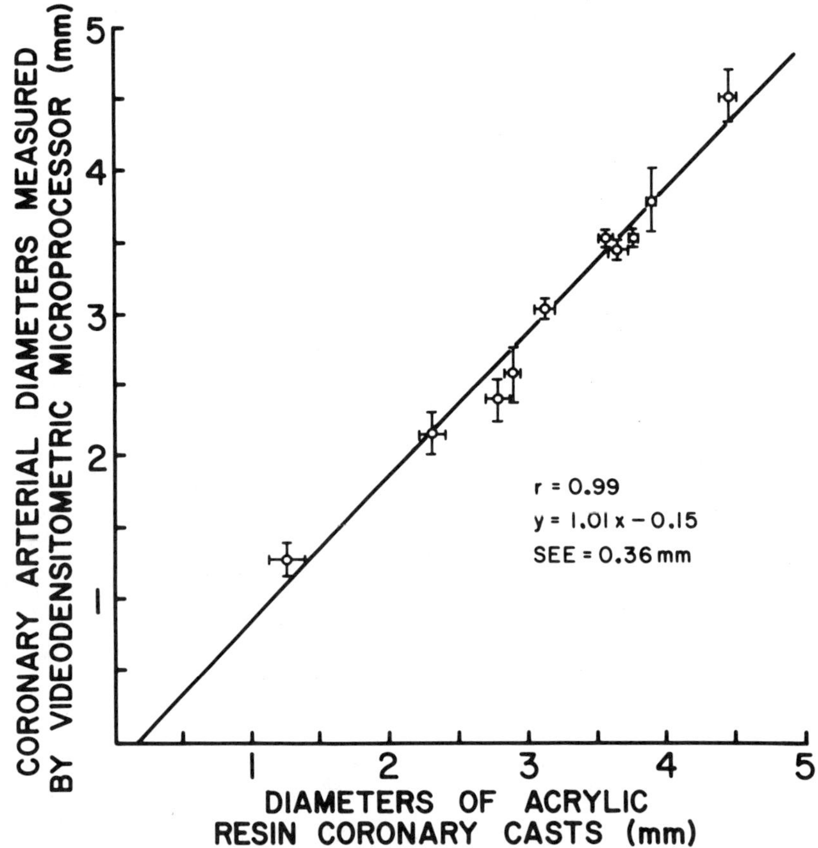

Fig. 37-9. Correlation between coronary artery diameters predicted by cinevideodensitometric analysis of coronary arteriograms and diameters measured by calipers of acrylic resin coronary casts from two postmortem human hearts. (From Silver, K.H., et al.: Cathet. Cardiovasc. Diag. **13**:291, 1987. With permission of Catheterization and Cardiovascular Diagnosis.)

mal arterial segments are commonly tapered or may be diffusely narrowed by atherosclerotic lesions, making selection of a truly normal segment difficult. Furthermore, we have found that selection of a normal segment by different observers is poorly reproducible,[24] whereas selection of a focally stenotic lesion is much more reproducible.

Absolute stenotic area may be a more useful predictor of the hemodynamic severity of a stenosis, because it is highly reproducible (Fig. 37-10),[24] and because slight changes in absolute stenotic area have profound hemodynamic effects, whereas comparable changes in the diameter of the normal segment have negligible effects.[30] The most important single determinant of the hemodynamic effect of a stenotic lesion is its cross-sectional area, since flow across a stenosis is inversely proportional to the second power of the cross-sectional area according to the Poiseuille relationship.[30] Although several other geometric rheologic variables influence blood flow through a stenosis, minimal cross-sectional area of the stenosis expressed as a ratio of unobstructed lumen area has been shown to be the most important variable in experimental studies in animals.[23]

CLINICAL APPLICATIONS OF CINEVIDEODENSITOMETRY

Cinevideodensitometric analysis of projected coronary arteriograms was initially developed as a research technique using mainframe computer systems with extensive computer memories. Subsequently a microprocessor system was designed in our laboratory and manufactured by Vanguard Instruments Corporation (Melville, N.Y.), which permits equally accurate densitometric measurements

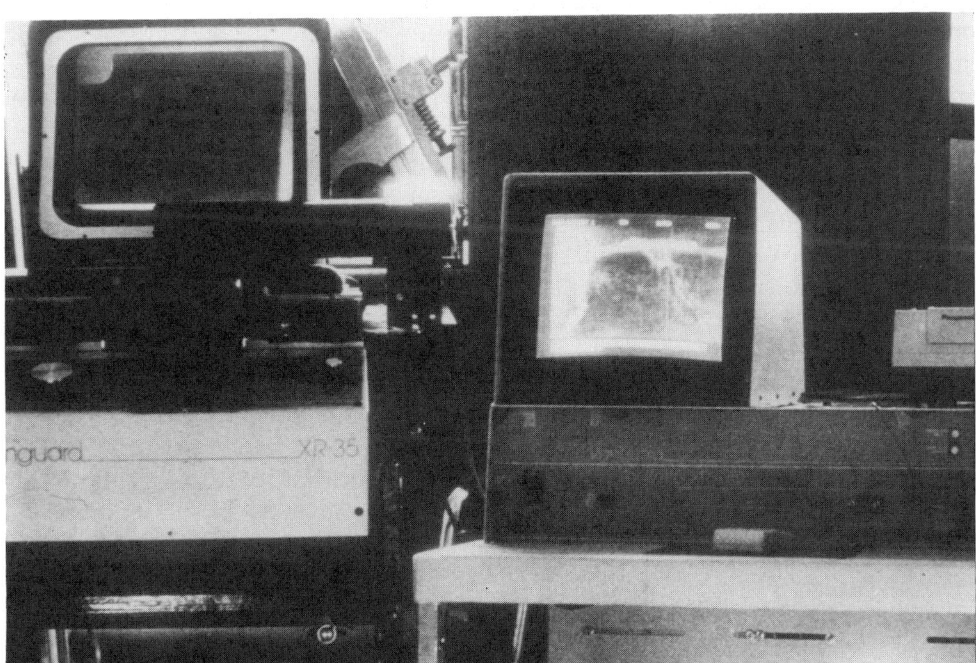

Fig. 37-10. Cinevideodensitometric microprocessor system attached to a cine film projector for quantitative analysis of conventional coronary arteriograms. (Courtesy Vanguard Instruments Corp., Melville, N.Y.)

without the major cost of a mainframe computer system or expensive service contracts. The microprocessor system requires considerably less computer memory and is preprogrammed for rapid measurement of absolute and relative coronary stenotic dimensions. The accuracy of the microprocessor has been demonstrated in radiographic phantom studies, and its reproducibility for analysis of projected angiograms has been evaluated.[28] The microprocessor system manufactured by Vanguard Instruments Corporation is an attachment to the Vanguard film projector (Fig. 37-10). The combination of a cine projector together with a dedicated coronary analyzer facilitates selection of individual cine frames for analysis and reduces analysis time considerably.

The following clinical applications of cinevideodensitometry have been studied in our laboratory: (1) quantitative measurements of regional myocardial blood flow to define the severity of flow-limiting lesions in patients with coronary disease at rest[26]; (2) studies of the hemodynamic significance of individual coronary stenotic lesions on regional myocardial perfusion during exercise[31]; (3) measurement of the rate of progression of coronary disease in patients undergoing serial coronary arteriography[32]; (4) quantification of the angiographic effects of coronary angioplasty[24]; (5) evaluation of criteria for optimal balloon size for coronary angioplasty based on cinevideodensitometric measurements of coronary arterial caliber[33]; and (6) and quantitation of the progression of coronary artery disease in patients following cardiac transplantation.[34]

Effect of Stenotic Lesions on Resting Myocardial Blood Flow

Few studies have been published describing the severity of coronary stenotic lesions that reduce regional myocardial blood flow either at rest or during exercise in patients with coronary artery disease. This issue is of major clinical significance, because defining the dimensions of flow-limiting stenosis would be useful for selecting stenotic lesions for surgical revascularization or angioplasty. Numerous experimental studies in anesthetized dogs have shown that distal myocardial blood flow remains normal as a coronary artery is gradually constricted, until a critical degree of stenosis is reached.[35-37] The luminal area must be severely reduced before distal blood flow falls, since flow is maintained at normal levels by autoregulatory vasodilatation of the distal vascular bed, until the stenosis is severe.[38,39] Vasodilatation of the distal vasculature lowers artery pressure distal to the lesion, increasing the pressure drop across the stenosis. This increased pressure gradient augments the driving pressure and maintains flow at normal or near-normal levels.

Few studies in patients have ever addressed the issue: What magnitude of stenosis limits myocardial flow at rest? Few techniques for measuring regional myocardial blood flow in patients have been available,[40,41] and caliper methods for quantifying severity of coronary stenosis have been relatively imprecise.[24] Smith and associates[42] recorded intraoperative ^{133}Xe clearance curves in patients during coronary artery bypass surgery and observed that myocardial flow was reduced distal to stenotic lesions greater than 80% reduction in diameter as measured from the preoperative coronary arteriogram with calipers.

In a study conducted in our laboratory,[26] 29 patients with isolated proximal lesions of the left anterior descending (LAD) coronary artery underwent regional myocardial blood flow determinations by intracoronary ^{133}Xe injected into the left main coronary artery. Regional blood flow rates were calculated from the ^{133}Xe clearance rates recorded with a multicrystal scintillation camera. Regional myocardial flow distal to stenotic lesions was expressed as a fraction of normal flow recorded in the circumflex arterial distribution to normalize for the effect of spontaneous variations in heart rate and systolic blood pressure between patients. Distal myocardial flow correlated with lesion cross-sectional area (r = 0.84) (Fig. 37-11), minimum lumen diameter (r = 0.84), and percent area stenosis (r = 0.70). Resting myocardial blood flow distal to proximal stenotic lesions was observed to remain normal until the degree of narrowing was severe. Reduced myocardial blood flow at rest was observed only for stenotic lesions with minimum stenotic areas less than 0.80 mm^2 (mean 0.34 ± 0.2 mm^2), which corresponds to a minimum calculated diameter less than 1 mm (mean 0.59 ± 0.3 mm). Percent stenosis, expressed as reduction in cross-sectional area, was greater than 85% (mean 94 ± 4%) for all patients with reduced distal flow.

Most of the patients with reduced flow at rest had unstable angina, and several had small collateral vessels to the LAD coronary artery from the right coronary artery. For patients with stenotic lesions ranging from 19 to 84% area reduction, distal regional blood flow was consistently normal.

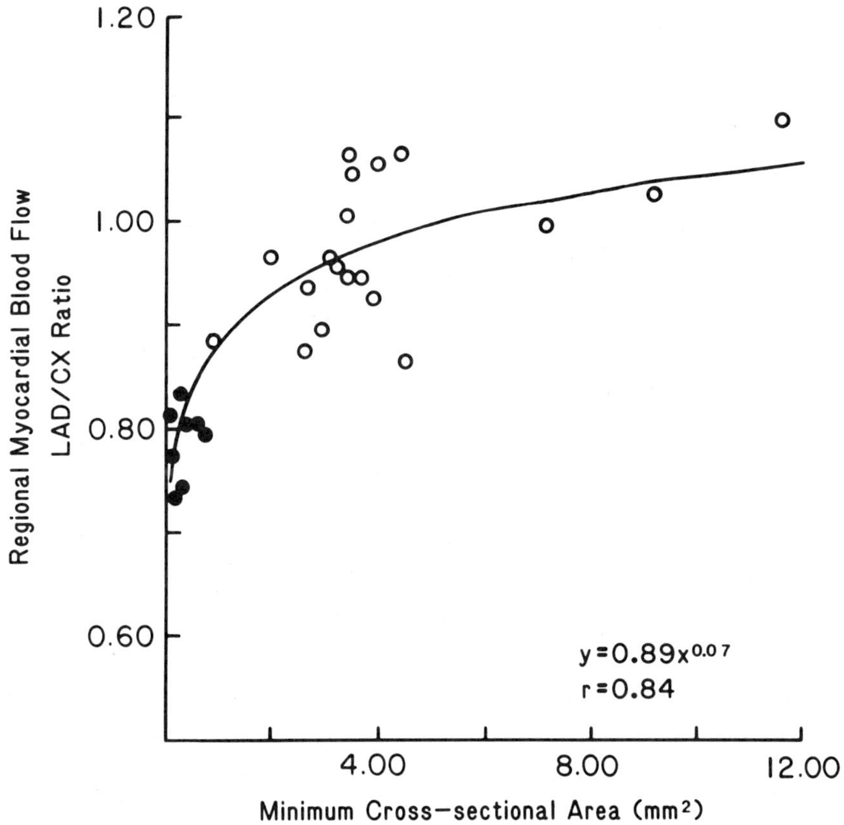

Fig. 37-11. Correlation between regional myocardial blood flow measured at rest by intracoronary ^{133}Xe clearance and stenotic cross-sectional area. Regional myocardial blood flow is expressed as a fraction of normal flow in the circumflex arterial distribution. (From Nichols, A.B., et al.: Circulation **74**:746, 1986. With permission of the American Heart Association.)

These results are consistent with the hemodynamic principle initially observed in laboratory animal models that regional myocardial blood flow remains normal until the degree of stenosis is severe. Studies in chronically instrumented dogs reported by Gould and associates[37] demonstrated that a diameter reduction of approximately 85% was required to reduce coronary blood flow. This degree of narrowing is equivalent to a 97% reduction in cross-sectional area and is comparable to the mean value of 94% area reduction observed for patients with reduced regional flow in our study.[26] Furthermore, the 80% reduction in diameter stenosis reported by Smith and colleagues[42] for patients with reduced flow measured by intraoperative xenon corresponds to 94% area stenosis and matches the magnitude of stenosis observed in our study. Our study demonstrates that cinevideodensitometric analysis of projected coronary arteriograms is capable of predicting which patients have reduced distal regional myocardial blood flow at rest.

Although other dimensional factors such as length of stenosis, eccentricity, and stenotic tapering have also been shown to have lesser effects on regional myocardial blood flow, percent reduction in cross-sectional area has been found to be the single most important determinant of blood flow through a stenotic artery in animal studies.[23] This pathophysiologic principle is based on the nonlinear relationship between regional blood flow and the stenotic dimensions described by the Poiseuille relationship in which regional flow is inversely proportional to the stenotic area squared. Since the primary measurement of cinevideodensitometric analysis is the cross-sectional area of the stenotic lumen, rather than relative diameter, cinevideodensitometry is suitable for assessing the hemodynamic severity of stenotic lesions. The dimensions observed for critical coronary stenotic lesions by intracoronary ^{133}Xe flow measurements in patients at rest correlate well with theoretic predictions based on fluid mechanics.[30]

Effect of Stenotic Lesions on Myocardial Perfusion During Exercise

Evaluating the severity of coronary stenosis that significantly impairs regional myocardial flow during exercise is considerably more difficult than measuring regional flow in patients during resting conditions. Very few techniques are available for measuring regional myocardial blood flow in patients during exercise. Furthermore, owing to wide variations in exercise levels, no single degree of coronary stenosis will define hemodynamic significance during exercise for all patients, since a lesion that is insignificant at a lower level of exercise may be significant at a greater level of exercise.

In a study conducted in our laboratory,[43] we demonstrated that regional myocardial uptake of ^{201}Tl in patients with coronary disease during exercise correlated well with regional myocardial blood flow measured during cardiac catheterization measured by the intracoronary ^{133}Xe technique during rapid atrial pacing to comparable pressure rate products achieved during exercise. This study confirmed in patients the principle that had previously been demonstrated in canine models: that regional ^{201}Tl uptake in the myocardium during exercise correlates highly with regional myocardial blood flow distal to stenotic lesions. Thus the heterogeneity of regional myocardial blood flow brought out by exercise is reflected in the regional heterogeneity of myocardial ^{201}Tl uptake quantified by computer regional analysis.

In 31 patients with isolated lesions of the LAD coronary artery, we studied the effect of severity of coronary stenosis on regional myocardial perfusion during exercise, as demonstrated by quantitative ^{201}Tl scintigraphy.[31] ^{201}Tl uptake in the distribution of the LAD coronary artery was expressed as a ratio of ^{201}Tl uptake in the circumflex arterial distribution, recorded in the left anterior oblique projection after symptom-limited treadmill exercise. Stenotic cross-sectional area, mean stenotic diameter, and percent area stenosis for each proximal stenotic lesion were measured by cinevideodensitometric analysis of the projected coronary arteriogram. ^{201}Tl uptake distal to lesions of the LAD coronary artery correlated significantly with absolute stenotic cross-sectional area ($r = 0.83$). For all 16 patients with reduced regional ^{201}Tl uptake during exercise, stenotic cross-sectional areas were less than 2 mm^2 (mean 0.9 ± 0.6 mm^2), and the stenotic diameters were less than 1.5 mm (mean 0.98 ± 0.4 mm). All patients with reduced regional flow during exercise had stenotic lesions greater than 70% area stenosis, which corresponds to 46% diameter stenosis. Regional ^{201}Tl uptake correlated poorly with percent area stenosis. Exercise-induced ^{201}Tl perfusion defects were shown to correlate best with the absolute dimensions of coronary stenotic lesions. This finding is consistent with the observation made in our laboratory[24] and by other investigators[29] that percent relative stenosis is an imprecise measurement due largely to variations in measurements of normal arterial segments.

Cinevideodensitometric analysis separated patients with exercise-induced regional flow abnormalities moderately well, but there was some overlap between the two patient groups. This overlap can be accounted for by variations in exercise level and by differences in lesion length and eccentricity that were not measured in the present study. While precise criteria for determining the hemodynamically significant lesions during exercise were not defined in the present study, the magnitude of flow-limiting stenotic dimensions was described.[31] The criteria of 2 mm^2 cross-sectional area of flow-limiting lesions was consistent with the observation reported by Logan[44] in a postmortem study of human atherosclerotic coronary arteries that resistance to coronary blood flow increases dramatically for stenotic lesions with minimal cross-sectional areas less than 2 mm^2. Further studies will be necessary to define the severity of coronary stenotic lesions that are flow limiting at different exercise work loads. Cinevideodensitometric analysis may provide an objective and uniform method for evaluating the hemodynamic significance of coronary stenotic lesions in individual patients, which may facilitate the selection of appropriate patients for coronary bypass surgery or coronary angioplasty.

QUANTIFICATION OF THE ANGIOGRAPHIC RESULTS OF CORONARY ANGIOPLASTY

Quantifying angiographic improvement in the degree of coronary stenosis following angioplasty with calipers has become widely utilized, but the accuracy of caliper measurements remains unproved. Following angioplasty, the margins of the dilated arterial segment are frequently indistinct because of possible edema formation in the arterial wall. Furthermore intimal dissections are often present, further limiting precise localization of the arterial wall. Lastly, the residual stenosis remaining after angioplasty is frequently eccentric, causing the minimal diameter to differ considerably in different radiographic projections. Finally, the sharpness of the luminal column of contrast medium is fundamentally limited by radiographic causes of unsharpness, including absorption unsharpness, focal spot penumbra, and Compton scatter. All of these causes of blurred arterial margins contribute to the difficulty of precisely measuring stenotic diameters before and after angioplasty with machinist calipers. We compared the accuracy of caliper and cinevideodensitometric measurements of coronary stenotic dimensions in radiographic phantom experiments and in coronary arteriograms of 30 patients recorded before and after coronary angioplasty.[24] Phantom studies were performed in contrast-filled Plexiglas cylinders, which were cineradiographed and analyzed by both techniques. To simulate eccentric lesions, solid Plexiglas rods were inserted into the contrast-filled cylinders displacing contrast medium in part of the Plexiglas cylinder and creating an eccentric annulus of contrast medium. Percent stenosis was calculated based on diameters measured by calipers or calculated from cinevideodensitometric measurements of cross-sectional areas. Cinevideodensitometric measurements correlated highly with actual percent reduction in cross-sectional area of the contrast-filled cylinders, whereas caliper measurements poorly estimated actual percent diameter reduction. Furthermore calipers caused a large systematic error in percent diameter reduction because of the limitation of caliper measurements to two dimensions. Cinevideodensitometric measurements were found to be more precise, reproducible, and accurate.

Videodensitometric profile curves generated by computer demonstrated a striking difference in the area under the density curves before and after angioplasty.[24] Cinevideodensitometric analysis in the 30 patients demonstrated a moderate fall in percent diameter stenosis following angioplasty with mean percent diameter stenosis of 70 ± 13% before angioplasty and 23.4 ± 15% after angioplasty. However, measurements of minimum cross-sectional area showed a substantial increase in stenotic cross-sectional area following angioplasty. The minimum cross-sectional stenotic area rose from 0.59 ± 0.5 mm^2 to 3.47 ± 1.6 mm^2. This five-fold increase in cross-sectional area implies that coronary flow reserve is markedly increased in the stenotic vessel following angioplasty, because coronary flow is inversely proportional to the minimum cross-sectional area squared, according to the Poiseuille relationship. Percent relative stenosis measurements failed to reflect this large increase in coronary flow capacity.

Cinevideodensitometric measurements are also used in our cardiac catheterization laboratory for selecting balloon sizes for patients undergoing coronary angioplasty. In a retrospective study of 120 patients undergoing coronary angioplasty, we found that oversized balloons frequently caused coronary dissections, whereas undersized balloons resulted in inadequate dilatation.[33] Balloons with inflated diameters less than normal arterial diameters often resulted in residual stenoses greater than 50% diameter reduction that were associated with a higher need for repeat angioplasty in the next few months. Balloon selection by visual estimates of the diameter of the normal arterial segment often resulted in oversizing or undersizing of balloons. Cinevideodensitometric measurements of normal arterial diameter facilitates optimal selection of balloon size for angioplasty and may reduce the frequency of complications resulting from overdilatation or under dilatation.

CONCLUSION

The studies reviewed in this chapter illustrate several of the clinical and investigative applications of cinevideodensitometric measurements of coronary stenotic lesions in patients with coronary artery disease. Practical advantages of cinevideodensitometry include its applicability for analyzing conventional 35 mm coronary arteriograms recorded in a single radiographic projection, its suitability for accurate measurements of coronary arterial dimensions from projected arteriograms with blurred margins, and its capacity for measuring eccentric stenotic lesions based on three-dimensional quantification of the amount of contrast medium in the stenotic lumen. Cinevideodensitometry was originally introduced as a research technique requiring expensive mainframe computer systems. The recent introduction of inexpensive dedicated microprocessor systems that provide rapid measurements of coronary stenotic dimensions will facilitate the introduction of quantitative coronary arteriography into clinical practice. Quantitative coronary arteriography may improve the management of patients with coronary artery disease by guiding evaluation of individual patients considered for coronary angioplasty or surgery, and by improving the planning and assessment of coronary angioplasty.

ACKNOWLEDGMENT

This work was supported by NHLBI grant HL-32906 from the U.S. Public Health Service, Bethesda, MD.

REFERENCES

1. White, C.W., Wright, C.B., Doty, D.B., Hiratza, L.F., Eastham, C.L., Harrison, D.G., and Marcus, M.L.: Does visual interpretation of the coronary arteriogram predict the physiologic importance of a coronary stenosis?, N. Engl. J. Med. **310:**819, 1984.
2. Detre, K.M., Wright, E., Murphy, M.L., and Takaro, T.: Observer agreement in evaluating coronary angiograms, Circulation **52:**979, 1975.
3. Zir, L.M., Miller, S.W., Dinsmore, R.E., Gilbert, J.P., Harthorne, J.W.: Interobserver variability in coronary arteriography, Circulation **53:**627, 1976.
4. DeRouen, T., Murray, J.A., and Owen, W.: Variability in the analysis of coronary arteriograms, Circulation **55:**324, 1977.
5. Vlodaver, Z., Frech, R., VanTassel, R.A., and Edwards, J.E.: Correlation of the antemortem coronary arteriogram and the postmortem specimen, Circulation **47:**162, 1973.
6. Grondin, C.M., Dyrda, I., Pasternac, A., Campeau, L., Bourassa, M.G., and Lesperance, J.: Discrepancies between cineangiographic and postmortem findings in patients with coronary artery disease and recent myocardial revascularization, Circulation **49:**703, 1974.
7. Robbins, S.L., Rodriguez, F.L., Wragy, A.L., and Fish, S.J.: Problems in the quantitation of coronary arteriosclerosis, Am. J. Cardiol. **18:**153, 1966.
8. Eusterman, J.H., Achor, R.W.P., Kincaid, O.W., and Brown, A.L.: Atherosclerotic disease of the coronary arteries, Circulation **26:**1288, 1962.
9. Vlodaver, Z., and Edwards, J.E.: Pathology of coronary arteriosclerosis, Prog. Cardiovasc. Dis. **14:**256, 1971.
10. Thomas, A.C., Davies, M.J., Dilly, S., Dilly, N., and Franc, F.: Potential errors in the estimation of coronary arterial stenosis from clinical arteriography with reference to the shape of the coronary arterial lumen, Br. Heart J. **55:**129, 1986.
11. McPherson, D.D., Kieso, R.A., Marcus, M.L., and Kerber, R.E.: Delineation of the extent of coronary atherosclerosis by high frequency epicardial echocardiography, N. Engl. J. Med. **316:**304, 1987.
12. Arnett, E.N., Isner, J.M., Redwood, D.R.,

Kent, K.M., Baker, W.P., Ackerstein, H., and Roberts, W.C.: Coronary artery narrowing in coronary heart disease: Comparison of cineangiographic and necropsy findings, Ann. Intern. Med. **91**:350, 1979.
13. Marcus, M.L.: The coronary artery in health and disease, New York, 1983, McGraw-Hill Book Co.
14. Campbell, F.W., and Maffei, L.: Contrast and spatial frequency, Sci. Am. **241**:106, 1974.
15. Christensen, E.E., Curry, T.S. III, and Dowdey, J.E.: An introduction to the physics of diagnostic radiology, Philadelphia, 1978, Lea & Febiger.
16. Spears, J.R., Sandor, T., Als, A.V., Malagold, M., Markis, J.E., Grossman, W., Serur, J.R., and Paulin, S.: Computerized image analysis for quantitative measurement of vessel diameter from cineangiograms, Circulation **68**:453, 1983.
17. Sandor, T., Als, A.V., and Paulin, S.: Cinedensitometric measurement of coronary arterial stenoses, Cathet. Cardiovasc. Diag. **5**:229, 1979.
18. Nichols, A.B., Gabrieli, C.O., Fenoglio, J.J., and Esser, P.D.: Quantification of relative coronary arterial stenosis by cinevideodensitometric analysis of coronary arteriograms, Circulation **69**:512, 1984.
19. Serruys, P.W., Reiber, J.H., Wijns, W., Brand, M., Kooijman, C.J., Katen, H.J., and Hugenholtz, P.G.: Assessment of percutaneous transluminal coronary angioplasty by quantitative coronary angiography: diameter versus densitometric area measurements, Am. J. Cardiol. **54**:482, 1984.
20. Simons, M.A., Kruger, R.A., and Power, R.L.: Cross-sectional area measurements by digital videodensitometry, Invest. Radiol. **21**:637, 1986.
21. Rutishauser, W.: Equipment for cinedensitometry from 35 mm film. In Heintaen, Paul H., editor, Roentgen, cine- and videodensitometry, Stuttgart, 1971, George Thieme Verlag.
22. Brown, B.G., Bolson, E., Frimer, M., and Dodge, H.T.: Quantitative coronary arteriography, Circulation **55**:329, 1977.
23. Young, D.F.: Fluid mechanics of arterial stenoses, J. Biomed. Eng. **101**:157, 1979.
24. Nichols, A.B., Berke, A.D., Schlofmitz, R.A., Watson, R.M., and Powers, E.R.: Comparison of cinevideodensitometric and caliper measurements of the efficacy of coronary angioplasty, J. Am. Coll. Cardiol. **9**:196A, 1987.
25. Reiber, J.H.C., Kooijman, C.J., Boer, A., and Serruys, P.W.: Assessment of dimensions and image quality of coronary contrast catheters from cineangiograms, Cathet. Cardiovas. Diag. **11**:521, 1985.
26. Nichols, A.B., Brown, C., Han, J., Nicoloff, E.L., and Esser, P.D.: Effect of coronary stenotic lesions on regional myocardial blood flow at rest, Circulation **74**:746, 1986.
27. Nicoloff, E.L., Han, J., Esser, P.D., and Nichols, A.B.: Cinevideodensitometric measurement of vessel dimensions from digitized angiograms, Invest. Radiol. **22**:815, 1987.
28. Silver, K.H., Buczek, J.A., Esser, P.D., and Nichols, A.B.: Quantitative analysis of coronary arteriograms by microprocessor cinevideodensitometry, Cathet. Cardiovasc. Diag. **13**:291, 1987.
29. Harrison, D.G., White, C.W., Hiratzka, L.F., Doty, D.B., Barnes, D.H., Eastham, C.L., and Marcus, M.L.: The value of lesion cross-sectional area determined by quantitative coronary angiography in assessing the physiologic significance of proximal left anterior descending coronary arterial stenosis, Circulation **69**:1111, 1984.
30. Brown, B.G., Bolson, E.L., and Dodge, H.T.: Coronary arteriography and the objective assessment of coronary artery pathology. In Kalsner, S., editor: The coronary artery, New York, 1982, Oxford University Press Inc.
31. Nichols, A.B., Schwann, T.A., Han, J., Esser, P., and Blood, D.K.: Determinants of the hemodynamic effects of isolated proximal coronary stenotic lesions on regional myocardial perfusion during exercise, J. Am. Coll. Cardiol. **7**:232A, 1986.
32. Shea, S., Sciacca, R.R., Esser, P.D., Han, J., and Nichols, A.B.: Progression of coronary atherosclerotic disease assessed by cinevideodensitometry: relationship to clinical risk factors, J. Am. Coll. Cardiol. **8**:1325, 1986.
33. Nichols, A.B., Berke, A.D., Smith, R.J., Schlofmitz, R.A., and Powers, E.R.: Selection of optimal balloon size for coronary angioplasty by cinevideodensitometric measurements (abstract), J. Am. Coll. Cardiol. (In press.)

34. Nichols, A.B., Rose, E., Smith, C.R., Smith, R.J., Drusin, R., Reison, D.S., and Powers, E.R.: Cinevideodensitometric quantification of coronary artery disease following cardiac transplantation (abstract), J. Am. Coll. Cardiol. (In press.)
35. Elzinga, W.E., and Spinner, B.: Hemodynamic characteristics of critical stenosis in canine coronary arteries, J. Thorac. Cardiovasc. Surg. **69**:217, 1975.
36. Furuse, A., Klopp, E.H., Brawley, R.K., and Gott, V.I.: Hemodynamic determinations in the assessment of distal coronary artery disease, J. Surg. Res. **19**:25, 1975.
37. Gould, K.L., Lipscomb, K., and Hamilton, G.W.: Physiologic basis for assessing critical coronary stenosis, Am. J. Cardiol. **33**:87, 1974.
38. Young, D.F., Cholvin, N.R., Kirkeeide, R.L., and Roth, A.C.: Hemodynamics of arterial stenoses at elevated flow rates, Circ. Res. **41**:99, 1977.
39. Gould, K.L., Lipscomb, K., and Calvert, C.: Compensatory changes of the distal coronary vascular bed during progressive coronary constriction, Circulation **51**:1085, 1975.
40. Klocke, F.J.: Coronary blood flow in man, Prog. Cardiovasc. Dis. **19**:117, 1976.
41. Cannon, P.J., Weiss, M.B., and Sciacca, R.R.: Myocardial blood flow in coronary artery disease: studies at rest and during stress with inert gas washout techniques, Prog. Cardiovasc. Dis. **20**:95, 1977.
42. Smith, S.C. Jr., Gorlin, R., Hermann, M.V., Taylor, W.J., and Collins, J.J., Jr.: Myocardial blood flow in man: effects of coronary collateral circulation and coronary artery bypass surgery, J. Clin. Invest. **51**:2556, 1972.
43. Nichols, A.B., Weiss, M.B., Sciacca, R.R., Cannon, P.J., and Blood, D.K.: Relationship between segmental thallium-201 uptake and regional myocardial blood flow in patients with coronary artery disease, Circulation **69**:310, 1983.
44. Logan, S.E.: On the fluid mechanics of human coronary artery stenosis, IEEE Trans. Biomed. Eng. **4**:327, 1975.

Chapter 38

Coronary Blood Flow Velocity During Angioplasty Using a Doppler Tip Balloon Catheter as a Guideline for Assessment of the Functional Result

Patrick W. Serruys, MD
Felix Zijlstra, MD
Yves Juillière, MD
Rene Koning, MD

Since the introduction of coronary angioplasty in 1977,[1] the procedure has gained increasing importance in the treatment of coronary artery obstructions. The immediate results of the procedure are usually assessed by coronary angiography and the residual pressure gradient. However, the change in luminal diameter of an artery following the mechanical disruption of its internal wall cannot always be assessed accurately from the detected angiographic contours.[2,3] Although the measured residual pressure gradient may have long-term prognostic value, it reflects only resting coronary hemodynamics.[4,5] The assessment of coronary flow reserve has recently been proposed as a better method of evaluating the functional consequences of a coronary obstruction.[6,7]

Intracoronary blood flow velocity measurements with a Doppler probe have previously been used to investigate regional coronary flow reserve, by measuring the maximal reactive hyperemia induced by pharmacologic vasodilation or by ischemia.[8-12] During angioplasty, maximal reactive hyperemia following each transluminal occlusion may be useful in assessing regional changes in coronary flow reserve resulting from the procedure.

STUDY POPULATION

Twenty-three patients undergoing elective coronary angioplasty for angina pectoris were studied. All patients had evidence of myocardial ischemia as indicated either by electrocardiographic (ECG) changes at rest or at exercise and/or positive exercise thallium scintigraphy. Informed consent was obtained for the additional investigations. All patients were studied without premedication, but their medical treatment (nitrates, calcium antagonists, and beta blockers) was continued on the day of the procedure. Patients with left ventricular hypertrophy, valvular heart disease, angiographic evidence of collateral circulation, anemia, polycythemia, or hypertension were excluded because these conditions may influence coronary flow reserve.[13-15]

METHOD

Intracoronary Blood Flow Velocity Measurements

A 20 MHz ultrasonic crystal mounted on the tip of the angioplasty catheter was used in all patients (Fig. 38-1). The Doppler crystal has a 1 mm diameter annulus with a 0.5 mm central hole. Two leads are soldered to the crystal and pass through the catheter between the original 0.5 mm lumen and a thin-walled tube that serves as a new 0.4 mm lumen (Fig. 38-2). The leads exit near the proximal Luer hub and are wired to a two-pin plug for connection to the pulsed Doppler instrument. The connector cable contains an integral toroidal isolation transformer that insulates the patient from the instrument and that also provides impedance matching for more efficient energy transfer. The new inner lumen extends from the Luer hub through the crystal providing a smooth unobstructed path for a guidewire. Blood flow velocity is measured from the catheter tip transducer using a range-gated 20 MHz pulsed Doppler designed especially for the purpose (Baylor College of Medicine). The master oscillator frequency of 20 MHz is pulsed at a frequency of 62.5 kHz. Each pulse is approximately 1 ms in width

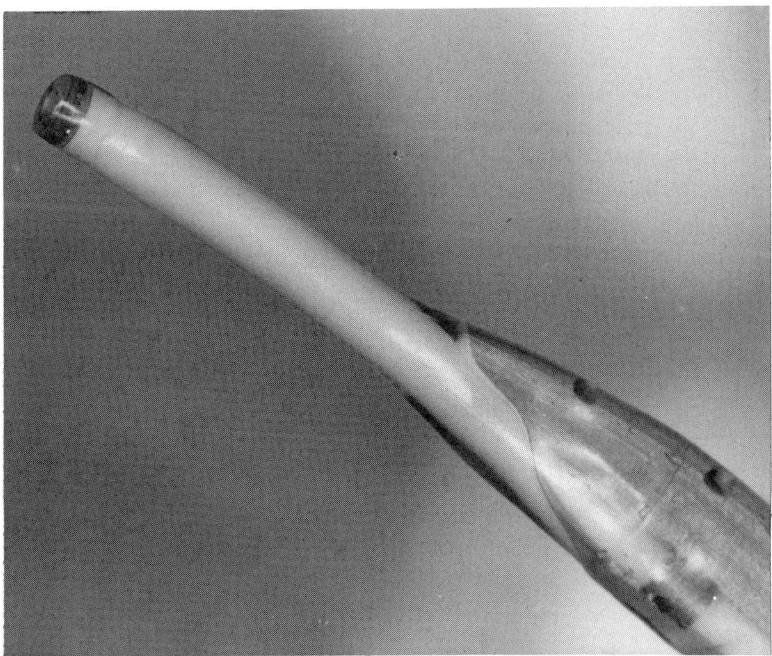

Fig. 38-1. Distal part of the angioplasty catheter showing the inflated balloon and the annular piezoelectric crystal end-mounted on the tip of the catheter.

and therefore contains 20 cycles of the master oscillator frequency. The parameters chosen (master oscillator frequency of 20 MHz and pulse repetition frequency of 62.5 kHz) allow velocities of up to 100 cm/second to be recorded at distances of up to 1 cm from the catheter tip. The sampling window was individually adjusted to obtain the most optimal signal, which (usually) resulted in a sampling window of 1.8 mm (range 1.5 to 2.2 mm).

The output of the pulsed Doppler is displayed as a frequency shift (f, kHz) that can be related to blood flow velocity by the Doppler equation: $f = 2F (V/c) \cos a$, where F is the ultrasonic frequency (20 MHz), V is the velocity within the sample volume, c is the speed of sound in blood (1500 m/second), and a is the angle between the velocity vector and the sound beam. Using an end-mounted crystal with the catheter parallel (± 20 degrees) to the vessel axis (cos a equals 1 ± 6%), the relation between the Doppler shift and velocity is approximately 3.75 cm/second/kHz.[28]

Previous calibration experiments in canine femoral and coronary arteries have shown that the measured Doppler shift frequency is proportional to volume flow measured by time collection.[8,9,12] Recently Sibley and associates[12] validated clinically and experimentally the ability of a similar catheter with an end-mounted piezoelectric crystal to provide accurate continuous on-line measurement of coronary blood flow velocity and vasodilator reserve.

In our laboratory, we verified the accuracy of each velocity probe by correlating velocity recorded with the Doppler probe in a 9F femoral sheath and the volume flow measured by a timed collection of blood from the side branch of the same sheath. Graduated flow rates (range 12 to 165 ml/minute) and the corresponding velocities (range 1.2 to 8.2 kHz) were obtained by incremental balloon inflation with the balloon positioned in the sheath. This simple model allows the assessment of the flow-velocity relation at different levels. As previously demonstrated, this relation is linear with correlation coefficients generally equal or 0.95,[8,9,16] but it underestimates true volume flow for flows over 150 ml/minute.[12] Flow rates of this magnitude, or velocities exceeding 7.5 kHz, were never encountered in this study population.

Protocol of the Investigational Procedure

A long guidewire (length, 315 cm; diameter, 0.014 inch) was passed through the coronary artery stenosis. A balloon catheter (Shiley Inc., Irvine, Calif.) with a Doppler probe at the tip was then advanced over the

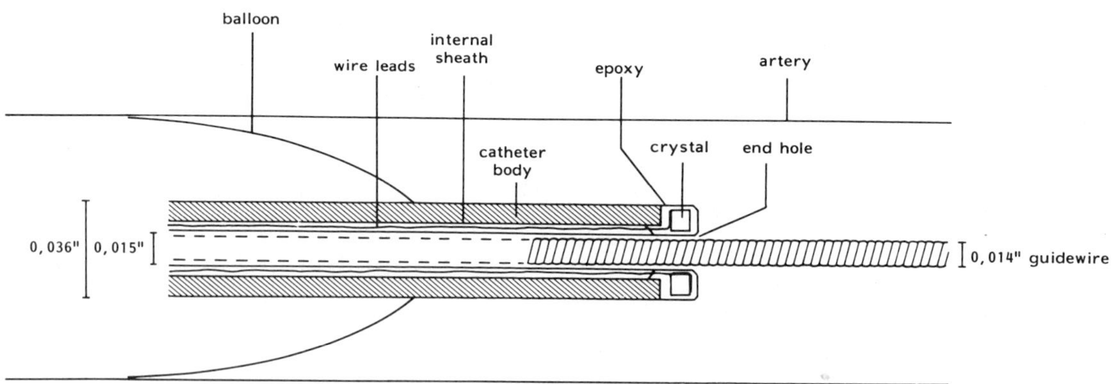

Fig. 38-2. Schematic cross-sectional drawing of Doppler tip angioplasty catheter with inflated balloon in an artery.

guidewire into the coronary artery to measure coronary blood flow velocity.

After recording the baseline intracoronary blood velocity in the proximal segment, the balloon was advanced across the stenosis and three to seven inflations with pressures up to 12 atm were used to dilate the stenosis. During and following each balloon inflation coronary blood flow velocity was recorded continuously with the Doppler probe situated across the stenotic lesion. Resting velocities before and after each procedure and those during reactive hyperemia immediately after balloon deflation were recorded and expressed in kilohertz (kHz).

A satisfactory functional result was considered to have been achieved if there was no further increase in reactive hyperemia. No additional dilations were performed then and coronary angiography was repeated after having removed the angioplasty catheter. The balloon diameter size used in this study varied from 2.5 to 3.5 mm. The cross-sectional area of the catheter with the balloon deflated was 0.68 mm^2 and its diameter was 0.93 mm.

Quantitative Analysis of the Coronary Artery

Coronary angiograms were performed in at least two, preferably orthogonal projections before angioplasty and the same projections were repeated after the procedure (Fig. 38-3A and B). The determination of coronary arterial dimension from 35 mm cine film was performed with the computer-based Cardiovascular Angiographic Analysis System (CAAS), previously described in detail.[17-19] In essence, boundaries of the relevant coronary artery segment are detected automatically from optically magnified and video-digitized regions of interest of a selected single cine-frame angiogram. The absolute diameter of the stenosis in millimeters (mm) is determined using the guiding catheter as a scaling device. This involves the automatic edge-detection of the boundaries of the catheter in situ and the comparison of this value with the actual diameter measurement of the catheter using a micrometer. Calibration of the diameter in absolute values (millimeters) is achieved by comparing the mean diameter of the guiding catheter in pixels with the measured size in millimeters.[20] To correct the detected contour of the arterial and catheter segments for pincushion distortion, a correction vector is computed for each pixel based on a computer-processed cine frame with a centimeter grid placed against the input screen of the image intensifier.[17] A computer estimation of the original arterial dimension at the site of the obstruction was used to define the interpolated reference area or diameter.[17,18] The interpolated percentage area stenosis and the minimal luminal cross-sectional area (in square millimeters) are then calculated from at least two, preferably orthogonal projections. The length of the lesion is determined from the diameter function on the basis of a curvature analysis.[17]

Statistical Methods

The statistical significance of the sequential changes in flow velocity (resting and hyperemic) observed during the procedure was assessed by variance analysis and Student's *t*-test for paired observations.

RESULTS

Clinical Data (Table 38-1)

The mean age of the 23 patients was 55 years (range 41 to 76 years), and 16 patients were men. Twenty-one patients had single vessel coronary disease and two patients had two-vessel disease. The investigated and dilated coronary artery was the left anterior descending (LAD) artery in 19 patients, the circumflex artery in 3 patients, and the right coronary artery in 1 patient. Left ventricular angiograms were made in right and left anterior

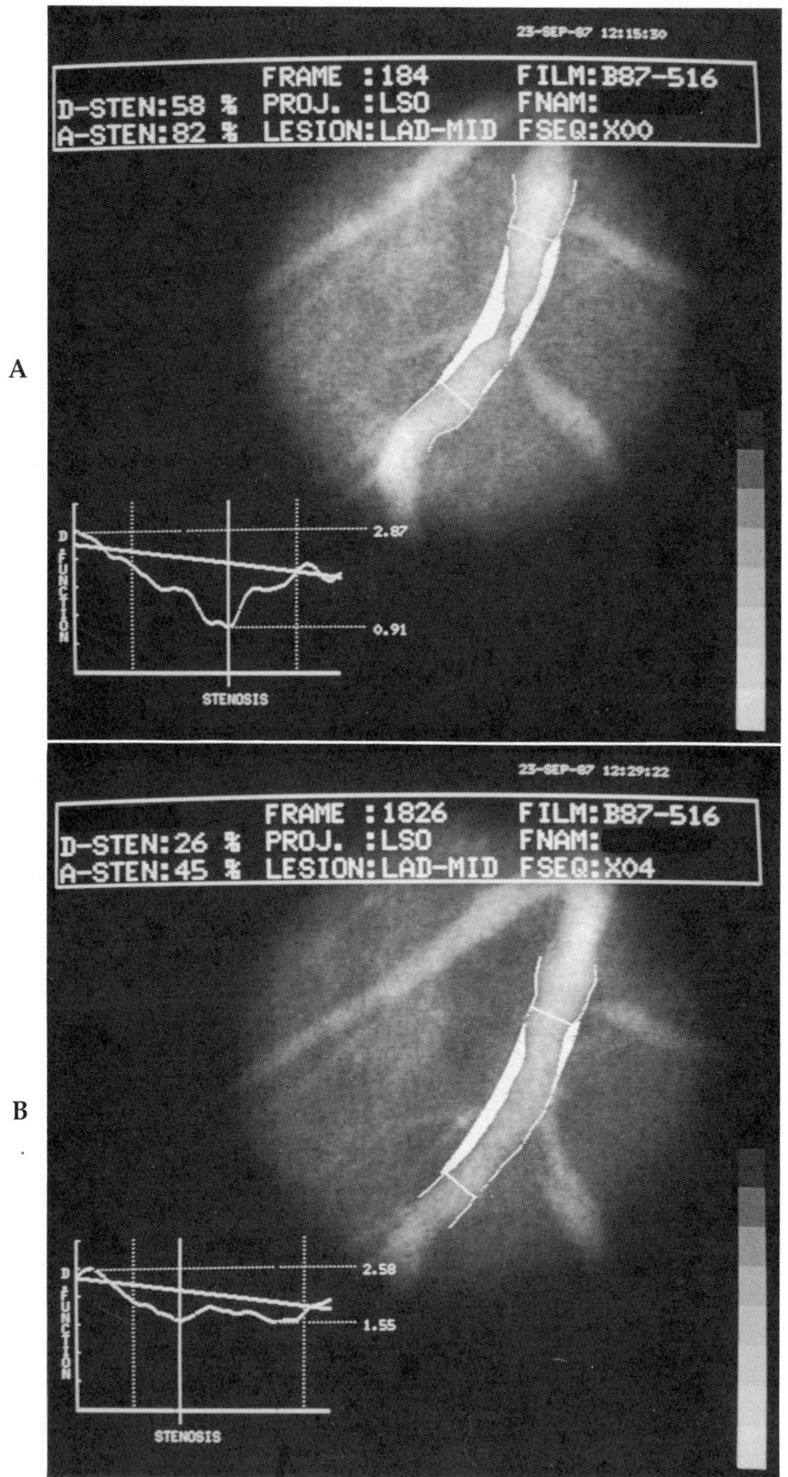

Fig. 38-3. See opposite page for legend.

oblique projections. All patients had normal systolic and diastolic wall motion and an ejection fraction of more than 55%. The length (mean ± SD) of the stenotic lesions was 6.3 ± 1.8 mm and did not change as a result of angioplasty. The mean number of balloon inflations was 4.3 per patient and ranged from 2 to 7 inflations. The angioplasty was successful in all patients. Five patients had small topical dissections of the dilated coronary artery segment after the procedure.

Quantitative Analysis of the Coronary Angiogram (Table 38-1)

The minimal luminal cross-sectional area (mean SD) increased from 1.1 ± 0.8 mm^2 to 2.6 ± 1.2 mm^2. Percentage area stenosis (mean ± SD) decreased from 83 ± 9% to 58 ± 14%. Percentage diameter stenosis (mean ± SD) decreased from 61 ± 10% to 36 ± 11%. The minimal luminal cross-sectional area before and after dilatation with the catheter across the lesion was estimated after subtraction of the cross-sectional area of the angioplasty catheter, with the balloon deflated (0.68 mm^2).

Intracoronary Doppler Shift During Angioplasty (Fig. 38-4A–D)

On the average, four dilatations were performed per patient with sequential mean inflation times of 54, 60, 63, and 68 seconds. The inflation pressure increased on the average for the four inflations from 7.6 atm to 10.4, 11.4, and 12.0 atm. Reactive hyperemia was maximal by 27 seconds (range 21 to 33 seconds) after deflation. The time to subsidence of hyperemia was 56 seconds (range 42 to 74 seconds).

Following each of the first three dilatations, both resting and hyperemic velocities increased (Table 38-2). On the average the velocities of the last two dilatations did not differ statistically, suggesting that the end result was already achieved by the third dilatation (Fig. 38-5). The ratios of peak hyperemic velocity to resting velocity for each inflation are reported in Table 38-3. When calculating"coronary flow reserve" using the peak hyperemic velocity and the resting velocity recorded before the first two dilatations, we observed a paradoxic decrease of the ratio from 3.69 ± 0.6 and 2.73 ± 0.5 to 1.88 ± 0.16 and 1.83 ± 0.21. This is due to the major increase in resting velocity whose values were very low before the first inflation, with the catheter across the undilated lesion. When this ratio is based on the resting velocity recorded after dilatation, the "coronary flow reserve" differed little from one inflation to the next, values ranging between 1.64 ± 0.21 and 2.2 ± 0.30. This absence of change was confirmed statistically by variance analysis. In other words, this ratio does not seem to be a useful functional guideline for PTCA, whereas the peak hyperemic velocity following successive balloon deflations shows a gradual and significant increase, leveling off in the majority of patients after the third dilatation.

DISCUSSION

The present study measures the changes of the intracoronary blood flow velocity during PTCA by means of a Doppler-tip balloon cath-

Fig. 38-3. Angiograms of a left anterior descending (LAD) coronary artery (left superior oblique projection) before **(A)** and after **(B)** angioplasty with superimposition of the automated contours at the coronary artery segment of interest. Beneath this is shown the diameter function of the detected contours of the coronary artery. The minimal lumen diameter *(vertical line)* and the interpolated diameter function *(horizontal line)* from which the reference diameter is derived are shown.

Table 38-1. Results of Quantitative Coronary Angiography

					Before PTCA			After PTCA				Before PTCA	After PTCA
Patient No.	*PTCA Artery*	*Balloon Size*	*Balloon Inflations*	*RA*	*MLCA (mm²)*	*DS (%)*	*AS (%)*	*MLCA (mm²)*	*DS (%)*	*AS (%)*	*RA (mm²)*	*Cor. MLCA (mm²)*	*Cor. MLCA (mm²)*
1	LAD	2.5	4	5.1	0.7	61	85	1.3	52	76	5.4	0.0	0.6
2	LC	2.5	5	5.1	0.9	56	80	1.4	48	73	5.6	0.2	0.7
3	LAD	2.5	4	3.7	0.4	66	88	1.4	43	67	4.6	0.0	0.7
4	LAD	2.5	5	6.2	1.3	53	77	1.2	49	73	4.6	0.6	0.5
5	LAD	3.0	5	6.4	0.7	66	88	1.2	48	73	4.6	0.0	0.5
6	LAD	3.0	4	6.7	0.7	55	77	2.0	32	54	4.3	0.0	1.3
7	LC	3.0	6	5.4	0.5	74	93	2.5	28	49	5.9	0.0	1.8
8	LAD	3.0	4	5.4	0.7	65	88	3.7	13	24	4.8	0.0	3.0
9	LAD	3.0	5	7.0	2.9	36	59	5.3	23	41	8.2	2.2	4.6
10	LAD	3.0	4	8.3	1.9	53	78	3.3	39	63	9.3	1.2	2.6
11	R	3.0	6	6.7	0.6	71	91	2.9	40	64	8.1	0.0	2.2
12	LAD	3.0	4	6.15	0.3	78	95	2.5	35	55	6.1	0.0	1.8
13	LAD	3.0	3	5.8	0.6	67	89	1.2	44	67	3.9	0.0	0.5
14	LAD	3.0	4	4.6	0.65	63	86	2.6	25	44	4.7	0.0	1.9
15	LAD	3.0	2	6.5	1.1	59	84	1.9	49	72	7.3	0.4	1.2
16	LAD	3.0	5	6.2	0.6	68	90	1.8	40	64	4.8	0.0	1.1
17	LAD	3.4	3	10.7	2.3	54	79	4.8	30	51	10.3	1.6	4.1
18	LAD	3.4	4	6.7	1.3	52	76	1.8	47	72	6.0	0.6	1.1
19	LAD	3.4	7	8.8	0.7	72	92	2.9	43	67	9.0	0.0	2.2
20	LC	3.4	4	11.0	3.3	48	72	4.1	34	56	9.5	2.6	3.4
21	LAD	3.4	4	6.5	1.6	47	72	3.5	30	51	7.5	0.9	2.8
22	LAD	3.4	4	5.4	0.3	74	93	3.0	18	32	4.5	0.0	2.3
23	LAD	3.4	4	7.6	0.9	63	86	3.5	22	40	6.4	0.2	2.8
Mean				6.6	1.1	61	83	2.6	36	58	6.3	0.5	1.9
±SD				1.8	±0.8	±10	±9	±1.2	±11	±14	±1.9	±0.8	±1.2

AS, Percentage area stenosis (%); Cor. MLCA, MLCA reduction due to the catheter across the lesion (mm²); DS, percentage diameter stenosis (%); LAD, left anterior descending coronary artery; LC, left circumflex coronary artery; MLCA, minimal luminal cross-sectional area (mm²); PTCA, percutaneous transluminal coronary angioplasty; R, right coronary artery; RA, reference interpolated area (mm²).

eter and the original purpose was to use this information as an on-line assessment of the functional result of the dilatation, with the PTCA catheter still across the stenosis. The technical innovation of this catheter is the combination of a diagnostic and therapeutic tool. Although the catheter is a first-generation prototype, it provides a unique opportunity to assess reactive hyperemia in awake human beings.

The poststenotic velocities recorded with the catheter across the lesion are low when

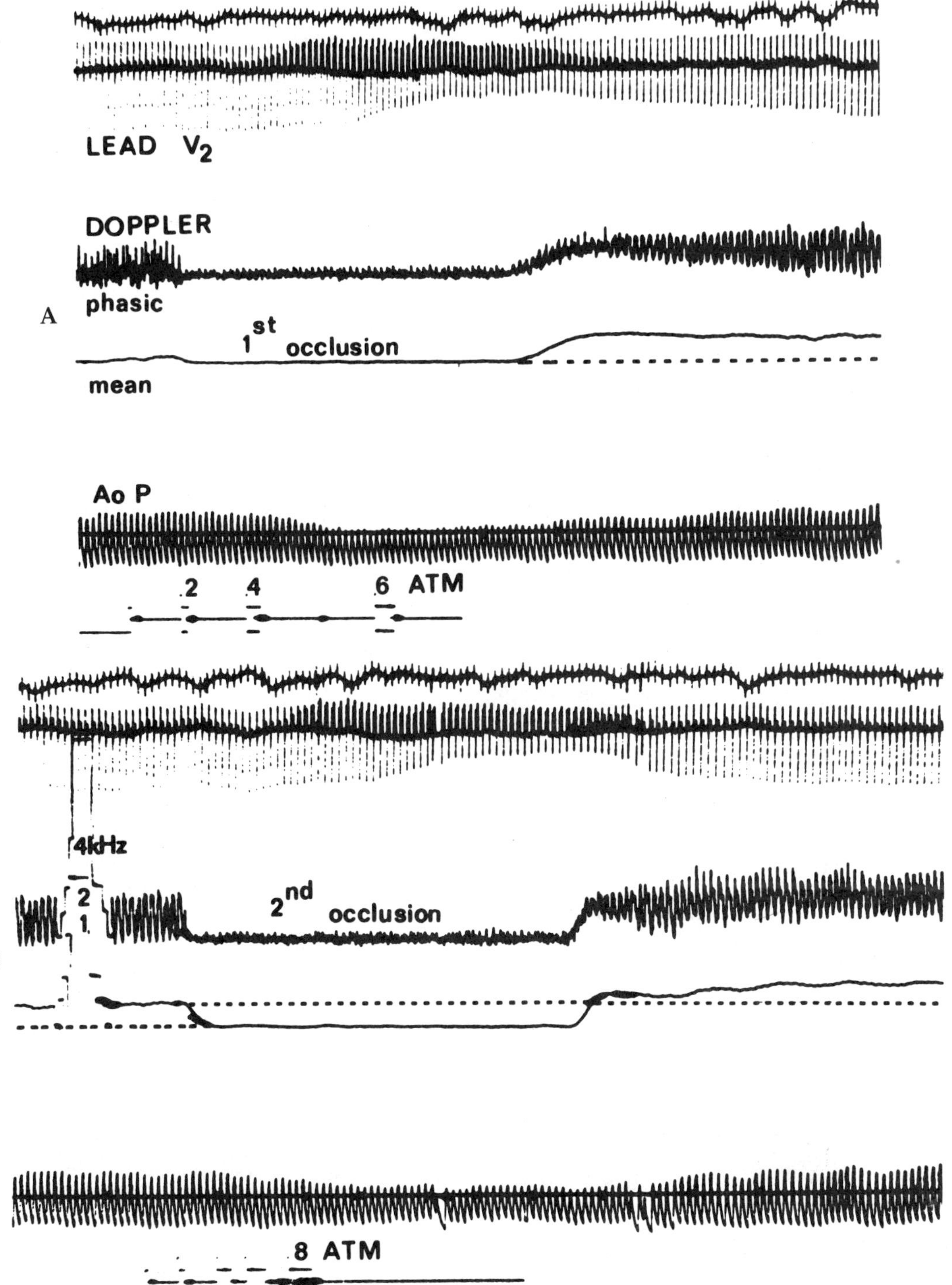

Fig. 38-4. Examples of mean and phasic Doppler signals before, during, and after balloon inflation. Reactive hyperemia occurs after balloon deflation. The precordial lead V shows ST-segment elevation. **A,** First transluminal occlusion using a balloon inflation pressure of 6 atm. **B,** Second transluminal occlusion using a balloon inflation pressure of 8 atm.

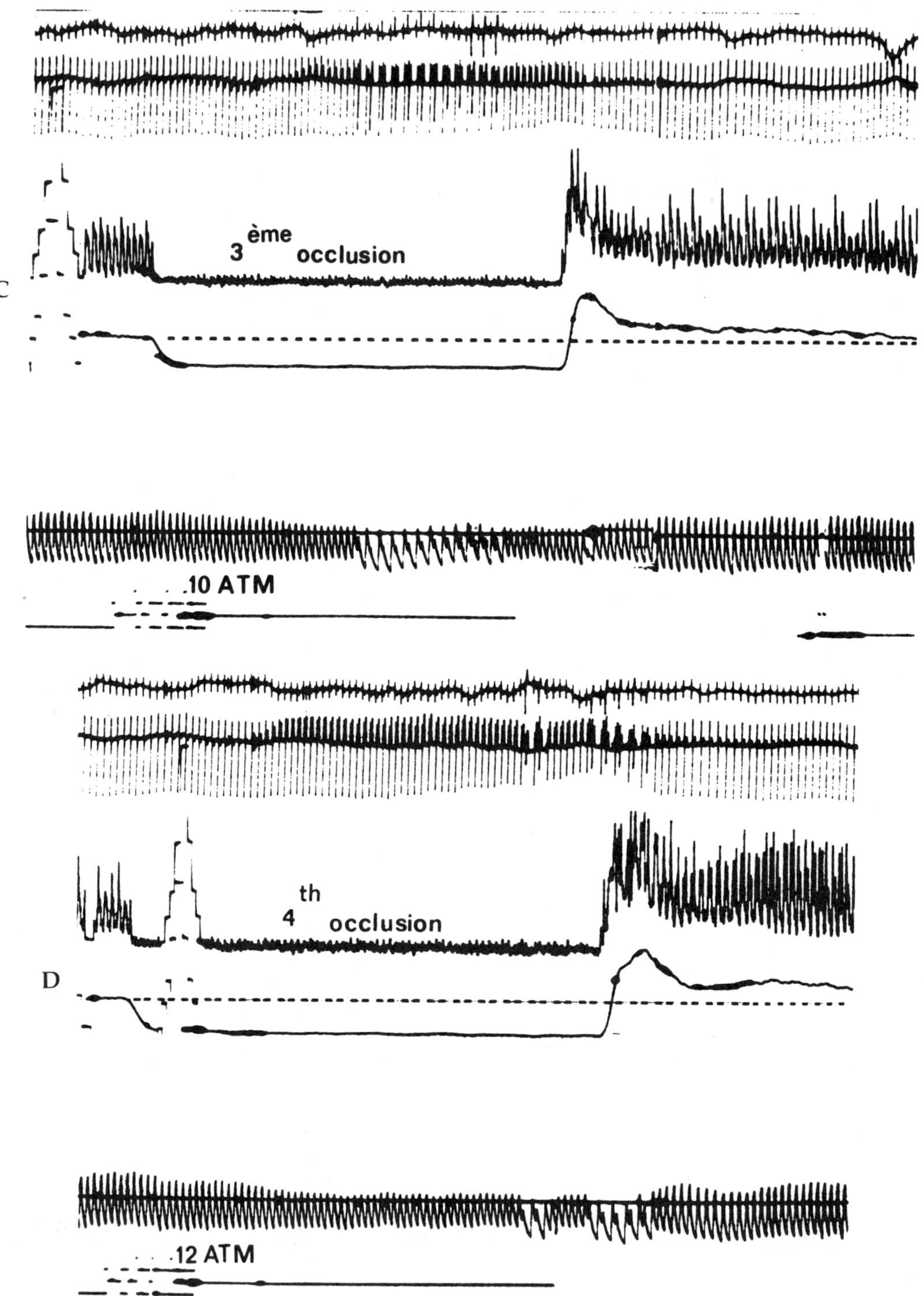

Fig. 38-4, cont'd. C, Third transluminal occlusion using a balloon inflation pressure of 10 atm. **D,** Fourth transluminal occlusion using a balloon inflation pressure of 12 atm.

Table 38-2. Doppler Shift (kHz) During Four Sequential Dilatations (Individual and Mean Data)

Patient	*Vb*				*Vh*				*Va*			
No.	*D1*	*D2*	*D3*	*D4*	*D1*	*D2*	*D3*	*D4*	*D1*	*D2*	*D3*	*D4*
1	1.65	1.54	2.00	3.00	1.54	2.00	1.00	2.00	1.54	2.00	1.00	2.00
2	0.10	0.60	0.40	0.70	0.40	0.90	1.50	0.70	0.30	0.50	0.60	0.50
3	0.18	0.12	0.87	—	0.81	1.25	1.19	—	0.18	0.87	0.56	—
4	0.50	0.62	0.62	0.75	1.43	1.25	1.68	1.43	0.62	0.56	0.62	1.06
5	0.12	0.44	1.06	1.12	0.69	1.31	1.44	1.12	0.50	1.00	1.25	0.81
6	0.56	3.75	2.00	2.19	4.62	3.19	3.37	2.31	0.75	2.00	2.00	1.56
7	0	0.25	0.25	0.31	0.56	0.31	0.81	0.56	0	0	0.25	0.25
8	0.12	0.12	1.12	0.81	0.25	0.56	1.37	1.87	0.12	0.12	0.50	—
9	0.62	0	0.56	0.50	0.62	0.81	1.06	2.43	0.62	0	0.75	1.25
10	0.12	0.87	1.18	1.25	1.06	1.62	2.81	3.25	0.81	1.25	1.18	0.56
11	0.12	0.37	0.62	0.75	0.56	0.75	1.06	0.93	0.56	0.56	0.43	0.37
12	0	0.12	0.37	0.50	0.25	0.94	0.88	0.48	0	0.62	0.37	0.50
13	0	1.00	1.80	—	0.27	3.15	2.61	—	0.09	2.34	2.43	—
14	1.00	1.57	0.92	0.71	1.71	1.14	1.14	1.28	1.57	1.14	0.85	1.00
15	0	0.92	—	—	1.42	1.07	—	—	1.1	0.71	—	—
16	0.5	0.57	1.50	1.71	1.07	1.78	2.14	2.71	0.64	1.42	2.00	2.42
17	1.06	1.25	2.75	—	2.18	1.68	5.50	—	1.25	1.12	2.87	—
18	0.90	0.95	0.65	0.95	1.30	1.05	1.50	1.35	1.20	1.05	1.00	1.25
19	0.50	1.81	1.62	1.50	2.06	2.12	1.93	3.18	1.81	1.68	0.75	1.75
20	0.10	0.10	0.15	0.65	0.35	0.60	0.35	1.10	0.15	0.50	0.30	0.70
21	0	0	0.75	1.06	0.50	1.00	1.18	2.25	0	0.25	0.50	1.25
22	0.37	1.18	1.43	1.18	3.00	1.81	2.12	2.43	0.87	1.37	1.25	1.06
23	0.37	0.56	0.50	0.81	0.56	0.75	1.06	2.00	0.43	0.75	0.50	0.93
Mean	0.39	0.81	1.05	1.08	1.18	1.35	1.71	1.76	0.66	0.95	1.00	1.07
± SE	±0.09	±0.17	±0.14	±0.15	±0.22	±0.16	±0.24	±0.19	±0.11	±0.13	±0.15	±0.14
	* (D1–D2)								* (D1–D2)			
	** (D1–D3)		NS (D3–D4)		* (D1–D3)		NS (D3–D4)		* (D1–D3)		NS (D3–D4)	

*D, Dilation; Va, resting velocity after dilatation; Vb, resting velocity before dilatation; Vh, peak reactive hyperemia. Variance analysis + paired t-test: * P <0.05; ** P <0.001; NS, not significant.*

compared with the previously published data that document values recorded proximal to the stenotic lesion.[12,16,21] Recently it has been suggested[22] that the "zero crossing" method underestimates poststenotic velocity, possibly because of disturbance of laminar flow and this may also explain the discrepancy between our results and those already published. The routine calibration of each Doppler probe by the timed blood volume collection from the femoral sheath (cross-sectional area, 6.9 mm^2) makes it unlikely that the in-

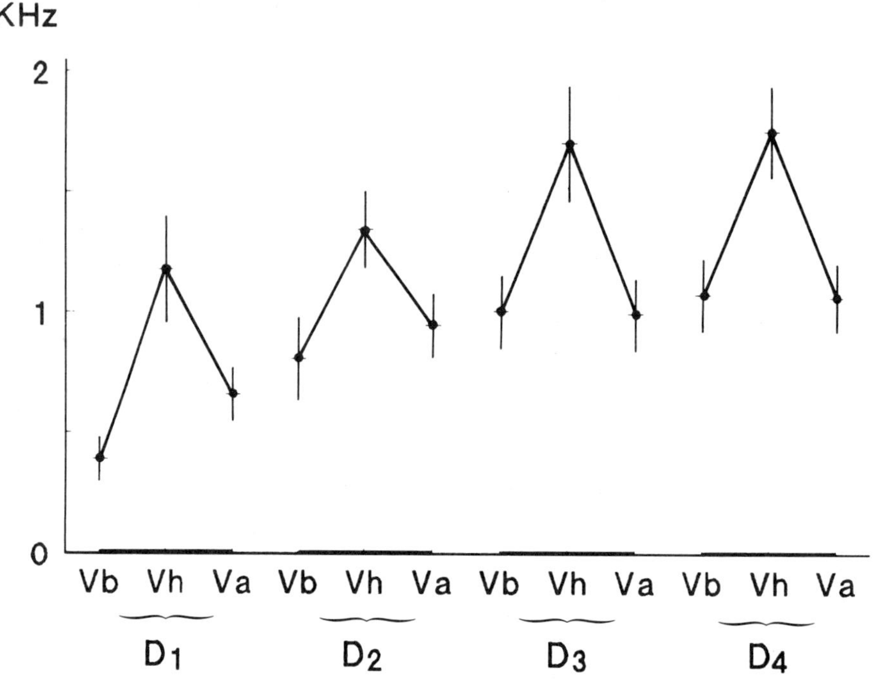

Fig. 38-5. Doppler shift (kHz, mean ± SE) during four sequential dilatations (D). (Vb, Resting velocity before dilatation; Vh, peak reactive hyperemia; Va, resting velocity after dilatation.)

tracoronary flow velocities recorded in this study with an end-mounted Doppler catheter are in error.

The duration of the hyperemia observed in all patients was longer than that in the previously reported literature.[11,13,23] However, in contrast to our results, these data were obtained after occlusion of normal arteries and after a shorter occlusion time (20 seconds maximal). Marcus and associates[23] have demonstrated that the duration of the hyperemic response increased progressively with increasing duration of occlusion.

Intracoronary blood flow velocity measurements with a Doppler probe have previously been used to investigate regional coronary flow reserve, assessing the maximal reactive hyperemia induced by pharmacologic vasodilation of ischemia.[8,12] During angioplasty, reactive hyperemia following each transluminal occlusion may be useful in assessing regional changes in coronary flow reserve resulting from the procedure. However, since coronary flow reserve is a ratio between maximal and resting coronary blood flow, any increase in resting flow results in a decrease of this ratio. This phenomenon was observed after the first two dilatations when the resting velocity preceding the inflation was used as the denominator of the ratio (peak hyperemic velocity/resting velocity). If the resting velocity following the deflation was used as the denominator, the ratio remained unchanged during four dilatations. This alternative is therefore useless as a functional guideline during the procedure. Since peak hyperemic velocity shows a gradual increase with successive dilatations that presumably reflects progressive enlargement of the lumen stenosis we attempted to correlate the cross-sectional area

Table 38-3. Ratios of Peak Reactive Hyperemia to Resting Velocity After Each Dilatation (Individual and Mean Data)

Patient No.	*Dilatation 1*		*Dilatation 2*		*Dilatation 3*		*Dilatation 4*	
	Vh/Vb	*Vh/Va*	*Vh/Vb*	*Vh/Va*	*Vh/Vb*	*Vh/Va*	*Vh/Vb*	*Vh/Va*
1	0.93	1.00	1.30	1.00	0.50	1.00	0.67	1.00
2	4.00	1.33	1.50	1.80	3.75	2.50	1.00	1.40
3	4.50	4.50	10.41	1.33	1.36	2.12	—	—
4	2.86	2.31	2.02	2.23	2.71	2.71	1.91	1.35
5	5.75	1.38	2.97	1.31	1.36	1.15	1.00	1.38
6	8.25	6.16	0.85	1.59	1.68	1.68	1.05	1.48
7	—	—	1.24	—	3.24	3.24	1.80	2.24
8	2.08	2.08	4.66	4.66	1.22	2.74	2.30	—
9	1.00	1.00	—	—	1.89	1.41	4.86	1.94
10	8.83	1.30	1.86	1.29	2.38	2.38	2.76	5.80
11	3.70	1.00	2.02	1.33	1.71	2.46	1.24	2.51
12	—	—	7.83	1.51	2.37	2.37	0.96	1.00
13	—	3.00	3.15	1.35	1.45	1.07	—	—
14	1.71	1.08	0.73	1.00	1.23	1.34	1.80	1.28
15	—	1.29	1.16	1.50	—	—	—	—
16	2.14	1.67	3.12	1.25	1.43	1.07	1.58	1.20
17	2.05	1.74	1.34	1.50	2.00	1.91	—	—
18	1.44	1.33	1.10	1.00	2.30	1.50	1.42	1.08
19	4.12	1.13	1.17	1.26	1.19	2.57	2.12	1.81
20	3.50	2.33	6.00	1.20	2.33	1.16	1.69	1.57
21	—	—	—	4.00	1.57	2.36	2.12	1.80
22	8.10	3.45	1.53	1.32	1.47	1.70	2.05	2.29
23	1.51	1.30	1.33	1.00	2.12	2.12	2.46	2.15
Mean	3.69	2.02	2.73	1.64	1.88	1.93	1.83	1.85
± SE	±0.60	±0.30	±0.55	±0.21	±0.16	±0.14	±0.21	±0.26

Va, Resting velocity after dilatation; Vb, resting velocity before dilatation; Vh, peak reactive hyperemia.

of the stenotic lesion "corrected" for the presence of the catheter across the stenosis, with the absolute value of the peak velocity during reactive hyperemia. Despite an orderly ranking of the two parameters no close correlation ($r = 0.41$) could be established. Ideally cross-sectional areas measured after each stepwise enlargement of the lumen by the gradual inflation of the balloon should have been correlated with the peak hyperemic velocity following the transluminal occlusion. Unfortunately, the poor quality of the coronary angiography performed with the PTCA catheter in the guiding catheter precludes quantitative analysis.

In the setting of PTCA, the absence of a precise mathematic relation between the peak hyperemic velocity measured after the last inflation and the post-PTCA "corrected" minimal lumen cross-sectional area is after all not so surprising. First, the changes in luminal size of an artery following the mechanical disruption of its internal wall may be difficult to assess by angiographic means.[2,3] The irregular shape with internal tears that fill with contrast medium to a variable extent will result in some overestimation of the true functional luminal size immediately following PTCA. Second, the extent of coronary atherosclerosis may be difficult to delineate angiographically. McPherson and co-workers[24] have documented that substantial intimal atherosclerosis resulting in diffuse obstructive disease, involving the entire length of an epicardial artery, is often present even when angiograms reveal only discrete lesions. As a consequence, relative measurements of stenosis severity are an inadequate approach to assessing the severity of coronary obstructions. In addition, the calculated cross-sectional area of the stenotic lesion after the subtraction of the cross-sectional area of the catheter (mean, 1.9 ± 1.2 mm^2; range, 0.5 to 4.6 mm^2) clearly suggests that the catheter is not only impeding the flow through the stenotic lesion, even after dilation, but might unpredictably disturb the velocity profile in the poststenotic segment.[16] Further miniaturization of the catheter may improve this major drawback. For all these reasons, the measurement of the peak velocity with this prototype first-generation catheter does not permit an accurate on-line prediction of the morphologic change of the stenotic lesion. However, during sequential dilatations the plateau observed in the peak hyperemic and resting velocity signals still provides valuable information that indicates that no further improvement in flow velocity can be expected from additional dilatations.

Some authors[25-27] have reported that angioplasty does not normalize coronary flow reserve. Clinical and experimental investigators have put forward several potential explanations for this phenomenon.

First, since coronary flow reserve is a ratio between maximal coronary blood flow and resting blood flow, any increase in resting flow results in a decrease of this ratio. However, several authors using the thermodilution technique in the coronary sinus or the great cardiac vein have reported comparable resting volume flows before and after angioplasty.[28,29]

Second, metabolic, humoral, or myogenic factors could potentially play a role in limiting coronary flow reserve after angioplasty. The metabolic derangements (lactate, hypoxanthine, potassium) caused by the angioplasty procedure seem quickly reversible,[28-30] and are therefore not likely to be of major significance in this regard. Although humoral factors such as thromboxane release[31] may influence vasoactive regulation in a specific subgroup of patients with complicated angioplasty, so far no scientific evidence has been presented for the persistence of humoral derangements after angioplasty. However, the long-standing reduction in perfusion pressure distal to the stenotic lesion may induce alterations in the complex mechanisms of autonomic coronary blood flow autoregulation.[32] A prolonged period may be needed before these abnormalities subside.

Finally, Bates and colleagues[32] postulated that the difference in coronary flow reserve in men with normal arteries and those who underwent revascularization is related to the atherosclerotic disease process, affecting the microvascular reactivity. In contradistinction, Wilson and associates[21] have shown in a human study that impaired coronary flow reserve is directly related to the severity of the stenosis. Cross-sectional area measured immediately after PTCA generally increased approximately threefold as a result of the procedure, but remained grossly abnormal and was generally less than half the diameter of the inflated dilating balloon.[33] In a previous study, our laboratory has established the relationship between cross-sectional area (OA) and coronary flow reserve (CFR)[19]; $CFR = 0.28 + 0.91\,(OA) - 0.039\,(OA)^2$. A measured cross-sectional area of 2.6 mm^2 after PTCA would correspond to an average coronary flow reserve of 2.4. However, if the catheter is taken into consideration, calculated coronary flow reserve is 1.86, consistent with the coronary flow reserve of 1.85 measured in this study. Therefore, this persisting reduction in cross-sectional area is by itself a sufficient explanation for the limited restoration of coronary flow reserve, although it does not exclude other contributing pathophysiologic mechanisms.

CONCLUSION

In the future, with further miniaturization of the device, the Doppler probe end-mounted on the tip of a balloon catheter may allow a more physiologic assessment of the angioplasty procedure. Following angioplasty, the coronary flow reserve is not restored to normal and the velocities remain relatively low, but their substantial improvement is consistent with the changes in coronary geometry brought about by angioplasty.

REFERENCES

1. Grüntzig, A.R., Senning, A., and Siegenthaler, W.E.: Nonoperative dilatation of coronary artery stenosis: percutaneous transluminal angioplasty, N. Engl. J. Med. **301**:61-68, 1979.
2. Block, P.C., Myler, R.K., Stertzer, S., and Fallon, J.T.: Morphology after transluminal angioplasty in human beings, N. Engl. J. Med. **305**:382-385, 1981.
3. Serruys, P.W., Reiber, J.H.C., Wijns, W., van den Brand, M., Kooijman, C.J., ten Katen, H.J., and Hugenholtz, P.G.: Assessment of percutaneous transluminal coronary angioplasty by quantitative coronary angiography: diameter versus densitometric area measurements, Am. J. Cardiol. **54**:482-488, 1984.
4. Leimgruber, P.P., Roubin, G.S., Hollman, J., Cotsonis, G.A., Meier, B., Douglas, J.S., King, S.B., and Grüntzig, A.R.: Restenosis after successful coronary angioplasty in patients with single-vessel disease, Circulation **73**:710-717, 1986.
5. Serruys, P.W., Wijns, W., Reiber, J.H.C., de Feyter, P.J., van den Brand, M., Piscione, F., and Hugenholtz, P.G.: Values and limitations of transstenotic pressure gradients measured during percutaneous coronary angioplasty, Herz **6**:337-342, 1985.
6. Hoffman, J.I.E.: Maximal coronary flow and the concept of vascular reserve, Circulation **70**:153-159, 1984.
7. Klocke, F.J.: Measurements of coronary blood flow and degree of stenosis: current clinical implications and continuing uncertainties, J. Am. Coll. Cardiol. **1**:31-41, 1983.
8. Cole, J.S., and Hartley, C.J.: The pulsed Doppler coronary artery catheter: Preliminary report of a new technique for measuring rapid changes in coronary artery flow velocity in man, Circulation **56**:18-25, 1977.
9. Hartley, C.J., and Cole, J.S.: An ultrasonic pulsed Doppler system for measuring blood flow in small vessels, J. Appl. Physiol. **37**:626-629, 1974.
10. Sibley, D., Bulle, T., Baxley, W., Dean, L., Chandler, J., and Whitlow, P.: Acute changes in blood flow velocity with successful coronary angioplasty (abstract), Circulation **74**(suppl 2): 193, 1986.
11. Sibley, D., Bulle, T., Baxley, W., Dean, L., and Whitlow, P.: Continuous on-line assessment of coronary angioplasty with a Doppler tipped balloon dilatation catheter (abstract), Circulation **74**(suppl 2):459, 1986.
12. Sibley, D.H., Millar, H.D., Hartley, C.J., and Whitlow, P.L.: Subselective measurement of coronary blood flow velocity using a steerable Doppler catheter, J. Am. Coll. Cardiol. **8**:1332-1340, 1986.
13. Marcus, M.L.: Physiological effects of a coronary stenosis. In The coronary circulation in health and disease, New York, 1983, McGraw-Hill Book Co.
14. Marcus, M.L.: Effects of cardiac hypertrophy on the coronary circulation. In The coronary circulation in health and disease, New York, 1983, McGraw-Hill Book Co.
15. Marcus, M.L., Doty, D.B., Hiratzka, L.P., Wright, C.B., and Eastham, C.L.: Decreased coronary reserve: a mechanism for angina pectoris in patients with aortic stenosis and normal coronary arteries, N. Engl. J. Med. **307**:1362-1366, 1985.
16. Wilson, R.F., Laughlin, D.E., Ackell, P.H., Chilian, W.M., Holida, M.D., Hartley, C.J.,

Armstrong, M.L., Marcus, M.L., and White, C.W.: Transluminal subselective measurement of coronary artery blood flow velocity and vasodilator reserve in man, Circulation **72:**82-92, 1985.

17. Reiber, J.H.C., Kooijman, C.J., Slager, C.J., Gerbrands, J.J., Schuurbiers, J.H.C., den Boer, A., Wijns, W., Serruys, P.W., and Hugenholtz, P.G.: Coronary artery dimensions from cineangiograms: methodology and validation of a computerassisted analysis procedure, IEEE Trans. Med. Imaging **MI-3:**131-141, 1984.
18. Reiber, J.H.C., Serruys, P.W., Kooijman, C.J., Wijns, W., Slager, C.J., Gerbrands, J.J., Schuurbiers, J.C.H., den Boer, A., and Hugenholtz, P.G.: Assessment of short- , medium- , and long-term variations in arterial dimensions from computer-assisted quantification of coronary cineangiograms, Circulation **71:**280-288, 1985.
19. Zijlstra, F., van Ommeren, J., Reiber, J.H.C., and Serruys, P.W.: Does quantitative assessment of coronary artery dimensions predict the physiological significance of a coronary stenosis?, Accepted for publication.
20. Reiber, J.H.C., Kooijman, C.J., den Boer, A., and Serruys, P.W.: Assessment of dimensions and image quality of coronary contrast catheters from cineangiograms, Cathet Cardiovasc Diagn **11:**521-531, 1985.
21. Wilson, R.F., Marcus, M.L., and White, C.W.: Prediction of the physiologic significance of coronary arterial lesions by quantitative lesion geometry in patients with limited coronary artery disease, Circulation **75:**723-732, 1987.
22. Kajiya, F., Ogasawara, Y., Tsujioka, K., Nakai, M., Goto, M., Wada, Y., Tadaoka, S., Matsuoka, S., Mito, K., and Fuwruara. T.: Evaluation of human coronary blood flow with an 80 channel 20 MHz pulsed Doppler velocimeter and zero-cross and Fourier transform methods during cardiac surgery, Circulation **74**(suppl 3):53-60, 1986.
23. Marcus. M.L., Wright, C., Doty, D., Eastham, C., Laughlin, D., Krumm, P., Fastenow, C., and Brody, M.: Measurements of coronary velocity and reactive hyperemia in the coronary circulation of humans, Circ. Res. **49:**877-891, 1981.
24. McPherson, D.D., Hiratzka, L.F., Lamberth, W.C., Brandt, B., Hunt, M., Kieso, R.A., Marcus, M.L., and Kerber, R.F.: Delineation of the extent of coronary atherosclerosis by high-frequency epicardial echocardiography, N. Engl. J. Med. **316:**304-309, 1987.
25. Johnson, M.R., Wilson, R.F., Skarton, D.J., Collins, S.M., and White, C.W.: Coronary lumen area immediately after angioplasty does not correlate with coronary vasodilator reserve: a video-densitometric study (abstract), Circulation **74**(suppl 2):193, 1986.
26. O'Neill, W.W., Walton, J.A., Bates, E.R., Colfer, H.T., Aueron, F.M., Le Free, M.T., Pitt, B., and Vogel, R.A.: Criteria for successful coronary angioplasty as assessed by alterations in coronary vasodilatory reserve, J. Am. Coll. Cardiol. **3:**1382-1390, 1984.
27. Wilson, R.F., Aylward, P.E., Talman, C.L., and White, C.W.: Does percutaneous transluminal coronary angioplasty restore normal coronary vasodilator reserve? (abstract), Circulation **72**(suppl 2):397, 1985.
28. Serruys, P.W., Piscione, F., Wijns, W., Harmsen, E., van den Brand, M., de Feyter, P., Hugenholtz, P.G., and de Jong, J.W.: Myocardial release of hypoxanthine and lactate during percutaneous transluminal coronary angioplasty: a quickly reversible phenomenon, but for how long? In Serruys, P.W.: Transluminal coronary angioplasty: an investigational tool and a nonoperative treatment of acute myocardial ischemia, doctoral dissertation, Rotterdam, 1986, Erasmus University.
29. Serruys, P.W., Wijns, W., van den Brand, M., Mey, S., Slager, C., Schuurbiers, J.C.H., Hugenholtz, P.G., and Brower, R.W.: Left ventricular performance, regional blood flow, wall motion and lactate metabolism during transluminal angioplasty, Circulation **70:**25-36, 1984.
30. Webb, S.C., Rickards, A.F., and Poole-Wilson, P.A.: Coronary sinus potassium concentration recorded during coronary angioplasty, Br. Heart J. **50:**146-152, 1983.
31. Peterson. M.B., Machay, V., Block, P.C., Palacios, I., Pithbin, D., and Watkins, W.D.: Thromboxane release during percutaneous transluminal coronary angioplasty, Am. Heart J. **1:**111-119, 1986.
32. Bates, E.R., Aueron, F.M., Le Grand, V., Le Free, M.T., Mancini, G.B.J., Hodgson, J.M.,

and Vogel, R.A.: Comparative long-term effects of coronary artery bypass graft surgery and percutaneous transluminal coronary angioplasty on regional coronary flow reserve, Circulation **72:**833-839, 1985.

33. Johnson, M.R., Brayden, G.P., Ericksen, E.E., Collins, S.M., Skaton, D.J., Harrison, D.G., Marcus, M.L., and White, C.W.: Changes in cross-sectional area of the coronary lumen in the six months after angioplasty: a quantitative analysis of the variable response to percutaneous transluminal angioplasty, Circulation **73:**467-475, 1986.

Chapter 39

Transcatheter Assessment of Coronary Artery Anatomy and Blood Flow

Robert A. Vogel, MD, FACC

Percutaneous transluminal coronary angioplasty (PTCA) requires that coronary anatomy and physiology be determined precisely. Improved diagnostic accuracy in these areas has been accomplished through the recent development of quantitative coronary arteriography and digital radiographic assessment of coronary flow reserve.[1-3] The former technique substantially reduces the observer variability associated with the visual assessment of stenosis severity and provides absolute dimensions of arterial segments. The latter technique provides regional information on coronary flow reserve assessed following pharmacologic vasodilation. Considerable debate continues to exist on the precise relationship between relative and absolute parameters of stenosis geometry and the effects of a stenosis on coronary blood flow.[4-7] Additionally, despite the help provided by quantitative arteriography and digital radiographic blood flow analysis in assessing the need for coronary angioplasty in individual instances, these techniques cannot be performed during the actual dilatation. Concomitant with the technologic explosion that has taken place over the past 10 years in coronary intervention, numerous new transcatheter diagnostic techniques are being developed for use during this critical period. Table 39-1 lists the various transcatheter techniques for the evaluation of coronary artery disease currently being studied. This chapter summarizes the principles associated with each technique, and provides detailed information on a closely related group of techniques that use electronic means for assessing coronary flow, myocardial perfusion, region of risk, and arterial cross-sectional area.

IMAGING TECHNIQUES

Direct angiographic visualization of the coronary arteries by means of contrast media injection through the guiding and balloon catheters remains the standard means for monitoring coronary anatomy during interventional procedures. This approach is, however, of limited value once the balloon catheter has been placed across the coronary stenosis. In this instance, some assessment of the stenosis

Table 39-1. Subselective Catheter Assessment of Coronary Arteries

Angiography
Angioscopy
Ultrasonography
Translesional gradient
Doppler velocity
Digital arteriographic flow
Impedance flow
Hydrogen perfusion
Flow/perfusion region-of-risk
Impedance cross-sectional area

is possible by noting the degree of notching in the silhouette of the inflated balloon. More accurate assessment of interventional success is accomplished radiographically following proximal withdrawal of the balloon catheter. Once this is done, the rate of contrast media clearance also provides a rough index of resting coronary blood flow. The utility of this is mostly limited to situations of markedly reduced or absent distal blood flow, with little information being provided under therapeutically successful conditions. Clearly, angiographic assessment of stenosis severity is limited during the dilatation process.

Another major limitation of angiography is its inability to assess atherosclerotic plaque rupture and the presence of intraluminal thrombus. Angioscopes of sufficient flexibility and small caliber have recently been introduced to enable direct visualization of the proximal coronary arteries.[8,9] Although most coronary angioscopy reported to date has been performed in the operating room in association with coronary bypass surgery, it is likely that percutaneous angioscopic techniques will become feasible in catheterization laboratories in the near future. Already, important information has been acquired in patients diagnosed with unstable clinical syndromes caused by endothelial ulceration and intraluminal thrombosis. Another proposed use for angioscopy employs automated color spectral analysis as a means for guiding laser angioplasty. Although it is unclear whether angioscopy will become part of routine diagnostic catheterizations, it is likely that important pathophysiologic information will be gained from its application. Also likely is its performance in conjunction with specialized coronary interventional procedures.

Both coronary angiography and angioscopy are unable to visualize the extramural structures. To assess the arterial wall, subselective catheters fitted with high-frequency ultrasonic crystals are now under development. These are generally fitted with rotating ultrasonic reflectors that enable the circumferential scanning of vascular segments in a radial fashion. This approach should prove especially helpful for assessing complex interventional circumstances, such as arterial dissection, as well as for obtaining direct information on the atherosclerotic pathophysiologic process.

TRANSLESIONAL GRADIENTS

Translesional gradients were previously measurable only under experimental conditions, but coronary angioplasty now allows the clinical measurement of this parameter of coronary stenosis physiology.[10-13] Patients with postdilatation gradients of less than approximately 20 mm Hg have been shown to have greater exercise tolerance and reduced incidence of restenosis. Close correlation between residual translesional gradient and digitally assessed coronary flow reserve has also been reported. In opposition to the assessment of coronary stenosis geometry, translesional gradients can be measured during the dilatation process. The value obtained is increased, however, by the presence of the catheter across the stenosis, as well as by elevated coronary blood flow. Some currently used dilatation catheter systems fail to provide any monitoring of distal coronary artery pressure. Measurements from those systems that are capable of monitoring distal pressure are less reliable when placed in small and/or distal vessels. Despite these problems, the assessment of residual translesional gradients remains clinically useful. High residual gradients portend poor clinical outcomes, although low residual gradients are not always followed by permanently successful results.

BLOOD VELOCITY AND FLOW

Although initial animal experiments reported close correlations of percent diameter stenosis and coronary flow reserve, more recent clinical studies have revealed more divergent findings. This is likely to be especially true under the complex conditions of coronary intervention, suggesting the need for the direct assessment of coronary flow reserve and absolute blood flow. Subselective balloon catheters have recently become available that can measure coronary blood velocity using Doppler techniques.[14,15] Although absolute coronary blood flow cannot be measured by this approach, coronary flow reserve can be determined by comparing blood velocities under pharmacologically induced hyperemic and baseline conditions. Papaverine, injected by the intracoronary route, has proved especially useful for this purpose, because it provides both near-maximal vasodilation and short duration of action.[16] Major advantages of this approach are that both phasic and mean blood velocity data are provided continuously and that injection of an indicator substance is not required. The technique is, however, sensitive to catheter position, and velocity measurements are significantly reduced when the catheter is located translesionally.

Coronary flow reserve can also be assessed using digital radiographic analysis of subselectively injected contrast media administered under hyperemic and baseline conditions.[17] This approach differs from the contrast medium appearance picture (CMAP) technique in its use of traditional indicator-dilution analysis. As with the former technique, data can be presented in color-coded parametric image format. The Doppler catheter and digital radiographic techniques for measuring coronary flow reserve are presently unable to measure absolute coronary blood flow. This limits their diagnostic utility because numerous conditions reduce flow reserve independently of epicardial stenosis. These include myocardial hypertrophy, prior myocardial infarction, coronary artery collaterals, vasoactive drugs, endothelial damage, and prolonged ischemia, as well as reduction in mean arterial pressure and elevation of heart rate and end-diastolic pressure. Coronary flow reserve also appears to be transiently reduced immediately following coronary dilatation. Clearly, flow reserve does not provide complete clinical assessment of stenosis severity, although it is generally true that a good physiologic result is strongly suggested by a postdilatation normal flow reserve value, whereas a low value does not preclude success.

ELECTRONIC TECHNIQUES

Four closely related techniques for assessing coronary artery anatomy and flow physiology are currently under development in our laboratory. These are designed to measure, respectively, absolute coronary blood flow, regional myocardial perfusion, region-of-risk, and arterial cross-sectional area. Each technique uses electronic principles that enable its eventual implementation using guidewire technology.

Absolute Coronary Blood Flow Measurements. The first of these is designed to measure absolute coronary blood flow, using impedance measurements and the Stewart-Hamilton indicator-dilution principle.[18] A standard angioplasty catheter has been modified with the addition of a third lumen that is used for infu-

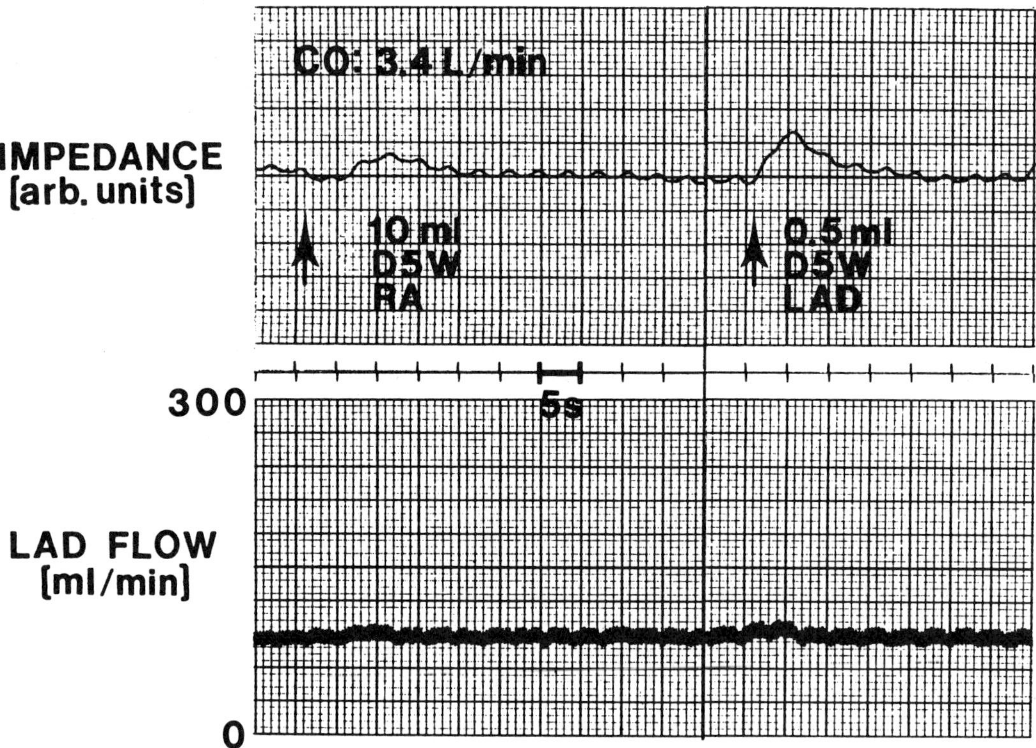

Fig. 39-1. *Top,* Impedance tracings obtained with a subselective angioplasty catheter positioned in a canine LAD coronary artery are shown. Arrows denote the onset of a 10 ml D_5W injection into the right atrium *(left)* and a 0.5 ml D_5W injection into the coronary artery through the catheter's proximal side port *(right).* The initial injection is used for in-situ calibration purposes and the latter injection for assessment of coronary blood flow. *Bottom,* Concomitantly measured left anterior blood flow determined by electromagnetic flowmeter is shown.

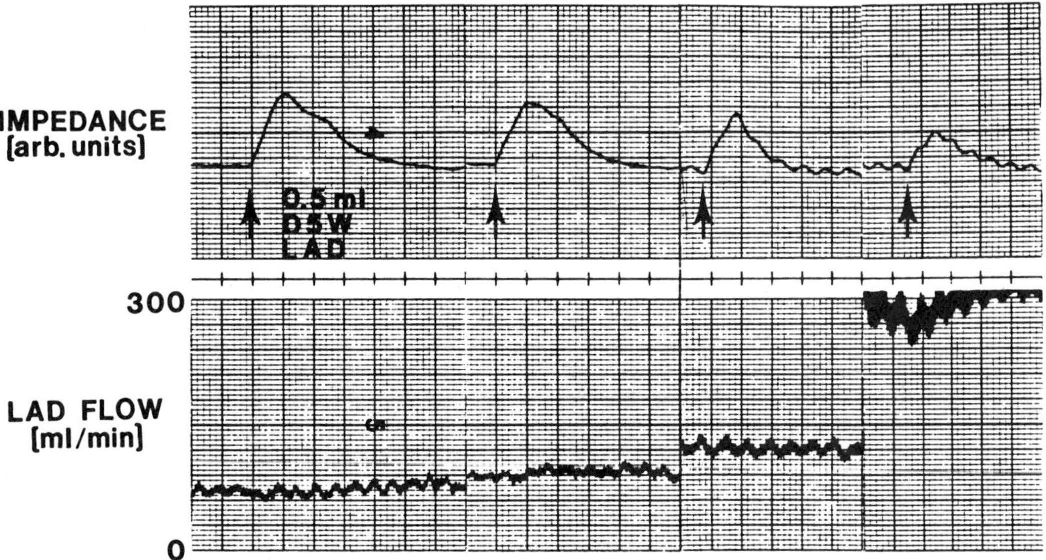

Fig. 39-2. *Top,* Four first-pass impedance tracings obtained with the catheter positioned in a canine LAD coronary artery. *Bottom,* Curve area diminishes as electromagnetically measured coronary flow increases.

sion of an indicator substance just proximal to the balloon. Four microelectrodes are positioned near the catheter's tip. Impedance is measured at a frequency of 50 kHz and a constant current of 10 μA between the two proximal and two distal microelectrodes spaced 2 mm apart. One-half milliliter of 5% glucose solution (D_5W) is injected over a 5-second period through the proximal port. The solution is hypotonic relative to blood, thereby causing an increase in impedance measurable at the microelectrodes. Absolute coronary blood flow is determined by inverse proportionality to the area under the impedance curves in a manner analogous to the determination of cardiac output using thermodilution methodology. The 3 cm distance between the proximal infusion port and the catheter's microelectrodes has been found to produce adequate mixing of the D_5W indicator and intrinsic blood flow. By the indicator-dilution principle, blood flow is determined at the site of introduction of the indicator substance. Subsequent arterial branching does not affect this determination, as long as adequate mixing is ensured. Because impedance measurements are affected both by blood conductivity and vessel volume, system calibration is currently performed in situ. A 10 ml bolus of D_5W is injected in the right side of the heart with simultaneous measurement of thermodilution cardiac output and coronary catheter impedance. Subsequent measurements of absolute coronary blood flow are calculated by the following equation:

$$\text{Coronary blood flow} = (\text{cardiac output}) \times (\text{cardiac output curve area}) \div 20\ (\text{coronary blood flow curve area}).$$

Validation of this principle was performed in a canine model using electromagnetic flowmeter data obtained from the left anterior descending (LAD) and circumflex coronary arteries in 67 instances and femoral arteries in 5 instances. Fig. 39-1 depicts impedance tracings obtained with the catheter positioned in a proximal LAD canine coronary artery, following reference injection into the right atrium *(left)* and into the coronary artery *(right)*. Cardiac output was measured by thermodilution in the initial instance. Fig. 39-2 depicts indicator dilution curves obtained in a canine LAD coronary artery under four different flow conditions ranging from 70 to 300 ml/minute. Note that the area under the dilution curve diminishes as flow increases. Fig. 39-3 depicts the correlation between measurements of absolute coronary and femoral artery flow obtained by the impedance catheter and electromagnetic flowmeter standard.

Measurement of Regional Myocardial Perfusion. The second transcatheter electronic technique is designed to measure regional myocardial perfusion using the Kety-Schmidt, inert gas washout principle.[19] Hydrogen-saturated saline is infused at a rate of 10 ml/minute for 30 seconds subselectively by means of a standard angioplasty catheter. High-impedance electrical potential (voltage) measurements are obtained from a platinum-tipped pacing catheter positioned in the pulmonary artery to monitor the effluent concentration of hydrogen during its washout phase. An example of such a tracing is depicted in Fig. 39-4, obtained in a canine preparation. In contrast to

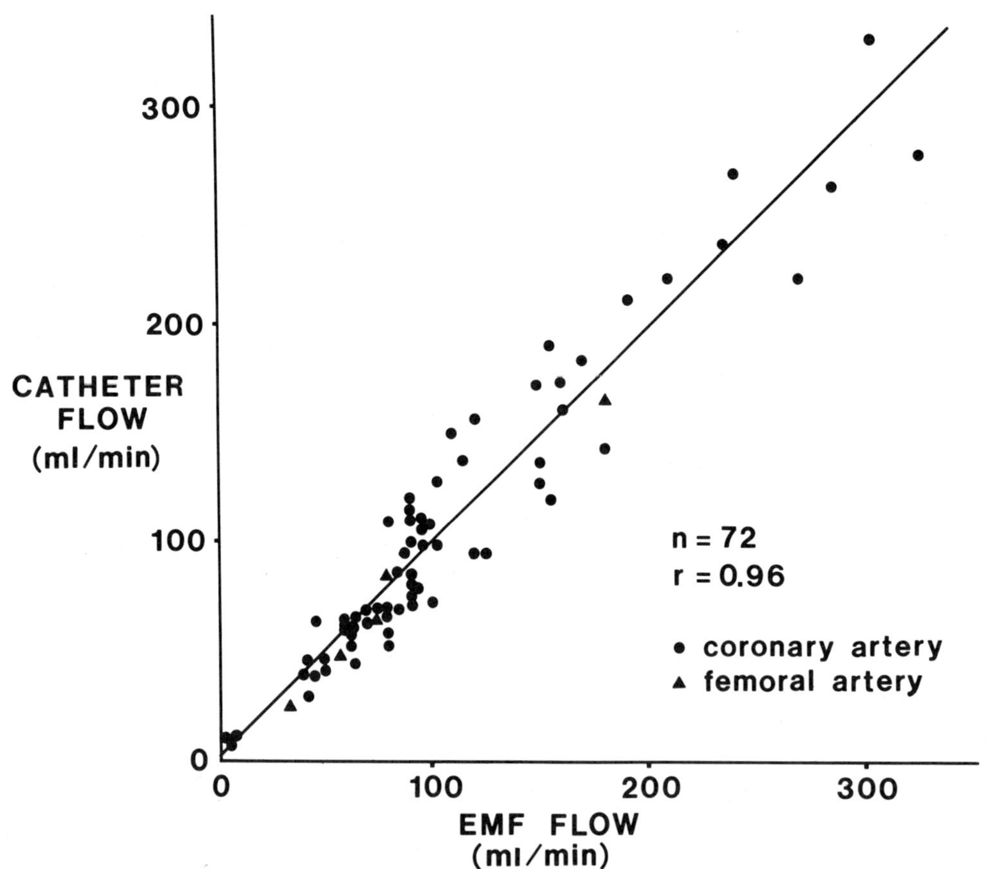

Fig. 39-3. Comparison of electromagnetic flowmeter and impedance catheter determinations of canine coronary and femoral artery blood flow.

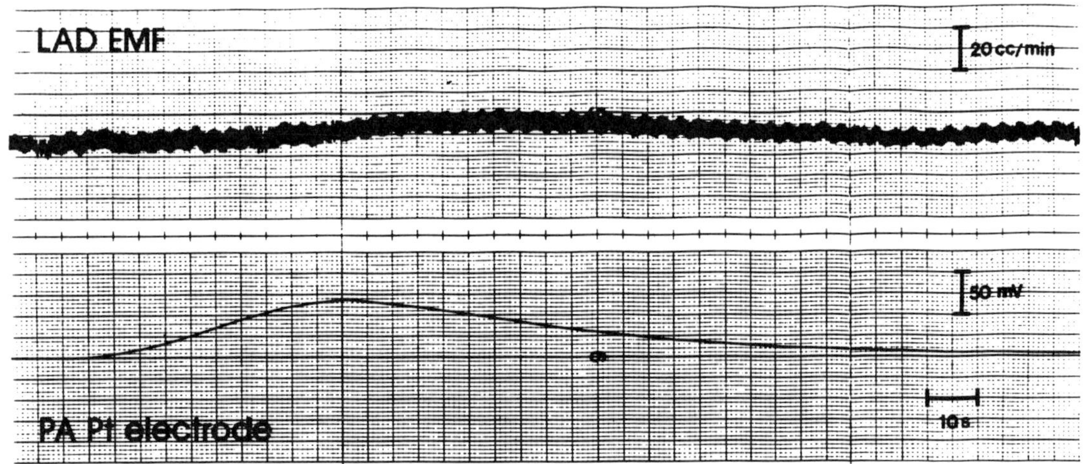

Fig. 39-4. *Top,* Electromagnetically measured canine LAD coronary artery blood flow and pulmonary artery platinum electrode catheter electrical potential measurements *(bottom)* are shown during subselective hydrogen infusion and subsequent washout.

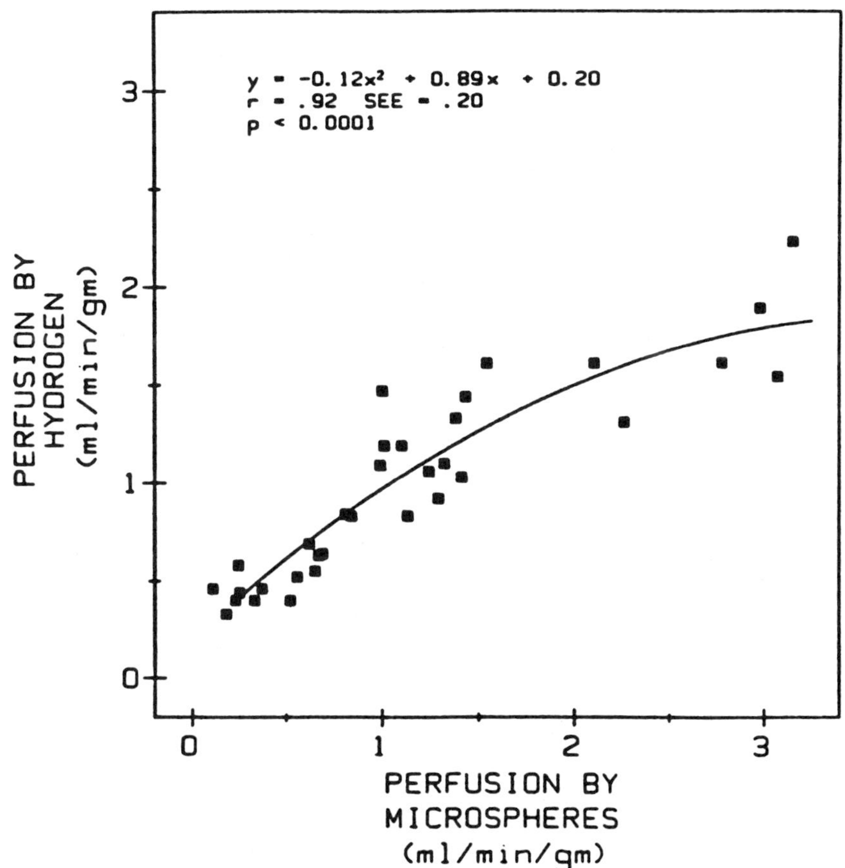

Fig. 39-5. Comparison of radiolabeled microsphere and subselective hydrogen perfusion estimations of regional myocardial blood flow.

previously utilized washout techniques, this approach uses selective administration of the inert gas tracer and nonselective detection. As with all washout techniques, it assumes that coronary blood flow remains constant during the measurement. This approach also requires that cardiac output remains constant. Validation of this approach was performed in a canine model using radiolabeled particles as a standard. Resultant data are depicted in Fig. 39-5. As with other reported washout techniques, some overestimation of low flow conditions and underestimations of high flow conditions were found.

Region-of-Risk Measurement. The combined abilities to measure absolute coronary blood flow and regional myocardial perfusion theoretically allow for the determination of region-of-risk, defined as the myocardial mass perfused by an individual coronary artery segment. Region-of-risk is calculated as coronary blood flow (ml/minute) ÷ regional myocardial perfusion (ml/minute/g). The theoretic validity of this approach was undertaken using simultaneous electromagnetic flowmeter determinations in subselective hydrogen washout analyses to determine region-of-risk, which was compared with staining and weighing

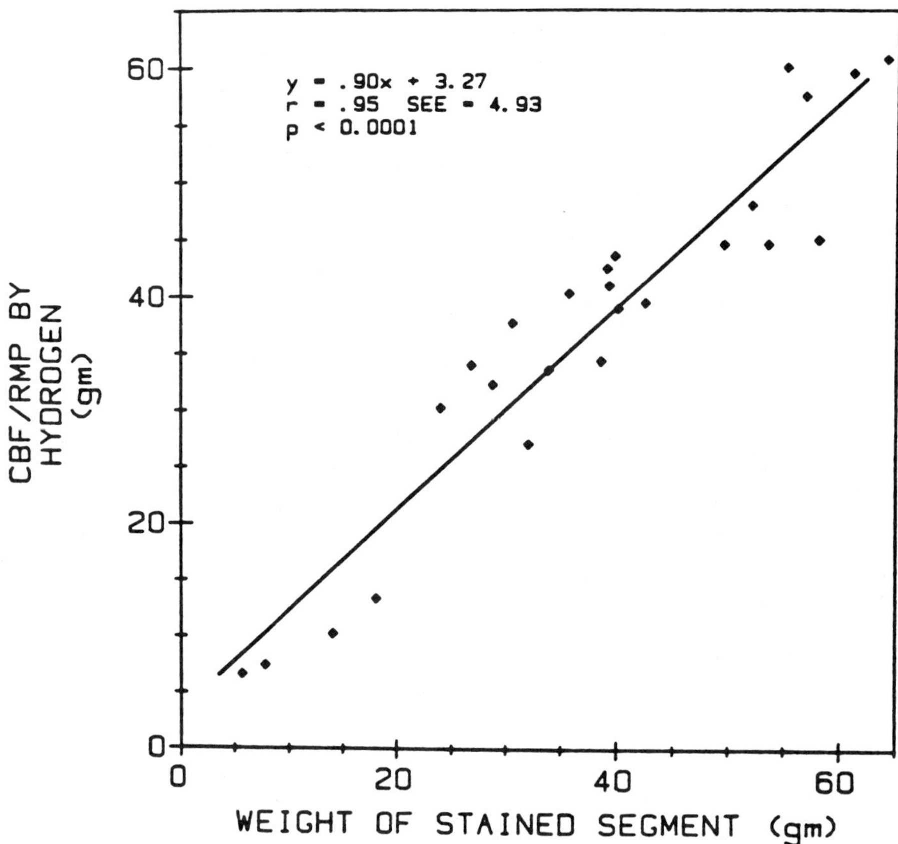

Fig. 39-6. Region-of-risk myocardial weight determined by sectioning, staining, and weighing are compared with the coronary blood flow/regional myocardial perfusion technique.

determinations.[19] A good correlation was found between the two determinations over a wide range of risk areas (Fig. 39-6). In the future, transcatheter measurements of blood flow and perfusion will allow assessment of the amount of viable tissue perfused by an individual coronary artery, a goal that has long eluded clinical cardiology.

Arterial Cross-Sectional Area Measurement. The last technology under development uses impedance principles to measure absolute arterial cross-sectional area.[20] As mentioned above, electrical impedance is affected by both arterial conductivity and vessel volume. The latter association has been used for online determinations of left ventricular volume. Similar principles are used for determination of arterial cross-sectional area utilizing the same impedance catheter designed for the determination of absolute coronary blood flow. Preliminary data suggests that a continuous recording of arterial cross-sectional area can be obtained by withdrawing the catheter's tip through a stenotic arterial segment. This principle is demonstrated in Figs. 39-7 and 39-8, which respectively depict a canine arterial preparation containing stenotic and dissected sections and associated impedance tracing. Three impedance tracings obtained by passage of the impedance catheter (left to right) at slightly different speeds are shown. Both the high-grade and low-grade stenoses are well-seen on the three impedance tracings that are not affected by the arterial dissection present. Guidewires fitted with microelectrodes are now being constructed for this pur-

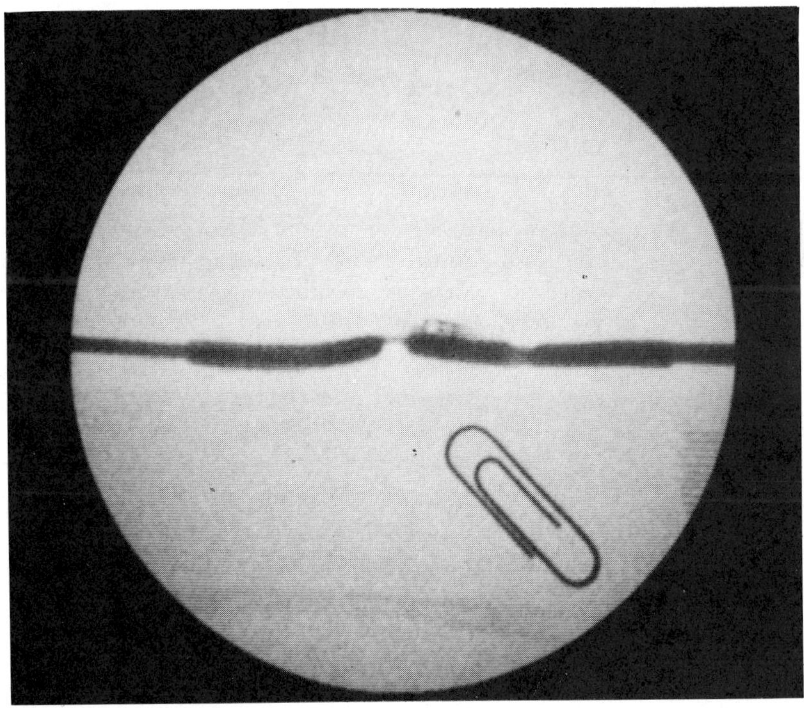

Fig. 39-7. An angiographic image of a canine artery phantom containing high-grade and low-grade stenoses. A small area of dissection is also shown.

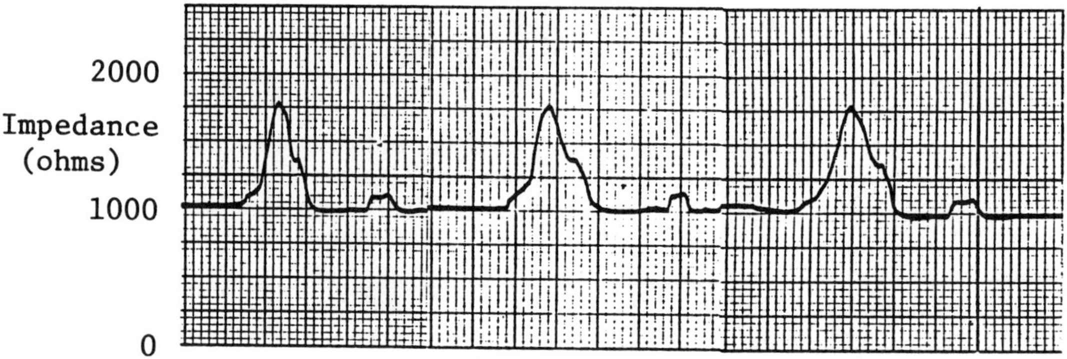

Fig. 39-8. Three successive impedance catheter transits (left-to-right) of the arterial phantom depicted in Fig. 39-7 are shown. Both the high-grade and low-grade stenoses are clearly visible.

pose. It is hoped that this will allow on-line measurement of absolute arterial cross-sectional area during the coronary intervention. This would provide objective assessment of the stenosis severity both before and after the dilatation.

CONCLUSION

Recent advances in interventional cardiology have pointed out substantial limitations of traditional arteriography in assessing coronary artery anatomy and physiology, especially during the dilatation process. Numerous new techniques are currently being developed to allow visualization of luminal and mural processes, parameters of relative and absolute coronary blood flow, regional myocardial perfusion, and regions-of-risk. It is possible that the analysis of coronary cross-sectional area may be performed in the future using nonangiographic techniques. The legitimate diagnostic demands and widespread use of coronary angioplasty make it likely that the more promising of these techniques will be clinically available in the near future.

REFERENCES

1. Brown, B.G., Bolson, E., Frimer, M., Dodge, H.T.: Quantitative coronary arteriography: estimation of dimension, hemodynamic resistance, and atheroma mass of coronary artery lesions using the arteriogram and digital computer, Circulation **55**:329, 1977.
2. Mancini, G.B.J., Simon, S.B., McGillem, M.J., LeFree, M.T., Friedman, H.Z., and Vogel, R.A.: Automated quantitative coronary arteriography: in-vivo morphologic and physiologic validation of a rapid method utilizing digital angiography, Circulation **75**:452-460, 1987.
3. Vogel, R.A.: The radiographic assessment of coronary blood flow parameters, Circulation **72**:460-465, 1985.
4. Klocke, F.J.: Measurements of coronary blood flow and degree of stenosis: current clinical implications and continuing uncertainties, J. Am. Coll. Cardiol. **1**:31-42, 1983.
5. Wilson, R.F., Marcus, M.L., and White, C.W.: Prediction of the physiologic significance of coronary artery lesions by quantitative lesion geometry in patients with limited coronary artery disease, Circulation **75**:723-732, 1987.
6. Zijlstra, F., van Ommeren, J., Reiber, J.H.C., and Serruys, P.W.: Does the quantitative assessment of coronary artery dimensions predict the physiologic significance of a coronary stenosis?, Circulation **75**:1154-1161, 1987.
7. LeGrand, V., Mancini, G.B.J., Bates, E.R., Hodgson, J.McB., Gross, M.D., and Vogel, R.A.: A comparative study of coronary flow reserve, coronary anatomy, and the results of radionuclide exercise tests in patients with coronary heart disease, J. Am. Coll. Cardiol. **8**:1022-1032, 1986.
8. Sherman, C.T., Litvack, F., Grundfest, W.S., Lee, M., Hickey, A., Chaux, A., Kass, R., Blanch, E.C., Matloff, J., Morganstern, L., Janz, W., Swan, H.J.C., and Forrester, J.: Demonstration of thrombus and complex atheroma by in-vivo angioscopy in patients with unstable angina pectoris, N. Engl. J. Med. **315**:913, 1986.
9. Forrester, J.S., Litvack, F., Grundfest, W.S., and Hickey, A.: A prospective of coronary disease seen through the arteries of living man, Circulation **75**:505-513, 1987.
10. Leiboff, R., Bren, G., Katz, R., Korkejl, R., and Ross, A.: Determinations of transstenotic gradients observed during angioplasty: an experimental model, Am. J. Cardiol. **52**:1311-1317, 1983.
11. O'Neill, W.W., Walton, J.A., Bates, E.R., Colfer, H.T., Aueron, F.M., LeFree, M.T., Pitt, B., and Vogel, R.A.: Criteria for successful coronary angioplasty as assessed by alterations in coronary vasodilatory reserve, J. Am. Coll. Cardiol. **3**:1382-1390, 1984.
12. Haraphongse, M., Tymchak, W., Burton, J.R., and Rossall, R.E.: Implication of transstenotic coronary pressure gradient measurement during coronary angioplasty, Cathet. Cardiovasc. Diagn. **12**:80-84, 1986.
13. Peterson, R.J., King, S.B., Fajman, W.A., Douglas, J.S., Gruntzig, A.R., Orias, D.W., Jones, R.H.: Relation of coronary artery stenosis and pressure gradient to exercise-induced ischemia before and after coronary angioplasty, J. Am. Coll. Cardiol. **10**:253-260, 1987.
14. Wilson, R.F., Laughlin, D.E., Ackell, P.H., Chilian, W.M., Holida, M.D., Hartley, C.J., Armstrong, M.L., Marcus, M.L., and White, C.W.: Transluminal subselective measurement of coronary artery blood flow velocity and va-

sodilator reserve in man, Circulation **72:**82, 1985.

15. Sibley, D.H., Millar, H.D., Hartley, C.J., and Whitlow, P.L.: Subselective measurement of coronary blood flow velocity using a steerable Doppler catheter, J. Am. Coll. Cardiol. **8:**1332-1340, 1986.
16. Wilson, R.F., and White, C.W.: Intracoronary papaverine: an ideal coronary vasodilator for studies of the coronary circulation in conscious humans, Circulation **73:**444, 1986.
17. Nisson, S.E., Elion, J.L., Booth, D.C., Evans, J., DeMarria, A.N.: Value and limitations of computer analysis digital subtraction angiography in the assessment of coronary flow reserve, Circulation **73:**562-571, 1986.
18. Vogel, R.A., Grines, C.L., McGillem, M.J., Beauman, G.J., and Mancini, G.B.J.: Impedance measurement of absolute coronary blood flow using a standard angioplasty catheter, Clin. Res. **35:**332A, 1987.
19. Grines, C.L., Mancini, G.B.J., McGillem, M.J., Gallagher, K.P., and Vogel, R.A.: Measurement of regional myocardial perfusion and mass using subselective hydrogen infusion and washout techniques: a validation study, Circulation. (In press.)
20. Martin, L.W., Meijboom, E., and Vogel, R.A.: Determinations of coronary artery diameter using impedance as measured by a standard angioplasty catheter, Clin. Res. (In press.)

Chapter 40

Application of Echocardiography to Catheter Balloon Valvuloplasty

Anthony N. DeMaria, MD, FACC
Thomas Wisenbaugh, MD
Mikel Smith, MD

The invasive interventional technique of catheter balloon valvuloplasty has resulted in a proportional, if unexpected, reliance on the noninvasive method of echocardiography. Thus the ability to perform valvuloplasty has increased the interventional cardiologist's interest in and reliance on the findings in the noninvasive laboratory. The contribution of echocardiography to valvuloplasty has taken several forms (Table 40-1). Echocardiography provides the first method by which to confirm the diagnosis and quantify the lesions of mitral and aortic stenosis. Echocardiography also allows the diagnosis of associated lesions that may determine the suitability of patients for catheter valvuloplasty. More importantly, particularly in regard to the mitral valve, morphologic characteristics of the echocardiogram are being shown to relate quite well to the potential for an excellent hemodynamic result following valvuloplasty. Echocardiography has been advocated and utilized by some to guide the valvuloplasty procedure by means of localizing the balloon itself. Of greater significance, echocardiography has provided an important tool for the detection of complications following valvuloplasty, as well as assessment of the effects in both the long and short term following the procedure. Therefore echocardiography now plays an integral role in the assessment of the patient undergoing balloon valvuloplasty.

QUANTITATION OF VALVE STENOSIS

Echocardiography has been demonstrated during the past several years to provide an excellent modality by which to quantify the severity of valvular stenosis.[1] A variety of echo imaging and Doppler velocity measurements can be performed that enable quantitation of both valvular gradient and cross-sectional area.[2] Although all echo maneuvers are potentially applicable to both mitral and

Table 40-1. Echocardiography in Catheter Balloon Valvuloplasty

Diagnosis and quantitation of lesion
Detection of associated abnormalities (regurgitation)
Evaluation of suitability for valvuloplasty
Guiding procedure
Detection of complications
Assessment of results
Long-term follow-up

aortic valves, certain assessments have been found to be of greater value with respect to specific valves.

Several methods exist to quantify the severity of mitral stenosis by echocardiography. The oldest method is based on the ability to visualize the cross-sectional area of the mitral valve. When images of the mitral valve leaflets are obtained in short-axis views, the area of the orifice can be easily planimetered, and these values have been shown to correlate quite well to either catheter or surgical measurements of the mitral valve area.[3] Such measurements are influenced by a variety of technical factors. The smallest orifice of the funnel-shaped mitral leaflets must be located and visualized. Excessive gain setting may obliterate some portion of the orifice by ultrasound reflectances. Angulation of the ultrasound beam to traverse the orifice tangentially may result in false estimates of its size. Therefore utilization of echo imaging techniques may not be suitable in some patients with mitral stenosis. Nevertheless, they provide an excellent modality for quantitation in the majority of patients with this lesion.

An alternate method for assessing the severity of mitral stenosis, and aortic stenosis as well, is provided by Doppler velocity measurements. Based on the Bernoulli equation: pressure gradient = 4 $(\text{velocity})^2$, the transvalvular flow velocity can be related to both the mean and the maximal gradient across the mitral valve during diastole.[4] For transaortic gradients, both maximal and mean gradients have been found to predict catheterization results well.[4,5] For transmitral gradients simultaneous measurements of mean gradient, in particular, have been shown to correlate quite well with catheterization pressure measurements. However, owing to influences of heart rate and cardiac output, a much superior estimate of the severity of mitral stenosis is the mitral valve area. An estimate of mitral valve area can be obtained using Doppler techniques by means of the pressure half-time approach.[6] Specifically, the time interval required for the velocity to fall to one half of the pressure equivalent is measured from the transmitral Doppler recording, and then divided into the empirical constant of 220 to achieve an estimate of mitral valve area (Fig. 40-1). Studies in several laboratories have demonstrated that the mitral pressure half-time method provides values of mitral valve area that correlate well with those derived by cardiac catheterization.[2,6]

Studies performed in our laboratory have demonstrated that both planed measurements of mitral valve orifice from two-dimensional (2-D) echo images and estimates of mitral valve area derived by the pressure half-time Doppler method yield values that correlate equivalently with catheterization-derived measures of mitral valve area in patients with native mitral valves.[2] However, of potential relevance to catheter balloon valvuloplasty, these studies have demonstrated that Doppler values are superior to those derived from planed echo images in patients who have undergone a previous mitral commissurotomy. The apparent explanation for this relates to scarring and distortion of the mitral valve leaflets following the commissurotomy procedure. It might be anticipated, therefore, that transmitral Doppler recordings could potentially provide a more accurate mechanism by which to evaluate the results of catheter bal-

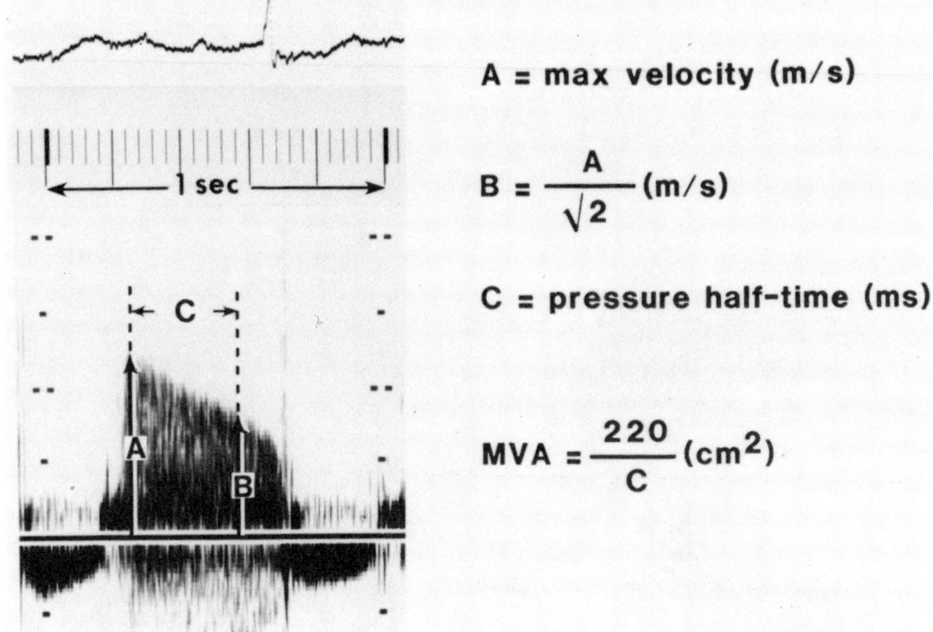

Fig. 40-1. Shown is the transmitral velocity trace obtained by continuous wave Doppler echocardiography in a patient with mitral stenosis. Velocity is plotted on the vertical axis, while time is on the horizontal axis. Pressure half-time is defined as the interval required for the maximal velocity (point A) to fall to one half of the pressure equivalent (velocity B). Mitral valve area can be obtained by dividing this interval in milliseconds into the empiric constant of 220.

loon valvuloplasty. However, few data are currently available regarding this issue.

As compared with the mitral valve leaflets, the aortic valve orifice is quite difficult to define by echocardiographic imaging because of multiple reflectances and the triangular shape of the valve.[7] Therefore the quantitation of aortic stenosis has focused on calculation of the transvalvular gradient by the Bernoulli equation utilizing continuous wave Doppler echocardiography (Fig. 40-2). More recently, studies have demonstrated that the continuity equation may be utilized to estimate aortic valve area.[8] This equation is based on the fact that the volume of blood flow through the left ventricular outflow tract must equal the volume of blood flow through the aortic valve orifice. Since volumetric blood flow equals the product of velocity and cross-sectional area, and since the velocity in cross-sectional area of the left ventricular outflow tract as well as the velocity of blood through the aortic valve orifice can be measured, one can therefore calculate the cross-sectional area of the aortic valve. Numerous studies have demonstrated the ability of Doppler echocardiography measurements of aortic valve severity to correlate well with catheterization determinations.

DETECTION OF ASSOCIATED LESIONS

A variety of lesions associated with the primary stenotic process may be detected by echocardiography (Table 40-2). Predominant

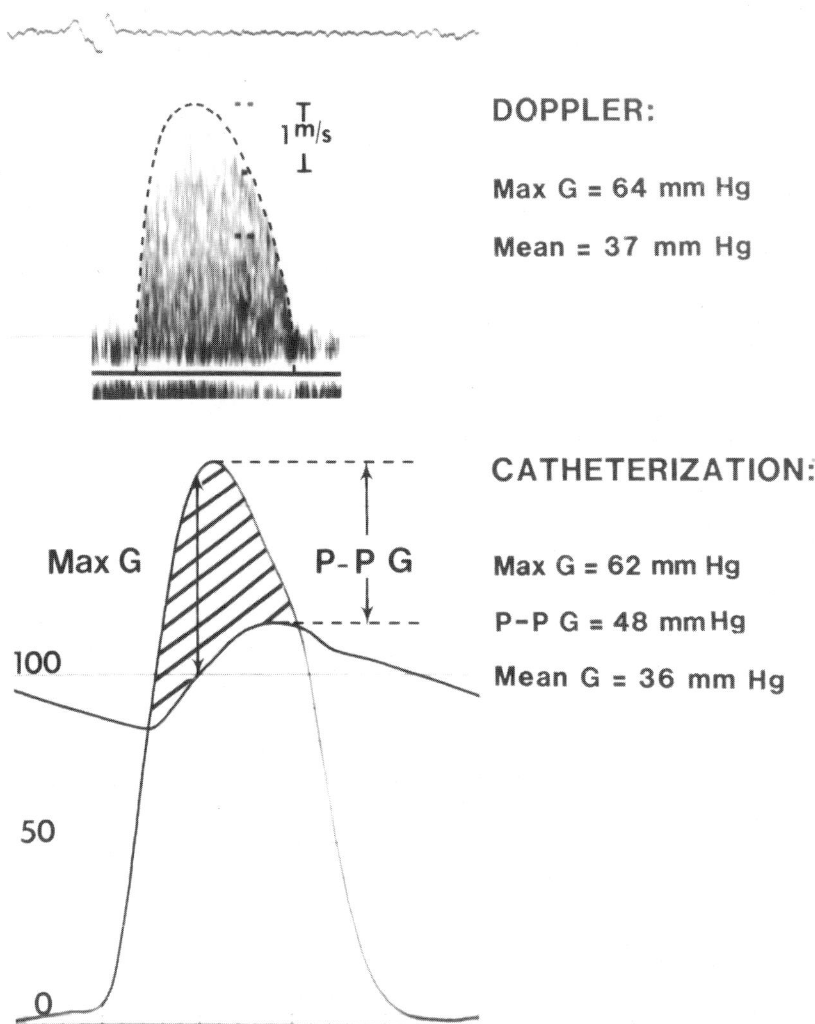

Fig. 40-2. Shown is the Doppler trace *(top)* and the pressure tracings at catheterization *(bottom)* in a patient with aortic stenosis. The aortic stenosis jet was recorded by continuous wave Doppler echocardiography in the ascending aorta with the transducer in the suprasternal notch. The maximal velocity is measured in meters per second at the greatest magnitude of the jet (here 4 m/second), while the mean gradient is taken as the average of gradients obtained at multiple intervals during systole. The maximal Doppler gradient correlates well with the instantaneous catheterization gradient (max G), but tends to overestimate the peak-to-peak gradient (P-PG) by catheterization. Mean gradients correlate best.

Table 40-2. Detection of Associated Abnormalities by Doppler Echocardiography in Catheter Balloon Valvuloplasty

Regurgitation
Additional lesions
Cardiac thrombi
Pulmonary hypertension
LV size and function

among these defects, of course, is the presence of valvular regurgitation. Since valvulotomy may result in the appearance of exacerbation of regurgitation, the determination that valvular insufficiency as well as stenosis is present is an important finding. The primary modality utilized to detect valvular regurgitation is Doppler recordings. Although both pulsed and continuous wave Doppler recordings can yield evidence of the lesion, as well as some indirect information about the relative hemodynamic consequences, the primary quantitative modality utilized at present is flow mapping. Thus, utilizing color Doppler flow imaging the regurgitant jet may be visualized, as well as the area of the jet plane. Several studies have demonstrated that the size of regurgitant jets visualized in this fashion relates in a general way to the quantitative severity of the lesion as assessed by cineangiography.[9] Echo images can also detect abnormalities of additional valves other than the primary stenotic lesion. Of greater significance, however, is the detection of intracardiac thrombi. Echocardiography has proved to be an effective method for the recognition of intraatrial thrombi when these masses have been centrally located with major intracavitary projection. However, echocardiography has thus far been less successful with thrombi involving the left atrial appendage. Recent studies have demonstrated that transesophageal echocardiography may provide superior sensitivity in the recognition of left atrial thrombi, and it is likely that this procedure may well play an important role in the evaluation of the patient with mitral stenosis who is being considered for catheter balloon mitral valvuloplasty. In regard to left ventricular thrombi, echocardiography provides an excellent modality for identification and assessment.

Echocardiography can, in addition to the above abnormalities, be utilized to assess left ventricular and left atrial size and function. Simple dimensional measurements of chamber size may be made in a variety of projections in the patient with a nongeometrically distorted left ventricle. In addition, 2-D echocardiography, particularly from the apical window, can enable visualization of the entire outline of the left ventricle in most patients. Measurements derived from such echocardiographic images utilizing either area-length or Simpson's approach may then be employed to derive measures of left ventricular size and ejection fraction. In regard to cardiac function and hemodynamics, echocardiography can be employed to assess pulmonary artery pressures. Thus, utilizing the Bernoulli approach in the patient with tricuspid regurgitation, or measuring the acceleration time of the pulmonary artery flow trace, can be employed to evaluate pulmonary artery pressures.

SUITABILITY FOR VALVULOPLASTY

Having identified a patient with mitral or aortic stenosis who does not have another lesion contraindicating catheter balloon valvuloplasty, one now turns to an assessment of the likelihood of a beneficial effect from this procedure. Echocardiography has been valuable in this regard, particularly as applies to the mitral valve. Thus a variety of morphologic criteria have been utilized to determine the likelihood of a favorable response to catheter

Table 40-3. Suitability of Doppler Echocardiography in Catheter Balloon Valvuloplasty Suitability

Morphologic Characteristics
- Mitral
  1. Valvular mobility
  2. Leaflet thickening
  3. Calcification
     a. Leaflets
     b. Commissures
  4. Subvalvular apparatus thickening and distortion
- Aortic
  - Bicuspid Valve

balloon valvuloplasty in the patient with mitral stenosis (Table 40-3). Four criteria have primarily been assessed: (1) mitral valve leaflet flexibility, (2) leaflet thickness, (3) calcification of the leaflets, and (4) thickening and distortion of the subvalvular apparatus in mitral stenosis. In regard to the flexibility of the mitral valve leaflets, motion of the midportion of the anterior leaflet has been primarily studied. The highly flexible leaflet will, in middiastole, exhibit considerable angulation of the midleaflet moving anteriorly and apically in the area that is not tethered at the base or tips. An estimate of flexibility has been attempted as the ratio of the height of such angulation to the length of the leaflet.[10] The thickness of the mitral valve leaflet has also been assessed in a semiquantitative fashion. Increased thickening in gradations of greater than 5 mm or greater than 8 mm have been applied. In addition, the presence of thickening involving a portion of the mitral valve leaflets or entire mitral valve leaflets have been assessed. Calcification has proved to be a more allusive criterion. The presence of highly dense reflectances within the mitral valve leaflets have suggested calcification, and have again been semiquantitatively assessed in terms of the amount of the mitral valve apparatus involved. Finally, thickening, shortening, and fusion of the subvalvular apparatus have been visualized by echocardiography, and indicate a poor prognosis for valvuloplasty. Thus far, these four criteria have been assigned values from 1 to 4+ indicative of greater degrees of abnormality. The higher the grade of morphologic distortion, the less likely one is to achieve an excellent hemodynamic result with valvuloplasty.

The assessment of mitral valve morphology as an indicator of the suitability for valvuloplasty continues to be evaluated. As with all other echocardiographic measurements, the tomographic nature of the technique makes it imperative that the entire mitral valve apparatus is scanned. Preliminary experience, however, has indicated that patients with heavily thickened, immobile mitral valve leaflets with substantial subvalvular apparatus thickening and shortening are unlikely to achieve good results with catheter valvuloplasty.

The aortic valve leaflets have been more difficult to visualize by echocardiography. Accordingly, comparable morphologic data have not yet evolved. However, it is possible that future observations may lead to greater insights on the use of echocardiography in judging the suitability of the aortic stenosis patient for catheter valvuloplasty.

DOPPLER ECHOCARDIOGRAPHY IN GUIDING CATHETER VALVULOPLASTY

It has been proposed that Doppler echocardiographic studies may be useful in the actual performance of catheter balloon valvuloplasty. Specifically it has been suggested that the ability of echocardiography to visualize the mitral valve apparatus might be useful in positioning of the balloons, determining whether or not movement occurs during inflation, and ensuring that the balloon occupies the entire valve orifice. Early reports have been conflicting in regard to the value of echo imaging in this capacity, and additional information will be required in the future.

Echocardiography clearly has a role, however, in detecting the complications of balloon valvuloplasty. Four specific complications can be considered: (1) valvular regurgitation, (2) torn leaflet-apparatus, (3) pericardial effusion, and (4) atrial septal defect. Doppler echocardiography has been shown to be of value in detecting each of these abnormalities. The performance of color flow mapping not only can detect the presence of regurgitation, but it can also help to localize the lesion. Torn leaflets or leaflet apparatus can be well visualized by echo imaging techniques. In regard to tearing of the valvular apparatus, this may be evidenced by either valvular regurgitation or multiple forward jets. We have observed at least one patient in whom two separate flow jets were seen emanating from the mitral leaflets in diastole following catheter balloon valvuloplasty. In this case, clearly a disruption of the valve apparatus had taken place, resulting in flow occurring through some area other than the central orifice. Pericardial effusion may occur with perforation of the heart, and again echocardiography provides the best technique for the recognition of this abnormality.

A specific word might be said in regard to atrial septal defect. The dilation of the foramen ovale was initially feared to have the potential of creating atrial septal defects. Indeed in our experience most patients have been observed to have at least some intraatrial flow following valvuloplasty. However, the flow as visualized by Doppler echocardiography has consisted of a very narrow stream and there is little evidence that significant shunting occurs to such small atrial septal defects. The potential for larger defects, however, can be well assessed by Doppler echocardiographic techniques.

EVALUATION OF THE EFFICACY OF BALLOON VALVULOPLASTY

Doppler echocardiography techniques provide the best method for assessing the efficacy of catheter balloon valvuloplasty. Direct invasive measurements may be performed immediately after the procedure, but may be influenced by factors attendant to the procedure itself such as alterations in cardiac output and perhaps the production of myocardial ischemia. Importantly, only Doppler echocardiography enables assessment of the results of valvuloplasty following stabilization of the patient and in repeat assessments during long-term follow-up. It is not surprising, therefore, that Doppler echocardiography will constitute the major evidence for long-term success of valvuloplasty in the Catheter Balloon Valvuloplasty Registry being sponsored by the National Institutes of Health.

As in the assessment of the severity of stenosis, Doppler echocardiographic techniques can be applied in a similar manner to assess the reduction in stenosis (Figs. 40-3, 40-4, and 40-5). Accordingly, calculations of transvalvular gradient and valve area can be performed for both mitral and aortic valves in the usual fashion. Studies performed in our laboratory in patients who had undergone open surgical commissurotomy as treatment for mitral stenosis have demonstrated that, although echo imaging and Doppler echocardiography are similar in their assessment of mitral stenosis in the native valve, Doppler measures of the transvalvular gradient may actually be slightly superior in patients following commissurotomy.[2] The explanation for this seemed to reside in the scarring and distortion of the mitral valve leaflets in the long term following commissurotomy. Whether similar findings would be present in the short term is uncertain. Indeed data on a small number of patients reported by Reid and associates[10] have suggested that Doppler assessment of the transmitral gradient is less

BALLOON VALVULOPLASTY

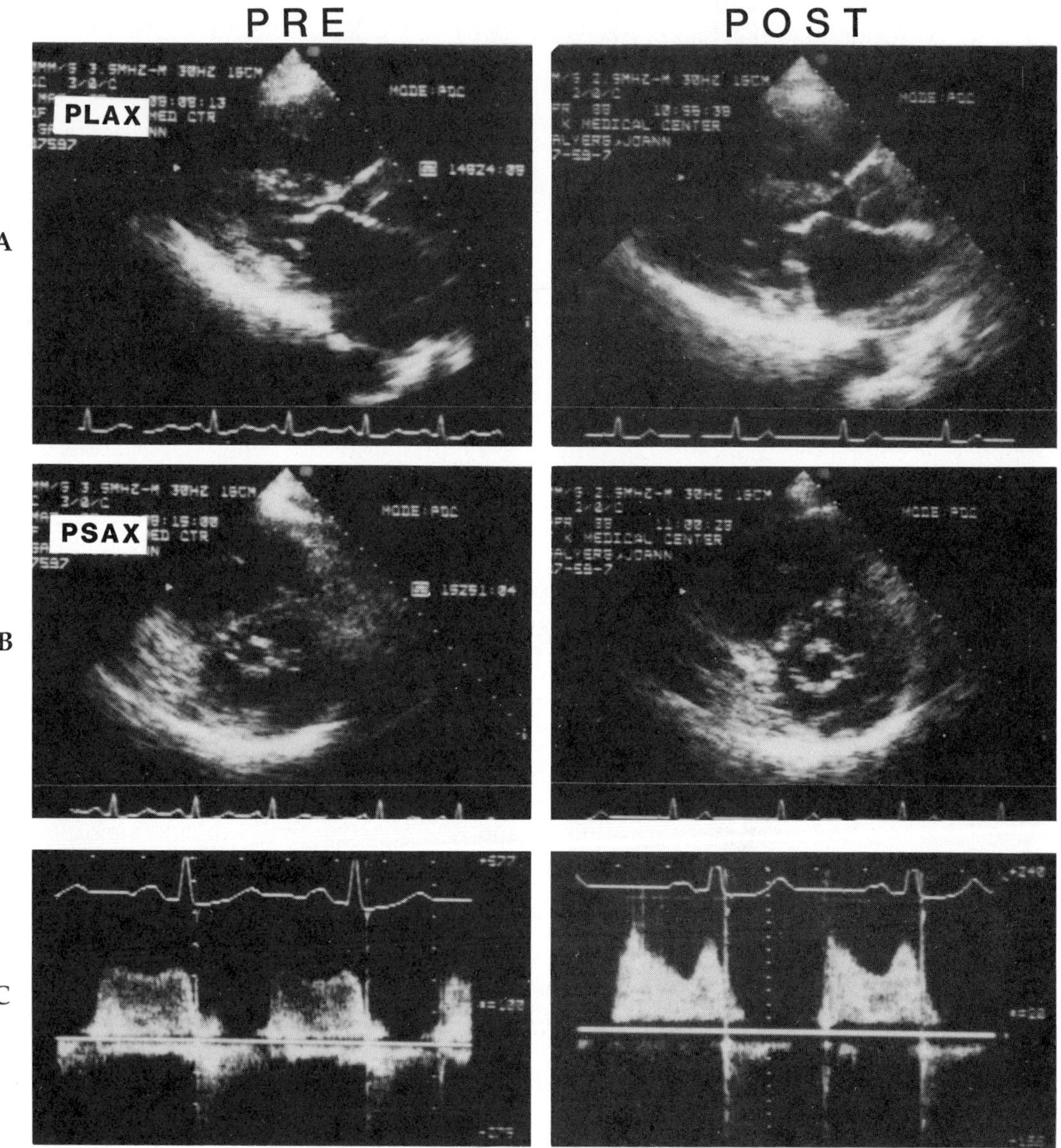

Fig. 40-3. A, The pre-procedure echocardiogram and the echocardiogram after balloon valvuloplasty obtained in the parasternal long axis view (PLAX) in a patient with mitral stenosis. The left ventricle is bigger and the mitral valve leaflet separation increased following valvuloplasty. **B,** Shown is the short-axis view of the mitral valve leaflets before *(left)* and after *(right)* balloon valvuloplasty. The mitral valve orifice is clearly larger after valvuloplasty. Importantly, an increase in the medial collateral diameter is indicative of separation along the commissures. **C,** Shown are the pre-procedure and post-procedure continuous wave Doppler transmitral velocity recordings in the same patient with mitral stenosis as seen in A and B. The prevalvuloplasty Doppler recording *(left)* shows a markedly reduced deceleration phase with velocities in excess of 2 m/second. Following balloon valvuloplasty *(right)* the deceleration phase is much more rapid, consistent with a decrease in pressure half-time and an increase in mitral valve area.

reliable after balloon valvuloplasty than is echo assessment of the planed mitral valve area. In regard to the aortic valve, data by Come and associates[11] have indicated that Doppler assessment of the severity of aortic stenosis remains as accurate in comparison with catheterization after valvuloplasty as before valvuloplasty.

As has been stated previously, Doppler echocardiography techniques provide an excellent modality for assessing the presence of valvular regurgitation. Such assessment can be performed not only immediately after the procedure, but during long-term follow-up. In addition, echo imaging can provide important information in regard to pulmonary hypertension by virtue of measurements of pulmonary artery systolic pressure obtained by the Bernoulli approach. Finally, echocardiography can provide additional important information regarding the status of left ventricular and left atrial size and function.

MECHANISM OF BENEFIT

Doppler echocardiographic studies may play an important role in assessing the mechanism of efficacy of catheter balloon valvuloplasty. Thus, in important studies by Reid and associates[10] a variety of measures of the mitral valve orifice were made from the short-axis projection on echocardiogram. The width of the mitral valve leaflets, as well as the angle formed at the junction of the two commissures of the anterior and posterior leaflets, were assessed both before and after valvuloplasty. The data from this study documented that the width of the mitral valve orifice increased following valvuloplasty, as did the angles for both commissures. Thus it was clear that catheter balloon valvuloplasty induced a freeing of fusion of the leaflets at the periphery that increased the width of the orifice, as well as the opening angles. These data were important in verifying that catheter balloon techniques were capable of separating fusion as the mechanism of increasing the orifice, rather than merely inducing stretching of the leaflets or even tearing or breaking of the apparatus.

CONCLUSION

Just as catheter balloon valvuloplasty is still in its infancy, the application of Doppler echocardiography techniques to this procedure is likewise evolving. Doppler echocardiography techniques have long played a central role in the diagnosis and quantitation of valvular heart disease, and will certainly continue to do so in the future. In addition to this information, Doppler echocardiography measures of value in determining the desirability of balloon valvuloplasty will include contraindications, such as left atrial thrombi, and measures of the suitability of a valve for this procedure. Utilizing available evidence, certain experienced laboratories are already selecting candidates for this procedure based on the morphologic characteristics of the mitral valve leaflets. Importantly, Doppler echocardiography will likely continue to provide the major method by which to assess the long-term results of the procedure. It appears certain, therefore, that whatever the role of catheter balloon valvuloplasty is in the future, it will be intimately intertwined with Doppler echocardiographic techniques.

REFERENCES

1. Smith, M.D., Kwan, O.L., and DeMaria, A.N.: Value and limitations of continuous-wave Doppler echocardiography in estimating severity of valvular stenosis, J. Am. Med. Assoc. **255:**3145-3151, 1986.
2. Smith, M.D., Handshoe, R., Handshoe, S., Kwan, O.L., and DeMaria, A.N.: Comparative accuracy of two-dimensional echocardiography and Doppler pressure half-time methods in assessing severity of mitral stenosis in patients with and without prior commissurotomy, Circulation **73:**100-107, 1986.
3. Henry, W.L., Griffith, J., Michaelis, L.L., McIntosh, C.L., Morrow, A.G., and Epstein, S.E.: Measurement of mitral orifice area in patients with mitral valve disease by real-time two-dimensional echocardiography, Circulation **51:**827, 1975.
4. Holen, J., Aasled, R., Landmark, K., et al.: Determination of pressure gradient in mitral stenosis with a non-invasive ultrasound Doppler technique, Acta Med. Scand. **199:**455-460, 1976.
5. Hatle, L., Angelsen, B.A., and Tromsdal, A.: Noninvasive assessment of aortic stenosis by Doppler ultrasound, Br. Heart J. **43:**284-292, 1980.
6. Hatle, L., Angelsen, B., and Tromsdal, A.: Noninvasive assessment of atrioventricular pressure half-time by Doppler ultrasound, Circulation **60:**1096-1104, 1979.
7. DeMaria, A.N., Bommer, W., Joye, J., et al.: Value and limitations of cross-sectional echocardiography of the aortic valve in the diagnoses and quantification of valvular aortic stenosis, Circulation **62:**304-312, 1980.
8. Skjaerpe, T., Hegrenaes, L., and Hatle, L.: Noninvasive estimation of valve area in patients with aortic stenosis by Doppler ultrasound and two-dimensional echocardiography, Circulation **72:**810-818, 1985.
9. Perry, G.J., and Nanda, N.C.: Recent advances in color Doppler evaluation of valvular regurgitation, Echocardiography **4:**503-513, 1987.
10. Reid, C.C., McKay, C.R., Chandraratna, P.A.N., Kawanishi, D.T., and Rahimtoola, S.H.: Mechanisms of increase in mitral valve area and influence of anatomic features in catheter balloon valvuloplasty in adults with mitral stenosis, Circulation **76:**628, 1987.
11. Come, P.C., Riley, M.F., McKay, R.G., and Safran, R.: Echocardiographic assessment of aortic valve area in elderly patients with aortic stenosis and changes in valve area after percutaneous balloon valvuloplasty, J. Am. Coll. Cardiol. **10:**115-125, 1987.

INDEX